The College of Physicians of Philadelphia

PORTRAIT CATALOGUE

Julie S. Berkowitz

With photographs by
Rick Echelmeyer

College of Physicians of Philadelphia
Philadelphia / 1984

Library of Congress Cataloging in Publication Data

College of Physicians of Philadelphia
The College of Physicians of Philadelphia portrait catalogue.

Includes indexes.
1. College of Physicians of Philadelphia—Catalogs.
2. Physicians—Pennsylvania—Philadelphia—Portraits—Catalogs. 3. Physicians—Portraits—Catalogs.
I. Berkowitz, Julie S., 1935- II. Title.
III. Title: Portrait catalogue. [DNLM: 1. Physicians—Pennsylvania—Portraits—Catalogs. WZ 140 AP4 c6c]
R315.C65 1984 016.61'0922 84-3206
ISBN 0-943060-03-6 Hardcover
ISBN 0-943060-04-4 Paper

Printed in the United States of America.

Contents

* * * * *

Acknowledgments

* * * * *

The College of Physicians of Philadelphia is grateful to Dr. Arthur M. Dannenberg, Sr., an active fellow for over 45 years. His generous donation provided the funds to support this portrait catalogue, and his energy and unflagging interest were an inspiration to everyone involved. The project was originally conceived by Mrs. Elizabeth M. Moyer, the recently retired curator of the Mütter Museum and College Collections, for whom the task of accessioning, conserving, displaying, and promoting the portraits was always a priority. College staff members who supplied research and compositional aid include Jean Carr, historical collections assistant; William F. Chaveas, executive director; Martha Jamison, publications manager; Barbara Kurimchak, historical collections assistant; Linda Mills, editorial assistant; Christine Ruggere, curator, historical collections; Gretchen Worden, curator, Mütter Museum and custodian, college collections; Edward Ciecko and Mary Jo Brown, work-study curatorial assistants; and Joan Bank, volunteer. Martha Jamison directed the design and production and coordinated the project with creativity and acute sensitivity to the content. Linda Mills lent expertise in editorial matters to make the text read more smoothly. Gretchen Worden worked untiringly to locate archival materials, to review the physicians' biographies, and to write an introductory essay. The work of Rick Echelmeyer, the photographer, bespeaks his superb technical skill and aesthetic sensibility.

Several consultants who offered expert opinions about the identity of the artists of 15 particularly puzzling and undocumented works include Darrell Sewell, curator of American art, Philadelphia Museum of Art; Joseph Amarotico, painting conservator, Pennsylvania Academy of the Fine Arts; and Ellen G. Miles, associate curator, National Portrait Gallery (and other staff members, including Robert Stewart, Monroe Fabian, Mona Dearborn, and Richard Doud).

There were numerous individuals from other medical and cultural institutions in Philadelphia who facilitated the availability of archival information and the accessibility to locations of art works, many of them in storage. They include Catherine Stover, archivist, Pennsylvania Academy of the Fine Arts; William T. Oedel, curator of paintings, and Carol Hevner, associate curator, Historical Society of Pennsylvania; Francis James Dallett, archivist, Paul Todd Makler, keeper of the art collections, and Maureen Parris, special assistant to the dean of the medical school, all at the University of Pennsylvania; Marianne Promos, head of the art department, Free Library of Philadelphia; Theresa Powers, director, audio-visual services, and Robert

T. Lentz, archivist, Thomas Jefferson University; Caroline Morris, librarian and archivist, Pennsylvania Hospital; Janet Evans, librarian, Academy of Natural Sciences; Ellen Calomiris, curatorial assistant, Independence National Historical Park; Richard M. Nelson, executive director, Philadelphia County Medical Society; and James Bilodeau, director of personnel, and Ann Preston, librarian, Drexel University. Others who offered support and advice were noted historians and authors of portrait catalogues: Maxwell Whiteman, *Paintings and Sculpture at the Union League of Philadelphia,* and Anthony N.B. Garvan and Carol Wojtowicz, *Catalogue of the Green Tree Collection,* of the Mutual Assurance Company.

The following art and archeological historians provided valuable biographical and historical information about specific artists and art works in the College's collections: H. Barbara Weinberg, Queen's College, City University of New York; Galina Gorokhoff, Museum of Fine Arts, Boston; Donald White, University Museum of the University of Pennsylvania; Gloria F. Pinney, Bryn Mawr College; Michael Panhorst, doctoral candidate, University of Delaware; Jane Myers, Munson-Williams-Proctor Institute; Lia Beretta, director, Italian Cultural Institute; Martin Bush, vice president, Wichita State University; Virginia Norton Naudé, sculpture conservator, and Linda Bantel, associate curator, Pennsylvania Academy of the Fine Arts; and Mary Mitchell, researcher, Lancaster, Pennsylvania. In addition, the following individuals supplied biographical information about their artist or physician relatives: Margaret Bye Richie, Rae Solowey, Russell Minton, Florence Wood Hacker, Sarah Wood Buchanan, Horatio C. Wood IV, and H. Curtis Wood, Jr. These artists kindly gave additional biographical information about themselves: Neil Kosh, Ila Junod Capolino, and William A. Smith.

Finally and with great affection, I must commend my husband, Henry, and children, Hank, Claire, and Laura, for being understanding and patient supporters of this project.

J. S. B., January 1983

The College of Physicians of Philadelphia: Talent and Treasure Since 1787

* * * * *

Founded in 1787, the year in which the Constitutional Convention met in this city, the College of Physicians of Philadelphia is the oldest extant organization of its kind in the United States. Patterned after similar academic bodies in Europe, this *collegium*, or gathering of professional workers in health science, was organized and nurtured by physician-citizens who participated in the birth and early growth of our nation. From its founding, the altruistic purpose of the College has been apparent; its motto, *Non sibi sed toti*—"Not for self but for all", denotes the high aim of its activities. The stately building of the College and its worldwide reputation make it a living shrine of American medicine. At the initial meeting on January 2, 1787, Dr. John Redman, first president, ordered "that the institution . . . be proclaimed to the world, and that all who are friendly to the progress of medical science . . . be invited to join in its promotion."

Attracting distinguished speakers from far and near through a series of endowed lectures, meetings of the College make available latest medical and surgical knowledge to members and guests. Clinicians and laboratory investigators in medicine and allied sciences gather to share information on current issues and research. Open to all interested persons, the stated lectureships and programs of the College sections—allergy, basic sciences, dermatology, geriatrics and gerontology, insurance medicine, ophthalmology, otolaryngology, Old Blockley, and medical history—provide stimulating sessions for kindred spirits in various fields. Through its quarterly journal, *Transactions & Studies*, first published in 1793 with Dr. Benjamin Rush as editor, a vast readership is reached throughout the world and exchanges are effected with other periodicals. The beauty and dignity of the College meeting rooms—Mitchell Hall, Cadwalader Hall, Thomson Hall, an attractive Fellows' Room, and the Gross, Hutchinson, Ashhurst, Norris, and Wood Rooms—blend tradition and comfort in gracious fashion.

Concerned with professional education since its inception, resources of the College today offer much to students and faculties of Philadelphia's six medical, two dental, two pharmacy, one veterinary, and medical technology and nursing schools in the Delaware Valley area. Basic science facilities, chemical and pharmaceutical organizations, and scientific publishing houses also use the services of its superb library. A revolving loan fund for interns and residents, administered under the aegis of a College committee, lends financial assistance to deserving young physicians in Philadelphia and its environs.

The College library, founded in 1788 by a gift of twenty-four books from Dr. John Morgan, is now one of the finest and largest in the world. Containing more than 300,000 volumes, it provides a teaching and research tool of great value to many users. Open to the public for reading and information, the library offers borrowing privileges to qualified persons. Its range of operation is local, regional, national, and international. Through current books and journals, indexes and abstracts, reference works and historical texts, interlibrary loans, and bibliographic, duplicating, and translating services, the library has a global outreach. The cost of this huge collection, its maintenance and continual growth, is obviously high. A journal-endowment plan, the S. Weir Mitchell Associates, begun in 1962, has attracted many who wish to help in this mission through personal or memorial contributions. Features of the library also include a medical documentation service—for searching, translating, and abstracting scientific literature; a rich historical collection—whose curator maintains a wide correspondence and reference role; and a cordial staff to accommodate readers in the building and borrowers from all states and many countries around the world. The book and periodical reading room, Packard-Krumbhaar Medical Historical Alcove, and other facilities in the College provide spaces conducive to scholarship amid comfortable surroundings. The Francis Clark Wood Institute for the History of Medicine is housed on the third floor. The present building, located at 19 South 22nd Street, was dedicated in 1909. Of English redbrick design by architects Cope and Stewardson, this edifice is the sixth home of the College since its establishment in the eighteenth century.

The Mütter Museum, dating from 1849, is one of the best and oldest of its kind in the world. A treasure trove of medical and surgical memorabilia, it is open to the public and offers an educational program of broad scope—including visits by students from art schools. The collections of portraits, drawings, anatomical models, pathological specimens, instruments, relics, medals, and badges of health interest are justly renowned. These College Collections are constantly augmented, moreover, through donations and purchase, and exhibits and displays are renewed frequently by the curator. The medicinal herb garden, situated in a restful setting beside the building, provides an oasis for the city visitor. This ornamental garden is maintained by the College women's committee and the Philadelphia unit of the Herb Society of America. A descendant of the tree of Cos, under which Hippocrates is said to have taught, is an arboreal delight.

A wide variety of scientific and social functions are held at the College each year. Professional workers meet with a common purpose here. The roster of resident, nonresident, honorary American, and foreign Fellows lists more than 1700 persons, diverse in background and geography but united in the goal of diffusing knowledge, promoting health, and alleviating suffering throughout the world.

The College of Physicians of Philadelphia, approaching its bicentennial, serves a useful, even vital, function in the scientific and humanitarian life of the medical community. Its members' aim, "Not for themselves but for all mankind," is repaid by professional accomplishment and satisfaction in this venerable institution of talent and treasure.

Fred B. Rogers, M.D.
Member, Editorial Committee, and former editor, Transactions & Studies
Past chairman, Committee on Mütter Museum and College Collections
The College of Physicians of Philadelphia

Introduction

* * * * *

The collection of oil paintings and sculptures at the College of Physicians of Philadelphia has been in the process of formation since the mid-19th century. These works represent a cross section of art historical styles prevalent in America and especially in Philadelphia from the late 18th century to the present. They range in format from large-scale, public works in the "grand manner" of portraiture, to the vastly more numerous private works in more intimate settings and scales. The artists range in reputation from the internationally celebrated to the most obscure and even the unidentified. Although the large majority of the subjects are Philadelphia physicians who were fellows (especially officers) of the College of Physicians, several portraits of local non-fellows and of non-Philadelphians are included. In addition, there are historical portraits of eminent ancient and Renaissance physicians and of 17th, 18th, and 19th century contemporary foreign physicians and scientists.

As is true with portrait collections in many public institutions, the collection as a whole is most noteworthy for its historical importance, the chief criterion for inclusion being the prominence of the subject. This is underscored by the large number of posthumous portraits, both original works and copies. Although this catalogue treats primarily the oil paintings and sculptures, the reader will observe that several works on paper—such as drawings, silhouettes, pastels, and the like—are included because of their historical or artistic importance or because they have been traditionally on display at the College. A few non-portraits are included for the same reasons.

The present volume is the first professional and extensively researched survey of the collection. Heretofore there had been numerous articles on special aspects of the collection and a few short catalogues. The latter, and also a more elaborate multi-volume catalogue of the entire college collections (1940), were essentially brief listings, often with omissions of basic information. Likewise, the facts in the *Catalogue of American Portraits,* a survey by the National Portrait Gallery in 1979, were based primarily on then-available College records; the *Catalogue* did, however, raise some questions about a few attributions and dates.

Extant documents, registration and archival records, and minutes of meetings are located in two separate departments of the College, and they were often found to be overlapping, contradictory, or fragmentary. In so many instances the fundamental facts—such as name of artist, date of work, name of donor, and date of donation—had never been recorded. Unfortunately, the one year allowed for the research and writing of the present catalogue did not grant sufficient time for examination of all the unsorted archival material. Nevertheless, this lack of accessible information is one of the *raisons d'être* for the new catalogue. It is gratifying that so much new information has been uncovered; this has resulted in the correction of several falsely attributed works, the identification of artists and assignment of dates of execution, the names of donors and dates of donation for many other works, and the raising of questions about still other works that remain problematical. It is to be hoped that this preliminary effort will be followed by additional research. If it becomes possible to catalogue the thousands of works on paper—photographs, prints, and drawings—which the college possesses, this may provide further clues to the sources for many of the portraits and also shed light on the history of the collection and its subjects.

There were several extremely helpful sources of information. Thanks to the existence of a catalogue of 1887 entitled *College of Physicians of Philadelphia Catalogue of Centennial Celebration Loan Collection of Portraits* and to the discovery of a handwritten *List of Portraits...Displayed in...the College, 1898-1915*, a terminus was provided for dating many works of art and many donations. A third source was the so-called Bradley File, a voluminous set of file-cards, negatives, and scrapbooks of photographs and letters compiled in the 1930s by Dr. William N. Bradley. His incredible "hobby" was to locate photographs of portraits of every physician known to have practiced medicine in Philadelphia up to his own time. His lists of related images and the photographs were important aids in making identifications of our own works. Other sources of information located just prior to completion of the manuscript for this catalogue were correspondence and bound volumes of College minutes; volumes 3 (1840-1856) through 11 (1929-1947) were especially informative in disclosing names of donors and dates of donation which hitherto had never before been listed in any College inventory.

As was mentioned above, the College owns several portraits that date from the late 18th and early 19th centuries. The rarest and most historically significant examples before 1830 include works in a variety of media: a Wedgwood relief medallion of John Fothergill (before 1787), the Joseph Sansom silhouettes of Abraham Chovet, Samuel Powel Griffitts, and John Redman (between 1790 and 1792), the Saint-Mémin drawing of John Monges (between 1798 and 1804), the Charles Willson Peale oil portraits of Baron Friedrich von Humboldt (1804) and Thomas Cooper (1819), the Rembrandt Peale encaustic and oil portraits of Joseph Gay-Lussac and Georges Cuvier (both ca. 1809-10), the George Miller wax relief of Adam Kuhn (1817), the G. P. Harding aquatint and water color copy of a 16th century portrait of Vesalius (1815), the William Rush plaster busts of Philip Syng Physick, Benjamin Rush, and Caspar Wistar (1812-13), the Joseph Wood oil miniature of William Gibson (1819), and the Thomas Sully oil portraits of Nathanial Chapman (1817) and Samuel Emlen (1828).

The College's collection of 53 sculpture portraits, which is about one-third as large as its collection of oil portraits, includes works in the following media: marble (12); bronze (7); plaster (31); and wax, ceramic, and fiberglass (one each). Several are obvious 19th century copies of ancient works, at least ten are known replicas of original works in other media, two are death masks, and one is a life mask. Fifteen works were given by individual fellows, eleven by the subject or family of the subject, two by a medical society, one by subscribers, two by the artist, ten by miscellaneous donors, and twelve by unknown sources. The vast majority of the figures are bust length; only two are full length, and nine are head-and-neck. Two are depictions of hands. The works range in size from a four-inch relief miniature of Fothergill to an eighty-six-inch monumental marble copy of an ancient statue of Aesculapius.

Most of the figures are shown in contemporary formal dress. A few are shown in military or ceremonial academic garb, and many are represented in the neoclassical manner with no drapery at all (12) or with ancient toga-like costumes. The three busts by William Rush and the Edward Stauch bust of George Bacon Wood combine two styles by having contemporary formal costume tied in toga-like folds at the bottom.

The sculptural styles and conceptions range from the more generalized and idealized neoclassical to the more individualized and idiosyncratic naturalistic. Therefore, the facial expressions show a corresponding range from the bland and neutral to the more personally revealing. Even so, a uniform air of dignity and high serious purpose pervades the group.

With the exception of the busts by William Rush, most of the outstanding portraits were made toward the second half of the 19th century and the early 20th century. There are not only works by many of the most prominent sculptors of the day but also some by obscure and unknown artists. The works include the portraits of Thomas D. Mütter by Peter Reniers; William E.Horner by Edward Dufrène; John Rhea Barton by Pasquale Romanelli; John Collins Warren by Robert Ball Hughes; George Bacon Wood by Edward Stauch and by Edward Dufrène; Georg Stromeyer by Friedrich Engelhard; Samuel David Gross by Joseph Obermeier; Henry Jacob Bigelow by Launt Thompson; William Pancoast by Castor Berbera (?); Edward B. Krumbhaar by A. Zellr; S. Weir Mitchell by William Ordway Partridge and by J. Otto Schweizer; Henry Beates, Horatio C Wood, W. W. Keen, James Tyson, and James Cornelius Wilson by Samuel Murray; Joseph Price and Louis Starr by Charles Grafly; and "Galienus," Samuel G. Morton, and Joseph Pancoast by unknown sculptors. Two outstanding non-portrait sculptural works are *Four Studies of the Progress of Fatigue in Athletes* by R. Tait McKenzie and *Girl with Basin* by Edward Fenno Hoffman III.

Although there are corresponding gaps in our knowledge of basic facts about the 143 oil paintings, there is now sufficient information to ascertain the manner in which most joined the collection. Fifty-seven were given by the immediate family or descendants of the subject, twenty-one by an individual fellow of the College, eleven by friends or a group of subscribers, ten by members of "the medical profession" or a medical society, eight by the collective fellows of the College, six by the subject, four by the artist, sixteen by miscellaneous donors, and ten by unknown sources. As with the sculptures, some of the paintings joined the collection as bequests. More than forty copies of earlier paintings or photographs are included in the collection, most of them posthumous works; in some cases the original sources are known, in others not.

The portraits represent a wide variety of styles and types from successive art historical periods, but they are remarkably uniform in many ways. As to portrait category, two are head-and-neck length, sixty-two are bust length, thirty are half length (to the waist), twenty-five are 2/3 length (to the knees), twenty-three are 3/4 length (mid-calf), and one is full length. They range in size from miniature to a canvas that measures seventy-three by forty-seven inches.

Most of the backgrounds are also of conventional type. Sixty-two have atmospheric backgrounds (a neutral or dark color suggestive of generalized space surrounding the subject) with no objects; another twenty include only a partial view of a chair. Outstanding works in these categories (not already mentioned among the early works listed above) are the portraits of William Potts Dewees and Robert Hare by John Neagle, Joseph Hartshorne by G. W. Pettit, Henry Neill by William Winner, Wharton Sinkler by Alice Roberts, Samuel Lewis and Charles D. Meigs by Samuel Waugh, Thomas Story Kirkbride by Howard R. Butler, Paul Beck Goddard by Edward Bowers, William F. Norris by Mihran Kevorkian, Ludwig Loeb by Julius Bloch, James Ewing Mears and Samuel W. Gross by Fannie Heberton, and Joseph Leidy and Frederick A. Packard by James L. Wood. Also exceptional are the drawings of John Herr Musser and William Osler by John Singer Sargent and that of R. Tait McKenzie by Violet Oakley.

There are forty-one portraits which contain one complete item of furniture, such as a table or desk with objects on it, or architectural detail, such as a wall or molding to suggest the interior of a room. Three portraits also display on a back wall framed paintings, of which one is recognizable as Rembrandt's *Dr. Tulp's Anatomy Lesson* (in Henry Rittenberg's portrait of Charles Hunter). An especially effective device in the portrait of John Hunter (after Sir Joshua Reynolds) by Anna Lea Merritt is the use of a niche cut into the back wall which expands the sense of depth in the room.

At least fourteen portraits utilize a strip or swag of drapery behind the sitter to lend a feeling of elegance and refinement to the setting, to suggest depth, and to show a graceful element of soft folds. Outstanding examples are in the portraits of William Shippen (after Gilbert Stuart) and Thomas Cadwalader by unknown artists, Nathaniel Chapman by Thomas Sully, Benjamin Rush (after Sully) by Adele von Helmbold, Thomas D.Mütter by Daniel Huntington, Louis A. Duhring and John H. Packard by Hugh H. Breckenridge, Nathan F. Mossell by Laura Wheeler Waring, and S. Weir Mitchell by Franz Dvorak.

Three other portraits include an architecturally unexplained column or pilaster in the background. The column once denoted the measure of man and often refers to classical erudition, moral strength, and high social status. The presence of both column and drapery exemplify a long tradition in portraiture, although their symbolic meanings were significantly reduced by the time of most of these works. One of the most effective portraits with a pilaster is that of Alfred Stillé by Bernard Uhle.

The most elaborately described interior space is found in the portrait of William Thomson by Thomas Eakins, in which the full-length seated figure is set back from the picture plane. A sense of receding space is accomplished by the artful placement and perspective rendering of the patterned oriental rug and desk and of the back wall with a framed ophthalmological chart affixed to it.

Only three paintings include a view into the outside. These are large-scale portraits in the traditional "grand manner" which show partial exterior views of sky or landscape and include swags of drapery with columns and parapets. These are the portraits of William Harvey (after Cornelius Jannsen) by Anna Lea Merritt, Philip Syng Physick (after Henry Inman) by Robert Reynolds, and John Ashhurst, Jr. by Adolphe Borie.

Not only are the background types conventional but also most of the iconographical attributes found in general portraiture appear. In addition to the column and drapery, a number of portraits show high-style period or contemporary furniture to suggest the social rank of the sitter. Outstanding portraits with fashionable furniture (in addition to some already mentioned) are those of Oliver Wendell Holmes by Sarah Whitman, Jacob Mendez Da Costa by Robert Vonnoh, D. Hayes Agnew by Bernard Uhle, and James Cornelius Wilson by Frank Linton.

A direct reference to education and scholarship is the presence of books and pamphlets found in more than thirty portraits. These items are usually placed on a desk or table or arranged in bookcases; sometimes the sitter holds the book. Since the titles are usually not legible nor the pages visible, the books symbolize general (not specifically medical) learning. Most often the sitter is not actively reading but has just paused to turn away from the open book or marks his place with a finger. Examples of outstanding portraits with books are those of Andreas Vesalius (after Titian [?]) by Adolfo Tagliaferri, George Bacon Wood by Bernard Uhle, S. Weir Mitchell by Robert Vonnoh, Francis R. Packard by Justin Pardi, and Edward B. Krumbhaar by Daniel Garber. In the portrait of Charles Caldwell attributed to Thomas Sully and in that of John A. Monges by an unknown artist, the titles are legible. The former shows two volumes of literary essays and natural history (indicating breadth of interest) and the latter, a volume from a medical encyclopedia.

Other generalized references to learning include the presence of desks, writing tables, inkstands and quills, sheaves of paper, and letters. None of the subjects is actually writing but instead seems to have paused for a moment. An example is the elaborate portrait of Benjamin Rush, seated at a writing table piled with closed and open books and writing equipment and with a portfolio bulging with papers in the foreground; he looks away from his work momentarily, his spectacles pushed up on his forehead. Parenthetically, at least thirty other sitters wear or hold spectacles, an outstanding example being the portrait of John Gibbon, Jr., by Charles Hopkinson.

The 143 oil portraits contain surprisingly few direct references to the sitter's actual profession. When present, these medical attributes are usually in the form of equipment resting near the sitter or in his hand but not being used actively. For example, in Huntington's portrait of Mütter the subject holds a sheaf of papers and is seated on a chair placed at a right angle away from a writing table, which displays letters, an inkstand and a large opened anatomical atlas with visible drawings; Mütter leans on the table but gazes in the other direction. The portrait with the most numerous references to medicine is that of John Hunter, who like Mütter leans on a writing table and looks off into the distance; his table is crowded with an inkstand, papers, a bell jar with specimens, closed books, and an open book with visible anatomical drawings. Behind him is a wall niche containing the bones of a giant. In Eakins's portrait of Thomson the physician holds an ophthalmoscope and there is an eye chart on the far wall. The portrait of Joseph G. Richardson attributed to Wilson shows a microscope next to the sitter. In Ben Solowey's portrait of Bernard P. Widmann the doctor is garbed in a white medical coat, holds a hospital chart, and is seated next to an X-ray tube. X-ray tubes appear also in the portraits of George Pfahler by Robert Susan and in the copy by Martha Fleck Brown. In John Johansen's portrait of Alfred Stengel the doctor wears a white laboratory coat and his hand rests on a stethoscope. In the portrait formerly identified as Benjamin Rush, the subject's hand rests on a skull, an infrequent symbol of the physician.

Costume is another important iconographical element in the oil portraits. The vast majority of sitters are shown in formal "business" suits. As mentioned above, two wear medical coats and three others wear military uniforms. Twenty-one wear ceremonial academic robes, most being described in sufficient detail to be identified as the robe of the president of the College of Physicians or of the university which granted the sitter a medical or honorary degree. Examples of outstanding portraits of sitters in academic robes (among those not already mentioned) are those of W. W. Keen by Robert Vonnoh, George E. de Schweinitz by Julian Story, William J. Taylor by Lazar Raditz, and T. Grier Miller by Charles Baskerville. The Richard H. Harte portrait by Leopold Seyffert shows the subject in both military and academic attire! There are six portraits whose sitters wear more unusual attire, including George Blumstein by Neil Kosh and Elliott H. Morse by Ila Junod Capolino (sport coats and slacks), Arthur V. Meigs by William Merritt Chase (a fur-trimmed coat), Roland G. Curtin by William Smedley (country attire, a Norfolk jacket, and knickerbockers), Katherine R. Sturgis by William A. Smith (a colorful cocktail dress), and the young George William Norris by John Lambert (a boutonnière in his lapel).

The overwhelming majority of sitters are shown in conventional standing or seated poses, with either neutral or reflective and thoughtful facial expressions. One exception is the informality of the portrait by Julian Story of George B. McClellan, who smokes a cigar. Interesting variations in furniture also create informality in two portraits by Daniel Garber, one of Charles W. Burr, who sinks back into a leather easy chair, and the other of William Zentmayer, who sits on a colorful, decoratively patterned, long cushion.

Only a few sitters penetrate the norm of reserve and sober demeanor in their facial expressions, by means of broad smiles or even by the hint of a smile. Subjects who appear with books or medical equipment often seem engrossed in related thoughts.

There are a few others whose faces express a more revealing aspect of their character. The portraits of William S. W. Ruschenberger by John Lambert and James Tyson by Joseph de Camp show men whose faces and bodies depict the physical and emotional toll of disease. Facial expressions in the portraits of William Thomson, S. Weir Mitchell (by Robert Vonnoh) and Horatio C Wood (by James L. Wood) register extreme introspection. In two other portraits the sitter is posed close to the traditional attitude of melancholy, with hand supporting forehead. Nathan F. Mossell's visage establishes eye contact with the viewer and confronts him directly with the intensity of his thoughts. In William Thomson's portrait of Jacob Solis-Cohen, the attitude is oblique but even more powerful; one hand grips the chair arm tensely, and the other hand places the tilted head partly in shadow so that the almost anguished gaze into the distance is localized in one mournful eye and intensified by brooding mouth and signs of advancing age throughout the face. Related attitudes of somber thoughtfulness are found in the portraits of John Hunter (by Anna Lea Merritt and by Charles Robert Leslie) and Benjamin Rush (by Adele von Helmbold), both of whom support their cheeks with their hands.

In conclusion, one may observe that for the most part the portraits follow the dictates of conventional, contemporary style in costume, pose, background elements, and facial expression. Except for the few that contain direct references to medicine or show unusual emotion, they are indistinguishable from comparable portraits of sitters from the worlds of business, government, and other professions. They fall in the category of commemorative works whose objective is to preserve the likeness of the sitter so that he will be remembered in the future for his worthiness of character and his contributions to society.

It must be remembered that the portraits at the College of Physicians were collected gradually, and until recent times their acquisition came under the direction of a succession of different committees which had little or no professional art expertise. The chief criterion for inclusion was the prominence of the subject, and the historical importance of the collection has long been recognized. Only a minority of works were commissioned by the College or by an individual or group with the express purpose of giving the work to the College. Most of the others were commissioned privately and many were copies of earlier works. Almost all donations were made singly by individuals; only a few single donors gave groups of portraits. Therefore, it can be seen that the collection in no way reflects the aesthetic policy of an individual collector or even of the institution itself. Although one may regret the absence of examples by a substantial number of well-known portraitists on the local and national scene, one admires the collection as a whole because it contains so many works of outstanding artistic merit, a tribute to the taste of those who commissioned the work and to the various departments within the College responsible for acquisition.

It is also important to consider the collection in the context of its location in the imposing setting of the College of Physicians building. By virtue of their sheer number and by their artful arrangement in the stately meeting rooms, library rooms, grand staircase, and halls of the College, the portraits are conspicuous and are accessible to fellows and visitors alike. Grouped together they serve as a reminder of the past and a statement of the present great tradition of medicine in Philadelphia. The sober and dignified faces of these distinguished physicians also serve as inspiration for the continuation of this tradition in the future.

Julie S. Berkowitz

The History of the Collection

* * * * *

The portraits are intimately connected with the history of the College itself. The circumstances of the collection's beginning, growth, documentation, care, and display reflect the College's basic purposes and activities over the past two hundred years.

This catalogue includes those portraits which are displayed within the College, either as permanent or temporary exhibits. With very few exceptions, these are the same works which have been traditionally included in lists of the College's portrait collections. Represented are all of the oil paintings, all of the statuary and nonmedallic bas-reliefs except for commercial reproductions, most of the original drawings in charcoal, pastel, or crayon, and most of the framed silhouettes.

The first recorded meeting of the College took place in 1787; the first recorded donation of a fellow's portrait was in 1850. One of the major reasons that so many years elapsed before the College began hanging portraits in its meeting rooms might have been because those rooms were rented for its first 76 years.

The meetings of the first five years were held in the Academy Building of the University of Pennsylvania at 4th and Arch Streets. There the College's library began with Dr. John Morgan's gift of 24 books in 1788. In 1791 the College moved to a second-floor room in the southeast corner of the American Philosophical Society's hall at 5th and Chestnut Streets, where it remained for almost 54 years. During much of that time the College's activities consisted of little more than its regular monthly meetings; the library had very few additions, the membership remained small (even being reduced to 18 in 1818), and the treasury was often very low as well.

The 1840s were a time of rejuvenation for the College. The purchase of Dr. John C. Otto's medical library in 1844 was the first large addition to the collections in many years. Continuing the search for larger quarters begun in the 1830s, the College finally found a meeting place across the street from Philosophical Hall in the newly erected building of the Mercantile Library on the southeast corner of 5th and Library Streets. After moving in 1845 to the airy, well-lighted room on the third floor, the fellows felt so much at home that for the first time the words, "Hall of the College," appear at the beginning of the minutes.

It was in this building that the College began acquiring its non-book collections. In 1849 Dr. Isaac Parrish convinced the other fellows that the College should establish a pathological museum, "to preserve noteworthy specimens for the education of their peers which might otherwise be lost to science."

It was also entered in the minutes of September 17, 1850, that "Mr. N. T. Harrison presented an engraved likeness of the late Dr. Joseph Hartshorne." This appears to be the first recorded donation of a fellow's portrait. The engraving was framed and hung in the meeting room, and the library committee was requested to "procure copies of such engraved likenesses of deceased fellows as have been published, for purpose of having them framed and suspended in the Chamber."

From the beginning, the College wished to enhance the dignity of the profession through the exemplary conduct of its fellows. Displaying the images of these respected colleagues was a natural and traditional expression of the College's high regard. In 1853 the College resolved to honor the memory of the late Dr. Nathaniel Chapman (a fellow and the first president of the American Medical Association) by obtaining his sculpture bust and an oil portrait. The wish preceded the deed by a number of years; the bust was acquired in 1868, and the handsome portrait by Thomas Sully arrived in 1910.

The implementation of the resolution to collect portraits was probably delayed by the continuing restrictions of rented facilities. In 1854, the College moved once more into rented quarters, this time to the "Picture House" of the Pennsylvania Hospital, near 8th and Spruce Streets. This building had been designed to hold the large Benjamin West canvases, such as *Christ Healing the Sick*, which had been presented to the hospital. The College continued its efforts to find a suitable property on which to settle, having established a building fund in 1849. In 1856, Dr. Thomas Dent Mütter began negotiating with the College concerning the donation of his immense teaching collection of surgical specimens and models. A major stipulation of the arrangement was that the collection must be housed in a fireproof building.

The potential donation of the museum, the recent acquisition of several large library collections, and the increasing success of the building fund proved to be an irresistible combination. The College signed the agreement with Dr. Mütter in 1858, construction of the building began on the northeast corner of 13th and Locust Streets in 1861, and the library and museum were installed in 1863. The impact of this move was tremendous. Most of the acitvities and organizational structure of the College as we know it today began after that date.

The first recorded non-print portrait to arrive after the move was, appropriately enough in light of the College's commitment to its heritage, the crayon portrait of its first president, Dr. John Redman, followed in the next two years by oil portraits of three other founders: Thomas Parke, William Shippen, Jr., and Thomas Chalkley James. Though the early years at 13th and Locust were not marked by a flood of portrait acquisitions, the eventual variety and breadth of the present collection was soon established. By the end of the first twenty-five years, the portrait subjects included figures associated with ancient medicine (Hippocrates), outstanding contributions to medical science (William Harvey), European medicine (Stromeyer, Dr. Nicolaes Tulp), and 18th century American medicine (Philip Syng Physick, Thomas Cadwalader). The portraits of beloved colleagues, such as Joseph Leidy and Samuel D. Gross, continued to form the heart of the collection. Service to the College seemed to be one of the factors determining which fellows' portraits were acquired. Officers of the College and committee members account for almost half of those portraits given before 1900.

The last relocation of the College was primarily a response to mounting pressures for more space which now came from two sources—the burgeoning library and museum collections. Having to choose between making extensive alterations to the old building or moving to a new site, the fellows reluctantly decided to leave their much-loved 13th and Locust Street building. Any regrets they felt were soon assuaged, because the new building was greatly to exceed the old in grandeur of design and accommodation of the College's needs. The cornerstone was laid in 1908 at the property on 22nd Street between Chestnut and Market, and the building was completed and occupied the following year. Then began the task of deciding where to hang the pictures.

The use of the portraits within the College emphasizes its continuing dedication to making the past a vital part of the present. Portraits are generally placed in the rooms with which the activities of the subjects were most strongly associated. The main room of the present College building, magnificently designed with a two-story ceiling to be the "hall of portraits," was named in honor of S. Weir Mitchell, one of the College's most distinguished fellows and a major fundraiser for the new home. Because the room is used for the general meetings of the fellowship, only the portraits of presidents or founders are placed there. Lack of space prevents the display of all of the eligible portraits inside the room. Some are placed as close to it as possible, such as the portrait of former president George Bacon Wood, which is in the hallway leading to Mitchell. The portraits of founding members Abraham Chovet, John Carson, and Benjamin Duffield, too small for the grandiose proportions of Mitchell Hall, are better suited to the lower ceilings in the library room nearby. With certain subjects, other considerations supercede their association as founders or presidents in determining placement. Former president John H. Ashhurst, Jr.'s, presence is required in the library reading room which is named after him; the elaborately carved two-story over-mantel contains a space specifically designed to accommodate his portrait. Founder James Hutchinson presides over the reception alcove on the first floor, which was originally furnished by contributions from his descendants.

The particular professional interest of the subject may also be taken into account when deciding where to hang a portrait. A number of the various local specialty groups, many of which were first organized in the College, continue to hold monthly meetings in rooms which are considered "theirs" by virtue of long association. In Thomson Hall, named after an outstanding Philadelphia ophthalmologist, the Philadelphia Academy of Surgery, the Pathology Society, the Neurology Society, and the College's section on ophthalmology meet under the close regard of many of their past members. Thomson Hall was also the "home" of the Philadelphia Roentgen Ray Society since its inception in the early years of this century. However, when its membership grew so large that the meetings had to be moved to Mitchell Hall, the portraits of radiologists, which the society had donated, followed them upstairs and now hang in the hallway and in the adjacent library room.

In addition to those previously mentioned, there are a number of other named rooms in the College which were furnished by family and friends of fellows. The Wood Room contains not only oil portraits and sculpture busts of George Bacon Wood and Horatio C Wood, but George Bacon Wood's bookcases and library, too. The Gross Library, specially designed to hold the personal library of Samuel D. Gross, displays his portrait and that of his son, Samuel Weissel Gross. In the Norris Room, more familiarly known as the periodicals room, a splendid grouping of portraits represents three physician members of the Norris family. The rest of the fellows' portraits are placed in the parts of the College where their greatest affection lay. In the library reading rooms are the men who supported the library through gifts of purchase funds or books. The museum houses those whose donations and interests are best represented in the anatomical and pathological collections.

The decisions about portrait locations are generally left to the discretion of the custodian of the College Collections. Specific suggestions made by donors, subjects, committee members, or other fellows are considered and usually followed if they are in accordance with the established guidelines and are aesthetically acceptable.

The presence or lack of documentation relating to the individual portraits is a result of the many changes in the past administration of the various collections. In the beginning, the officers took care of all of the College's business, including supervising the library, collecting the dues, paying the rent, and arranging and recording the meetings. In 1834 a standing committee on the library was created to take over that responsibility from the officers. Everything that was given to the College before 1863, whether a book, print, or curio (except for the cabinet of pathological specimens, which had its own curator), fell under the library committee's jurisdiction. The presentation of a gift was usually recorded in the general College minutes, which is often the only accurate source for dates of donation and names of donors, since committees were not required to keep minutes until the early 1880s. In 1863 the Hall Committee was set up to take care of the building and all College property which was not otherwise provided for. This came to include the statuary and anything which was hung or fastened to the walls, such as framed pictures, certificates, and commemorative plaques. The library continued to list the portraits in its card catalogue, but the Hall Committee made all the arrangements for framing, repair, cleaning, and labeling.

This division of responsibilities continued until 1935, when the College appointed a new committee to take care of all the collections which were not specifically part of the library or the museum but which had been presented to the College as a whole. This included all of the oil portraits, sculptures, medals, memorabilia, and silver. The chairman and members of the new committee were to be the same as those of the Mütter Museum Committee, and the curator of the museum became the Custodian of the College Collections. One distinction was made regarding the prints and photographs: those which were framed and hanging on the walls were considered part of the College Collections; those which were unframed belonged to the library. In 1980, all of the framed prints and photographs remaining in storage or on the walls of the library, museum, and College offices were unframed in order to prevent further damage from dirt, light, and acidic framing materials and they were transferred to the library.

There were inherent problems in keeping records of the collections. By the time the portraits were turned over to the College Collections Committee, the existence of earlier files was often forgotten, and basic information such as the names of donors and dates of donation was never transferred to the new files kept in the museum. Additional information on the collections has recently been found in files which would not ordinarily have been considered as likely sources. For example, the Building Committee for the 1909 relocation became involved with the art collections while making arrangements for certain rooms which were to be furnished by donations from the families or friends of fellows and named in their honor. Correspondence in these files contained previously unrecorded facts concerning several important pieces. These unanticipated discoveries lead to speculation that the answers to many remaining mysteries may eventually be found in the College archives. However, consolidation of the collections under a single committee has much improved the record-keeping practices since 1935.

The present condition of the portraits reflects the application of various conservation techniques. The conservators known to have been used by the College are typical of those generally available until fairly recently to private institutions and individuals. Since there were very few special programs providing graduate-level training in conservation until the last twenty years, almost all paintings conservators of the past began as practicing artists who had a special interest in restoration. Many did careful and competent work according to accepted contemporary practices and technology. It is only with sophisticated modern examination techniques that we can judge their efforts.

Correspondence and committee minutes identify fourteen different private conservators used by the College since 1904; the names of those who did the earlier work have not been found. Of the named conservators, most referred to themselves as "artist-restorers" or were known to be active artists. Half worked on only one painting; five of the others were responsible for 77 of the total 92 restorations. Approximately two-thirds of the oil portraits have had at least one treatment since joining the collection.

The earliest reference to the care of a specific portrait appears in the College minutes of 1868, when the Hall Committee was authorized to have the portrait of Dr. Chovet cleaned and framed. In 1886 it was noted that the painting was separating from its canvas and it was ordered repaired. In 1921 the same painting was "fully restored and relined"; today it is again in need of a thorough cleaning. The conservation history of this painting illustrates some of the problems encountered in the rest of the collections. Since this 18th century painting did not arrive at the College until 1867, it is not unreasonable to surmise that it probably had some sort of treatment before coming to the College. Of its subsequent conservation at the College, no information was recorded as to the identity of the restorer, how it was cleaned, the nature of the 1886 repair, or what the 1921 restoration involved. This creates problems for conservators having to deal with the effects of earlier treatments, and every effort is now made to get complete treatment records for each piece sent out for conservation.

The practices of varnishing paintings and applying new supports for the canvases represent the most frequent treatment recorded for the College's portraits. Removing and replacing old varnish and linings may cause undesirable changes in the original painting. When overdone, cleaning and retouching paintings can result in a portrait in which no original surface is left and the intent of the artist is barely discernible. This is the case in a number of the College's portraits, particularly those which have been in the collection for a long time and have undergone several restorations.

It is not known whether there was any professional conservation treatment of the sculpture. Almost all of the plaster busts are coated with several layers of paint or whitewash. In some cases, this was done to cover a dirty surface. At other times, it reflected an attempt to make a plaster bust look like bronze by applying a matte brown or metallic finish. This was occasionally done by the artist and is an integral part of the piece. Often, however, it was done in order to give an inexpensive plaster cast the appearance of the more expensive metal cast. As fashions changed, a plaster which had been painted brown to imitate bronze might get a new coat of white paint so that it would look "marble" again, or vice versa.

In 1978 the Women's Committee of the College funded a major sculpture conservation project which had been suggested by the museum's curator, Mrs. Elizabeth M. Moyer, and which was directed by a professional sculpture conservator. All of the marble busts and bronze pieces were treated. In 1982, the plaster busts of Benjamin Rush, Philip Syng Physick, and Caspar Wistar by William Rush were completely conserved for display in the special Rush exhibit at the Pennsylvania Academy of the Fine Arts. Eventually, when funds become available, it is intended that the conservation of the plasters be continued until all are relieved of their present detail-obscuring coatings.

The portrait collection of the College of Physicians is probably typical of those in private institutions in terms of its care and documentation. Fortunately, the fellows and staff have always showed special interest in the art collections, even though their formal training lay elsewhere. Increasingly professional standards for the management of the art works have been set and consistently supported by the College.

This catalogue shows the many reasons why the portrait collection of the College of Physicians of Philadelphia is worthy of notice: for the outstanding achievements of the subjects, for the famous artists whose works are represented, and for the way it reveals the College's history and accomplishments. But the collection's real significance was best expressed by William Osler at the presentation of S. Weir Mitchell's portrait in 1890:

> *To join the noble group which graces this hall is one of the greatest honors which can be conferred upon a member of our profession.*

Gretchen Worden
Curator, Mütter Museum, and
Custodian, College Collections

Note

* * * * *

The portraits are arranged alphabetically according to the surnames of the subjects. Dimensions are given in inches, in order of height and width (height, width, and depth for sculpture). The paintings were measured from the front surface, inside edge of the frame, unless otherwise noted. Numbers at the end of technical descriptions refer to the accession code of the College of Physicians. In the portrait descriptions, the terms "right" and "left" are from the spectator's point of view, unless otherwise stated, e.g., "his right hand holds a book". Names of female artists are given first by their professional names (how known publicly and how they signed their work) and then, in certain cases, by their married names, if they were sometimes listed that way in biographical directories.

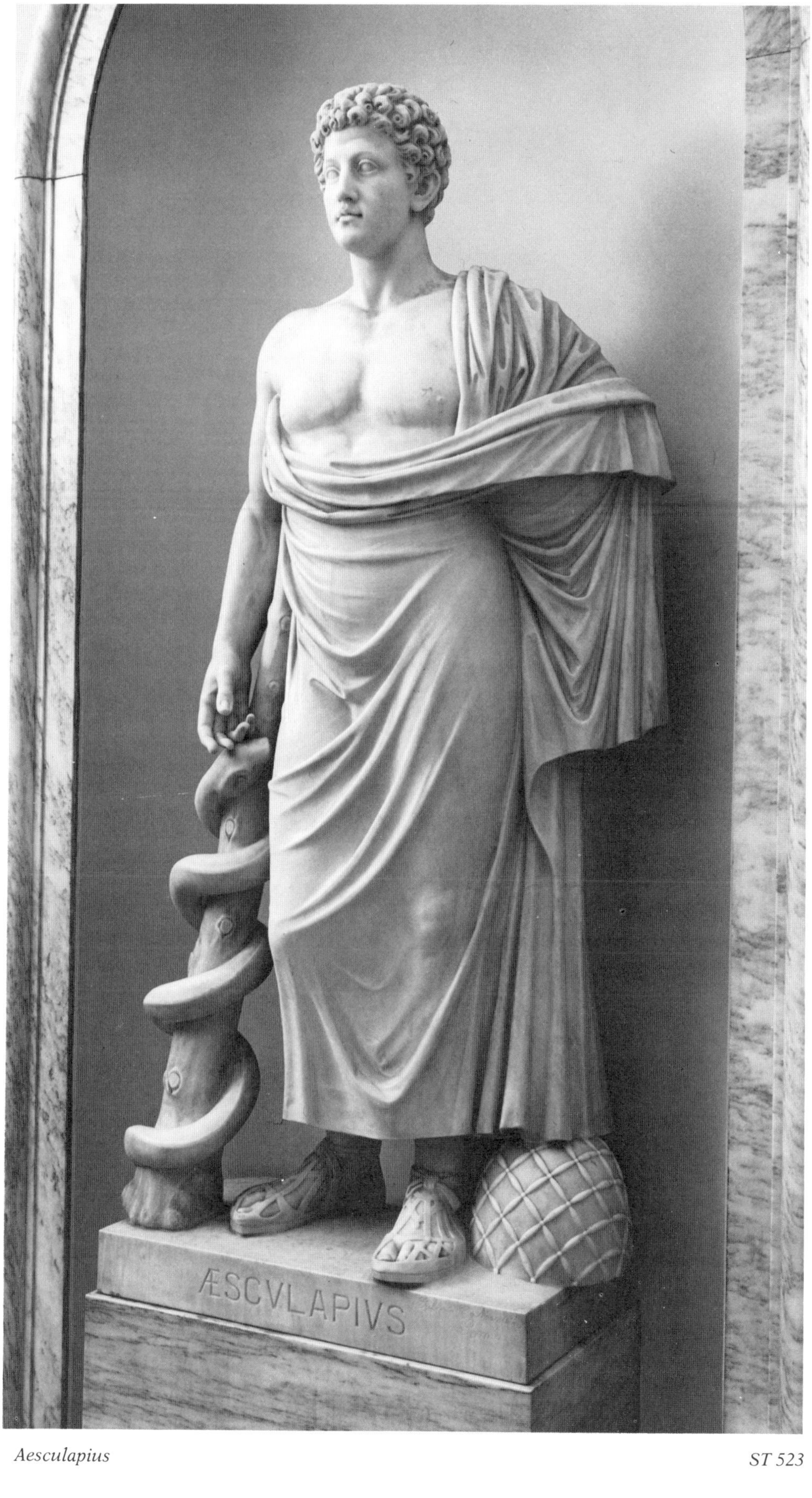

Aesculapius *ST 523*

The Portraits

* * * * *

Aesculapius

Differing versions of the origin of the Greco-Roman hero and god of healing, Aesculapius, range from Homer's description of him as a mortal ("the blameless physician") to the assertion of Pindar and Hesiod that he was the son of Apollo and Coronis. Since he not only healed the sick but recalled the dead to life, it was believed that Zeus killed him to eliminate the possibility that men might escape death altogether. The cult probably originated in Triccia in Thessaly and then spread throughout Greece and Rome to Asia Minor. Aesculapius first achieved real prominence at Epidaurus, where his sanctuary included a temple, theater, gymnasium, altars, and pits, as well as a tholos, stoa, and propylon. The central feature of the cures was the ritual of incubation. Also important was the use of therapeutic diet, baths, and exercise supplemented by auto-suggestion and miracles of faith. The Aesclepieia, festivals for Aesculapius, consisted of hymns, processions, and sacrifices. His descendants, called Aesclepiadae, were orders of priests whose knowledge of medicine was regarded as a sacred secret. In sculptures and coins, Aesculapius usually appears as a mature, long-haired, bearded man, although occasionally beardless and younger. His most common attributes are the staff and the snake that is often coiled around it; the snake was a sacred symbol of regeneration, and it had the power of discovering healing herbs. Aesculapius is sometimes shown seated on a throne with a cock, dog, or scroll.

Artist: Carlo Manetti (d. 1929)

Marble; 86 x 43 x 20 1/2; base integral with sculpture, 4 7/8 x 37 5/8 x 20 3/4; resting on marble pedestal 28 3/4 in. high; inscribed, "Aesculapius," on center of front base and signed on right front of base, "Galleria C. Manetti/ Roma." According to a letter dated May 3, 1982, in the files of the College of Physicians of Philadelphia from the firm of C. Manetti, the firm was founded by Carlo Manetti in 1897 and specialized in the manufacture and sale of marble museum copies and original works. The statue of Aesculapius was carved by Carlo Manetti and is a copy of a statue of Aesculapius in the Vatican, dated 150 A.D. Presented by Dr. Richard H. Harte (q.v.), 1911. ST 523.

Aesculapius is shown full length, larger than life size, the head and body frontal. He stands with his weight on his left foot, the right leg bent at the knee, and the right foot pulled back. The head is covered with ringlets that frame the face; there are large blank eyes, a straight nose, and very full curving lips. The square face is youthful except for a single furrow in the forehead. The massive chest is bare, and the powerful right arm hangs down with fingers curved and resting on the head of a serpent; the left arm is hidden by the drapery. A classical garment is draped over the left shoulder and arm, with horizontal folds bunched over the chest and diagonal folds crossing from hips to knees. The sandals are intricately strapped and tied. The attributes include a staff placed under the right arm; a serpent twisted around the staff; and an omphalos, or navel, a hemispherical form with a raised grid interlaced over its exterior. The smooth surface of the marble shows no tool marks. The drapery has a "wet" look, which allows the bodily forms under the costume to be visible. The huge dimensions and superhuman proportions, the posture, and the attributes give the figure an appropriately commanding presence. The copyist has made the face of his statue more frontal and squarer than the original in the Vatican; the body was made on an even more massive scale.

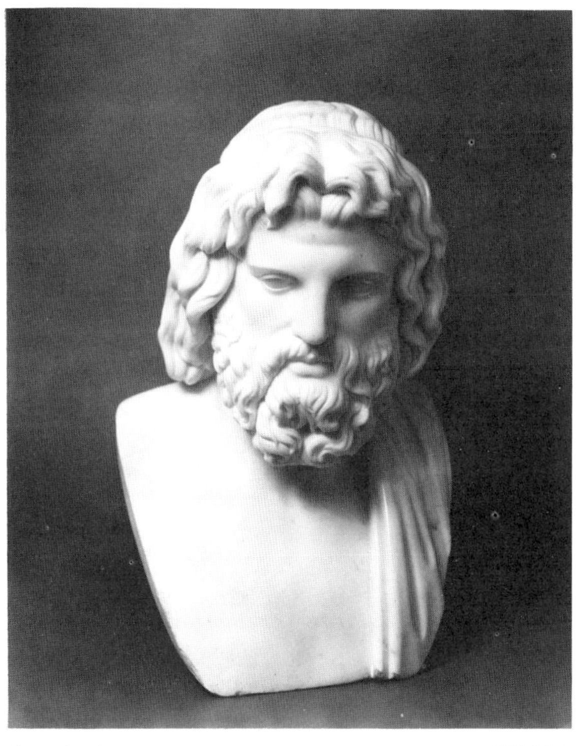

Aesculapius *ST 505*

Artist: Unknown

Marble; 21 1/2 x 14 x 13 1/2; not signed or dated. No base. Presented by Dr. John B. Roberts, 1910. *ST 505*

Probably a 19th century copy or interpretation of an ancient sculpture, this bust has a frontal torso and head turned slightly to the left. The hair is wavy and of shoulder length, parted in the center, and indented by a narrow fillet. The widely spaced, deepset eyes gaze downward. The broad-bridged nose comes close to the full lower lip. The upper lip is covered by a long moustache that joins the side whiskers to the beard. A narrow piece of drapery falls in vertical folds over the left shoulder. The marble surface is very smooth except for the deeply carved strands of hair. The torso is not really described anatomically and is relatively small in proportion to the head, which is larger than life size. The idealized features and blank expression are characteristic of this type.

David Hayes Agnew (1818-1892)

Dr. Agnew, an outstanding surgeon and anatomist, was born in Lancaster County, Pennsylvania, and graduated from the medical department of the University of Pennsylvania in 1838. After spending his early years in general practice with his father in the country, he returned to Philadelphia to establish a more rewarding career. In 1852 he began to teach practical anatomy and operative surgery at the Philadelphia School of Anatomy and he was appointed surgeon at the Philadelphia, Wills Eye, Pennsylvania, and Orthopaedic Hospitals. In 1862 he became demonstrator of anatomy and assistant lecturer in surgery in the medical department of the University of Pennsylvania. In 1871 he succeeded to the senior chair of surgery and in 1877 he was named the first John Rhea Barton Professor of

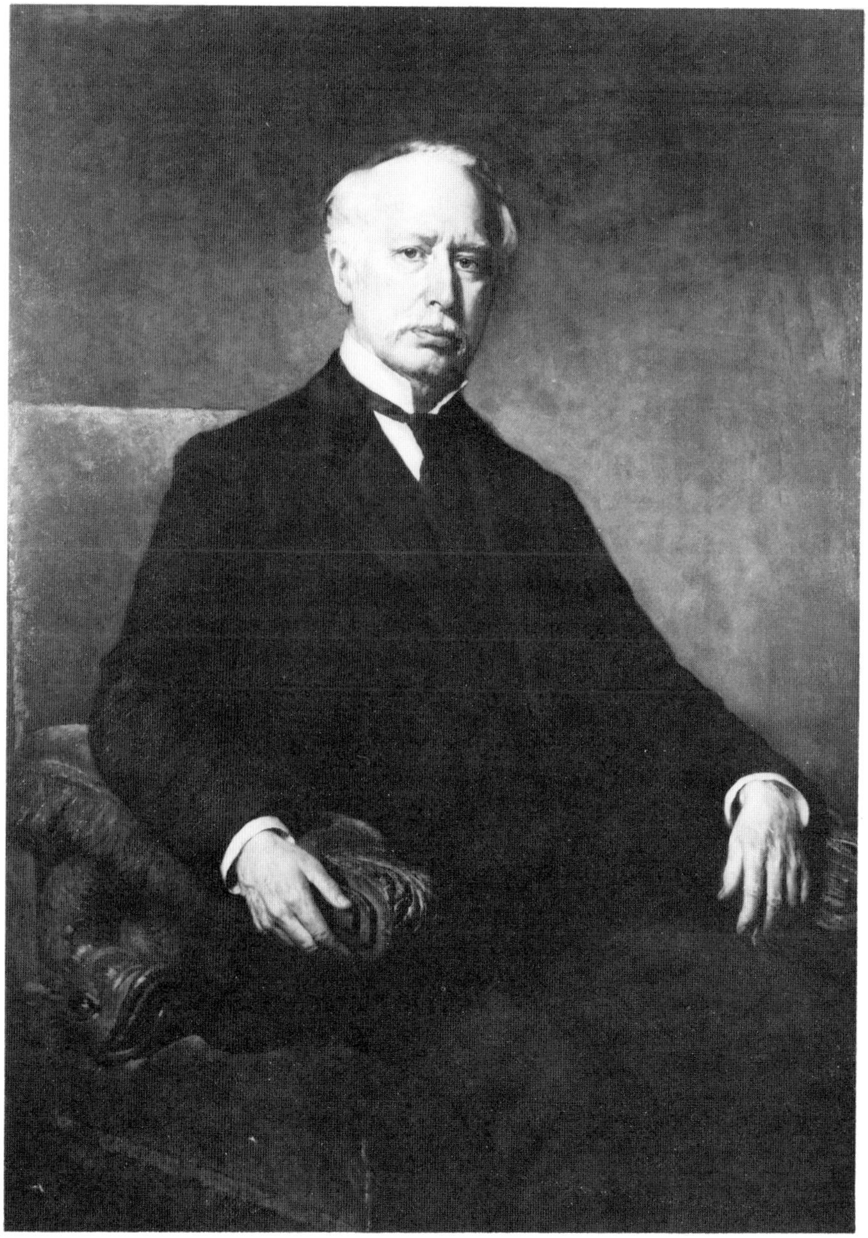

David Hayes Agnew *PA 7*

Surgery. This post he held until 1889. A leader in his profession, he served as president of the American Surgical Association, the Philadelphia Academy of Surgery, the Philadelphia and Pennsylvania Medical Societies, and the College of Physicians of Philadelphia (1889–92). He was also a member of the American Philosophical Society. Agnew was a prolific author. Among his sixty-six titles are *Anatomy in its Relation to Medicine and Surgery* (1859–64) and his chief work, *Treatise on the Principles and Practice of Surgery* (three volumes, 1878-83). He was an exceptional teacher. His masterful lectures on surgical anatomy were always crowded with students who appreciated his clarity and precision, and his clinical teaching was enhanced by sound judgment and didactic methods of description. He is shown in both these roles in Thomas Eakins's celebrated painting of 1889, *The Agnew Clinic,* which was commissioned by members of the undergraduate medical classes at the University of Pennsylvania upon Agnew's retirement and presented to the University at commencement. Because of his expertness in the treatment of gunshot wounds, Agnew was named the chief consultant when President James Garfield was mortally wounded in 1881. Through a sense of duty he attended the President loyally for three months, even though he at once recognized the hopelessness of the case.

Artist: Bernard Uhle (1847–1930)

Born in Chemnitz, Saxony, Uhle came to the United States in 1851. He studied art at first with his father and then at the Pennsylvania Academy of the Fine Arts and at the Munich Academy. He traveled to Europe twice in the late 1870s to study the old masters in Italy, Germany, and France. During the early part of his career he specialized in photography. Later he opened a portrait studio in Philadelphia and was in constant demand. He was an instructor in portrait painting at the Pennsylvania Academy from 1886 to 1890.

Oil on canvas; 51 1/2 x 37 1/2; signed and dated lower left, "B. Uhle/1889." Presented by members of the medical profession, 1890. Exhibited at The Art of Healing: Medicine and Science in American Art, *Birmingham Museum of Art, 1981.* *PA 7*

Agnew is shown three-quarter length, seated in an armchair set at an angle to the picture plane. His body is turned to the right, the head turned to the left and tilted slightly sideways. The arms rest on the chair arms, the right hand lightly grasping the chair arm, the left hand hanging loosely over the chair arm. The exceptionally high-fashioned Empire-style chair is upholstered in yellow-green velvet, has a fringed apron, carved dolphin arm supports and leafy handholds. The atmospheric background is gray, darker at the top. Agnew has white hair and a long white moustache. His crinkled blue eyes look out in the direction of the head turn. His eyebrows are knitted, and there are puffy circles under the eyes. He has a long nose, full lips, and a ruddy complexion. His costume consists of a white shirt with standup collar, black necktie, and black vest, coat, and trousers. The configuration of the body beneath the costume is suggested. The meticulously painted surface is smooth and the forms have sharply-defined contours. The facial expression is serious, determined, and direct. The posture, erect but not stiff, is suffused with great energy. The entire figure is vibrantly alive, suggesting Dr. Agnew's well-known strength, confidence, and imperturbability.

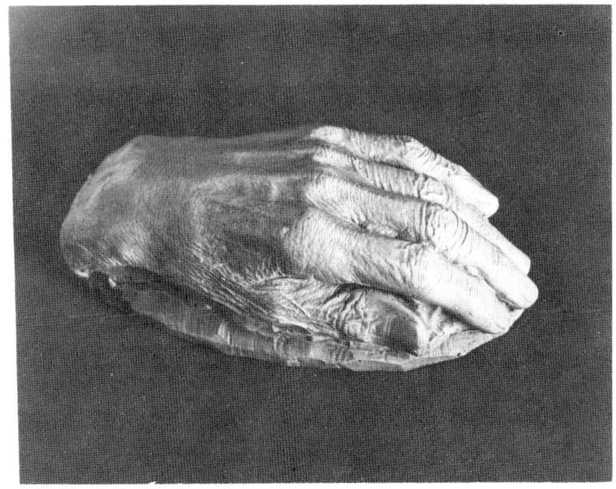

Hand of David Hayes Agnew *ST 17838.97*

Artist: Attributed to Samuel Aloysius Murray (1870–1941)

The son of an Irish stonemason, Murray was born and educated in Philadelphia. In 1887 he entered the Art Students' League of Philadelphia, where he studied with Thomas Eakins. Murray not only became Eakins's favorite pupil, but eventually was his assistant, trusted friend, and lifelong companion. They shared a studio together for many years and each did portraits of the other and of his family. They collaborated on several public monuments. Eakins secured a faculty position for Murray at the Philadelphia School of Design for Women, where he was instructor in modeling from life and lecturer in anatomy. He exhibited his naturalistic sculpture at the National Academy of Design in 1892–93 and at the Pennsylvania Academy of the Fine Arts frequently between 1892 and 1933. His prizes include honorable mention at the World's Columbian Exposition in Chicago in 1893, gold medal at the Philadelphia Art Club (1894), honorable mention at the Pan-American Exposition in Buffalo (1901), and a silver medal at the Louisiana Purchase Exposition in St. Louis (1904). Murray was commissioned to do several monumental public sculptures, including ten terra-cotta prophets for the Witherspoon Building in Philadelphia and bronze full-length portraits of Commodore John Barry, Dr. Joseph Leidy, Admiral George Wallace Melville, Monsignor William Corby, and Senator Boies Penrose. Other important public works include marble pedimental reliefs and a colossal bronze *Winged Victory* for the

Pennsylvania State Memorial at Gettysburg National Military Park, a life-size bronze figure of *Sorrow* for the Alfred O. Deshong Memorial in Chester, Pennsylvania, and a life-size bronze figure of Christ for the Bishop Shanahan Memorial, St. Patrick's Cathedral, Harrisburg, Pennsylvania. In addition, Murray was sought after for his portrait busts, physicians being a favorite subject. He made busts of more than 19 physicians, some in more than one version. His only one-man exhibition during his lifetime was held at the Pennsylvania Academy in 1896 under the auspices of the Fairmount Park Art Association. An exhibition of the Murray collection owned by the Hirshhorn Museum and Sculpture Garden in Washington was held in 1982.

Plaster cast, painted buff; 8 1/2 x 3 3/4 x 3 1/4; not signed or dated. Identified as the work of Murray by the Bradley File. Dr. Bradley's attribution is probably correct, because he not only befriended Murray and Mrs. Thomas Eakins in the 1930s, but had his portrait done by both Murray and Susan Eakins. According to a note in the files of the College of Physicians of Philadelphia, Bradley stated that the cast was made in 1892 by Murray and that Eakins was present at the time. It was presented in 1940 by Dr. E. Vernon Mastin, grandson of Dr. Claudius H. Mastin, to whom Dr. Agnew's daughter had given the sculpture in 1893. It was shown at the exhibition, The Art of Healing: Medicine and Science in American Art, *Birmingham Museum of Art, 1981.* *ST 17838.97*

The cast shows Dr. Agnew's left hand and wrist. As he was large and ambidextrous, it is not surprising that the hand shows great strength and size, despite the subject's advanced age. The irregular surface of the sculpture suggests an anatomical structure underneath the slack, wrinkled skin.

Harrison Allen (1841-1897)

Allen was descended from a 17th century Philadelphia Quaker family. He began his studies with a year in dentistry, followed by an M.D. degree from the University of Pennsylvania in 1861. During the Civil War he was an assistant surgeon in the U.S. Army. His teaching career spanned over thirty years at the University of Pennsylvania, where he occupied the chairs of comparative anatomy and zoology in the auxiliary department of medicine and of the institutes of medicine in the medical department. He also had positions at the Philadelphia Dental College, Wills Eye Hospital, and St. Joseph's Hospital. Though of retiring personality, he was a leader in several professional societies. He was president of the American Laryngological Association, the Association of American Anatomists, and the American Association of Naturalists. He was vice-president of the Pathological Society of Philadelphia, fellow of the College of Physicians,

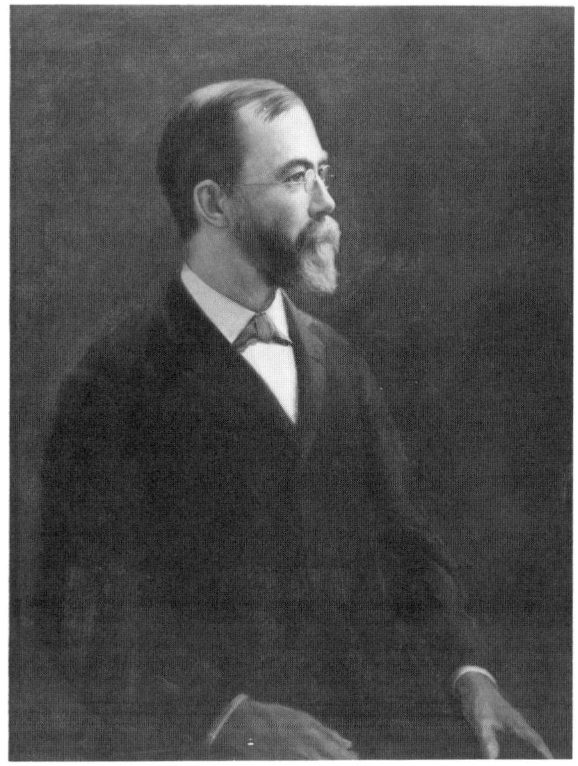

Harrison Allen *PA 86*

and member of the American Philosophical Society. A prolific author, he wrote more than 97 works, ranging from *Monograph on the Bats of North America* to the textbooks, *Outlines of Comparative Anatomy and Medical Zoology* and *A System of Human Anatomy.*

Artist: Anna Margaretta Archambault (1856-1956)

Descended from an ancient and titled French family, Miss Archambault was born in Philadelphia, the daughter of a steam-engine designer and founder of the Kensington Iron Works. She studied art at the Pennsylvania Academy of the Fine Arts and in Paris, portrait painting at the Académie Julien, and miniature painting with Mme. de Billemont-Chardain. In addition to her large portraits, her miniatures are widely known, notably those of Presidents Warren G. Harding and Calvin Coolidge. She was an active director and board member of the Philadelphia School of Miniature Painting and of the Pennsylvania Miniature Society. At the Pennsylvania Academy of the Fine Arts she was on the Fellowship Board between 1903 and 1914 and exhibited in the annual watercolor and miniature exhibitions intermittently between 1905 and 1946. Her prizes included the Miniature Painters' Medal of Honor in 1922, the Emily Drayton Taylor Gold Medal in 1939, and the Howell Tracy Fisher Memorial Prize in 1940. She served on committees for the Philadelphia Sesquicentennial and Chicago Columbian expositions, and she wrote the book, *Art, Architecture and Historic Interests in Pennsylvania.*

Oil on canvas; 341/2 x 261/4; signed and dated lower left, "Archambault 1917." Presented by friends of the subject, 1918. Closely resembles the James L. Wood portrait of Allen at the University of Pennsylvania, painted in 1900 from a photograph. PA 86

Allen is shown half-length. His body is turned slightly to the right, the head almost profile to the right, the hands resting on the legs. The background is greenish-brown. He has dark gray hair brushed across the top of his head, side-whiskers, a full moustache, and a pointed beard. His brown eyes look straight ahead through metal-rimmed spectacles. He wears a white shirt, a blue-gray striped necktie, and a dark blue-gray suit. Even though the portrait was not painted from life, the pose conveys Dr. Allen's reticence and intellectual force as he sits quietly and meditatively staring off into space, avoiding contact with the viewer.

Astley Paston Cooper Ashhurst (1876-1932)

Born in Philadelphia, the son of the illustrious surgeon, Dr. John Ashhurst, Jr. (q.v.), Dr. A.P.C. Ashhurst was named after the renowned English surgeon, Sir Astley Paston Cooper. From the University of Pennsylvania he received the A.B. degree in 1896 and the M.D. degree in 1900, graduating first in his class. His teaching appointments at the University included prosector to the associate professor of applied anatomy (1904-11), instructor in surgery (1911-20), and professor of clinical surgery in the Graduate School of Medicine (1912-32). He was surgeon to the Episcopal, Children's, German (now Lankenau) Hospitals, and to the Philadelphia Orthopaedic Hospital and Infirmary for Nervous Diseases, and he headed the gynecological dispensary at the Pennsylvania Hospital. He served with distinction during World War I as director of Base Hospital No. 34, recruited from Episcopal Hospital, and also as chief of the surgical service at Walter Reed General Hospital. He wrote, in addition to numerous articles, *Surgery: Its Principles and Practice for Students and Practitioners*. He was a fellow of the College of Physicians and other societies.

Artist: Erwin Frank Faber (1866-1939)

Born in Philadelphia, Faber studied with his father, Hermann, a famous artist and teacher. He was equally well known as a portrait painter and as a medical illustrator. He served for more than twenty years as an instructor in pathological drawing at the medical school of the University of Pennsylvania, after having observed methods used at the Mayo Clinic, Rockefeller Institute, and in Vienna. He collaborated with his father and his brother Ludwig in illustrating George A. Piersol's *Human Anatomy* (1908), Gwyllm G. Davis' *Applied Anatomy* (1910), and Ross Hall Skillern's *Nose and Throat.*

Oil on canvas; 341/2 x 291/2; not signed or dated on the front. Written on the back of the canvas, "E.F. Faber/Dr. A.P.C. Ashhurst". Presented in 1937 by the Philadelphia Academy of Surgery, which purchased the portrait from the artist in that year. The Bradley File gives the date of 1937 for the painting. It probably was painted after a photograph. The portrait closely resembles a photograph of Ashhurst in "Medical Memories: An Account of Events and Personalities that I Saw and Heard as a Medical Student at the University of Pennsylvania 1895-1899," by George William Norris. PA 103

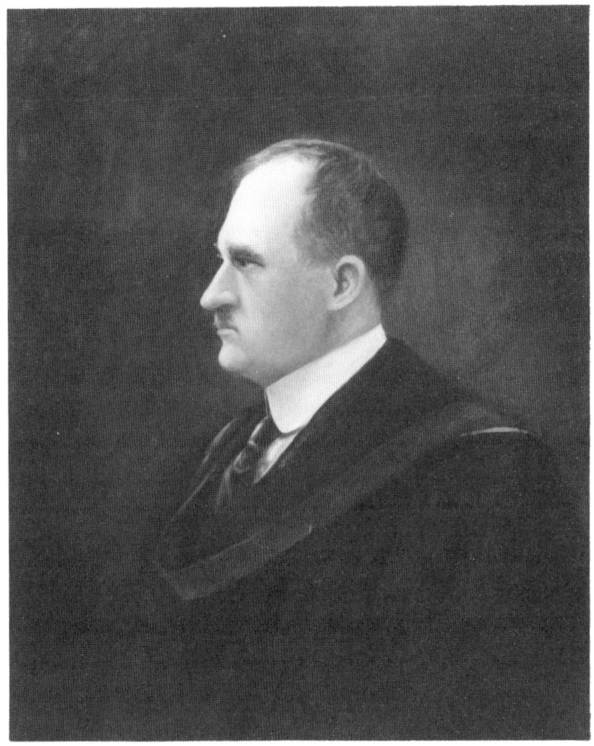

Astley Paston Cooper Ashhurst PA 103

Ashhurst is shown bust length, the body turned three-quarters to the left, the head in profile. The background is a warm mottled brown. The hair and brush moustache are brown, the blue eyes look straight ahead. The nose is long, with its tip pointed down toward the tightly closed, frowning lips. The subject wears a white shirt, a necktie with two-tone gray pattern, a brown suit coat, and a black academic robe whose mantle is decorated with a green border and a thin strip of red. The surface of the portrait is painterly in the background and costume, more smoothly brushed in the head. The construction of the head is moderately solid and three-dimensional. Although the rendering is naturalistic and the features are very individualistic, the subject does not engage the viewer and lacks energy and vitality.

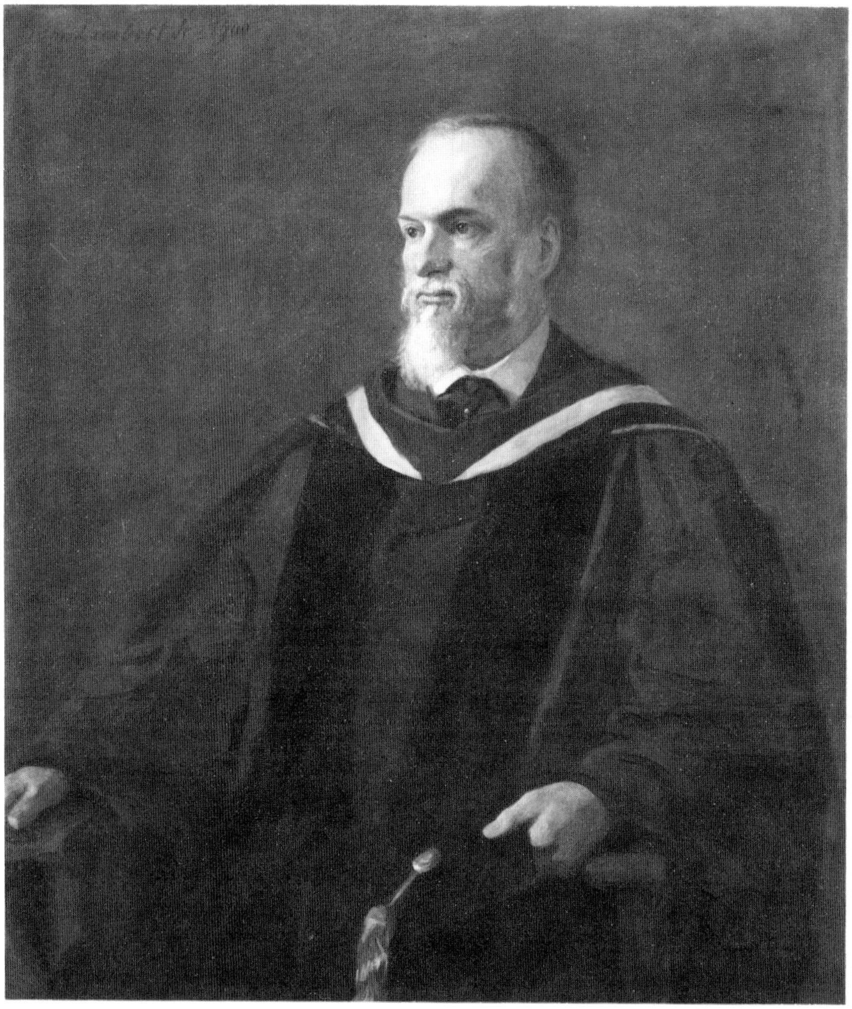

John Ashhurst, Jr. *PA 12*

John Ashhurst, Jr. (1839-1900)

Born in Philadelphia, Ashhurst was the descendant of English forbears who came to America in 1801. He showed such intellectual promise early in life, that at the age of fourteen he entered the University of Pennsylvania, where in his junior year he received the highest average grade ever theretofore attained by any student. He received the A.B. degree in 1857, and the A.M. and M.D. degrees in 1860. He forsook further study in Europe in order to enlist in the U.S. Army, serving as assistant surgeon in the Civil War to 1865. After the war he was appointed attending surgeon to the Episcopal and Children's hospitals. He became professor of clinical surgery at the University of Pennsylvania in 1877 and served as John Rhea Barton Professor of Surgery from 1889 to 1900. He was expert in orthopedic, vascular, and plastic surgery and was admired for his faultless judgment, thoroughness of detail, and coolness during emergencies. He was a passionate bibliophile and bequeathed his medical collection to the College of Physicians. A noted author, he wrote *Injuries of the Spine* (1865), edited Erichsen's *Science and Art of Surgery* (1869), wrote *Principles and Practice of Surgery* (1871), collaborated in Lippincott's *Medical Dictionary* (1897), and was an editor of the *American Journal of the Medical Sciences* and the *International Encyclopedia of Surgery*. Ashhurst was also a leader in professional societies. He served the College of Physicians as president from 1898 to 1900. He was president of the Pathological Society of Philadelphia, vice president of the Philadelphia Academy of Surgery, and vice president of the American Surgical Association. He was a member of the American Philosophical Society.

Artist: John Lambert, Jr. (1861-1907)

Lambert was born in Philadelphia and received a Certificate of Proficiency in the Arts from the University of Pennsylvania in 1883. He also studied at the Pennsylvania Academy of the Fine Arts, the Art Students League of New York, and abroad in Paris, under Lucien Olivier Merson and Lucien Doucet. A prominent portrait painter, he exhibited his works at the Academy, the Art Club of Philadelphia, the Corcoran Gallery in Washington, the Society of American Artists in New York, the Chicago Art Institute, the Carnegie Institute in Pittsburgh, and in Boston and Worcester, Massachusetts. He also exhibited at many of the national expositions. His works are included in many public and private collections. He was a member of the jury at the St. Louis Exposition in 1904. An inheritance of $1,000,000 changed his life-style and allowed him to travel widely. Contemporary newspaper accounts give poignant reports of his being hospitalized for a retinal inflammation, supposedly caused by the glaring sunlight of Spain, where he worked in the summers. He spent a good part of the last year of his life in a dark room in Pennsylvania Hospital. This treatment failed to save his eyesight. Lambert was devoted to the Academy and served as a board member and vice president of its Fellowship. He bequeathed a fund of $50,000 to the Academy for the purchase of works exhibited at the Academy annuals by promising young artists. In 1930 there was a memorial exhibition of his works at the Academy.

Oil on canvas; 39 1/2 x 34 1/4; signed and dated upper left, "John Lambert, Jr. 1900." Presented by Fellows of the College, 1900. *PA 12*

Ashhurst is shown two-thirds length, with head and body turned to the left. He is seated, arms resting on chair arms, his left hand holding a black mortarboard with gold tassel. The atmospheric background is a warm brown. His gray hair is thin, as are the white moustache and pointed beard. The large brown eyes look straight ahead in the direction of the head turn. The long thin face is accentuated by the sunken cheeks. The costume consists of a white shirt, a black tie with pearl pin, a black coat, and a black academic robe whose mantle has a green V with white and red stripes. The costume is broadly brushed, with little suggestion of the subject's body. The head is painted in more exact detail with smaller brush strokes and is rendered in solid, three-dimensional forms. The expression is wistful. The luminous eyes are sad and the corners of the mouth are turned down. The painting has a predominantly soft quality. There are no hard lines.

Artist: Adolphe Borie (1877–1934)

Born in Philadelphia, Borie graduated from the Lawrenceville School in 1895 and the University of Pennsylvania in 1899. He studied art at the Pennsylvania Academy of the Fine Arts and at the Royal Academy in Munich. A consistent exhibitor in local and national exhibitions, he received the Carol Beck gold medal at the Pennsylvania Academy (1910), the silver medal at the Panama-Pacific Exposition in San Francisco (1915), the Isaac N. Maynard portrait prize at the National Academy of Design (1917), a silver medal at the Sesquicentennial in Philadelphia (1926), a bronze medal at the Corcoran Gallery (1926), a gold medal at the Philadelphia Art Club (1928), and the Harris bronze medal at the Art Institute of Chicago (1928). He belonged to the Academy of National Arts, the Fellowship of the Pennsylvania Academy as board member and vice president, the National Society of Portrait Painters, and the Art Club of Philadelphia.

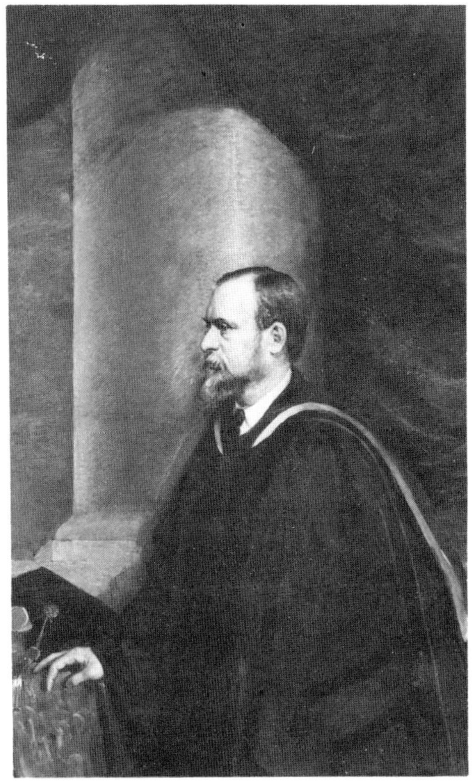

John Ashhurst, Jr. *PA 55*

Oil on canvas; 71 x 46; signed and dated lower right, "Adolphe Borie, 191[?, last digit indecipherable]." Presented by the children of Dr. Ashhurst, 1912. Obviously not painted from life, this portrait combines features found in two earlier depictions: a profile bust length portrait by James L. Wood (signed and dated 1901, from a photograph) at the University of Pennsylvania and the John Lambert half-length portrait with academic attire, at the College of Physicians of Philadelphia; it could be a composite. *PA 55*

Ashhurst is shown two-thirds length, standing, body turned three-quarters to the right, head in almost full profile. His right hand rests on a parapet covered with red cloth. The elaborate outdoor setting includes maroon drapery falling in swags from the upper left corner to the middle right border. A huge stone column is situated behind and to the left of the figure. A mortarboard and scroll are seen on a stone wall or parapet. At the upper left side there is an area painted blue as if to represent sky. The subject has brown hair and grayish-brown sideburns, a moustache, and a pointed beard; his brown eyes look straight ahead. He wears a white shirt, a black tie, and a black academic gown with two green stripes on the voluminous sleeves and green, white, purple, and red trim on the hood. The mortarboard is black with a gold tassel. The painter has used two styles here. The costume and drapery are depicted by broad, fluid strokes and have a flat appearance while the face, hair, hands, and column are rendered by short, choppy, painterly brush strokes that give a well-modelled, three-dimensional appearance. Though the space is somewhat ambiguous, the composition is ambitious and dramatic, and it is one of the few in the College of Physicians collection that hints at the out-of-doors. The figure, however, is made subservient to the grandeur of the setting.

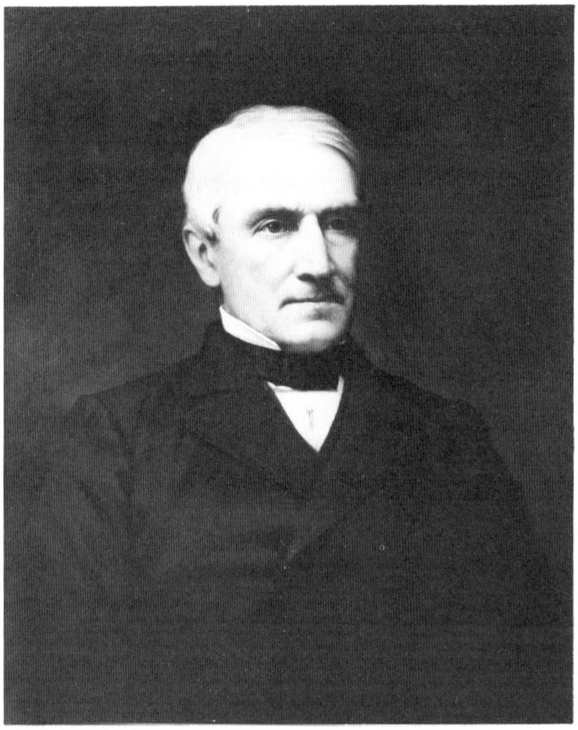

John Light Atlee PA 43

John Light Atlee (1799-1885)

Descended from a distinguished English family, Atlee's great-grandparents came to this country in 1733. Dr. John Atlee was born in Lancaster, Pennsylvania, where his medical education began with apprenticeship to a local doctor. He received the M.D. degree from the medical department of the University of Pennsylvania in 1820. His eminent sixty-five year career in both general and surgical practice was carried out in his native city. At Franklin and Marshall College he was professor of physiology and anatomy, trustee, and recipient of an honorary LL.D. degree. He was a founder and president of the Lancaster County Medical Society, the Pennsylvania Medical Society, and the American Medical Association. He was an associate fellow in the College of Physicians of Philadelphia and an honorary member of the Gynecological Society of Boston. Although he performed almost every surgical operation then extant, he was known best for his work in obstetrics and gynecology. At a time when ovariotomy was in great disfavor he successfully revived this procedure in 1843 and performed it in 78 cases with a mortality rate of only 18%. A public-spirited figure, Atlee was also very active in local educational and humanitarian causes. He helped inaugurate the state system of free public education, served as director of the Lancaster County School Board, and was a founder of the normal school at Millersville. He was an officer in the House of Refuge, the Bishop Bowman Church Home, the Home for Friendless Children, and the State Lunatic Asylum at Harrisburg.

Artist: Fanny Darrach (Mrs. Hart Darrach)

Oil on canvas; 29 1/4 x 24 1/4; not signed or dated. Documented as a portrait by Fanny Darrach (Mrs. Hart Darrach) by the College Minutes of 1886, vol. 6, p. 169. Presented by the subject's son, Dr. Walter F. Atlee, 1886. According to a letter in College of Physicians files from Rebecca J. Beal (author of Jacob Eichholtz: Portrait Painter of Pennsylvania, *Philadelphia, 1969), this is probably the portrait of John Light Atlee lent by the College to the Lancaster Historical Society's* Loan Collection of Historical and Contemporary Portraits *in 1912.* *PA 43*

Atlee is shown bust length, his body and head turned slightly to the right. The atmospheric background is dark greenish-gray above and warm brownish-gray below. The silver-gray hair sweeps horizontally across the forehead. The deepset, large brown eyes look out in the direction of the head turn. The aquiline nose is very wide at the bridge. The wide mouth has thin pursed lips. The rectangular face has a square jaw, cleft chin, and strong shadows under the eyebrows and nose. The subject wears a white shirt with stand-up collar and shirt stud and a black bow tie; his vest and double-breasted coat are dark brown with precisely tailored seams, lapels, and buttonholes. The surface of the portrait is smoothly brushed. The head and body are rendered naturalistically, with three-dimensional solidity. The surgeon's posture is erect, almost stiff. His gaze averts the viewer and his somber facial expression is accentuated by the knitted brows and tight lips.

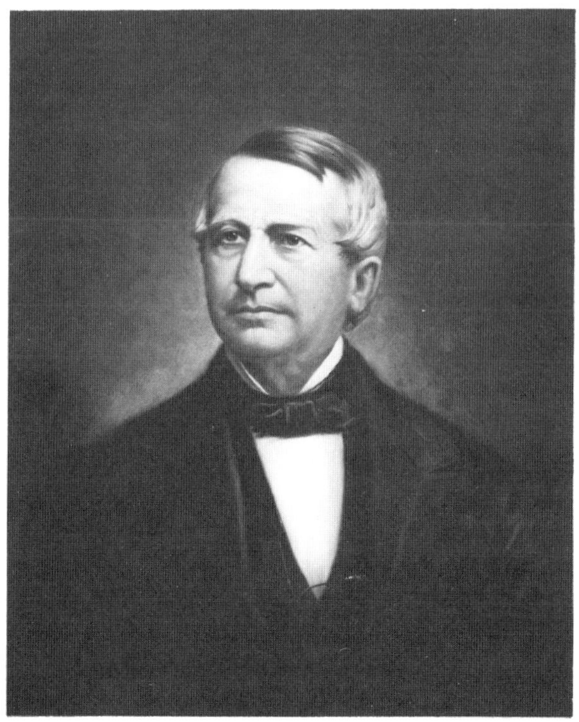

Washington Lemuel Atlee PA 41

Washington Lemuel Atlee (1808-1878)

The youngest brother of John Light Atlee (q.v.), Dr. Washington Lemuel Atlee was born in Lancaster, Pennsylvania, and lived with his grandparents from the age of seven, after the death of his father. Unhappy at his placement in a dry goods store, he began to study medicine with his brother. He earned the M.D. degree from Jefferson Medical College in 1829. After ten years of private practice in Lancaster, where he was a founder of the Lancaster County Medical Society, he became professor of medical chemistry at the University of Pennsylvania and held this post from 1844 to 1852. He was president of the Pennsylvania Medical Society and vice-president of the American Medical Association. He was a founder of the American Gynecological Society. Atlee had assisted his brother, John (q.v.), at the latter's first ovariotomy and he, too, became a successful champion of this procedure despite violent opposition from his colleagues, including some who called him a "dangerous man" and a "murderer." He wrote numerous articles on the surgical treatment of fibrous ovarian tumors and sarcoma of the uterus. His most important work was *General and Differential Diagnosis of Ovarian Tumors with Specific Reference to the Operation of Ovariotomy*, published in 1872.

Artist: Stephen James Ferris, Jr. (1835-1915)

Born in Plattsburgh, New York, Ferris studied with Christian Schussele, Samuel Waugh, and John Sartain at the Pennsylvania Academy of the Fine Arts, where he exhibited almost annually from 1855 and where he was made an associate in 1860 and an academician in 1871. He exhibited in Paris and London, as well as in most of the prestigious exhibitions in America. He received the Fortuny Prize for the best portrait of the artist in Rome in 1876. He was an instructor in the School of Design and was a founder of the Philadelphia Sketch Club and the Philadelphia Society of Etchers. He was also active with the Artists Fund Society and the Art Club of Philadelphia. He is said to have executed more than 2000 portraits, some of which were for illustrations in Ridpath's *Histories*.

Oil on canvas; 29 1/4 x 24 1/2; not signed or dated. Documented as a portrait by Stephen Ferris in the College Minutes of 1888, vol. 6, p. 330. Presented by the family of Dr. Atlee, 1888. According to a letter in the College of Physicians files from Rebecca J. Beal (see John Light Atlee), this is probably the portrait of Washington Lemuel Atlee lent by the College of Physicians to the Lancaster Historical Society's Loan Collections of Historical and Contemporary Portraits *in 1912.* *PA 41*

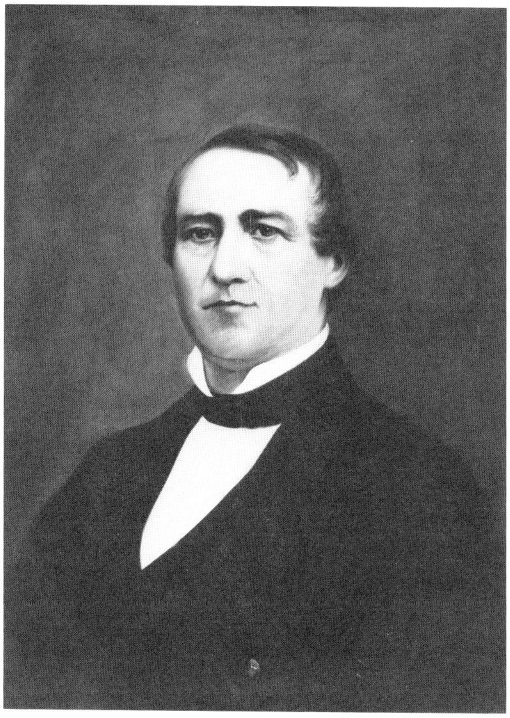

Washington Lemuel Atlee *PA 92*

Dr. Atlee is shown bust length, body frontal and head slightly to the left. The atmospheric background is medium brown at the top, warm yellowish-brown at the center, and dark brown below. Atlee's gray-brown hair sweeps across his forehead, forming pointed curls at the temples. His blue-gray eyes look straight ahead in the direction of the head turn. His long nose points down to a wide, full-shaped mouth; his round-shaped face has a round chin and florid complexion. Atlee wears a white shirt with turned-up collar, a black bow tie, a black vest, and a black coat with wide lapels; spectacles hang from a strap around his neck. The paint surface of this portrait is smoothly brushed. The subject's head is solidly rendered in three dimensions; the costume is flatter, and there is no sense of underlying bodily forms. The sturdy neck and breadth of shoulders make him appear physically commanding. His facial expression is dignified, though somewhat bland.

Artist: Unknown

Oil on canvas mounted on board; 23 x 17 1/2; not signed or dated. Presented by Mrs. George W. Conover, 1907. College records add the cryptic information that this portrait was "copied in Japan from a small photograph." *PA 92*

Dr. Atlee is shown bust length; his head and body are turned to the left. The background is green. He has dark brown hair brushed across his forehead. His gray eyes look straight ahead. His wide nose is bulbous, and his wide mouth has an exaggeratedly thin upper lip so close to the mouth that a large space is left between mouth and round chin. The subject wears a white shirt with stand-up collar and a black bow tie, vest, and coat. The surface of portrait is smoothly brushed. The rendering of the face deviates from anatomical accuracy; the body is flat, and the costume fades away into the background, not unlike some contemporary photographs. Although the head is in a similar position to the previous portrait of Dr. Atlee, the effect is comparatively wooden and without vitality.

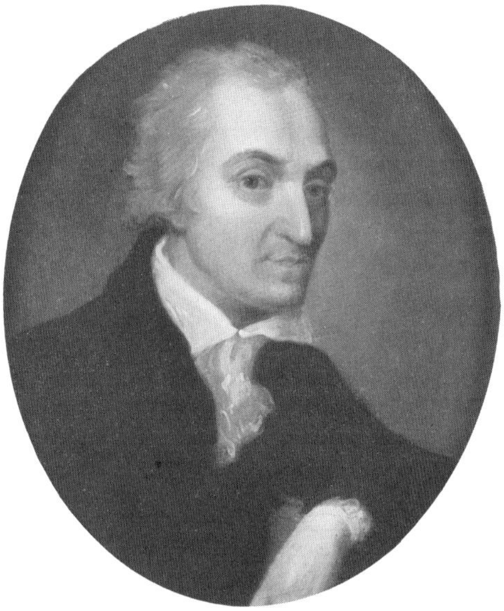

Benjamin Smith Barton *PA 100*

Benjamin Smith Barton (1766-1815)

Often called the father of American materia medica, Barton studied medicine at the College of Philadelphia (later the University of Pennsylvania) under Dr. William Shippen, Jr., and at the Universities of Edinburgh, London, and Göttingen. The last-named granted him an M.D. in 1789. While at Edinburgh he received the Harveian prize from the Royal Society and this made him a member. While a student in Philadelphia, he joined his uncle, David Rittenhouse, on a surveying expedition to western Pennsylvania. This trip sparked a lifelong interest in natural history and in the American Indian. In 1789 he was appointed professor of natural history and botany at the College of Philadelphia. He succeeded Dr. Griffith (q.v.) in the chair of materia medica and then Dr. Benjamin Rush (q.v.) as professor of the theory and practice of medicine. Barton's published works include books and articles on zoology, botany, natural history, the American Indian, archeology, and materia medica. Many of these works appeared in the *Transactions of the American Philosophical Society*. In 1805 he started to publish *The Medical and Physical Journal.* He was a member of the Imperial Society of Naturalists of Moscow, the Danish Royal Society of Sciences, the Linnaean Society of London, the Society of Antiquaries of Scotland, and the College of Physicians of Philadelphia.

Artist: Unknown

Oil on wood; oval miniature, 7 7/8 x 6 5/8. Typewritten note on back of painting says, "Benjamin Smith Barton, M.D./ 1766-1815/painted on wood after W. Haines, presented by Hampton L. Carson, Esq. 1920." Other College of Physicians records, the Bradley file, and College minutes of 1929 give the donation date as 1929, which should be considered correct. William Haines (1778-1848) was a prominent English engraver and portraitist who, according to the Dictionary of National Biography, *worked in Philadelphia at some time between 1800 and 1805, when he painted several portraits including one of Dr. Barton. The copy at the College of Physicians was formerly the property of Dr. Joseph Carson (1808-1876).* *PA 100*

Barton is shown bust length, his body turned slightly to the right, the head three-quarters to the right and tilted downward slightly. The left hand holds a small book. The brown atmospheric background is lighter to the right of the head. The subject has gray hair with white highlights, brushed back from the forehead. Under light brown eyebrows, the brown eyes, shifted to the left, gaze out toward the viewer. The prominent nose is long and thin, the tip pointing down toward the pursed mouth. The costume consists of a white shirt with collar pointed down, a frill, lace cuffs, and a buttoned black coat with M-notched lapel. The surface of the portrait is smoothly painted, with occasional visible brush strokes in the highlights. The three-dimensional depiction of the head is not conspicuous. The costume appears flat. The facial expression is one of tension and seriousness.

John Rhea Barton (1794-1871)

The son of Judge William Barton and nephew of Dr. Benjamin Smith Barton (q.v.), John Rhea Barton was born in Lancaster, Pennsylvania. He received the M.D. degree from the medical department of the University of Pennsylvania in 1818 and became surgeon, first at the Philadelphia Almshouse in 1818 and then at the Pennsylvania Hospital in 1823. His reputation as an outstanding surgeon was established as early as 1827, when he published *On the Treatment of Anchylosis by the Formation of Artificial Joints*. His name is linked with the "Barton bandage," a muslin strip wrapped in a figure-eight to support the mandible, and the "Barton fracture," which refers to his paper of 1838, *Views and Treatment of an Important Injury of the Wrist, a Modification of the Colles's Fracture of the Lower End of the Radius above the Wrist Joint.* He introduced bran dressings for the treatment of compound fractures. In his memory his widow, Susan Ridgway Barton, donated $50,000 to the University of Pennsylvania to endow a professorship in the principles and practice of surgery.

Artist: Pasquale Romanelli (1812-1887)

Born in Florence, this sculptor was the father and grandfather of artists. He was the student of L. Pampaloni and chief student and collaborator of Lorenzo Bartolini. His public monuments and other work can be found at the Uffizi Gallery and Santa Croce in Florence, and in Arezzo, Ferrara, and Montreal as well as in England, Russia, and the

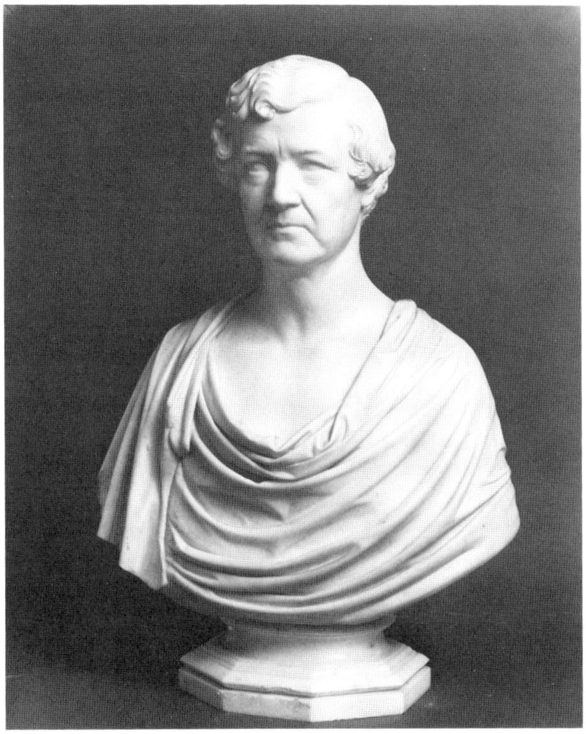

John Rhea Barton *ST 504*

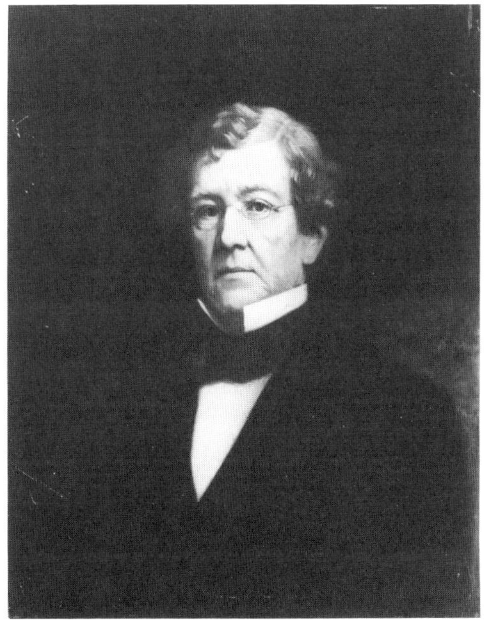

John Rhea Barton *PA 66*

United States. He exhibited a work in the Pennsylvania Academy of the Fine Arts Annual exhibitions from 1857 to 1860. His most famous works were portraits of Prince Demidoff and Napoleon, which Romanelli completed after the death of his master, Bartolini. He made at least three portrait busts of Bartolini. Other works by Romanelli in Philadelphia are the statues *Benjamin Franklin* at the University of Pennsylvania, and *Franklin and His Whistle* at the Union League of Philadelphia.

Marble; 24 3/4 x 20 5/8 x 12 1/2; resting on hexagonal base 4 in. high; signed and dated on back of base, "P. Romanelli F./Firenze, 1854." Presented by Barton's granddaughters, Mrs. John Astor and Mrs. Frank Lawrence, 1914. *ST 504*

Barton is shown bust length, the head and torso frontal. The full head of wavy hair is curled thickly on the forehead and over the ears. The large eyes, which have lightly incised irises and puffy lower lids, look straight ahead. There are deep furrows in the forehead and next to the nose and mouth. The mouth is small, the lips are tight. The head is square. The subject wears a toga whose deep, U-shaped folds fall over the right shoulder. The marble surface is very smooth. Although the conception is neoclassical, the features of the solidly constructed head are individualized and resemble other images of Dr. Barton. The facial expression is dignified and impassive.

Artist: Attributed to Adele von Helmbold, after Gordigiani

Adele von Helmbold studied intermittently at the Pennsylvania Academy of the Fine Arts between 1880 and 1900. She exhibited portraits and still lifes at nine annual exhibitions of the Academy between 1890 and 1904 and at seven Art Club of Philadelphia exhibitions between 1891 and 1904.

Oil on canvas; 29 1/4 x 23; not signed or dated. Included in the College of Physicians' Centennial Celebration Loan Collection of Portraits *of 1887 was a portrait of Barton owned by Mrs. E. S. Willing. The artist was listed as Gordigiani, presumably Michele Gordigiani (1830–1909), a portrait painter of international renown; this portrait is unlocated. Included in the College of Physicians of Philadelphia Inventory of 1898–1915 and subsequent lists was a portrait of Barton. The artist is listed as Miss von Helmbold and the painting is said to be a copy of one by Giordiani [sic]; it was presented by Mrs. E. S. Willing, daughter of Dr. Barton, in 1893.* *PA 66*

Dr. Barton is shown bust length, with body and head turned slightly to the left. The head is tilted slightly downward. The background is very dark greenish-black; the reddish back of an upholstered chair is seen on the right. The steel-gray hair is thick and wavy on top and at the ears, with one curl on the forehead. The blue eyes look through metal-rimmed spectacles directly at the viewer. Compared with the sculpture by Romanelli, the mouth is wider, with fuller lips, and the head is more rectangular. There are deep lines next to the nose and mouth. The subject wears a white shirt with stand-up collar and a black neckcloth, waistcoat, and coat. The background and costume are very smoothly painted, dark, and flat. In contrast, the head is constructed solidly in three-dimensional, well-modulated planes. The style is painterly, with visible brush strokes in the pink and cream highlights, violet and gray middle tones, and dark green and brown shadows. Dr. Barton's expression is serious, dignified, and in direct regard of the viewer.

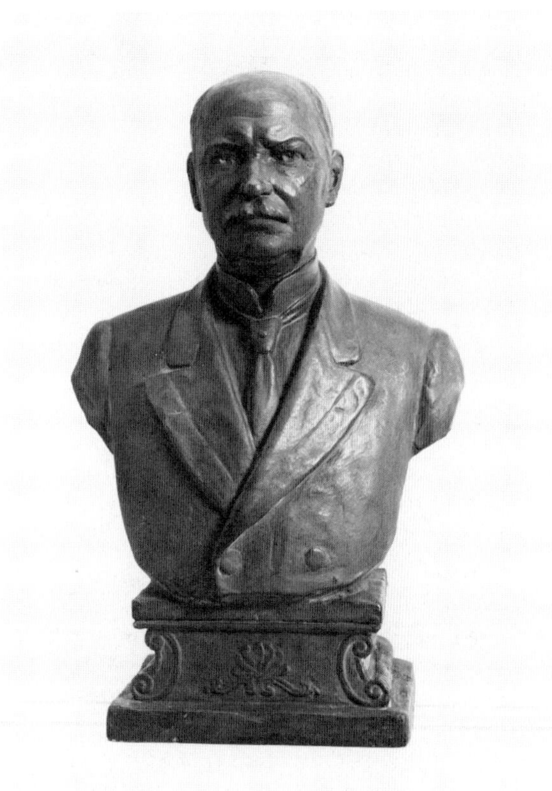

Henry Beates *ST 556*

Henry Beates (1857-1926)

Beates was born in Philadelphia, the son of a wholesale purveyor of drugs. He was an outstanding medical student at the University of Pennsylvania, where he received the M.D. degree in 1879. He was known best for his efforts to raise the standards of medical education. As a student he was chosen to participate in a joint faculty-student decision to extend the three-year course in medical education to four years. He was later appointed a member of the first state board of medical examiners in 1893 and was its president until 1911. For two years he served as president of the National Confederation of State Medical Examining and Licensing Boards. He was a fellow of the College of Physicians of Philadelphia. He received an honorary D.S. degree from Washington and Jefferson College in 1911.

Artist: Samuel Aloysius Murray (1870-1941)

For biography, see page 3.

Plaster, painted bronze color; 16 x 10 1/2 x 6 3/8; rectangular base, integral with sculpture, 3 1/4 in. high in front; signed and dated on rear, below shoulders, "To my friend/Dr. Beates/Saml Murray/July/1912." Shown at annual exhibition of the Pennsylvania Academy of the Fine Arts in 1913. Murray made another bust of Beates in 1912. Presented by Dr. William N. Bradley, 1943. *ST 556*

Dr. Beates is shown bust length, body frontal, head turned very slightly to the right. The partly bald head has flat strands of hair at the sides. The narrow eyes, with irises and pupils carved, look straight ahead. They are crowned by very long, S-curved eyebrows. The wide mouth is surmounted by a brush moustache. The square face has high cheekbones, long, thin ears, and an asymmetrical jowl and chin line. The subject wears a shirt with stand-up collar, a thin necktie with tie pin, and a double-breasted coat. The surface of this naturalistic sculpture is rather smooth, with subtle gradations of modelling and texture, which give a solid, anatomical construction to both head and body. The subject looks serious and dignified as he gazes directly and steadfastly toward the viewer. The base is unusually decorative, with a palmette flanked by volutes at the front.

Henry Jacob Bigelow (1818-1890)

The leading New England surgeon of his time, Bigelow was born in Boston, the son of Dr. Jacob Bigelow, first professor of materia medica at Harvard Medical School. Henry Bigelow received his degrees from Harvard, the A.B. in 1837 and the M.D. in 1841, and also studied in Paris and London. He was professor of surgery at Harvard from 1849 until 1882, when he was made professor emeritus. He was a pioneer in surgical pathology and was one of the earliest physicians to advocate the use of ether. In 1852 he excised the hip joint for the first time in America. In 1861 he demonstrated the accessory Y-ligament of the capsular ligament of the hip joint. In 1869 he wrote a classical treatise, *Mechanism of Dislocations and Fractures of the Hip, with the Reduction of the Dislocation by the Flexion Method.* He was equally famous for his method of crushing stones in the bladder and evacuating the fragments in one operation. He fought bitterly against Charles W. Eliot, president of Harvard University, who considered Bigelow intolerant and dogmatic for opposing vivisection, coeducation in medical school, and acceptance by visiting staff of fees collected from private patients treated in the hospital. He was an associate fellow of the College of Physicians.

Artist: Launt Thompson (1833-1894)

Born in Ireland, Thompson was brought to Albany, N.Y., where he studied anatomy with a physician and then spent nine years as a student and assistant in the sculpture studio of Erastus Dow Palmer. In 1857 he opened a studio in New York City, starting modestly with cameo portraits and idealized reliefs. He progressed quickly, becoming an associate of the National Academy of Design in 1859 and a full academician in 1862. His career was enhanced immeasurably through his friendship with William Waldorf Astor and his marriage to the sister of the

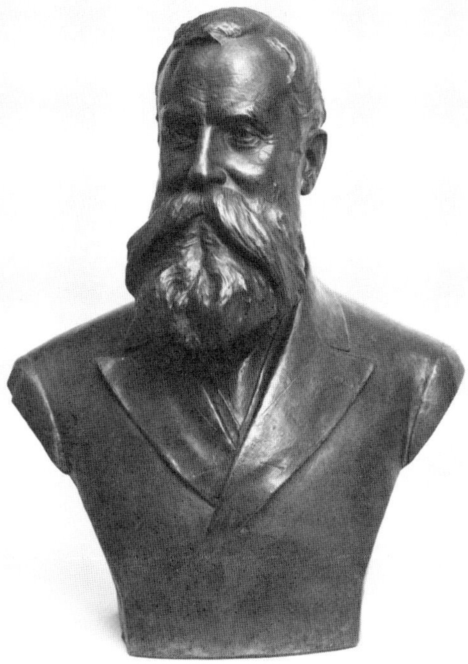

Henry Jacob Bigelow *ST 538*

Episcopal Bishop of New York, through whom he met the social elite. Thompson is best known for his vigorous portrait busts and full-length statues of prominent social, military, and political subjects such as Generals John Sedgwick and Winfield Scott, Admiral Dupont, Abraham Pierson, Edwin Booth in his role as Hamlet, and William Cullen Bryant. His portrait of Napoleon I was widely acclaimed at the Paris Exposition of 1867. After two trips to Rome and Florence in the late 1860s and 1870s, his brilliant career started to deteriorate, as he apparently underwent a personality change. Eventually he had to be committed to a mental hospital, where he died.

Bronze; 28 x 22 1/4 x 14; no base; signed and dated on rear of shoulders, "Lau Thompson/c/8 [?; 2nd digit not legible]"; "Gorham Mfg Co Founders N.Y.," inscription on bottom of right side. A replica is at Johns Hopkins University School of Medicine. Donor and date of donation not recorded.
ST 538

Dr. Bigelow is shown bust length, frontal torso, head turned to the left and tilted slightly downward. His hair is flat and wavy. His narrow eyes have deep crinkles in the corners and look out in the direction of the head turn. The slender nose and hollow cheeks are almost unnoticeable because of the long moustache and massive square beard, which projects forward five inches from the neck. The expansive torso is clothed in a shirt with high standing collar, a neckcloth with large round stick pin, a vest, and a coat with wide lapels. Bigelow's reputation for physical vigor, dramatic personality, and fashionable dress are well portrayed. The bust is over life size, with naturalistic rendering of body and costume by a solid, three-dimensional technique. The projections into space, especially of the beard, produce dramatic contrasts of light and shade on the irregularly tooled bronze surface. As a result of the size and technique, the subject displays a commanding and almost aggressive appearance.

Plaster, painted white; 28 1/2 x 22 x 14; no base; signed and dated on rear of shoulders, "Lau Thompson/c/8 [?; second digit not legible]"; replica of the above. Paper pasted on back of the sculpture states "Presented by Mr. Isaac [last name illegible], November [date illegible], Replica of a bust of / Dr. Henry C. [sic] Bigelow." College minutes of November 5, 1884, acknowledge presentation of sculpture by Isaac Hinckley. *ST 512*

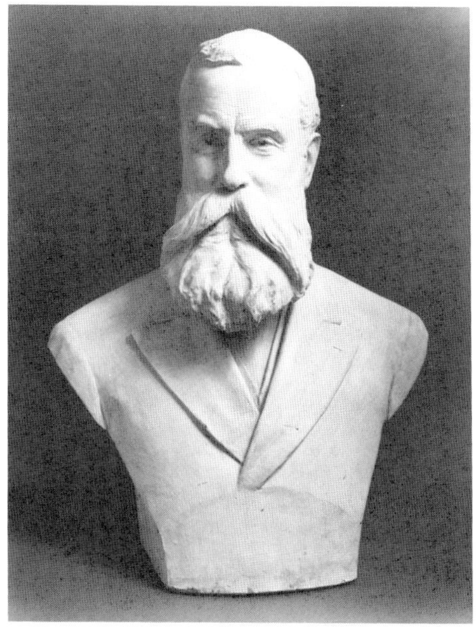

Henry Jacob Bigelow *ST 512*

George Isaac Blumstein (b. 1904)

Born in Philadelphia, Blumstein attended Temple University and received the M.D. degree from its school of medicine in 1929. At Temple he was successively instructor (1932); associate in medicine (1943–49); assistant professor of medicine (1950–56); associate professor of medicine (1957–64); chief, clinic of allergy and applied immunology (1964–74); clinical professor of medicine and immunology (1964–75); and emeritus professor (1975). At the Albert Einstein Medical Center he was associate in medicine and chief of allergy (1952–60) and attending in allergy (1960–65). Blumstein is certified by both the American Board of Internal Medicine and the American Board of Allergy and Immunology. He was president of the Philadelphia Allergy Society. He served the American Academy of Allergy as chairman of its section on allergy, member of the advisory board of the research

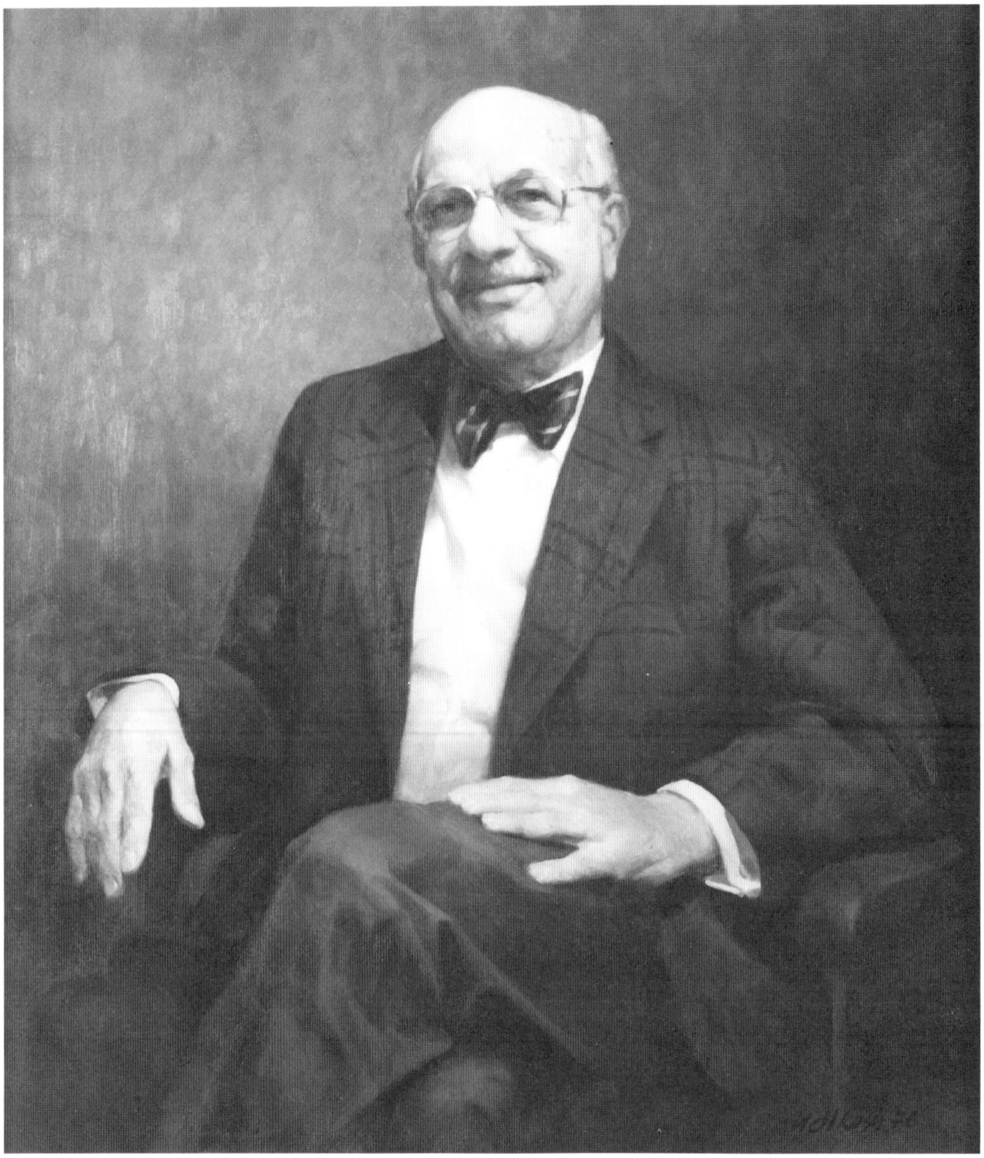

George Isaac Blumstein *PA 135*

council committee, treasurer, and president (1961–62). He was chairman of the Subspecialty Board of Allergy. At the College of Physicians of Philadelphia he was chairman of the S. Weir Mitchell Associates Committee, member of Council, vice president, president (1970–72), and chairman of the planning committee. He was vice-president of the section on allergy of the Pan American Medical Association. His writings include more than forty articles on such topics as the diagnosis, measurement, and treatment of allergy to food, pollen, and ragweed; hay fever; asthma; atopic dermatitis; nasal polyps; and anaphylaxis. With his son, Dr. Charles G. Blumstein, he wrote the chapter on drug reactions in Conn and Conn's *Current Diagnosis* (1971). He was on the editorial advisory board of the *Skin and Allergy News* and *Family Practice News*. He was given the Distinguished Service Award of the American Academy of Allergy in 1970 and in 1979 was honored by the Pennsylvania Medical Society for fifty years of medical service.

Artist: Neil Kosh (b. 1926)

Kosh was born in St. Clair, Pennsylvania. He attended Oberlin College. He received the B.F.A. and the B.S. in Education degrees from Temple University in 1954 and the M.F.A. degree from Temple in 1956, where he held a teaching fellowship. He served in the Navy during World War II and in the Army during the Korean War. At Temple he has taught drawing, painting, modelling, the science and technique of painting, and art education. He was chairman of the art department from 1963 to 1982 and director of the Temple University Program Abroad, at the Villa Caproni in Rome, from 1973 to 1975. Kosh is best known for his figure studies and portraits, including many of physicians. He has exhibited at group shows at the Pennsylvania Academy of the Fine Arts, the Philadelphia Art Alliance, the Butler Institute of Art, the San Diego Museum, the Springfield, Massachusetts, Museum of Fine Arts, the University of Delaware, Rosemont and Moravian Colleges, and the Woodmere Art Gallery in Philadelphia, where he has won first prize, Best-of-Year, and Purchase prizes. He has had one-man shows at the Woodmere Gallery, the Pearl Fox Gallery in Melrose Park, and the Paley Cultural Center at Temple University.

Oil on canvas; 35 1/2 x 39 1/2; signed and dated lower right, "Neil Kosh '76." Presented by Dr. George I. Blumstein, 1976. *PA 135*

Dr. Blumstein is shown three-quarters length, body slightly to the left, head slightly to the right and tilted upward. He is seated in a gray armchair placed at an angle of 45 degrees to the picture plane. The legs are crossed at the knees. The forearms rest on the chair arms, right hand pendent, the left hand on the thigh. The background is composed of mottled pink and green strokes, lighter on the left, darker on the right, and more muted toward the bottom. The subject has a high forehead with white hair at the sides of the head and a white brush moustache. His brown eyes look slightly upward through metal-rimmed glasses. He has a broad nose, a wide mouth with a full lower lip which emphasizes his expansive smile, a wide jaw, and a cleft chin. There are creases under his eyes and next to his nose and mouth. He wears a white shirt, a bright green and white striped bow tie, a single-breasted plaid sport coat with a green background and thin olive and red stripes, brown trousers, and gold cuff links. The surface of the portrait is painterly, with carefully placed but visible brush strokes including red accents throughout. The head and hands are rendered in solid, three-dimensional anatomical forms. There is a suggestion of the body underlying the costume. Although the pose is conventional, the choice of costume, affable smile, and lack of attributes create an informal, unpretentious portrayal; yet the impact on the viewer is forceful because of the subject's erect and energetic posture, kindly facial expression, and optimistic, confident demeanor.

Thomas Bond (1712-1784)

One of the foremost medical men of the 18th century, Bond was born in Calvert County, Maryland, and studied medicine under Dr. Alexander Hamilton in Annapolis and then in Paris. He established a general medical and surgical practice in Philadelphia with his brother, Phineas. Benjamin Franklin's *Autobiography* credits Bond with being the driving force behind the founding of the Pennsylvania Hospital. In 1766, Bond delivered at that hospital the first series of clinical lectures given in the United States. He was a member of the original board of trustees at the College of Philadelphia (later called the University of Pennsylvania) and was involved in establishing its medical school in 1765. He was a founder of the American Philosophical Society in 1768, a volunteer to the Committee of Safety in 1776, and the president of the Humane Society of Philadelphia in 1780.

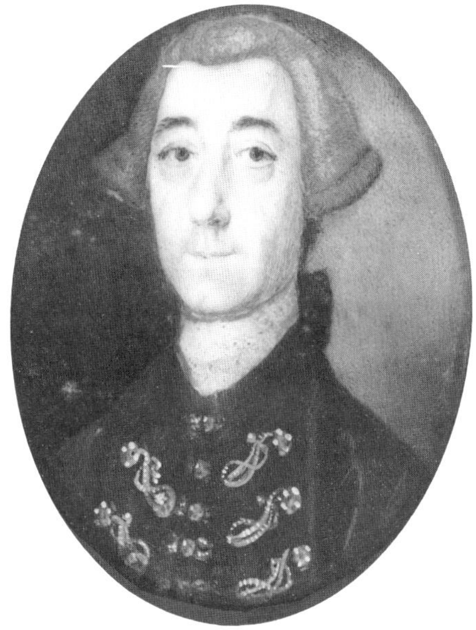

Thomas Bond *PH 574, PA 105*

Artist: Unknown

Water color on ivory; oval miniature, 2 x 1 1/2; not signed or dated. Presented by Dr. D. Sergeant Pepper from the estate of Dr. William Pepper, 1948. *PH 574, PA 105*

Dr. Bond is shown bust length, head and body turned slightly to the left. The background is medium brown on the left, lighter brown on the right. The gray wig has two formal curls at the ears and probably a queue in the back; a black ribbon can be seen at the nape of the neck. The blue eyes look toward the viewer. The nose is long and bulbous, the mouth small, with thin, pursed lips. The chin is square. The costume consists of a white stock, a dark brown waistcoat, and a brown coat with decorative gold frog closures. Although the well-drawn head is rendered sensitively in a smooth paint style, neither head nor body has solid, three-dimensional depth. Shadows, such as those under the eyes, consist of fine gray hatching, with brown overlying lines. The artist has succeeded in portraying the subject's elongated face and delicate constitution noted by several biographers.

Charles Walts Burr (1861-1944)

Descended from pre-revolutionary New Jersey Quakers and Irish Presbyterians, Burr was one of several nationally known Philadelphia neuropsychiatrists. After graduating from the University of Pennsylvania in 1883 and its medical school in 1886, he became assistant to Dr. S. Weir Mitchell (q.v.) at the Philadelphia General Hospital and was associated with Dr. Wharton Sinkler (q.v.) and Dr. William Osler (q.v.) at the Orthopaedic Hospital. From 1901 to 1930 he occupied the chair of psychiatry at the University of Pennsylvania School of Medicine and was consultant to many other hospitals. He was president of the Philadelphia Neurological Society, the Philadelphia Pathological Society, the

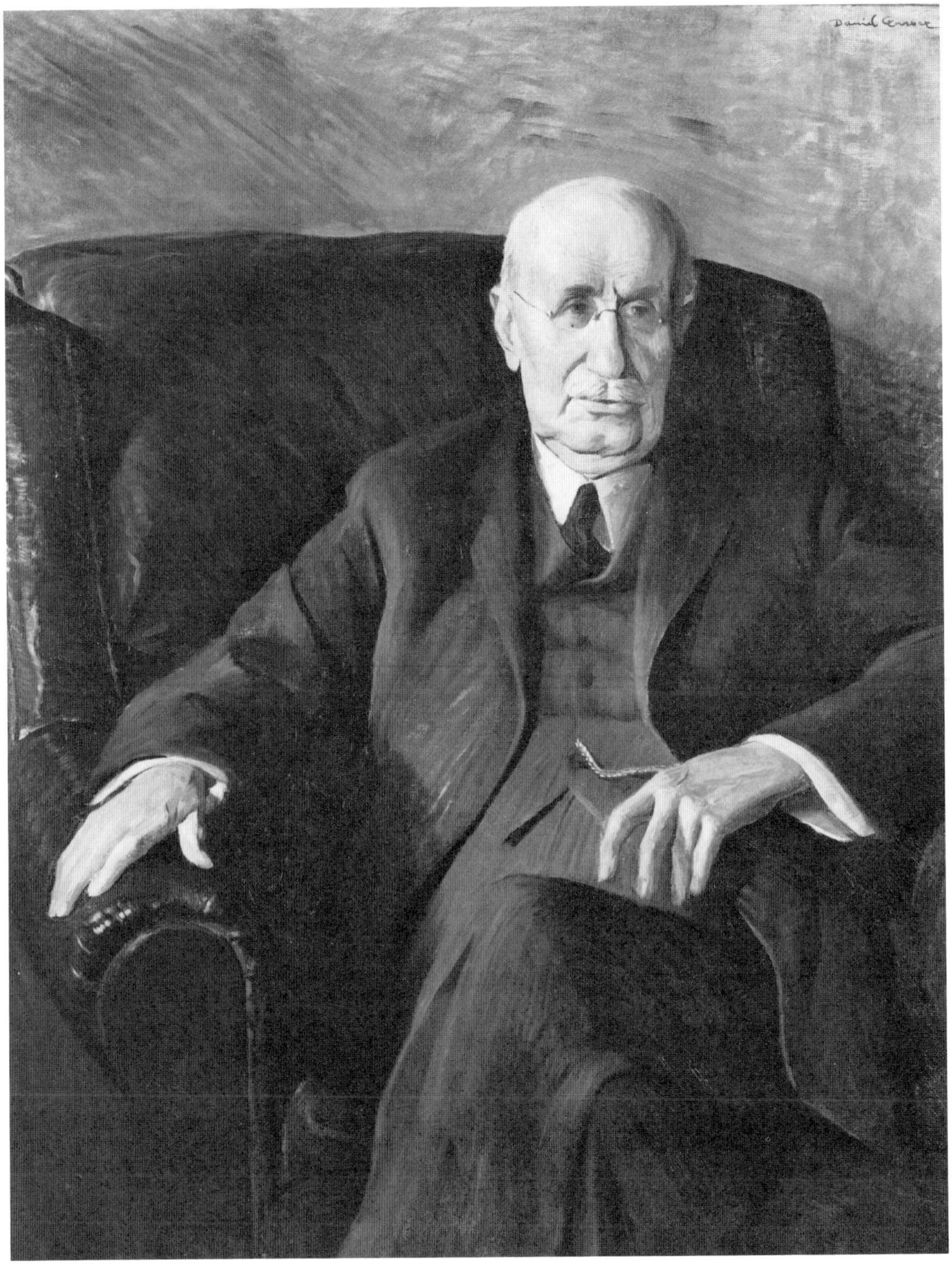

Charles Walts Burr PA 102

Philadelphia Psychiatric Society, and the National Eugenics Research Society. He was a trustee of the Episcopal Academy and of the University of Pennsylvania, where he received a Doctor of Science degree. He was awarded the Strittmatter Medal. A man of broad interests, he was a fellow and honorary librarian at the College of Physicians of Philadelphia, an active member of the Dickens Fellowship of Philadelphia, the American Philosophical Society, the Franklin Inn Club, the Numismatic and Antiquarian Society of Philadelphia, and the Philobiblon Club. Greatly interested in the welfare of promising students, Dr. Burr often subsidized their education and guided their careers.

Artist: Daniel Garber (1880–1958)

Born on an Indiana farm, Garber's forbears were Pennsylvania-German immigrants who came to America in the mid-18th century. His first art instruction was at the Cincinnati Art Academy in 1897, at a time when Frank Duveneck and other German-trained artists exerted influence there. He continued at the Pennsylvania Academy of the Fine Arts from 1899 to 1905, under Thomas Anshutz, William Merritt Chase, and Cecilia Beaux; while a student he won the Toppan Prize in 1903 and Cresson Traveling Fellowship in 1905, which enabled him to study in London, Florence, and Paris. Upon his return to Philadelphia he taught at the Philadelphia School of Design for Women for a short time and then joined the faculty of the Pennsylvania Academy, where he remained a beloved teacher and distinguished artist for forty-two years. Garber was best known for his impressionist canvases of lyrical color, especially his landscapes of Bucks County, and for his genteel, domestic figure studies. Garber was an aggressive exhibitor and a consistent prize winner; he was an artist of national reputation, and his works are owned by prominent museums across the country. At the National Academy of Design he was made an academician in 1913 and won prizes in 1909, 1915, 1917, 1922, and 1923. At the Pennsylvania Academy he won the Lippincott Prize in 1911, the Stotesbury Award in 1918, the Temple Gold Medal in 1919, the Locust Club Medal in 1923, the Gold Medal of Honor in 1929, the Sesnan Gold Medal in 1937, the Pennell Medal in 1942, and popular prizes in 1933, 1940, and 1941. He won the Clark Prize at the Corcoran Gallery in 1910, 1912, and 1921, the Potter Palmer Gold Medal at the Art Institute of Chicago in 1911, the Gold Medal at the Panama-Pacific Exposition in San Francisco in 1915, the Gold Medal of the Art Club of Philadelphia in 1923, and prizes at the Carnegie International Exhibition in 1924 and 1933. He painted a mural for the Pennsylvania Building at the Sesquicentennial exhibition in 1926. Important one-man exhibitions of his work were held at the Philadelphia Art Alliance in 1918 and 1924, the Macbeth Gallery in New York in 1925 and 1931, the Tricker Galleries in New York in 1938, the Norfolk Museum of Arts and Science in 1940, the Woodmere Gallery, Philadelphia, and the Corcoran Gallery in 1942, the American Academy of Arts and Letters in 1948, and the Pennsylvania Academy of the Fine Arts in 1945 and 1980 (the exhibition catalogue of the latter show provided many of these facts).

Oil on canvas; 39 x 31; signed upper right, "Daniel Garber." Presented by the friends of Dr. Burr, 1938. On the back of the canvas is written, "Portrait of Charles Walts Burr/Born Nov. 16, 1861/Elected Fellow of College Physicians, 1892/ Painted by Daniel Garber/October, 1938." PA 102

The figure is shown at three-quarter length, seated in a large brown leather easy chair, with legs crossed and arms resting on rolled chair arms. The background consists of diagonal streaks of yellow-green, orange, tan, white, and brown. The head is bald except for a white fringe at the sides. The blue-gray eyes look out toward the spectator through metal-rimmed spectacles whose magnification blurs the eyes. The long nose is accentuated by the downward tilt of the head. Age is described by deep lines above and below the white moustache and on the forehead, by the jowls, and by loose skin at the neck. The subject wears a white shirt, a black necktie, a three-piece gray suit, and a watch chain. The impressionistic style of rapid strokes produces a painterly surface which suits the relaxed posture, kindly facial expression, and direct, almost conversational pose. The head has been depicted as solidly three-dimensional. There is a suggestion of the torso underlying the costume. The artist has succeeded in capturing his subject's confident and generous nature.

Thomas Cadwalader (1707?-1779)

The son of 17th century Welsh settlers, Cadwalader studied medicine first in Philadelphia with an uncle and then at Rheims and in England under William Cheselden. On his return to Philadelphia he established a large medical practice and was active in civic affairs. According to Dr. Caspar Wistar (q.v.) he "made dissections and demonstrations for the instruction of the elder Dr. Shippen and some others who had not been abroad." About this time (1730 or 1731), he made inoculations against smallpox and was associated with Benjamin Franklin in establishing the Philadelphia Library. It is said that he performed the first truly scientific autopsy in this country (1742). *An Essay on the West India Dry Gripes with the Method of Preventing and Curing that Cruel Distemper. . .* , published by Franklin in 1745, was one of the earliest medical monographs issued in this country. He was one of the original members of the Philadelphia Medical Society and a vice president of the American Philosophical Society. He was a trustee of the Academy of Philadelphia (later the College of Philadelphia, now the University of Pennsylvania). He was a member of the Philadel-

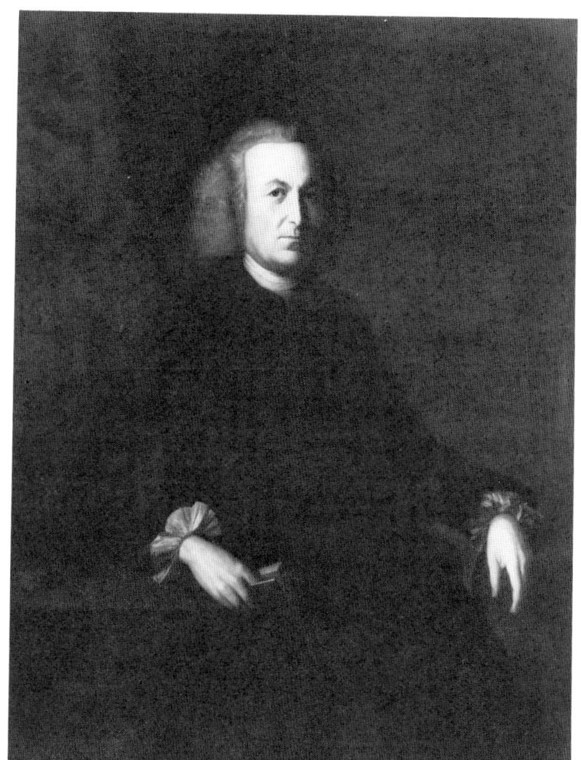

Thomas Cadwalader PA 70

phia Common Council and the Provincial Council. He is said to have helped Dr. John Morgan (q.v.) in his work as director-general of the American military hospitals.

Artist: Unknown

Oil on canvas, mounted on wood; 49 1/4 x 39 1/4. Copy after portrait by Charles Willson Peale, 1772, owned by Capt. John Cadwalader (U.S.N., ret.). Presented by John Lambert Cadwalader, Esq., 1881. Probably a middle to late 19th century copy; resembles a portrait of Cadwalader at Pennsylvania Hospital. *PA 70*

Dr. Cadwalader is shown two-thirds length, with body and head turned slightly to the right. He is seated in a Queen Anne-style armchair, his legs spread apart. His left arm rests on the chair arm, the hand hangs over the edge. His right arm rests on a table; his hand holds a book, the index finger marking the place. The background on the right is grayish-green atmospheric space. On the left maroon drapery hangs down to a table that is covered in green fabric and has a small wooden oval box on its top. The subject has a high forehead surmounted by a full, gray, frizzed, chin-length wig. His blue eyes look out toward the viewer. The tip of his long, thin nose points downward toward the wide mouth and thin, pursed lips. The jaw is square. The subject wears a white stock, a long black waistcoat buttoned in rippling folds over a paunchy abdomen, a long, black, unbuttoned coat without a collar, white ruffled cuffs, black breeches, and black stockings. The surface is painted smoothly, with no visible brush strokes; the edges are hard. The hands and face appear more solid and three-dimensional than the body. The subject engages the viewer with a serious, confident, determined expression, as though he had paused for a moment in his reading.

Charles Caldwell (1772-1853)

Born in North Carolina, the son of Irish Presbyterians who immigrated in 1752, Caldwell received the M.D. from the medical department of the University of Pennsylvania in 1796. In the same year he was elected a member of the American Philosophical Society and of the College of Physicians of Philadelphia. Dogmatic and aggressive, he aroused the enmity of his former mentor, Benjamin Rush (q.v.), over the causes of yellow fever, and he never received appointment in the medical department of the University. However, he was elected to the chair of geology and philosophy of natural history. He served as surgeon under George Washington in the Whiskey Rebellion of 1794. He edited *The Port Folio*, a leading literary journal. He left Philadelphia and helped to found the medical department of Transylvania University in Lexington, Kentucky, where he was professor of materia medica from 1818 to 1837. In 1837 he was instrumental in founding the Louisville Medical Institute, later merged into the University of Louisville, and was professor of materia medica. His literary writings number more than two hundred.

Artist: Attributed to Thomas Sully (1783-1872)

An illustrious painter of portraits, miniatures, and historical scenes, Sully was the son of English actors who brought him to Charleston, South Carolina, from Horncastle, Lincolnshire, in 1792. His earliest instructors were painters of miniatures in Richmond, Virginia. Later, he watched Henry Benbridge and John Trumbull paint his own portrait and then spent three weeks in Boston with Gilbert Stuart, who advised him to go to London. In 1808, after Sully had settled in Philadelphia, patrons provided him with funds for study in England, where he studied with Benjamin West, Henry Fuseli, and most importantly, with the prominent portraitist, Sir Thomas Lawrence. Upon his return to Philadelphia and during his long career, Sully did almost 500 subject paintings, but he was best known for the more than 2000 portraits of the leading social and political figures in Philadelphia and other East Coast cities. One of his greatest honors was to paint the recently crowned Queen Victoria in London in 1838. In 1812 he was elected an academician at the Pennsylvania Academy of the Fine Arts. He declined an invitation to become the Academy's president but he exhibited work there between 1811 and 1868. In 1922 the Academy held an exhibition of his portraits. He also exhibited at the National Academy of Design, where he was an honorary professional member between 1827 and 1852. From 1819 to 1847 Sully was associated with James Earle, a carver, in a commercial gallery that sold American and foreign works of art. Sully kept an almost complete documented list of his portraits, known as *A Register of Portraits Painted by Thomas Sully*, and wrote a treatise titled *Hints to Young Painters and the Process of Portrait Painting*. This was prepared in 1851, revised in 1871, and published in 1873.

Oil on canvas; 29 x 24 1/4; not signed or dated. Donor and date of donation are unrecorded. At the College of Physicians' Centennial Celebration Loan Collection of Portraits *in 1887, the owner of this portrait was listed as the College of Physicians and the artist was listed as "unknown"; at the Pennsylvania Academy's* Loan Exhibition of Historical Portraits *(1887-88), the owner was listed as the College of Physicians and the artist was listed as "anonymous"; the 1898-1915 Inventory of the College of Physicians of Philadelphia lists it as "artist unknown." Although no documents at the College of Physicians of Philadelphia relate to this work, various inventories starting in the 1930s credit it to Sully, and the same attribution was given in 1965 by* The Art of Philadelphia Medicine *exhibition at the Philadelphia Museum of Art. The work is not mentioned in Sully's* Register of Portraits. *The portrait has had extensive cleaning and repainting, especially over the face. The*

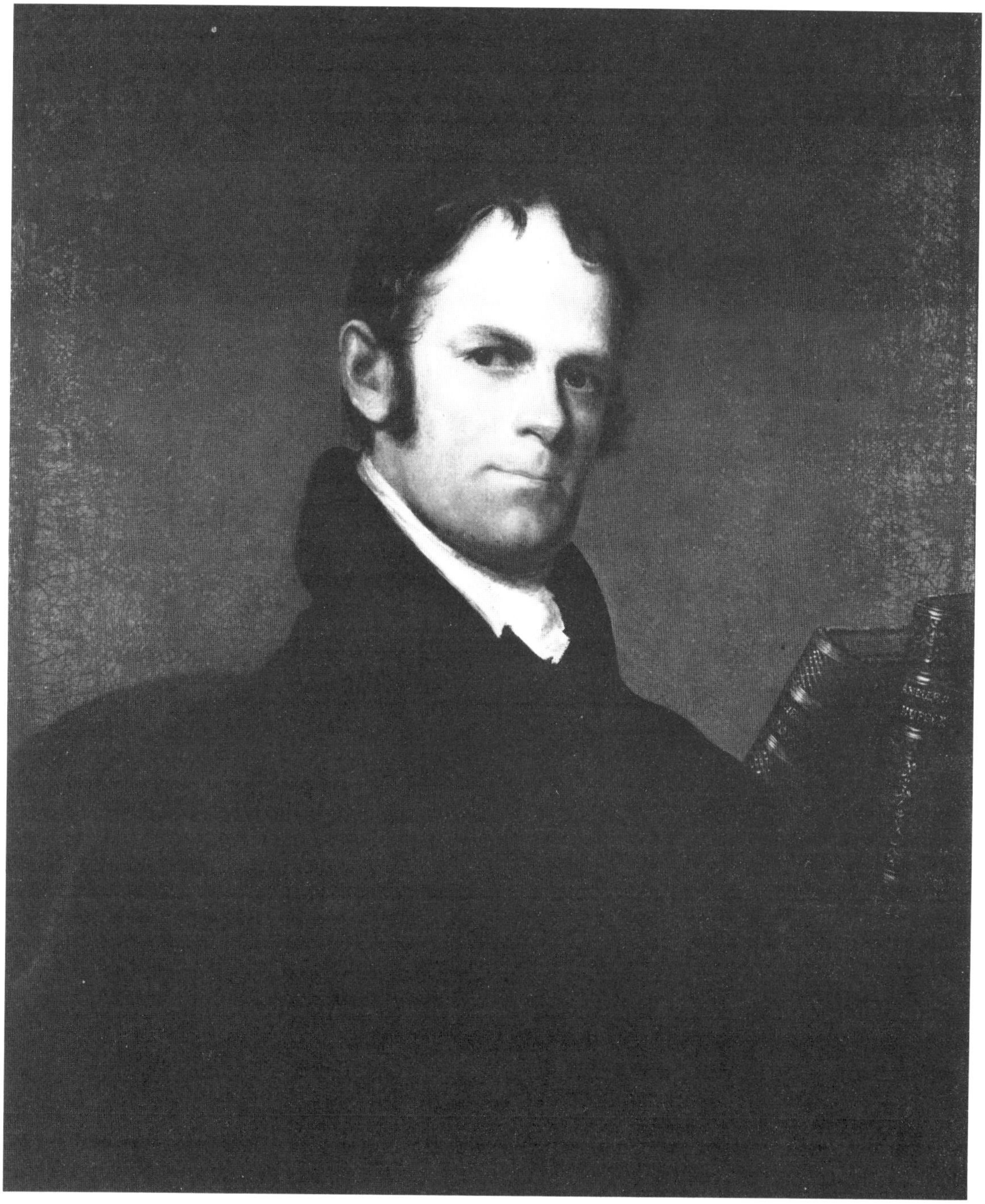

Charles Caldwell

PA 49

stretchers are old and probably contemporary with the subject. Of three experts who recently examined the painting, one is of the opinion that it is not by Sully, one was non-committal, and one felt that it could probably be "attributed to" Sully because of the dash of the pose with its characteristic elongated neck and tilt of the head and the paint quality in the neckcloth and collar. Fine as the painting is, it cannot be positively identified as a work by Sully without further research. *PA 49*

Dr. Caldwell is shown bust length, body and head turned to the right, head tilted slightly downward. He is seated in a red upholstered armchair. Next to his left shoulder are two books bound in green with gold lettering, "Warton's Pope" and "Smellie's Buffon VII"—intended, no doubt, to underscore Caldwell's breadth of interest. The reference is to the *Essay on the Writings and Genius of Pope* by the critic and poet Joseph Wharton and to W. Smellie's translation of Georges Louis Leclerc Buffon's multivolume *Histoire Naturelle* . . . . The atmospheric background is warm greenish-umber. The subject has dark brown hair with several curly strands on his high forehead and long side-whiskers, brown eyes which look out just past the spectator, a wide mouth, thin lips, and a round chin. He wears a white neckcloth and a black double-breasted, high-necked coat. The painterly style of the portrait has visible brush strokes, especially on the hair and face; the head is rendered as a three-dimensional, solid structure. The costume, though more smoothly and flatly painted, has wrinkles in the coat, suggestive of fabric puckered over the underlying body. The attentive facial expression and expansive torso portray the commanding physical presence for which Caldwell was known.

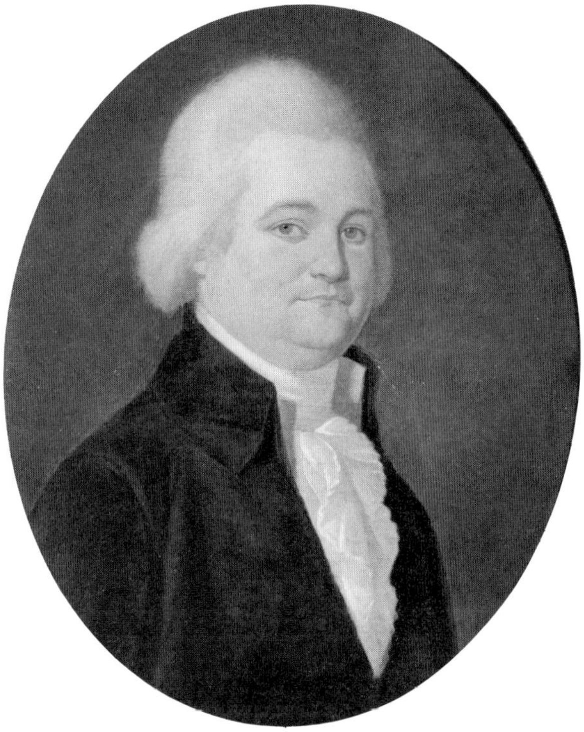

John Carson *PA 111*

John Carson (1752–1794)

Born in Philadelphia and the son of Irish immigrants from County Antrim, Carson was graduated from the College of Philadelphia (later the University of Pennsylvania) in 1771 and received his medical degree from the University of Edinburgh in 1776. After his return to Philadelphia he was made attending physician at the Philadelphia Dispensary. He was one of the original junior founding fellows of the College of Physicians of Philadelphia, a member of the American Philosophical Society, surgeon of the First Troop Philadelphia City Cavalry, and one of the first two physician-members of the Hibernian Society. He was trustee of the University of Pennsylvania from 1791 to 1794 and was elected to the chair of chemistry in 1794.

Artist: Unknown

Oil on canvas; oval, 23 x 19 1/4; not signed or dated. Presented by the estate of Joseph Lapsley Wilson, grandson of Dr. Carson, in 1932. In the College of Physicians' Centennial Celebration Loan Collection of Portraits *(1887), a portrait of Dr. Carson was included, owned by Mrs. Elizabeth Febiger Wilson, the artist listed as "unknown." The portrait at the College of Physicians of Philadelphia was included in* The Art of Philadelphia Medicine *Exhibition, Philadelphia Museum of Art (1965), labeled "attributed to Rembrandt Peale." Problems surrounding this painting include the observation that the subject looks older than 42, his age at death, whereas if the painting had been done from life by Rembrandt Peale, the artist would have been no older than 16. The painting has been so extensively overcleaned and repainted that little of the original surface remains. Careful reading of correspondence from descendants in the College of Physicians files reveals that the family had two copies made by Albert Rosenthal (1863–1939, q.v.), one larger and one smaller. The larger one, located at the University of Pennsylvania, is rectangular, and although showing the same pose, differs in details of costume, hair, and facial features. An inscription on the back of this Rosenthal large copy says, "Painted for Hampton L. Carson (for the University of Pennsylvania) by Albert Rosenthal from an original painting owned by Captain R. Lapsley Willson. . . ." The location of the smaller copy is unknown. Correspondence in the College of Physicians files also gives rise to doubt that the painting at the College of Physicians of Philadelphia is the original painting by Peale and indicates that many family portraits have been widely distributed among the heirs of Joseph Lapsley Wilson. The extensive overcleaning and repainting almost precludes making an attribution on the basis of style.* *PA 111*

Dr. Carson is shown bust length, with head and body turned to the right. The background is very warm reddish-sienna. The subject has thick, almost wooly, gray hair that is chin length and brushed back from his face. Light blue-gray eyes look out of the corners to gaze at he observer. The nose is small, the lips are thin. The florid round face has a double chin. The subject wears a white stock, a white shirt with frill, a yellow high-collared waistcoat, and a dark brownish-black coat with high collar and no lapels. In its present state the surface of the painting has visible brush strokes, especially the green, gray, and blue shadows in face and hair. The head is solidly structured, and there is some feeling for the underlying mass of the body beneath the costume. The lack of animation in the face is probably due to extensive restoration.

Nathaniel Chapman (1780–1853)

Born in Fairfax County, Virginia, Chapman began his medical studies privately in Virginia and continued them under Benjamin Rush (q.v.) in Philadelphia. In 1801 he graduated with honors from the medical school of the University of Pennsylvania and completed his studies in London and Edinburgh. From 1813 to 1850 he was professor of materia medica at the University of Pennsylvania and later served as professor of theory and practice of medicine. In 1817 he founded the Medical Institute of Philadelphia, the first post-graduate medical school. He was also clinical lecturer at the Philadelphia Almshouse, later known as the Philadelphia General Hospital. He was president of the Philadelphia Medical Society for six successive yearly terms. In 1847 he was elected by acclamation the first president of the American Medical Association. He was president of the American Philosophical Society and a fellow of the College of Physicians of Philadelphia. In 1820 he was editor of the *Journal of Medical and Physical Sciences.* He was author of *Elements of Therapeutics and Materia*

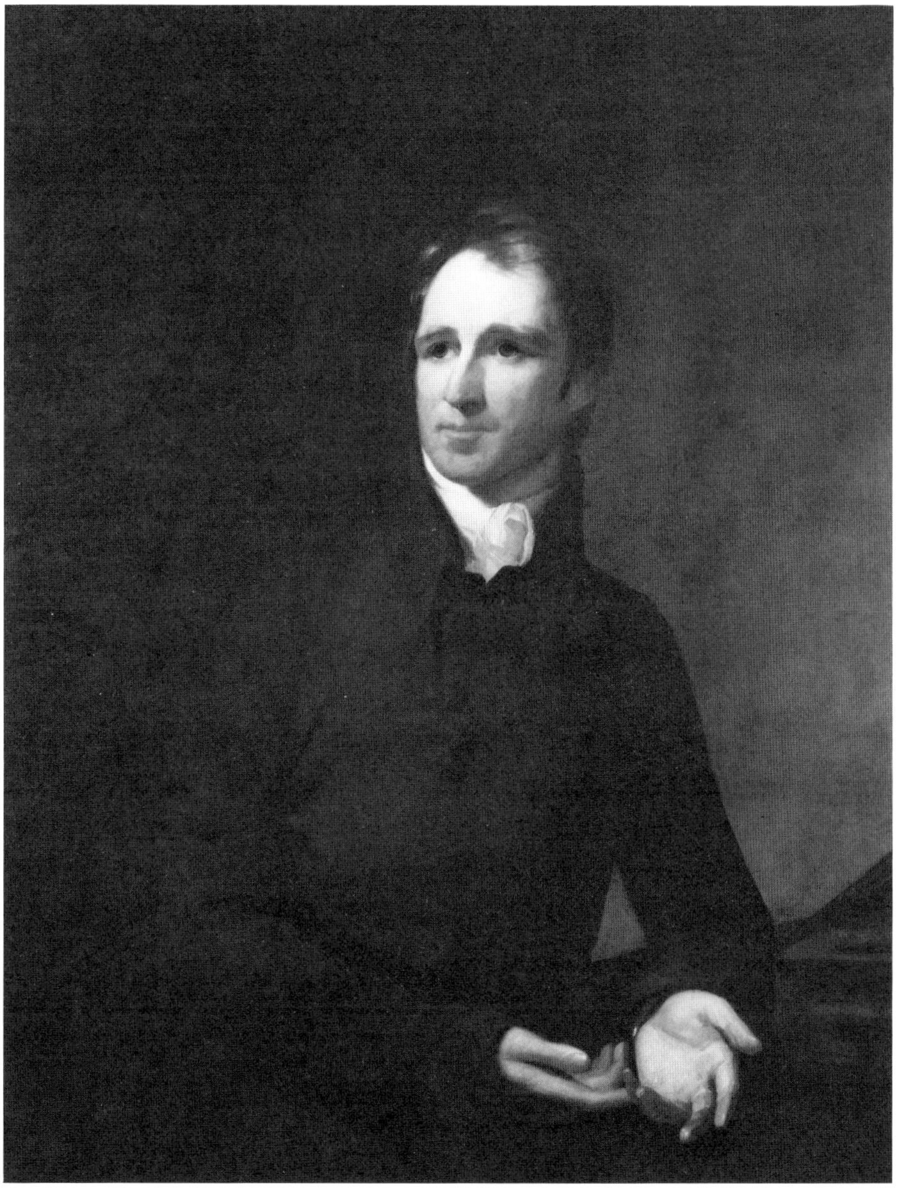

Nathaniel Chapman *PA 40*

Medica (1827), *A Compendium of Lectures on the Theory and Practice of Medicine* (1846), and other important books. At his death, the College of Physicians of Philadelphia resolved to procure a "Bust and Portrait" to commemorate Dr. Chapman's distinguished career.

Artist: Thomas Sully (1783–1872)

For biography, see page 18.

Oil on canvas; 41 x 32 1/4; signed and dated on back of relined canvas, "TS/1817." Listed in Sully's Register of Portraits *as having been begun April 14 and completed July 1, 1817. Engraved by John Neagle and by C. Goodman and R. Piggot. Sully painted Chapman again in 1848, a three-quarter length portrait at the University of Pennsylvania, from which Samuel Bell Waugh made in 1859 a bust-length copy that is at the American Philosophical Society. The portrait belonging to the College of Physicians of Philadelphia was shown at its* Centennial Celebration Loan Collection of Portraits *(1887); in that catalogue the owner is listed as Dr. Henry C. Chapman; the College's portrait was also shown at the* Sully Memorial Exhibition, *Pennsylvania Academy of the Fine Arts (1922), at the American Medical Association convention in Philadelphia (1957), and at* The Art of Philadelphia Medicine *exhibition, Philadelphia Museum of Art (1965). Presented by Mrs. Henry Cadwalader Chapman, 1910, in memory of Professor Henry Cadwalader Chapman, grandson of Nathaniel Chapman; copied by Mr. Phillip in 1936 for Mr. Van Antwerp Lea.* *PA 40*

Dr. Chapman is shown half-length, the body frontal, the head turned to the left. He stands with his weight leaning on his left forearm, which rests on a table covered with green cloth and three books. The right arm crosses the body so that the hands come together with palms up, almost an explanatory gesture. Behind the figure on the left is a diagonal area of reddish-brown drapery. Dimly visible on the right upper half are the outlines of bookshelves lined with books; the background color below is a light brown. The subject has medium brown hair with a few strands brushed on his forehead. His deepset large gray eyes, which look to the left, have strong shadows under the brows. The prominent nose has a wide bridge and broad tip turned downward. The costume consists of a white neckcloth and a dark brown double-breasted coat. This is a romantic style of portraiture with soft edges, subtle gradations of light and dark, expressive gesture, and touseled hair. The surfaces of the face and hands are painterly, with visible brush strokes, while the costume is smoothly painted but with loose, fluid strokes. The figure is energetic, lively, and in motion with a turn of the head and gesture of the hands, as though in animated conversation with an unseen visitor. Chapman is said to have been a man of great charm, exuberant vitality, and genial wit.

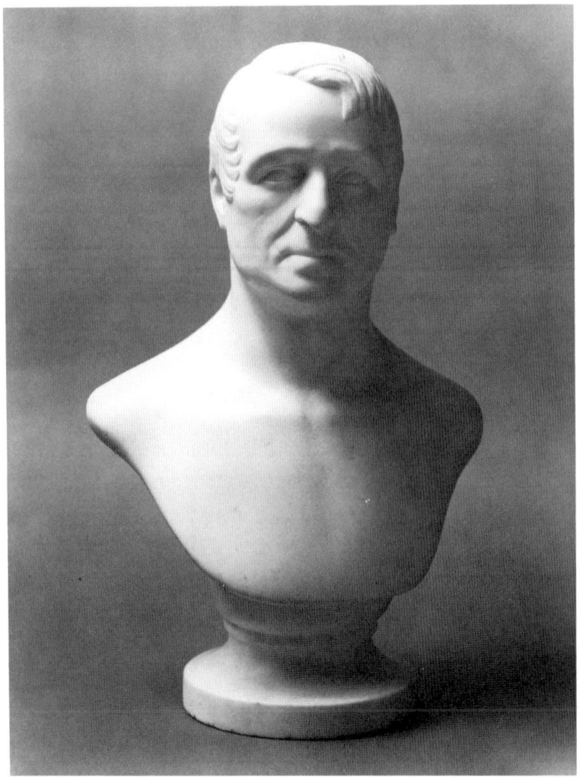

Nathaniel Chapman *ST 545*

Artist: Unknown

Marble; 19 x 12 1/4 x 8; circular base integral with sculpture, 3 1/2 in. high in front; not signed or dated. Presented by William S. Vaux, Esq., 1868. *ST 545*

Dr. Chapman is shown bust length, with frontal torso and head turned slightly to the left. The hair consists of wide, differentiated strands brushed toward the cheeks and with bangs above the left eye. The eyebrows are long and flat. The eyes, with pupil and iris incised, look straight ahead. The nose is elongated, with a flat, drooping tip. The small mouth has pursed lips. The jaw line is wide and the chin is pointed. The shape of the face is square, in contrast with the more oval shape in Sully's painting of Chapman. Despite the idiosyncratic nose, the sculpted portrayal is idealized and neoclassical in concept, with its stylized hair, nude bust, and neutral, bland expression.

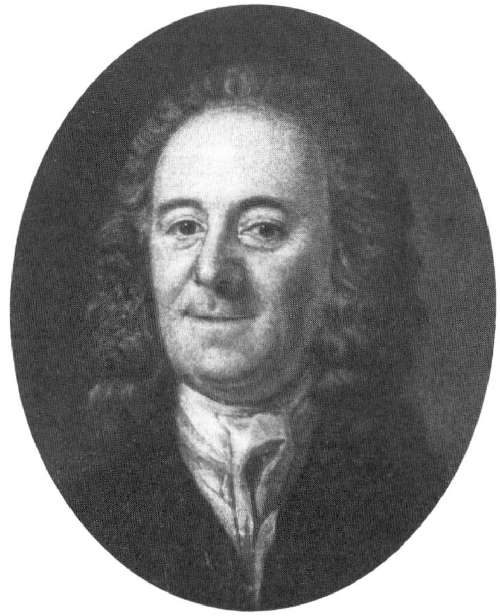

Abraham Chovet *PA 56*

Abraham Chovet (1704–1790)

The only founder of the College of Physicians of Philadelphia born outside of America, Chovet was born in England. Although his parentage and education are unknown, by 1732 he had published in London *A Syllabus, or Index, of all the Parts that enter the Composition of the Human Body*. To illustrate the twelve lectures described in this work, he created wax anatomical models. From 1734 to 1736 he was demonstrator of anatomy for the Company of Barber-Surgeons in London. Perhaps because of professional notoriety concerning a bizarre scheme to keep alive a hanged criminal, Chovet left London and practiced anatomy in Barbados and Jamaica. It is not known why Philadelphia was his next destination, but by 1774 he was a professional and social success there, delivering lectures in anatomy for both medical and lay audiences, including prominent political, clerical, and social dignitaries. By 1777 he had collected an anatomical museum for his dried specimens and wax models and had built an amphitheater for his lectures. His wax models were so widely admired that after his death they were purchased from his heirs by the Pennsylvania Hospital. Later they were transferred to the University of Pennsylvania but were mostly destroyed in a fire in 1888. Chovet was more than eighty years of age when the College of Physicians was established. It was considered a singular honor for this elderly doctor to be a senior founder.

Artist: Unknown

Oil on canvas; oval, 16 3/4 x 14 3/4. Presented by Mrs. L.C. Hay, 1867. Included in College of Physicians' Centennial Celebration Loan Collection of Portraits *(1887); also in* Loan Exhibition of Historical Portraits, *Pennsylvania*

Academy of the Fine Arts (1887–88), where artist is suggested as "C.W. Peale (?)." It is definitely not by Peale, but could perhaps be by an English or English-trained artist who was a contemporary of the subject. *PA 56*

Dr. Chovet is shown head and neck length, body frontal, head turned slightly to the left. The dark brown atmospheric background is lighter on the right. The gray, shoulder-length wig has curls which frame the face. The brown eyes gaze straight ahead toward the viewer. The wide mouth has lips parted in a smile. The full, oval face has a double chin. The subject wears a white stock and a neckcloth, a white waistcoat, and a black coat. In spite of the damaged state of the portrait, it is apparent that the paint surface probably was smoothly brushed originally. The head is well formed, although the portrayal is somewhat primitive anatomically, since the nose is turned more to the side than the eyes and mouth. Chovet's sparkling eyes and cheerful smile give him a pleasant expression and suggest his outgoing personality.

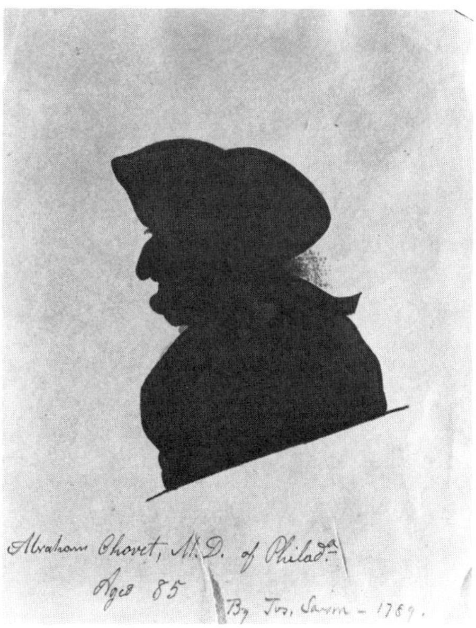

Abraham Chovet *PH 293*

Artist: Joseph Sansom (1767–1826)

According to an article by Charles Coleman Sellers ("Joseph Sansom, Philadelphia Silhouettist," *Pennsylvania Magazine of History and Biography*, vol. 88, October, 1964), Sansom was an amateur silhouettist whose life was devoted to travel, literature, and the arts. After his marriage to Beulah Biddle in 1798 he spent three years traveling in Switzerland and Italy. Upon his return to Philadelphia he designed a series of medals to commemorate important events in American history. In recognition, he was elected to the American Philosophical Society and his portrait by Charles Willson Peale was placed in the Society's museum. The Historical Society of Pennsylvania owns a manuscript book of thirty-four silhouettes by Sansom entitled *An OCCASIONAL COLLECTION of PHYSIOGNOMICAL SKETCHES Chiefly North Americans, and drawn from the life; designed to preserve the characteristic features, personally, mentally, or officially [of] REMARKABLE PERSONS, and the endeared Memory of PRIVATE FRIENDS or PUBLIC BENEFACTORS, with professional Notices &c. PHILADELPHIA, 1790, 91, & 92.* Under each profile the artist has written in ink the name and sometimes an identification, the city, and age of the subject. The table of contents lists the subject's height ("tall" or "short"), place of birth, and dates. This valuable tabulation lists many silhouettes which had been sold from the collection before it came to the Historical Society. It is known that several items in the original collection were copied by Thomas Gilpin, George Vaux, and August Edouart (q.v.). In the preface Sansom confusingly states that the silhouettes are "defective in regard to relative proportions, being drawn from memory, without the use of a scale." Whether drawn from life or from memory, they were painted freehand, without the use of mechanical devices, and are exuberant and sometimes flamboyant in character.

Silhouette; black ink on cream colored paper; 4 7/8 x 3 7/8; written in black ink below silhouette, "Abraham Chovet, M.D. of Philadª/Aged 85"; written in pencil in another hand, below the name of the subject, "By Jos. Sansom — 1789"; the date of 1789 is incorrect because this is one in a group done in 1790–92). This silhouette is missing from the Historical Society book, but is mentioned in its table of contents with the information, "short, London. 1704–1790." There is a copy in the Gilpin collection. If the age of 85 is correct (Sansom gives Chovet's dates correctly and Chovet was 85 in 1789), perhaps this is one silhouette which was done from memory, or perhaps Chovet was actually 86, and it could have been done the year of his death. Presented by Hampton L. Carson, 1910. *PH 293*

Chovet is shown bust length, profile to the left. His large hooked nose, recessed lips, and jutting chin appear almost caricatural, but the profile agrees with a description of him in his old age when he lacked teeth. Details include eyelashes, and there are dots at the neck to indicate hair. The subject wears a cocked hat turned up at the brim, a hair ribbon, and a coat. The contours of this silhouette are drawn in heavy black lines and are filled in with a black wash of varying degrees of opacity.

Portrait of "Christ" [Insane Patient]

Artist: Unknown

Oil on canvas; 13 1/2 x 11 1/2; signed and dated lower right, "Maurer, 1890." Presented by Mrs Daniel E. Hughes, through Dr. T.H. Andrews, 1902. This portrait presents unsolved problems of identity. A letter in the files of the College of Physicians of Philadelphia, said to have been on the back of the painting and dated November 4, 1902, was addressed to Dr. Andrews. It describes the painting as the work of an artist named Benjamin Fox, who was a patient in the "insane wards" at Philadelphia Hospital in 1892 and 1893. He imagined that he was Christ and painted himself as Christ; he gave the painting to Dr. Hughes. His age as

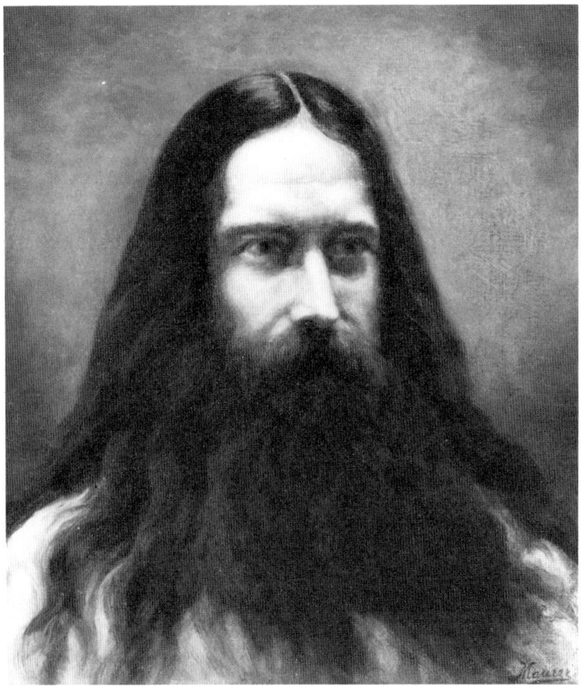

"Christ" [Insane Patient] PA 42

stated in the hospital records and in a reference to a newspaper article corresponds exactly with that of one Benjamin B. Fox, who studied at the Pennsylvania Academy of the Fine Arts in 1882, 1883, 1884, and 1888, and won the Charles Toppan First Prize in the annual exhibition of 1888. However, when the painting was cleaned at a later date, the signature, "Maurer, 1890," was revealed. This is two years before Fox was supposed to have painted his work. There have been many artists named Maurer. This painting could possibly be the work of Charles Maurer (1844–1931), a well-known portraitist in Philadelphia. A newspaper photograph shows him at the age of 83, standing in front of a recent self-portrait. Interestingly, the head is in the same position as that in the College's portrait; moreover, the subject wears a beard and moustache, and has a similarly shaped nose and head. More research must be done on this painting to establish whether any connection existed between Benjamin Fox and any artist named Maurer. PA 42

"Christ" is shown bust length, torso frontal, head turned to the right. The atmospheric background is gray, lighter around the head, darker in the corners. The subject has long, dark brown hair, parted in the center, flowing over his shoulders to meet the long beard and moustache. The deepset blue eyes look out in direction of the head turn. The long, slender face is creased by lines in the forehead and cheeks. The subject wears a white shirt or robe. The surface of this portrait is painterly, with visible brush strokes which define carefully modelled planes; the edges of forms are soft. The head is constructed in an anatomically solid, three-dimensional style. The contemplative, almost mysterious facial expression is most apparent in the eyes, which are unfocused and in deep shadow, and in the mouth, which is completely hidden by the beard and moustache.

Richard Alsop Cleeman (1840-1912)

Cleeman was born in Philadelphia and received all his higher education at the University of Pennsylvania. He received the A.B. in 1859 and the M.A. and M.D. degrees in 1862. He served in the military department of Episcopal Hospital and in the U.S. Army Hospital in Nicetown from 1862 to 1864. In the course of his career Dr. Cleeman was physician to the Philadelphia Dispensary, St. Mary Hospital, and the Church Home for Children. In addition to holding membership in numerous medical societies, he was alumni manager of the University Hospital, member of the Board of Health, director of the Board of Charities and Correction, president of the State Quarantine Board of Pennsylvania, and manager of the Pennsylvania Institute for the Instruction of the Blind. He was secretary of the American Philosophical Society and was secretary of the College of Physicians of Philadelphia from 1879 to 1885.

Artist: Attributed to Anna Jurgens

Plaster, painted buff; 19 1/2 x 12 3/8 x 10 7/8; base is integral with sculpture, 2 in. high; not signed or dated. Included in College of Physicians of Philadelphia Inventory of 1898–1915, with the artist listed as Anna Jurgens. Presented by heirs of Dr. Cleeman, 1912. ST 540

Dr. Cleeman is shown bust length, the head and torso frontal. He has smooth, close-cropped hair. The deepset eyes with carved irises and pupils look straight ahead. A long moustache covers the upper lip and meets the square jaw. The ears protrude from the long, narrow face. The subject is dressed in a shirt, tie, and coat. The wooden expression and lack of convincing anatomical structure may be due in part to incomplete restoration of the sculpture.

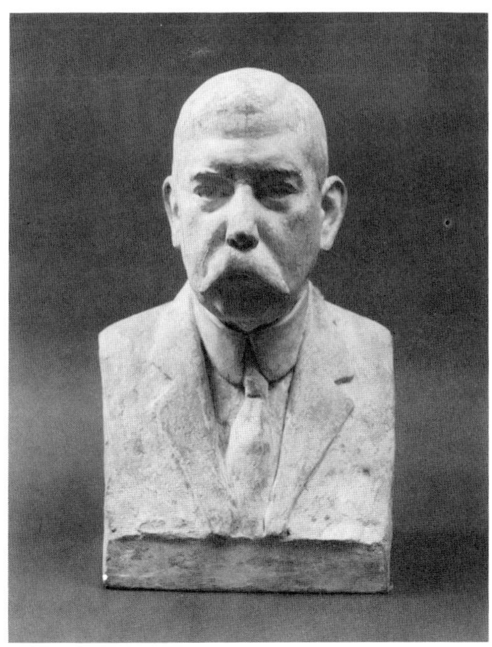

Richard Alsop Cleeman ST 540

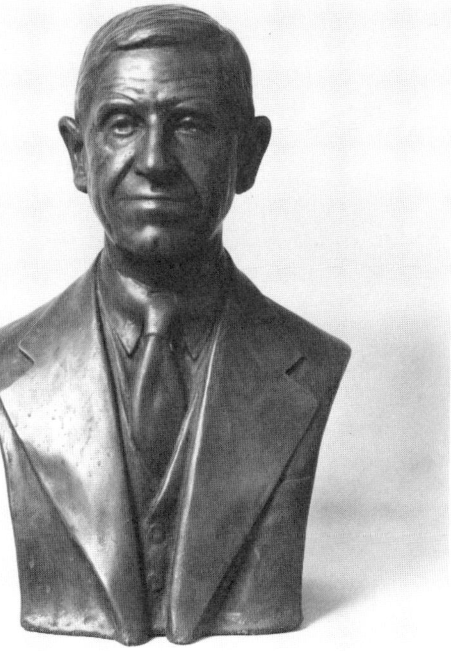

George Morrison Coates *ST 569*

George Morrison Coates (1874–1960)

Dr. Coates was descended from Quaker ancestors who preceded William Penn to this country. He received his degrees from the University of Pennsylvania, the A.B. in 1894 and the M.D. in 1897. He began the study of laryngology with Dr. Francis R. Packard (q.v.) at the Pennsylvania Hospital and with Dr. Walter Roberts at the Philadelphia Polyclinic and College for Graduates in Medicine. When the latter institution merged with the graduate school of medicine at the University of Pennsylvania, he was appointed professor and chief of service of otolaryngology. He also held those positions in the school of medicine and the Hospital of the University of Pennsylvania. A leader in his specialty, Dr. Coates was president of the American Laryngological Association, the American Otological Society, the American Laryngological, Rhinological and Otological Society, and the American Academy of Ophthalmology and Otolaryngology. He received the Newcomb Award of the American Laryngological Association in 1943, the Award of Merit of the American Academy of Ophthalmology and Otolaryngology in 1946, and the Gold Medal Award of the American Otological Society in 1949. He was editor-in-chief of the A.M.A. *Archives of Otolaryngology*, co-editor with Dr. I. S. Ravdin of the American edition of *Kirschner's Operative Surgery*, co-editor with Dr. Chevalier Jackson of *The Nose, Throat and Ear and Their Diseases*, and editor of the five volume international reference work, *Otolarygology*. He served on the library committee of the College of Physicians of Philadelphia.

Artist: Luigi Maraffi (b. 1890)

An immigrant to Philadelphia in 1903, Maraffi was born in Aversa, Italy. He studied sculpture first at the Fleisher Art Memorial and then at the Pennsylvania Academy of the Fine Arts at irregular intervals between 1910 and 1918. He was an outstanding pupil of Charles Grafly (q.v.) and won the Cresson traveling scholarship in 1914 and 1915 and the Stewardson sculpting prize in 1915. He was a frequent exhibitor at annual exhibitions of the Pennsylvania Academy of the Fine Arts between 1914 and 1929.

Plaster, painted bronze color; 21 3/4 x 14 1/2 x 10 3/4; no base; signed and dated in recessed area on right side, "Luigi Maraffi/194 [?, last digit illegible]." Presented by Dr. Alan Shuster, 1968. *ST 569*

Dr. Coates is shown bust length, torso frontal and head turned very slightly to the left. His smooth hair is brushed across his head. There are deep lines in forehead, cheeks, corner of eyes, and chin. The small, close-set eyes, with pupils and irises carved, stare straight ahead. The wide mouth has a jutting lower lip. Large ears protrude from the side of the head. The subject wears a shirt, a necktie, a buttoned vest, and an open suitcoat with wide lapels. The surface of this naturalistic portrait is smooth. The facial expression is serious and somewhat quizzical, because of the jutting lip and the lines in the forehead, as though the eyebrows were raised.

Thomas Cooper (1759–1839)

A political activist, freethinker, educator, lawyer, and physician, Cooper was born in London and educated at Oxford University. He subsequently studied both law and medicine, attending anatomical lectures in London and taking care of patients in Manchester. Feeling encumbered by conservative reaction to his revolutionary views, he removed to America in 1794, settling near his friend, Joseph Priestley, in Northumberland, Pennsylvania. He practiced law and medicine in this location and served as a judge in Luzerne County. From this post he was removed "for arbitrary conduct" by radical factions in the state government. This is ironic, since he had previously been sentenced to prison for sedition for siding with the Jeffersonian Democrats. Returning to science and education, he filled the chair of chemistry at Carlisle (now Dickinson) College from 1811 to 1815 and was professor of applied chemistry and mineralogy at the University of Pennsylvania from 1815 to 1819. He was elected a member of the American Philosophical Society and received an honorary M.D. from "a University of New York." Then he became professor of chemistry, mineralogy, and political economy at the South Carolina College (now the University of South Carolina) and served as president

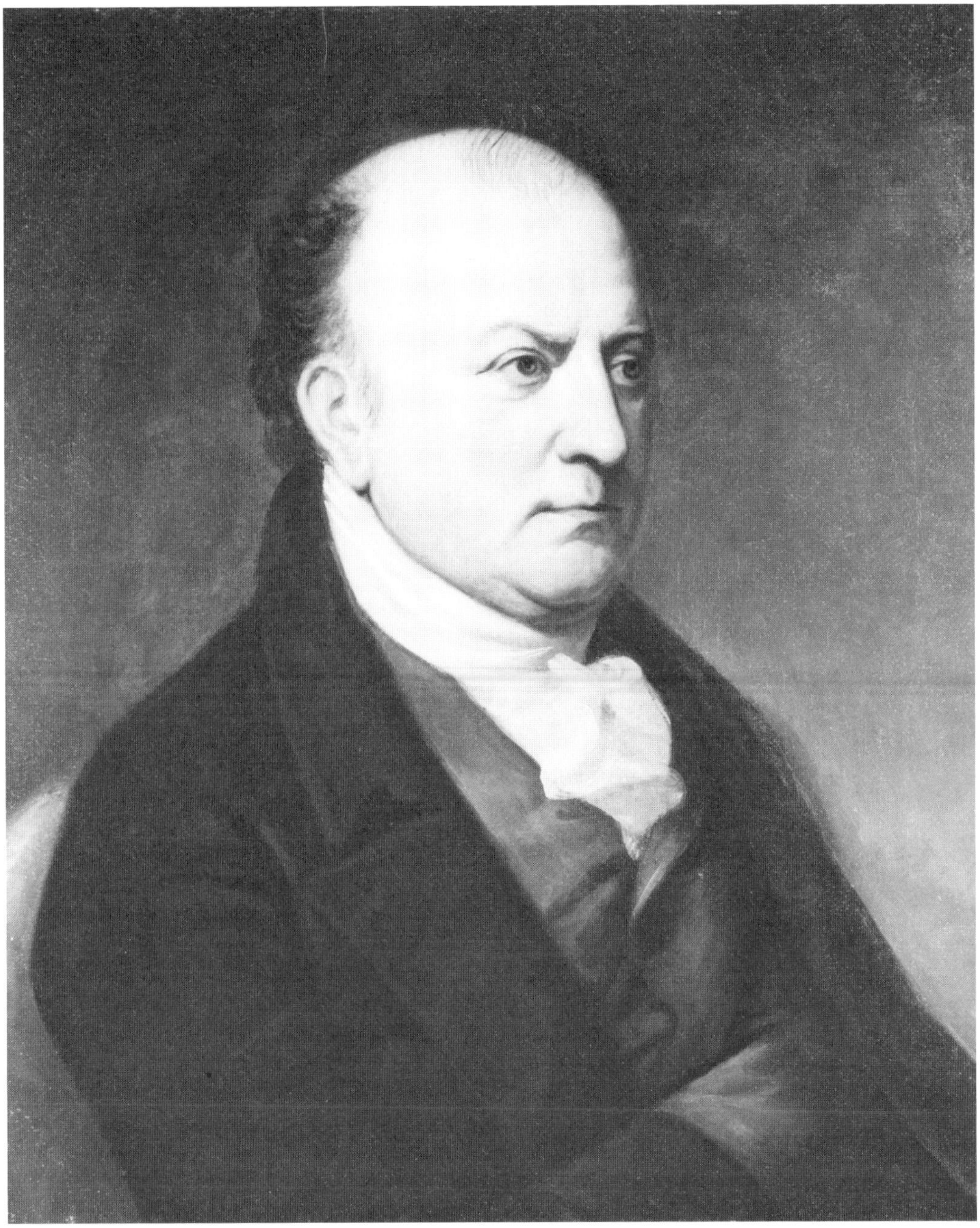

Thomas Cooper PA 67

of the college from 1821 to 1834, when he was dismissed for unpopular views but was given an honorary L.L.D. He was active in establishing the first medical school and first insane asylum in the state. He was a prolific writer of political pamphlets, textbooks, and scientific writings for popular consumption, most notably his description of Priestley's discoveries.

Artist: Charles Willson Peale (1741–1827)

An illustrious artist, naturalist, inventor, and organizer of cultural institutions, Peale was the eldest son of a country schoolmaster in Queen Anne's County, Maryland. The main support of a widowed mother, he combined the trades of saddle and chaise maker, silversmith, and clock and watch repairer, as well as amateur sign and portrait painter. His first instruction in art was given by John Hesselius from 1762 to 1763. Subsidized by a group of Maryland gentlemen who sent him to London to study painting under Benjamin West from 1766 to 1769, Peale acquired a sophisticated style of portraiture as well as expertness in miniature painting and mezzotint. First in Maryland and then later in Philadelphia, where he moved in 1778 after having served three years in the Continental Army, Peale became a sought-after portraitist and a painter of political allegories. His portraits of George Washington and other military heroes were immensely popular. In 1782, by adding a skylighted room to his house, he became the proprietor of a picture gallery. This developed into a full-fledged museum and picture gallery in 1786, first located at the American Philosophical Society building and then in the second floor of the State House (Independence Hall). Here he exhibited and lectured on his portraits of distinguished Americans which eventually numbered more than 250, many of which are located at Independence National Historical Park today. He also showed preserved animals in natural habitat displays, but the chief object of public interest was the skeleton of a mastodon which had been exhumed under his direction. Peale guided the establishment of several artists' organizations—the short-lived art school of 1791, the Columbianum art school and exhibition (which lasted only from 1794 to 1795), and finally, with the help of a group of artists and influential laymen, the Pennsylvania Academy of Fine Arts in 1805. Here Peale's own work was exhibited from 1811 to 1828. He never accepted outside students but his ideas on painting were passed on to Peales of the second and third generations through several of his seventeen children who became artists.

Oil on canvas; 22 1/2 x 18 3/4; dated 1819 in Charles Coleman Sellers' Charles Willson Peale *(Philadelphia: American Philosophical Society, 1947). No donor or date of donation is recorded. The portrait was located at Peale's Philadelphia Museum gallery from 1819 until 1854, when it was sold to "Ogden" at an auction of the Gallery's portraits (according to an annotated copy of the auction catalogue found at the Historical Society of Pennsylvania). It entered the College of Physicians' collection between 1854 and 1887 when it was shown at the College's* Centennial Celebration Loan Collection of Portraits, *listed as owned by the College. It was also shown at the* Loan Exhibition of the Historical Portraits, *Pennsylvania Academy of the Fine Arts (1887–88), the* Exhibition of Portraits by Charles Willson Peale, James Peale, and Rembrandt Peale, *Pennsylvania Academy of Fine Arts (1923), and at* The Art of Philadelphia Medicine, *Philadelphia Museum of Art (1965). PA 67*

Dr. Cooper is shown bust length, with head and body turned to the right. He is seated in a red upholstered armchair. His right arm reaches across his body, the hand apparently being under his waistcoat. The atmospheric background is umber, lighter on the right. His bald head has a few sparse hairs on top and a fringe of curly brown hair at the sides. His extraordinary eyebrows form a cyma curve with dark shadows underneath. His blue eyes, which look straight ahead in the direction of head turn, have deep shadows below. Under the small, tightly closed mouth there is a double chin. The wide, round face has a florid complexion. The subject wears a white stock, a white jabot, a gray waistcoat, and a black coat with M-notched lapels. The meticulously painted surface of this portrait has smooth brush strokes. Although the body is only suggested beneath the costume, the head is well modelled as a solid, three-dimensional anatomical structure, with strong linear contours and contrast of light and shade. The pinched mouth and curved eyebrows lend a degree of pugnacity to the serious expression. The viewer feels tension, energy, and a sense of the living presence of the subject.

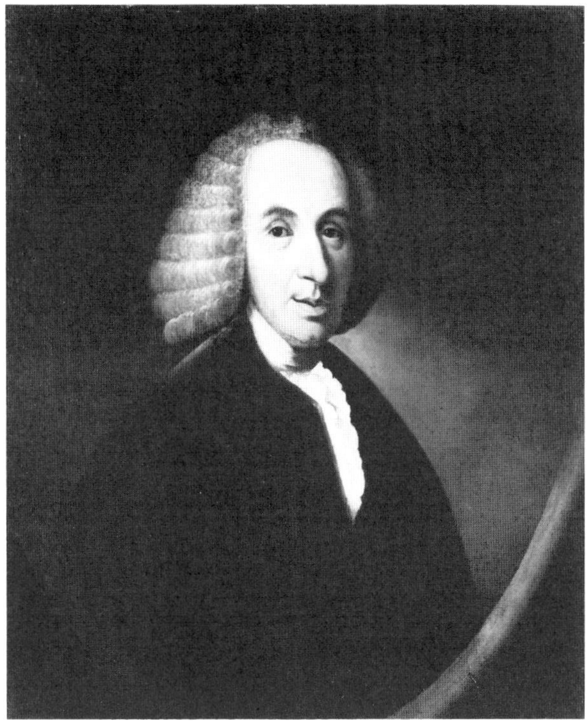

William Cullen *PA 48*

curved eyebrows lend a degree of pugnacity to the serious expression. The viewer feels tension, energy, and a sense of the living presence of the subject.

William Cullen (1719-1790)

An eminent eighteenth century teacher, Cullen was born in Hamilton, Scotland, the son of a factor to the Duke of Hamilton. His education was interspersed with varied experiences. While at Glasgow University he was also the pupil of a physician. Then, after working as surgeon on a merchant ship, he assisted an apothecary in London. After two sessions at the Edinburgh Medical School, he worked as a surgeon in Hamilton and finally received the M.D. at Glasgow in 1740. His career as a teacher began at Glasgow, where he was one of the two earliest independent lecturers in chemistry in Britain. He also taught theory and practice of physic, botany, and materia medica. He was elected to the chair of medicine in 1751. Four years later he removed to Edinburgh to become the professor of chemistry. He also gave clinical lectures at the infirmary and then presented formal lectures in materia medica. In 1768 he was made professor of theory and practice of medicine. He was president of the Edinburgh College of Physicians from 1773 to 1775 and was instrumental in founding the Royal Society of Edinburgh and the Royal Medical Society. This distinguished teacher was a prolific author of treatises on medicine and chemistry.

Artist: Unknown

Oil on canvas; 29 1/2 x 24 1/2. Presented by Dr. Cullen to Dr. Caspar Wistar (q.v.) and bequeathed to the College of Physicians of Philadelphia by Mrs. Mifflin Wistar, date unrecorded. When shown at the College of Physicians' Centennial Celebration Loan Collection of Portraits *in 1887, the painting was still owned by Mrs. Wistar; when included in the College of Physicians Inventory of 1898 to 1915, it was owned by the College. Probably it was painted from life by a British artist.* *PA 48*

Dr.Cullen is shown bust length, with body turned to the right and head slightly to the right. The setting is a *trompe l'oeil* porthole device, an illusionistic half-round moulding for an oval frame. The four corner spandrels are dark brown. Cullen's wig is chin-length with horizontal rows of tight, formal curls. The arched brown eyebrows surmount very dark brown eyes which gaze straight ahead toward the spectator. The tip of the long, bumpy nose points down to a full mouth, slightly askew; the lips are parted in a smile. The subject wears a white stock and shirt frill, a black waistcoat, and a black single-breasted coat with no lapels or collar. The surface is smooth, with no visible brush strokes. The costume is flat and there is no sense of the underlying body mass. The head is solid and three-dimensional but has a primitive appearance because the features are misaligned. This effect may be the result of faulty restoration and overpainting.

Roland Gideon Curtin (1839-1913)

Of Puritan and noble Irish ancestry, Curtin was born in Centre County, Pennsylvania, and received his M.D. degree in 1866 and Ph.D. degree in 1871 from the University of Pennsylvania. His posts at the University Hospital included chief of the medical clinic, assistant to the professor of clinical medicine, lecturer on physical diagnosis, and physician from 1887 to 1896. He was also associated with Philadelphia, Presbyterian, Howard, Maternity, Rush, Douglass, and St. Timothy's Hospitals. He was an active committee member or officer of the following: the Centennial Exposition and the Inter-

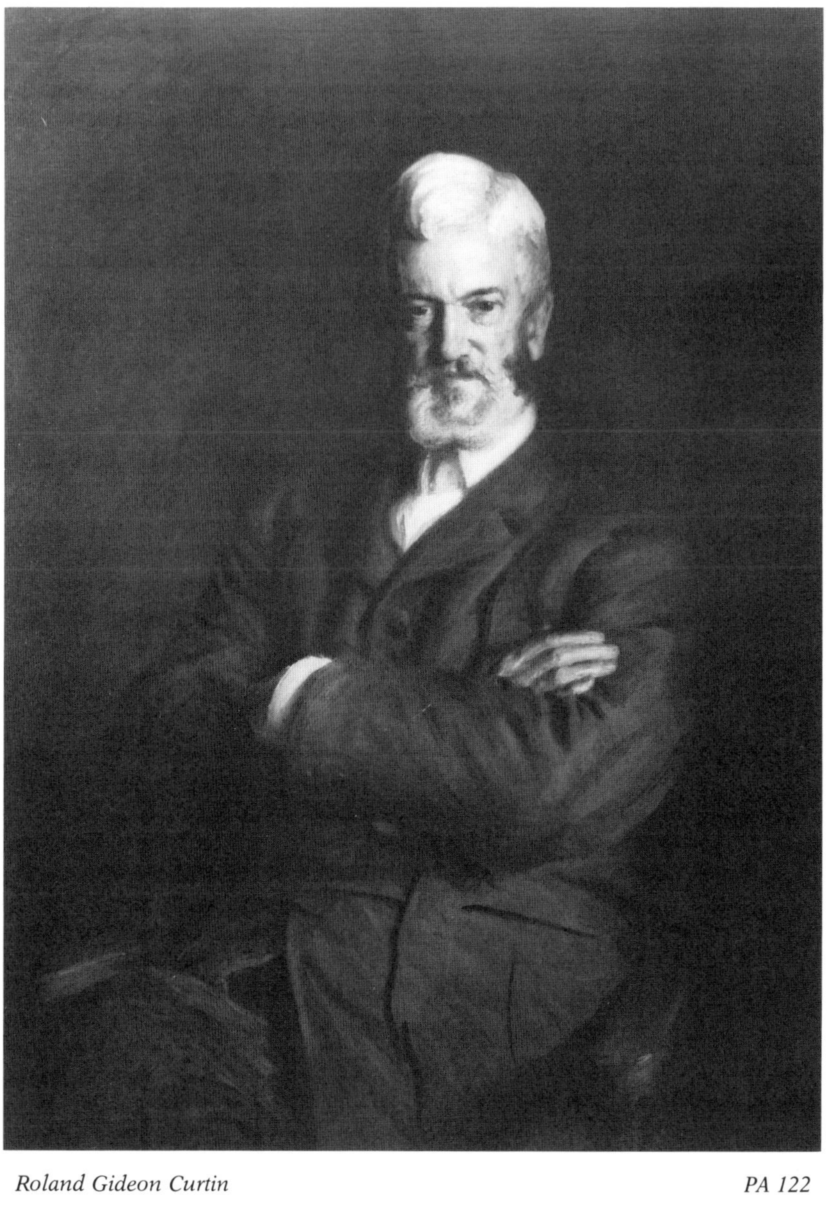

Roland Gideon Curtin *PA 122*

national Medical Congress, Philadelphia (1876); the international congress in Washington (1887); the world's congress at the Chicago Exposition (1893); and the Pan-American medical congresses. He was president of the medical board of Philadelphia Hospital, the Association of Hospital Surgeons and Physicians of Philadelphia, the Philadelphia County Medical Society, the Philadelphia Medical Club, and the American Climatological Society. He was an active member of the College of Physicians of Philadelphia and many other medical, scientific, art, historical, genealogical, and patriotic societies. To recognize his devoted service to the various alumni organizations of the University of Pennsylvania, the Philadelphia Alumni Society of the Medical Department of the University of Pennsylvania created the Roland G. Curtin scholarship for sons of alumni physicians desiring to study medicine.

Artist: William Thomas Smedley (1858-1920)

Born in Chester County, Pennsylvania, this painter and illustrator studied art at the Pennsylvania Academy of the Fine Arts in 1877 and then with Jean Paul Laurens in Paris. He opened a studio in New York in 1880 and exhibited widely in the United States and the Paris salons. He exhibited at the National Academy of Design intermittently between 1881 and 1898 and was made an associate in 1897 and an academician in 1905. His membership in the following societies shows the range of his artistic interests: the National Academy of Design, Society of American Artists, American Water Color Society, National Society of Mural Painters, National Institute of Arts and Letters, Society of Illustrators, National Association of Portrait Painters, Artists' Aid Society, and the Century Association. His awards include the Evans Prize, American Water Color Society (1890); bronze medal, Paris Exposition (1900); bronze and silver medals, Pan-American Exposition, Buffalo (1901); Proctor Prize (1906); and Carnegie Prize (1916), National Academy of Design. In addition to painting in oil, Smedley was a well-known illustrator for *Harper's* and other periodicals. In 1882 he accompanied surveyors, including the Marquis de Lorne, to western Canada to illustrate their work for the publication *Picturesque Canada.*

Oil on canvas; 38 1/2 x 29; signed and dated upper left, "W.T. Smedley, 1905." Purchased from the artist's widow by her cousin Dr. Malcolm C. Guthrie, who sold it to the Medical Society of the University of Pennsylvania, which gave it to Dr. Smedley's daughter, Miss Mary C. Curtin, who presented it to the College of Physicians of Philadelphia in 1953. Exhibited at the Art Club of Philadelphia (1905) and at Carnegie Hall (1905). *PA 122*

Dr. Curtin is shown two-thirds length, with body and head turned slightly to the left, head tilted down. He is seated in a plain, wooden chair, with his arms folded across his chest and his legs crossed. The background is dark brown on the right and center, medium brown on the left. The subject has thick white hair, dark gray eyebrows and side-whiskers, and a light gray beard. The brown eyes look down and have deep circles underneath. The long, thin face has a slender, bumpy nose, hollow cheeks, and a small mouth. He is dressed in the country attire which he usually wore during his annual vacation at his bungalow at Bear Lake, Luzerne County, where the portrait was painted. He wears a white shirt, no necktie, a Norfolk sporting jacket, and knickerbockers. The painterly surface of this portrait shows animated brush strokes both in the costume and in the solidly constructed, three-dimensional head; there is masterful use of brown in all its varieties. The subject has been caught in an introspective, thoughtful mood. His expression is serious. His upper body sinks back into his chair, and his folded arms and downward gaze set a barrier between him and the viewer.

Georges Léopold Chrétien Frédéric Dagobert Cuvier (1769-1832)

The great naturalist, comparative anatomist, and paleontologist was born at Montbéliard, Württemberg (later annexed to France); he was the son of a minor military officer. After spending four years at the Hohen Carlsschule in Stuttgart, he became tutor to a noble family in Normandy. His tutorial duties were light and they allowed him to spend much time in botanical studies and animal dissections. These provided the basis for the paper he presented to the scientific community soon after moving to Paris in 1795, in which he marked a new stage in the study of invertebrates by adding new classifications. In that year he also began teaching as professor of zoology at the École Central du Panthéon and as assistant professor of animal anatomy at the Muséum d'Histoire Naturelle, becoming titular professor there in 1802. He later added work in public and educational administration to his scientific activities of studying, and he organized the natural history collections of the Museum, then the world's largest institution devoted to scientific research. His great contribution to the study of animal anatomy was to apply systematically structural comparison throughout the entire animal kingdom. His arrangement of animal species and higher groups in an order determined by anatomical principles and general relationships made his work in animal taxonomy the standard manual for most of the 19th century. His researches in fossil quadrupeds formed the basis for all subsequent studies in vertebrate paleontology. Besides his classic works in general zoology and comparative anatomy,

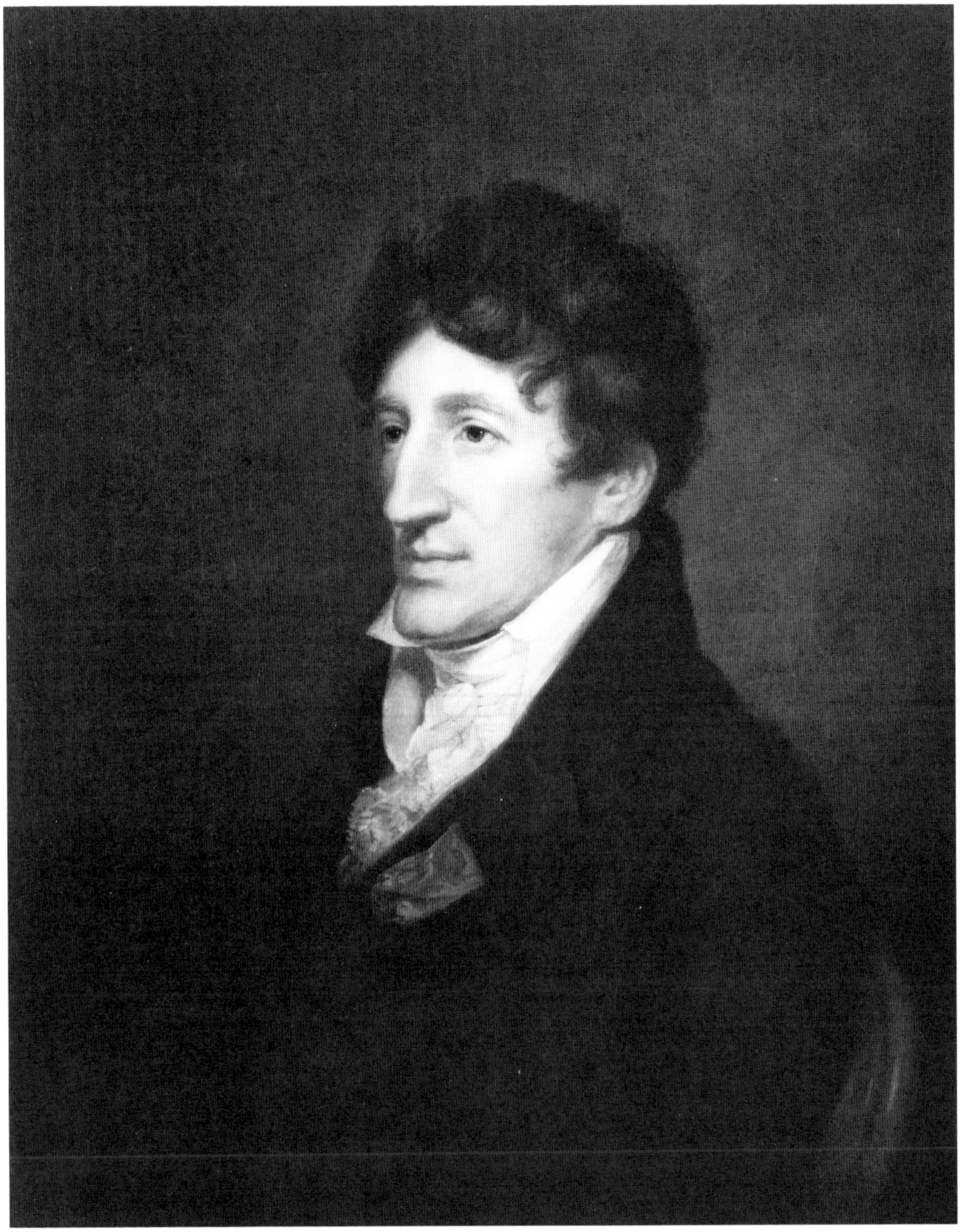

Georges Léopold Chrétien Frédéric Dagobert Cuvier *PA 35*

he also published extensively in the history of science. For services to his country as an administrator, he was made a baron in 1819, an officer in the Legion of Honor in 1824, and was nominated peer of France in 1831.

Artist: Rembrandt Peale (1778–1860)

Rembrandt Peale, second son of Charles Willson Peale (q.v.), was a painter of portraits, historical scenes, and miniatures. He was born in Bucks County, Pennsylvania. At the age of thirteen, while studying with his father, he started to paint portraits. By the age of seventeen he was so adept that George Washington was persuaded to sit for him. The result was the first of many portraits of Washington, including the celebrated "Porthole" portrait, but was the only one done from life. In London in 1802 while exhibiting items from his father's museum, Peale attended classes at the Royal Academy and also studied with Benjamin West. After returning to Philadelphia to earn his living as a portrait painter, Peale became one of the founders of the Pennsylvania Academy of the Fine Arts, where he was elected an academician in 1812 and served on the board of directors from 1811 to 1813. In 1808 and again in 1809–1810 he was in Paris, where he made portraits of many distinguished Frenchmen for his father's museum. In Philadelphia in 1811 he entered six portraits in the first annual exhibition of the Society of Artists of the United States. When his first attempts at ambitious historical painting were not well received, he removed to Baltimore to found a museum of art and natural history in 1814. He persisted in the genre of history, and his *Court of Death* (1820, Detroit Institute of Art) became a huge financial success because he took it on tour and charged admission fees to the public, who flocked to see it. This yielded him the means to open studios in New York, Boston, and Philadelphia, and to make two additional trips to Europe. He was an original member of the National Academy of Design and was president of the American Academy of Fine Arts in New York. He published *Notes on Italy*, *Peale's Graphics*, and *Portfolio of an Artist*. His final years were spent in reproducing likenesses of Washington and traveling about the country giving lectures on life portraits of Washington.

Oil on canvas; 27 1/2 x 22 1/4; written on back of relined canvas, "original portrait of the distinguished Baron Cuvier, painted at Paris by Rembrandt Peale." Although Cuvier did not have the title until 1819, the portrait dates from Peale's first trip to Paris in 1808; a letter of introduction (located at the American Philosophical Society) of Rembrandt Peale to Cuvier was written by Charles Willson Peale on April 21, 1808, in which he requests the scientist to sit for a portrait so that it could be placed "Amongst the eminent characters which I have been collecting for a series of years, and which is now a valuable part of my museum." In a second letter dated November 12, 1808, C. W. Peale notes that Rembrandt Peale has brought back from Paris "seven excellent portraits," including that of Cuvier. No donor or date of donation is recorded. The portrait was sold to L. H. Newbold at an auction of portraits from Peale's Philadelphia Museum Gallery in 1854 (according to an annotated copy of the auction catalogue located at the Historical Society of Pennsylvania). It entered the collection of the College of Physicians between 1854 and 1887, when it was shown at The Centennial Celebration Loan Collection of Portraits *and was listed as owned by the College. It was also shown at the Pennsylvania Academy's* Loan Exhibition of Historical Portraits *(1887), its* Exhibition of Portraits by Charles Willson, James, and Rembrandt Peale *(1923), and* The Rembrandt Peale Exhibition *at the Municipal Museum of the City of Baltimore (1937). PA 35*

Cuvier is shown bust length, body and head turned to the left, head almost in profile. The atmospheric background is a warm greenish-brown, lighter around the head and darker near the rounded chair back, which is upholstered in red. The subject has thick, reddish-brown hair with carefully arranged curls brushed onto his face. The long prominent nose has a large bump on the bridge. The narrow gray eyes look straight ahead in the direction of the head turn. The narrow mouth is wide, the lips full and red. The chin juts forward and the cheek bones are high. The figure wears a white shirt with stand-up collar, a white neckcloth tied into a bow, and a white shirt frill. The yellow waistcoat has a high stand-up collar. The high-necked black coat has an M-notched lapel on which there is a red ribbon decoration that bears a silver pin. The paint surface is smooth, and the anatomical structure of the head and body is solid and three-dimensional. The portrayal is romantic: the forms have soft edges, dazzling highlights, and deep shadows. The subject has artfully touseled hair and he gazes thoughtfully into the distance, averting eye contact with the viewer. These devices lend his coarse, almost common features an aura of meditative self-assurance to match the elegance of his costume.

Jacob Mendez Da Costa (1833-1900)

Born in St. Thomas of a Portuguese family long resident in London, Da Costa was educated in Dresden and took his medical degree at Jefferson Medical College in 1852, when he was chosen as demonstrator for Dr. Thomas Mütter (q.v.). He completed his studies in Paris, Prague, and Vienna. After his return to Philadelphia his first position was as lecturer in physical diagnosis at the Summer Association for Medical Instruction; he also held private courses in physical diagnosis and clinical medicine. At Jefferson Medical College he was instructor, clinical lecturer, chairman of the theory and practice of medicine (1872-91), and finally professor emeritus. He was also physician to the Episcopal, Philadelphia, Jefferson, Children's, and Pennsylvania Hospitals. In 1857 he took an active part in organizing the Pathological Society of Philadelphia, over which he presided from 1864 to 1867. He was president of the College of Physicians (1884-85 and 1895-98). He was one of the original members of the Association of American Physicians and its president in 1897. He was a member of the American Philosophical Society and other scientific and historical societies. His early medical papers dealt with pathology and clinical medicine, especially enteric fever and valvular and functional diseases of the heart. His *Medical Diagnosis*, published in 1864, is considered a masterpiece among textbooks. He was awarded the honorary LL.D. by Jefferson College, the University of Pennsylvania, and Harvard University.

Artist: Robert William Vonnoh (1858-1933)

A well-known impressionist painter of portraits, figures, and landscapes, Vonnoh was born in Hartford, Connecticut, and studied at the Massachusetts Normal Art School in Boston. He continued his studies abroad in two trips, first from 1881 to 1883, when he studied the figure at the Académie Julien in Paris under Gustave Boulanger and Jules Joseph Lefebvre, and again in 1887 to 1891, when he concentrated on landscapes. In America he became an influential teacher. In Boston he taught at the Cowles Art School and the School of the Museum of Fine Arts. At the Pennsylvania Academy of the Fine Arts he was principal instructor in portrait and figure painting in 1891 to 1895, 1912, and 1918 to 1921. During the 1890s he worked on portrait commissions in Philadelphia, New York, and Chicago, and on landscapes in Old Lyme, Connecticut. Vonnoh was a member of the Society of American Artists, an academician of the National Academy of Design (1906), chairman of the board of the League of American Artists, and a member of many other art organizations in the United States and in Paris. He served on many local and international art juries. He and his second wife, the

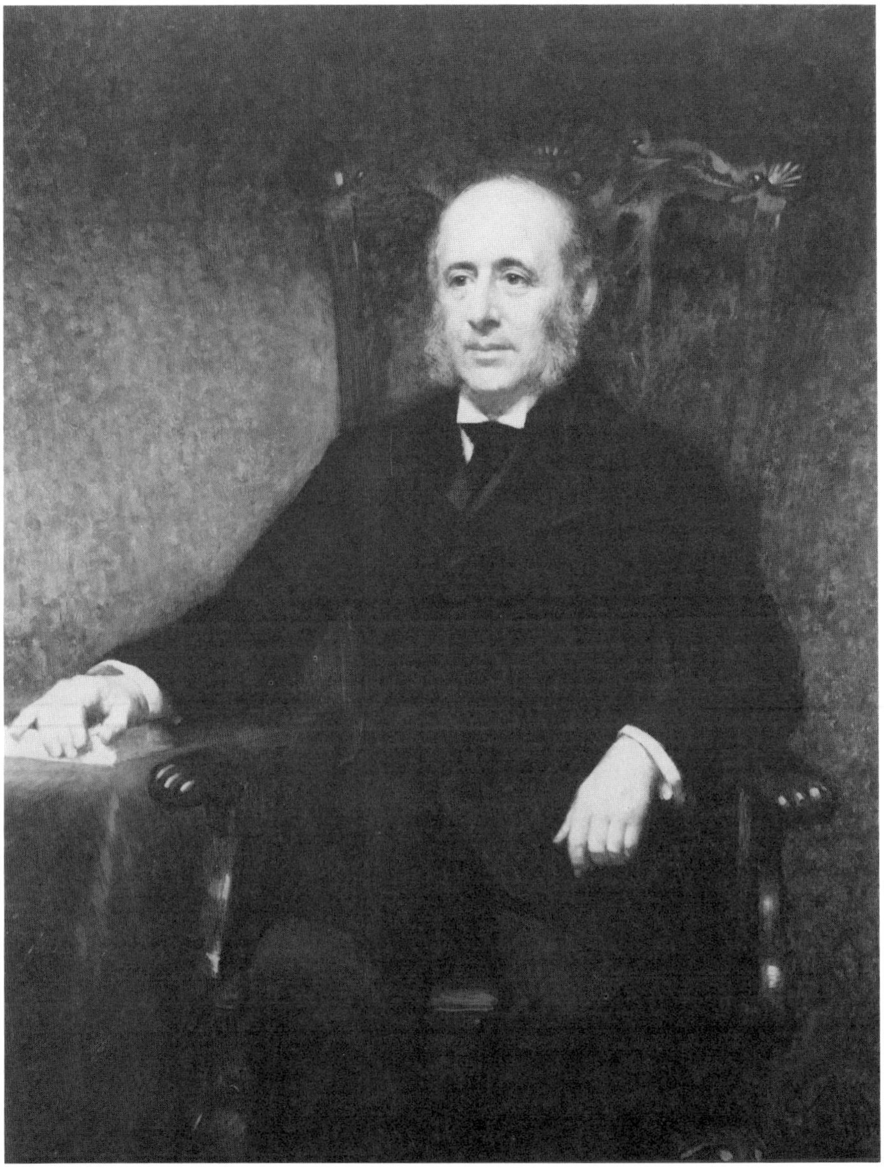

Jacob Mendez Da Costa *PA 10*

sculptor Bessie Potter Vonnoh, lived in France from 1907 to 1911. His awards include honorable mention at the Paris Salon (1899); bronze medals at the Paris Expositions (1889, 1900); Proctor portrait prize, National Academy of Design; gold medals at the Charleston and Panama-Pacific Expositions; and medals in Boston, Buffalo, and Chicago. His work is owned by important museums and institutions. Retrospective exhibitions of his work were held in New York at the Ainslie Gallery (1923) and at the Durand-Ruel Gallery (1926).

Oil on canvas; 49 1/2 x 39 1/2; signed and dated lower right, "Vonnoh/ Phila/1893." Shown at the annual exhibition of the Pennsylvania Academy of the Fine Arts, (1893-1894). Presented by Fellows of the College of Physicians in 1894, after a meeting held in January, 1892, at the home of Dr. S. Weir Mitchell (q.v.), at which a resolution was approved by admiring colleagues of Da Costa for funds to be raised for two portraits, one for the College of Physicians of Philadelphia, and the other for Jefferson Medical College, both to be painted by Robert Vonnoh. *PA 10*

Dr. Da Costa is shown three-quarters length, the body frontal, the head turned slightly to the left. He is seated in a high-backed, ornately carved Chippendale-style armchair. His left arm rests on the chair arm, left hand pendent. His right arm rests on the surface of the table covered with brown cloth, while his right hand toys with the pages of a book. The background is composed of mottled strokes of green-umber. The subject's head is bald, with gray hair at the sides, and chin-length side-whiskers. Beneath dark gray eyebrows, the brown eyes look to the left, in the direction of the head turn. The elongated face has a delicately regular nose and mouth. He wears a white shirt with turned-down collar, a black necktie, a black double-breasted frock coat, and dark gray trousers. The impressionistic, painterly surface of the portrait has all-over small brush strokes, except for the costume, which is more broadly brushed. The head and hands show solid, three-dimensional contruction. There is a suggestion of the body underlying the costume. Although the subject is frontal and centrally placed, there is a curious contradiction in emphasis. With acutely observed characterization, the artist has given unusual attention to the chair, whose shell-carved cresting rail

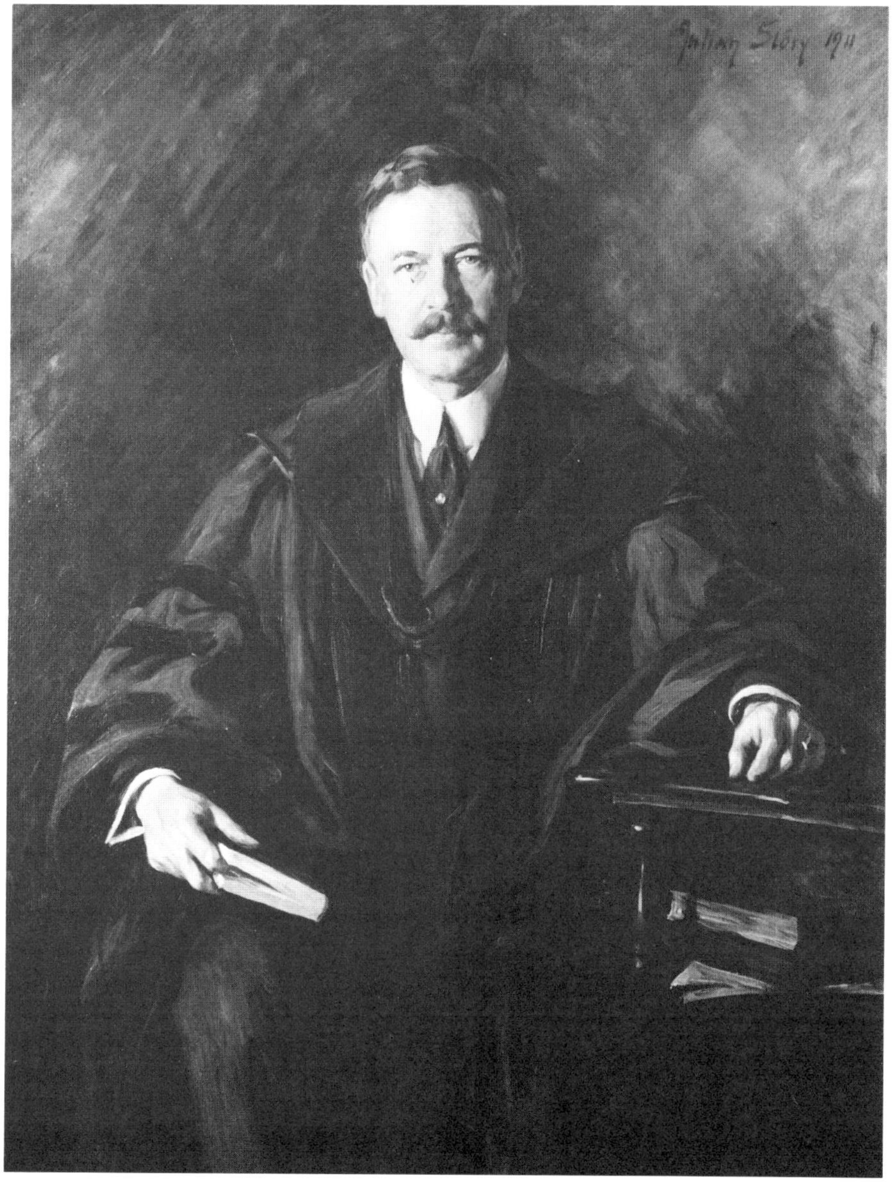

George Edmund de Schweinitz *PA 31*

rises above and almost engulfs the subject, whose slender stature, sidewards glance, and irresolute gesture with the book, give him an appearance of frailty and a musing, meditative air. Dr. James C. Wilson's memoir of Da Costa mentions "the refinement of his daily life, a delicacy of feeling that sometimes seemed carried to an extreme and the modesty with which he bore unusual honors. . . ."

George Edmund de Schweinitz (1858–1938)

Descended from distinguished Huguenot and Silesian ancestors, de Schweinitz spent his boyhood in Bethlehem, Pennsylvania. In 1876 he received the A.B. from Moravian College (of which his father was president) and the M.D. from the University of Pennsylvania in 1881. From 1883 to 1885 he was prosector of anatomy for Dr. Joseph Leidy (q.v.). His professional appointments include ophthalmologist to Orthopaedic Hospital and Infirmary for Nervous Diseases, ophthalmic surgeon to Philadelphia General Hospital, professor of ophthalmology at Philadelphia Polyclinic and College for Graduates in Medicine, clinical professor and then professor of ophthalmology at Jefferson Medical College, and chair of ophthalmology at the University of Pennsylvania from 1902 to 1924. He received an honorary degree from the University in 1914 and was a trustee in 1924. He was president of the College of Physicians of Philadelphia (1910–12), the American Medical Association (1922–23), the American Ophthalmological Society (1916), and the International Congress of Ophthalmology (1922). Professional awards include honorary degrees from Moravian College, University of Michigan, and Harvard University and research prizes and medals from the College of Physicians of Philadelphia, the Société Française d'Ophtalmologie, the American Medical Association, the National Society for the Prevention of Blindness, and the American Ophthalmological Society. He was awarded the Huguenot cross. He belonged to the American Philosophical Society and was on the board of directors of the Library Company of Philadelphia. Outstanding among his contributions to medical literature is *Diseases of the Eye*, which was written at the suggestion of William Osler (q.v.) and was published in 1892. The book went through ten editions.

Artist: Julian Story (1857–1919)

The son of a poet and sculptor, William Wetmore Story, Julian Story was born at Walton-on-Thames, England, and studied at Eton. He received the A.M. degree at Oxford in 1879. He studied art in Florence under Frank Duveneck and in Paris under Gustave Boulanger and Jules Joseph Lefebvre. He exhibited principally in Paris, London, Berlin, and America. His honors include awards at the Paris salon of 1889, gold medal at the Berlin Exposition of 1891, medals at the Paris expositions of 1899 and 1900, silver medal at the Pan-American Exposition in Buffalo in 1901, and an award at the San Francisco Exposition of 1915. He was made a chevalier of the Legion of Honor of France in 1901, and his salon picture of 1898 was bought by the French government. He was a member of the Society of American Painters in Paris, the Society of American Artists of New York, and the London Society of Portrait Painters. He died in Philadelphia in 1919.

Oil on canvas; 49 1/4 x 39; signed and dated upper right, "Julian Story 1911." Presented by Rudolph Ellis, 1911.
PA 31

De Schweinitz is shown three-quarter length. The body and head are frontal but the head is tilted slightly to the right. He is seated with the right hand resting on his thigh; he is holding a book and marking the place with his index finger. The left hand rests on a table top, below which is a shelf with books and papers. The background is painted in streaky shades of brown—dark on the left, medium on the lower right, and light on the upper right. The subject has light brown hair and a pointed moustache; his blue-green eyes look straight ahead at the viewer. The regular features and tall, lithe figure caused one colleague to refer to de Schweinitz as a "Norse warrior." He wears a white shirt and a brown necktie with tie tack. There is a ring on the left hand. He wears a gray academic robe with a green mantle, three green stripes on the sleeves, and dark green panels at the front. The style of painting is fluid throughout, but is controlled, so that the head and hands are well constructed and there is a sense of the three-dimensional body underlying the costume, which has deep folds. The attentive expression and erect posture, as well as the glance toward the viewer, give the subject an air of self-assurance and ease.

William Potts Dewees (1768–1841)

Descended from early Swedish settlers at Delaware Bay and from the English founders of Pottstown, Dewees worked in the offices of an apothecary and physician before attending medical lectures at the University of Pennsylvania (1887–89), where he received a baccalaureate degree in medicine. With the encouragement of Dr. Benjamin Rush (q.v.), he removed his obstetrical practice from Abington, Pennsylvania, to Philadelphia, where he established a very successful career at a time when most deliveries were performed by midwives. As there was no formal university training in the subject, Dewees gave systematic instruction in his office. He received the M.D. from the University of Pennsylvania, writing a thesis titled *An Essay in the Means of Lessening Pain and Facilitating Certain Cases of Difficult Parturition.* He was disappointed at not having been made the first professor of midwifery at the University when the subject was finally introduced in 1810. Then he was forced to retire to the country for five years because of pulmonary tuberculosis. When he regained his health, he returned to Philadelphia and became associated with the Medical Institute, was elected to the American Philosophical Society, and was finally appointed adjunct professor of obstetrics (1825), then professor (1834). The next year, at the height of his powers, he fell victim to a cerebral hemorrhage and was forced to resign. His textbook, *A Compendious System of Midwifery*, published in 1824, is regarded as the first authoritative American work on the subject.

Artist: John Neagle (1796–1865)

Neagle was born in Boston to parents who were from Philadelphia. His modest training in art took place in Philadelphia, where he had a few months of study with Pietro Ancora, a teacher of drawing; with Thomas Wilson, a coach and ornamental painter; and with Bass Otis, the portraitist and printmaker. Except for brief trips to the South, Neagle spent his entire career as a painter of portraits in Philadelphia. The two main influences on the development of his facile style were Thomas Sully (his father-in-law) and Gilbert Stuart, whom he visited briefly in July, 1825. Stuart did Neagle the honor of sitting for a portrait, and while painting, Neagle "drank deeply at the fountain of Stuart's genius." His reputation was established in 1827 by the exhibition at the Pennsylvania Academy of the Fine Arts of his most celebrated painting, *Pat Lyon at the Forge*, a full-length portrait of a notorious blacksmith. Neagle was active as an exhibitor and an administrator at the Academy, where he was an associate, academician, and member of the board of directors (1830–31), and at the Artists' Fund Society, where he was a founder and president from 1835 to 1844. In 1828 he was elected an honorary member of the National Academy of Design. Although he also did landscapes, Neagle was most renowned for his portraits of members of society, professional persons, actors, and artists. These works are located in many important museums and cultural institutions in Philadelphia and other cities. There was an exhibition of his portraits at the Academy in 1925. Neagle was also interested in professional theory and practice and owned an outstanding collection of engravings and drawings.

Oil on canvas; 22 x 17. Presented by Dr. I. Minis Hays, 1885. In the College of Physicians' Centennial Celebration Loan Collection of Portraits, *1887, the artist's name is omitted. In the College of Physicians Inventory of 1898–1915 and in subsequent inventories, the artist is listed as Neagle. A recently discovered label, old and torn, on the back of the painting reads, "artist—Naegle [sic]/authority—his son/ G—gle" (Garrett Neagle, son of the artist, did certify another painting in the College collection; see note on Robert Hare). Two experts who recently examined the portrait thought that in spite of overcleaning and repainting in some areas, the deft style of painting resembles that of Neagle and that the frame and stretchers are contemporary with the subject. Neagle painted another portrait of Dewees located at the University of Pennsylvania.* *PA 50*

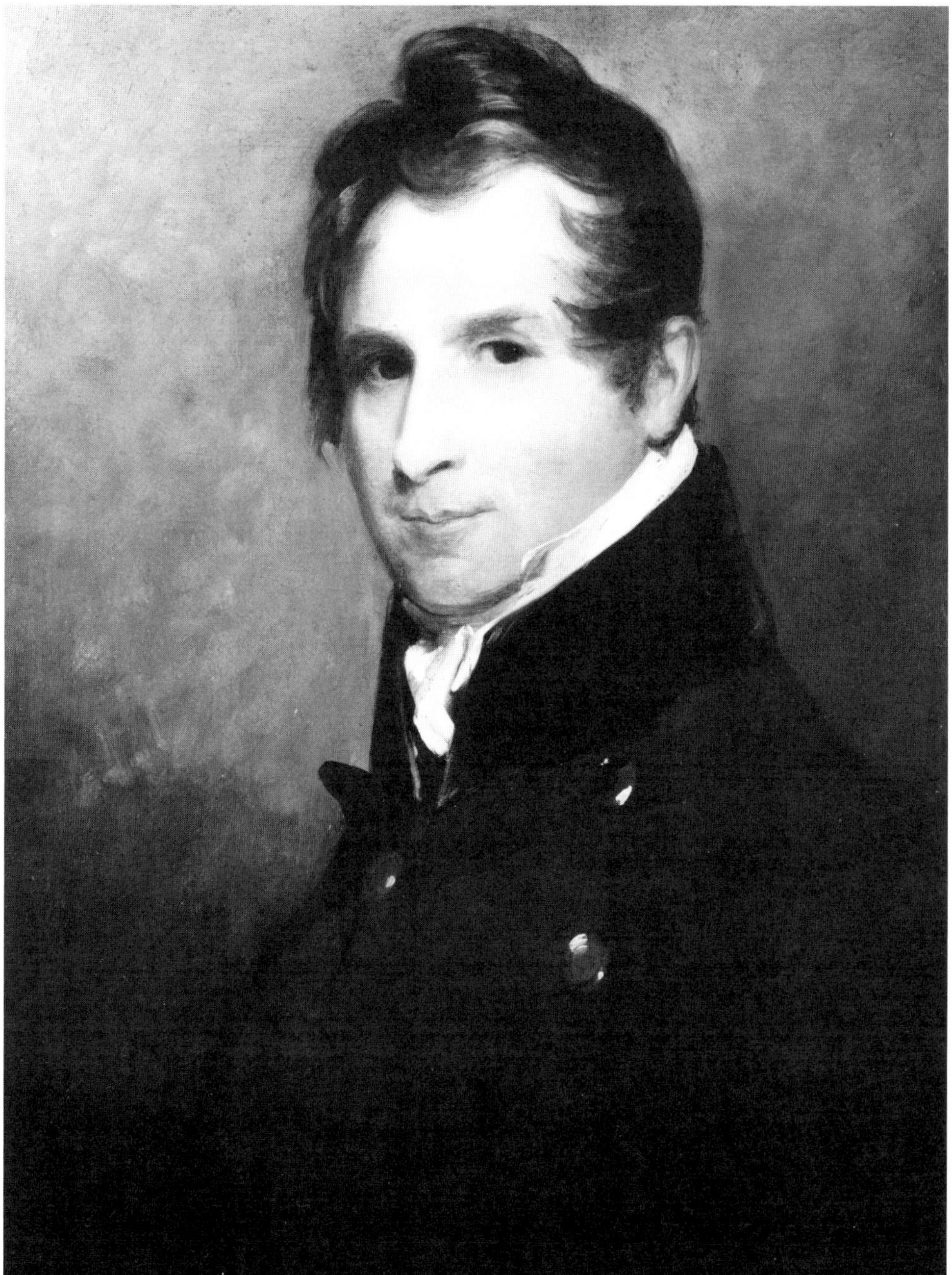

William Potts Dewees *PA 50*

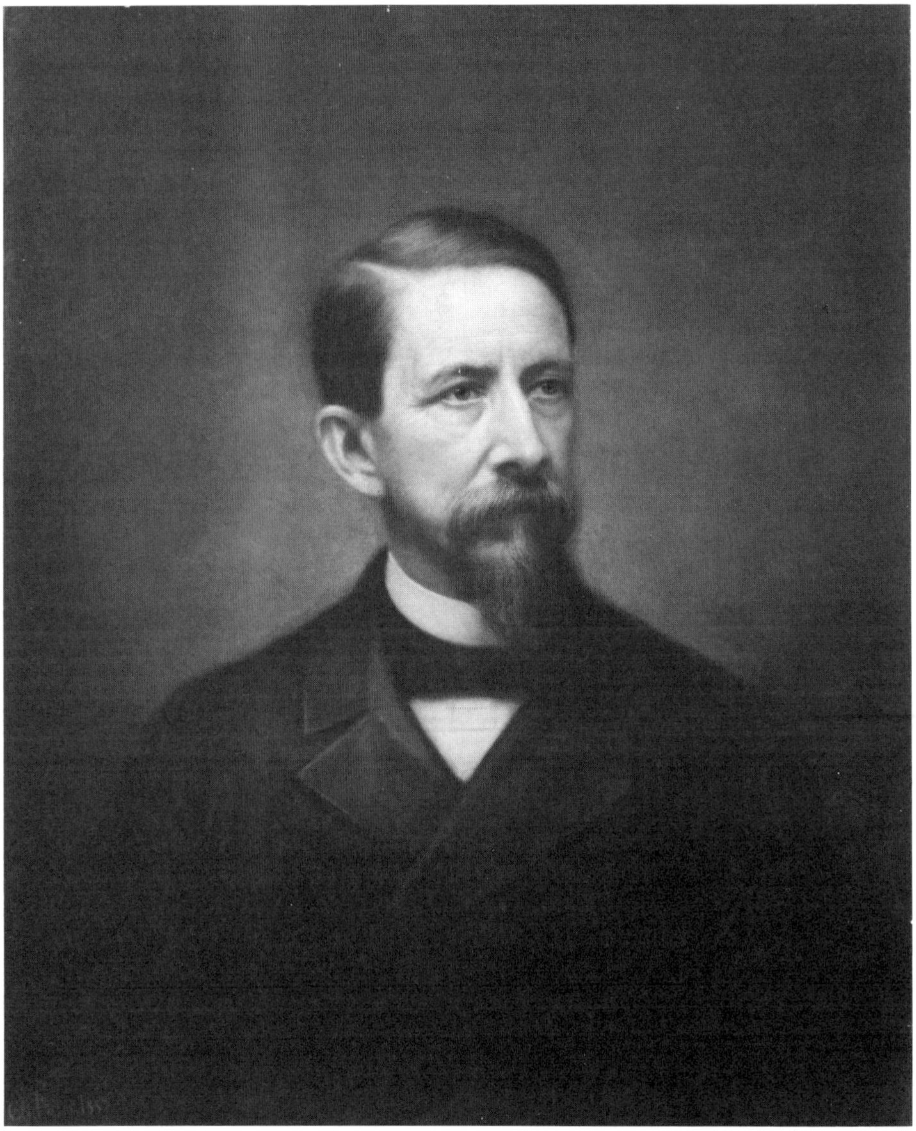

Thomas Murray Drysdale *PA 143*

Dewees is shown bust length, body turned three-quarters to the left. The head is turned slightly to the left and tilted slightly down. The atmospheric background consists of scumbled strokes of medium-toned greenish-brown above and darker strokes below. He has thick, dark brown hair, with several strands brushed onto his forehead. His blue eyes look out of the corners to the right, in the opposite direction of the head turn. The oval face has a straight nose and a well-shaped mouth, with pursed lips, round chin, and pink cheeks. Dewees wears a white shirt with a stand-up collar, a white neckcloth, and a dark brown double-breasted coat with high collar and brass buttons. The surface of the portrait is painterly, with visible brush strokes throughout. The head is constructed with solid, three-dimensional anatomical forms. The costume is comparatively flat, with no sense of the underlying body. The conception is romantic, with soft edges, blurry outlines, and strong contrasts of light and shadow. Although he does not regard the observer, the subject radiates a feeling of energy, vitality, and movement, as though he had just turned his head to look at something.

Thomas Murray Drysdale (1831–1904)

Drysdale was born in Philadelphia and was descended from Scottish Presbyterian Covenanters. As a youth he worked in a drug shop in order to learn pharmacy. He studied medicine with Dr. Washington Lemuel Atlee (q.v.) while a student at the University of Pennsylvania, which granted him the M.D. degree in 1852. He was Atlee's assistant for ten years and married his daughter, Mary. He was professor of chemistry at the Wagner Free Institute of Science, professor at the Franklin Institute, and consulting surgeon at Girard College. During the Civil War he was surgeon to the First Regiment, Infantry. He was president of the Philadelphia County Medical Society, president of the Pennsylvania State Medical Society, vice president of the American Academy of Medicine, and president of the Obstetrical Society of Philadelphia. He was a fellow of the College of Physicians of Philadelphia. He was famous in his day for a diagnostic technique which consisted of testing the fluid formed by ovarian cysts.

Artist: Stephen James Ferris, Jr. (1835–1915)

For biography, see page 9.

Oil on canvas; 30 x 25 (actual size); signed and dated lower left, "S.J. Ferris 1887." Presented in 1981 by William J. Jedlick, who had received it 15 years previously from an unidentified individual. *PA 143*

Drysdale is shown bust length, the body frontal, and the head turned to the right. The background is dark brown at the top and sides and warm yellow-brown at the center. The subject has light brown hair brushed across his high forehead and greenish-hazel eyes which look in the direction of the head turn. The full brown moustache and long, pointed beard hide the upper lip. The almost ascetic, slender face has a long thin nose. The subject wears a white shirt with a high, stand-up collar, a black bow tie, and a black double-breasted coat. The surface of the portrait is smoothly brushed. The naturalistic rendering presents a solidly constructed head. The body appears flat under the costume, which seems to melt into the background. There is an all-over reticence in both the style of painting and the expression. The edges of forms are soft, the colors are muted, and the facial tones are comparable to those of the background. The subject's gaze, directed away from the viewer, is thoughtful, quiet, and unassertive.

Benjamin Duffield (1753–1799)

Duffield was born in Bucks County, a descendant of English ancestors who had settled in Pennsylvania in 1682. He received the M.A. degree from the College of Pennsylvania in 1771. His medical training included study in the office of John Redman (q.v.), attendance at the lectures of William Shippen,Jr. (q.v.) and John Morgan (q.v.), and study in Edinburgh. After the Revolutionary War, during which he was surgeon in charge of a military hospital in Reading, he established a large practice in Philadelphia and gave lectures on obstetrics. He was physician at the Yellow Fever Hospital at Bush Hill and physician to the Walnut Street Prison. He was a member of the American Philosophical Society and one of the original junior founders of the College of Physicians. It is thought that he devised the College seal and its motto: *Non sibi sed toti* (not for oneself but for all).

Artist: Unknown

Oil on canvas; 14 1/2 x 11 3/4. Presented by Dr. John Neill, 1867. Shown at the College of Physicians Centennial Celebration Loan Collection of Portraits *(1887), the Pennsylvania Academy of the Fine Arts* Loan Collection of Historical Portraits *(1887–88), and the Philadelphia Museum of Art,* The Art of Philadelphia Medicine *(1965).* *PA 58*

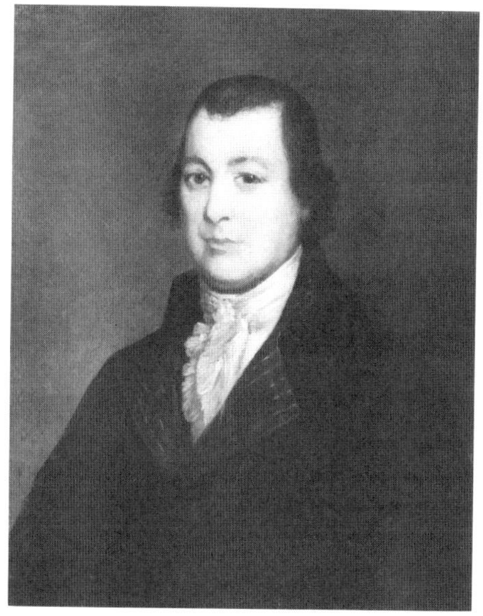

Benjamin Duffield *PA 58*

Duffield is shown bust length, with head and body turned slightly to the left. The gray-brown atmospheric background is darker on the right. He has dark brown, collar-length hair; brown eyes that look toward the spectator; and a small nose and mouth. He wears a white stock and shirt frill, a gray waistcoat with tan stripes, and a black coat with wide lapels. The paint surface is smooth. The costume is rendered convincingly, with a suggestion of the underlying body mass. The head, which may have suffered from damage and overpainting, seems anatomically primitive—the features are aligned frontally, although the head is turned slightly to the side.

Louis Adolphus Duhring (1845–1913)

Born in Philadelphia of educated and prosperous German and Swiss parents, Duhring was raised in an environment of culture. After spending three years at the University of Pennsylvania, he enlisted in the U.S. Army and then graduated from the medical department of the University in 1867. After fifteen months as intern at Philadelphia (Blockley) Hospital, he spent two years studying dermatology in Berlin, Paris, London, and, especially, Vienna (under the brilliant Ferdinand Hebra). After his return to Philadelphia he opened a dermatologic practice and organized the Dispensary for Skin Diseases, with which he was associated from 1870 to 1890. He was affiliated with the University as lecturer on skin diseases (1871), clinical professor (1876), professor (1890), professor emeritus (1910), and recipient of an honorary LL.D. (1912). He was also a visiting dermatologist at the newly opened dermatology department at Blockley from 1876 to 1887. His *Atlas of Skin Disease*, published in 1876, and *Practical Treatise in Diseases of the Skin*,

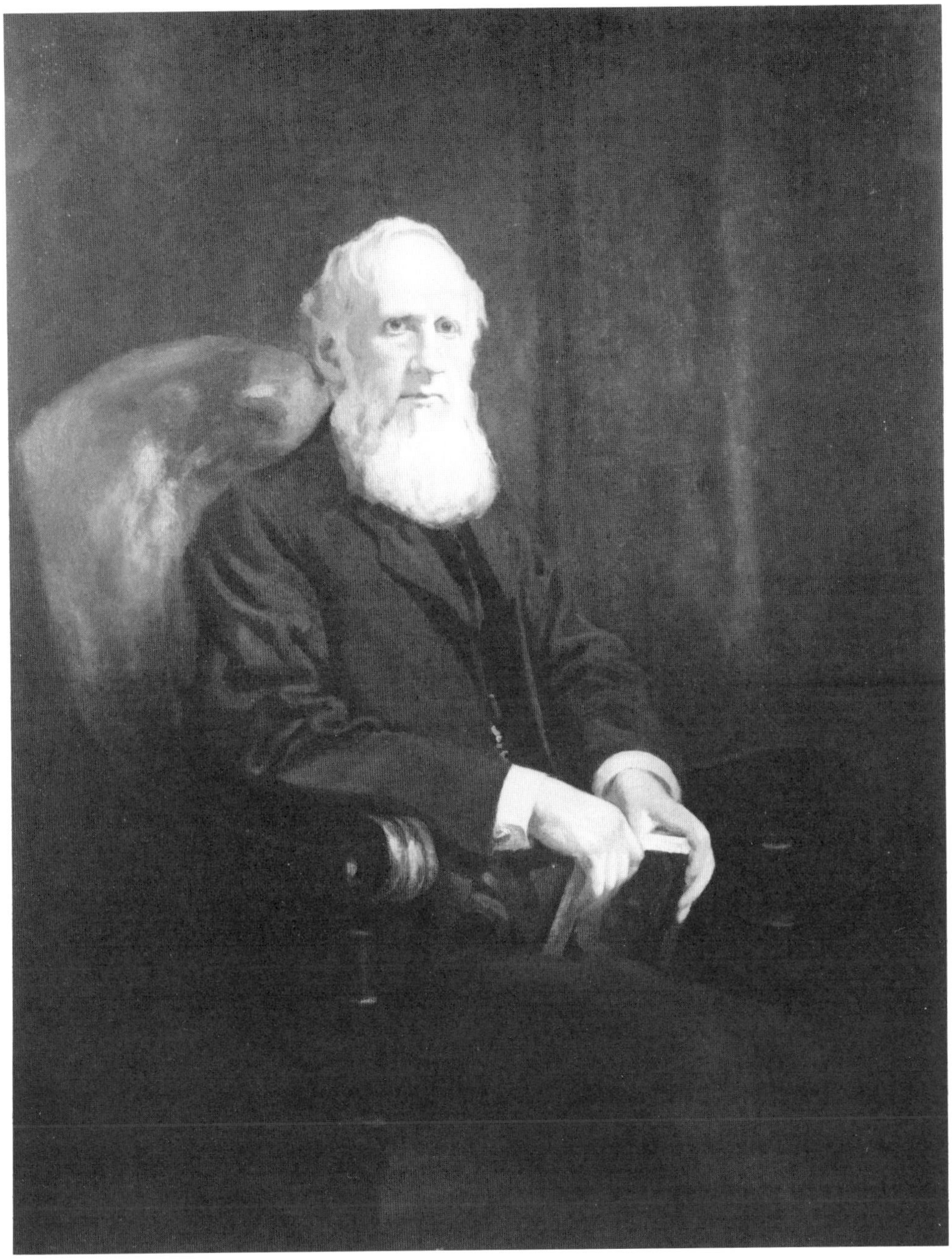

Louis Adolphus Duhring *PA 60*

published in 1877, were the first textbooks on the subject and established him as the leading dermatologist in America. A series of articles between 1884 and 1891 on the disease group that he called "dermatitis herpetiformis" led to its being renamed "Duhring's Disease." He wrote the chapter on cutaneous diseases in Pepper's *System of Medicine* and two volumes of *Cutaneous Medicine*, a projected encyclopedic work. An active fellow of the College of Physicians, he bequeathed one-sixth of his considerable fortune of $1,250,000 to the College library.

Artist: Hugh Henry Breckenridge (1870–1937)

The son of a cabinetmaker in Leesburg, Virginia, Breckenridge studied at the Pennsylvania Academy of the Fine Arts, starting in 1887; this began an association that lasted fifty years. He spent a year in Paris on a Cresson traveling scholarship, studying with William Adolphe Bouguereau, Gabriel Ferrier, and Lucien Doucet. Upon his return to Philadelphia, he served the Pennsylvania Academy as instructor from 1894 to 1937 and as curator of the school from 1907 to 1908. He operated a summer school with Thomas Anshutz from 1900 to 1918. He served as director of the department of fine arts at the Maryland Institute at Baltimore in 1919 and opened the Breckenridge School of Art in East Gloucester, Massachusetts, in 1920. He was a prolific exhibitor at large annual exhibitions at the Academy, the Art Institute of Chicago, the St. Louis Art Museum, and many of the national expositions. He served on more than fifteen art juries, including the municipal art jury of Philadelphia. He was an associate member of the National Academy of Design. The style of his paintings varied from early impressionistic landscapes, to academic portraits, to late abstract and intensely colored compositions. He was a steady winner of prizes, including honorable mention at the Paris Exposition (1900), bronze medal at the Pan-American Exposition in Buffalo (1901), gold medal at the Art Club of Philadelphia (1907), gold medal at the Panama-Pacific Exposition in San Francisco (1915), $1000 Clark prize, and bronze medal at the Corcoran Gallery (1916). The Pennsylvania Academy awarded him the Stotesbury prize (1919), the Academy gold medal (1919), and the Sesnan gold medal (1920). Major exhibitions of his work were held at the Pennsylvania Academy (1934), the Philadelphia Art Alliance (1938), and the Valley House Gallery in Dallas (1967). His work is found in many important public and private collections in Philadelphia and other cities.

Oil on canvas; 52 1/4 x 40 1/4. Commissioned from Breckenridge by resolution of Fellows of the College in appreciation of Dr. Duhring's generous bequest and in honor of his memory. Presented in 1915 (hence dated between 1913 and 1915). Probably painted after a portrait by Leopold Seyffert (1904, University of Pennsylvania) in which the head, body position, and costume are similar. According to visual evidence in the portrait and photographic documentation of the original work, at some time this painting was enlarged at the bottom, although most of the details are obscured through paint loss and varnish bloom. *PA 60*

Duhring is shown three-quarter length, with head and body turned three-quarters to the right. He is seated, with his arms leaning on the chair arms and both hands holding a book which rests on his thighs. Behind him on the right and center are brown draperies with vertical folds. On the left there is dark brown atmospheric space. His armchair, which is set at an angle to the picture plate, has a high, round upholstered back, volute handholds, and turned baluster arm supports. The subject has long strands of white hair combed over his high forehead and white side whiskers with a long, full, rounded beard. His blue eyes gaze out into the distance in the direction of his head turn. The tip of his straight nose is a sharp accent in an otherwise slender and delicate face. He wears a white shirt that is hidden except for the cuffs. He has a black vest, coat, and trousers and a gold watch fob. The surface has painterly, short brush strokes in the head, hands, and furniture carving. The costume is painted more fluidly, with a sense of the underlying bulk of the body. The posture is erect. The facial expression is sober, as if the sitter were lost in thought. At the time of the portrayal Duhring was in almost continuous poor health, possibly because of a constricting band of the ileum found at autopsy, which may have been responsible for the neurasthenic symptoms that first developed in 1885. He had grown progressively reclusive as close members of his family died and he isolated himself from society.

Robley Dunglison (1798-1869)

Born in Keswick, England, Dunglison was apprenticed to a local practitioner and then studied medicine in Paris, Edinburgh, and London. In the last-named city he was licensed by the Royal College of Surgeons and the Society of Apothecaries; he began practice in 1819. In 1824 he received a medical degree from the University of Erlangen. In the same year, soon after appointment as physician-accoucheur at the Eastern Dispensary, he was offered a chair of medicine at the University of Virginia, at the invitation of Thomas Jefferson. He accepted the appointment there and performed the Herculean task of teaching anatomy, physiology, surgery, materia medica, pharmacy, and the history of medicine. During his nine-year stay at Virginia he was an intimate friend and physician to both Thomas Jefferson and James Madison, and he published his *Medical Dictionary* and *Human Physiology*, a pioneering work. In 1833 he accepted the chair of materia medica, therapeutics, hygiene, and medical jurisprudence at the University of Maryland. While at Maryland he published *General Therapeutics and Materia Medica* and *Elements of Hygiene,* another pioneering work. In 1836 he was induced to come to Jefferson Medical College to occupy the chair of the institutes of medicine, created expressly for him. Throughout his more than thirty years at Jefferson, he endeavored to elevate the standards of the medical curriculum and to eliminate debilitating competition between faculty members and between medical schools. Dunglison was also physician to the Philadelphia Hospital, where his lectures were especially well attended. His prolific writing continued in the form of articles, translations, addresses, editing, biographical notices, lectures, and the books, *Medical Student, or Aids to the Study of Medicine, New Remedies,* and the *Practice of Medicine*. Often called "the father of American physiology," Dunglison had a reputation as a teacher and scholar which secured him more than a hundred testimonials, including an honorary LL.D. from Jefferson and an honorary M.D. from Yale. He was a Fellow of the College of Physicians, vice-president of the American Philosophical Society, and vice-president of the Institution of the Blind and of the Training School for Idiots.

Artist: Attributed to Thomas Sully (1783-1872)

For biography, see page 18.

Oil on canvas; 29 1/2 x 24 1/2; signed and dated on back of relined canvas "TS/1868." Presented by Dr. Jonathan E. Rhoads and Dr. Lewis C. Scheffey (q.v.) in 1957. This painting is attributed to Sully on historical documentation only; the portrait has been so thoroughly overcleaned and repainted that virtually nothing remains of the original

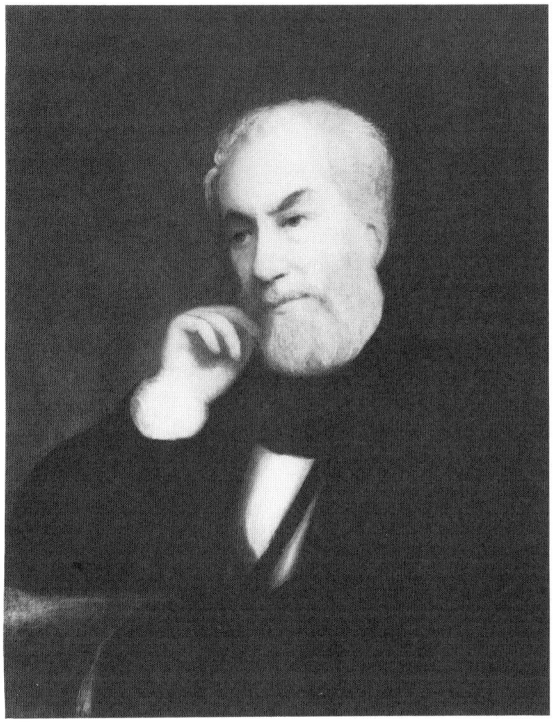

Robley Dunglison *PA 125*

surface. Sully's own Register of Portraits 1801–1871 *lists a portrait of "Dr. Dunglison, for the M.F.S. of Prest," 30 x 25, 1868. Dunglison was president of the Musical Fund Society of Philadelphia from 1856 to 1869, and Sully was vice president of the Society from 1860 to 1873 and was official portraitist of its presidents. According to several contemporary Board members of the Society, the portraits of Dunglison and 21 others remained in the possession of the Society until 1957, when 18 of them were sold. Apparently they were offered first to descendants of the subjects. The donors of the Dunglison portrait recall purchasing it from the Dunglison family. College of Physicians council minutes and the College Collections committee minutes from 1957 onward refer to the portrait as a portrayal of Dunglison by Thomas Sully. Shown at* The Art of Philadelphia Medicine *exhibition, Philadelphia Museum of Art, 1965.* *PA 125*

Dr. Dunglison is shown bust length, with body to the left, head to the left and tilted down. His right arm is bent at the elbow with upper arm resting on a green cloth-covered table. His right hand is raised to his chin, fingering his beard. The atmospheric background is brownish-green. Dunglison's hair, side-whiskers, moustache, and rounded beard are blondish-gray with pale green highlights. Under dark eyebrows raised in a quizzical arch, his narrow blue eyes look down in the direction of the head turn. He has a straight nose and a wide mouth with full lower lip. He wears a wide black neckcloth, a white shirt, a black waistcoat, and a black coat. The black straps hanging from his neck could be from a monocle. The surface of the portrait is smoothly brushed except for the head and hands, which are formed of short, choppy, fussy, overworked strokes. Although the head and hands have been constructed solidly, the features are soft and blurry, with an unsettling and pervasive use of pale green shadows. The costume is flat and lacks details, and there is no sense of underlying body forms. The facial expression is serious, the gesture contemplative.

Artist: Auguste Edouart (1789–1861)

Born in Dunquerque, France, Edouart served with the French army until 1813, when his family was ruined in the aftermath of the French Revolution. He went to England, where he tutored in French and tried his hand at animal portraits, some of which were made of hair. Accepting a challenge to make better "shades," he showed an aptitude for silhouettes that opened the way for a successful career, even though his efforts were snubbed by colleagues and friends. He traveled all over England, Ireland, and Scotland, making 50,000 silhouettes in ten years. He took his art seriously and in 1835 published a book titled, *A Treatise on Silhouette Likenesses by Monsieur Edouart, Silhouettist to the French Royal Family, and patronised by His Royal Highness the Late Duke of Gloucester, and the principal Nobility of England, Scotland, and Ireland.* In 1839 Edouart arrived in America, where he prospered by making silhouettes of most of the famous men of the day, even though he had to compete against the newly introduced daguerrotype. In America he visited Boston, Washington, Saratoga, New Orleans, Philadelphia (1843), Louisville, Lexington, Charleston, and New York. He embarked for England on the *Oneida* in 1849, but the ship was wrecked off the Island of Guernsey and many of the scrapbooks which contained duplicates of all of his silhouettes were lost. Ten of the British and six of the American volumes were saved, out of a total of fifty. Broken in health and spirit, he spent the rest of his days near Calais.

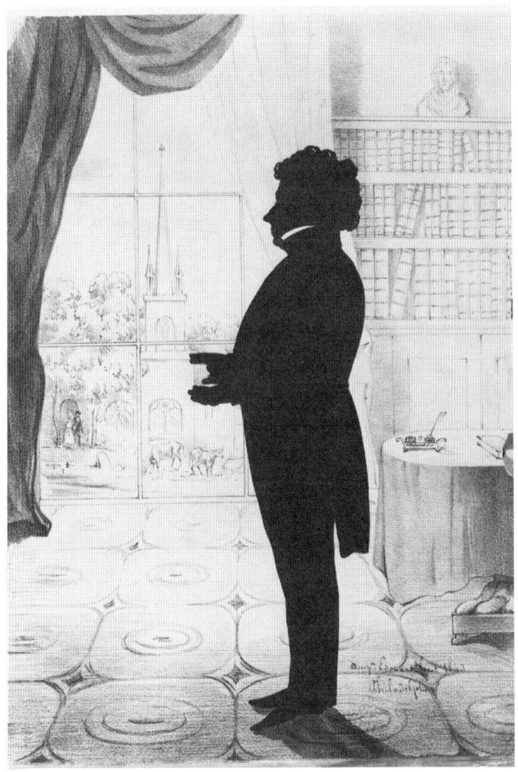

Robley Dunglison *PH 118*

Black paper silhouette, pasted to a lithograph of an interior scene on buff-colored paper; 11 1/8 x 7 7/8; signed and dated lower right, "Augst Edouart fecit 1843/Philadelphia." Presented by Dr. Richard H. Dunglison, son of the subject, in 1875. Dunglison's image is similar to that in another silhouette made by Edouart in 1843 in which the subject is identified by name and profession. *PH 118*

Dr. Dunglison is shown full length, profile to the left. He is standing with his arms bent at the elbow, his hands reaching out beyond his body. The lithographic setting is a library. There are draperies at the window, bookshelves with three rows of books and a bust on the top shelf, a pedestal table covered with a cloth on which are placed an ink stand and a book, and a rug with oval pattern. The view through the window includes a church, two human figures, two cows, and foliage. The subject has collar-length curly hair. The meticulously cut profile includes eyelashes, a prominent nose, and a slightly receding chin. Girth is emphasized by the round abdomen. The subject wears a shirt with stand-up collar, a waistcoat, and a double-breasted, cutaway frock coat with an M-notched collar. The variety of tonalities in the shading creates interest in the stock setting. The figure seems planted on the ground by means of the shadow below his feet. His costume is rendered sensitively by the details of tailoring shown in a fine gray line. Edouart's characteristic white collar is a separate piece of white paper inserted into a slit cut into the neck.

Guillaume Dupuytren (1777-1835)

Born near Limoges, France, Dupuytren was the second of nine children of a poor solicitor. He graduated from the Collége de La Marche, a Jesuit school in Paris, in 1794. He studied medicine at the École de Santé in Paris, where he was outstanding enough to be appointed prosector in charge of autopsies and was soon giving his own course of lectures in pathology. In 1812 he was appointed to the chair of operative surgery at the Hôtel Dieu, and in 1814 he became chief surgeon. Although he had a choleric and abrasive personality and was avaricious and self-aggrandizing, even his enemies admitted his outstanding contributions to surgery. He was the first to excise the mandible (1812) and to treat torticollis by subcutaneous section of the sterno-mastoid muscle (1822). He was one of the first to drain a brain abscess and to remove the uterine cervix for cancer. He was the first to describe the lines of skin tension and to classify burns by the degree of depth. He was renowned for his surgery of aneurysms, for the extraction of cataracts, and for the treatment of hydrocele, rectovaginal and rectovesical fistulas, and other conditions. He wrote extensively about orthopedic problems, especially fracture of the fibula and congenital dislocation of the hip. A collection of his lectures, *Leçons orales de clinique chirurgicale faites à l'Hôtel Dieu de Paris*, reveals the variety and range of his interests. He

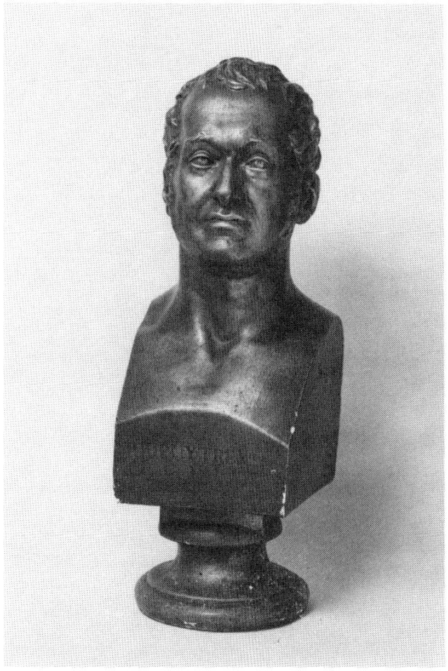

Guillaume Dupuytren *ST 553*

was an indefatigable worker and amassed a great fortune. His annual load of patients, including outpatients, was estimated at 10,000. He was awarded a baronetcy by Louis XVIII and was appointed surgeon to King Charles X.

Artist: Unknown.

Plaster, painted a mottled bronze and black; 21 3/4 x 10 1/4 x 11; figure integral with base, 5 3/4 in. high; not signed or dated. "Dupuytren" inscribed on front of sculpture. Presented by Dr. Ludwig Loeb, 1940. *ST 553*

Dupuytren is shown over life-size, head-and-neck length, the body frontal, the head tilted very slightly to the right. Thick strands of hair have been brushed toward the rounded face. There are long side-whiskers below the ears. The eyes, which have carved irises and pupils, look upward. The tip of the long nose points down toward the mouth, which has thick lips with exaggerated curves. The neck is thick, the torso compressed. The surface of this portrait is smooth, no tool marks being visible. The head is moderately well constructed. The size of the head and neck are disproportionately large in relation to the abbreviated torso. Though the intention of the artist was probably to suggest a neoclassical style, the features are not idealized and the facial expression resembles a sneer.

Samuel Emlen (1789-1828)

Born in Chester County, Pennsylvania, a descendant of one of the oldest Quaker families, Emlen studied medicine as a house-pupil of Dr. — Parrish and received the M.D. degree from the University of Pennsylvania in 1812. He spent the next two-and-one-half years studying and traveling in England, Ireland, Scotland, France, and Holland. After his return to Philadelphia he was elected physician and

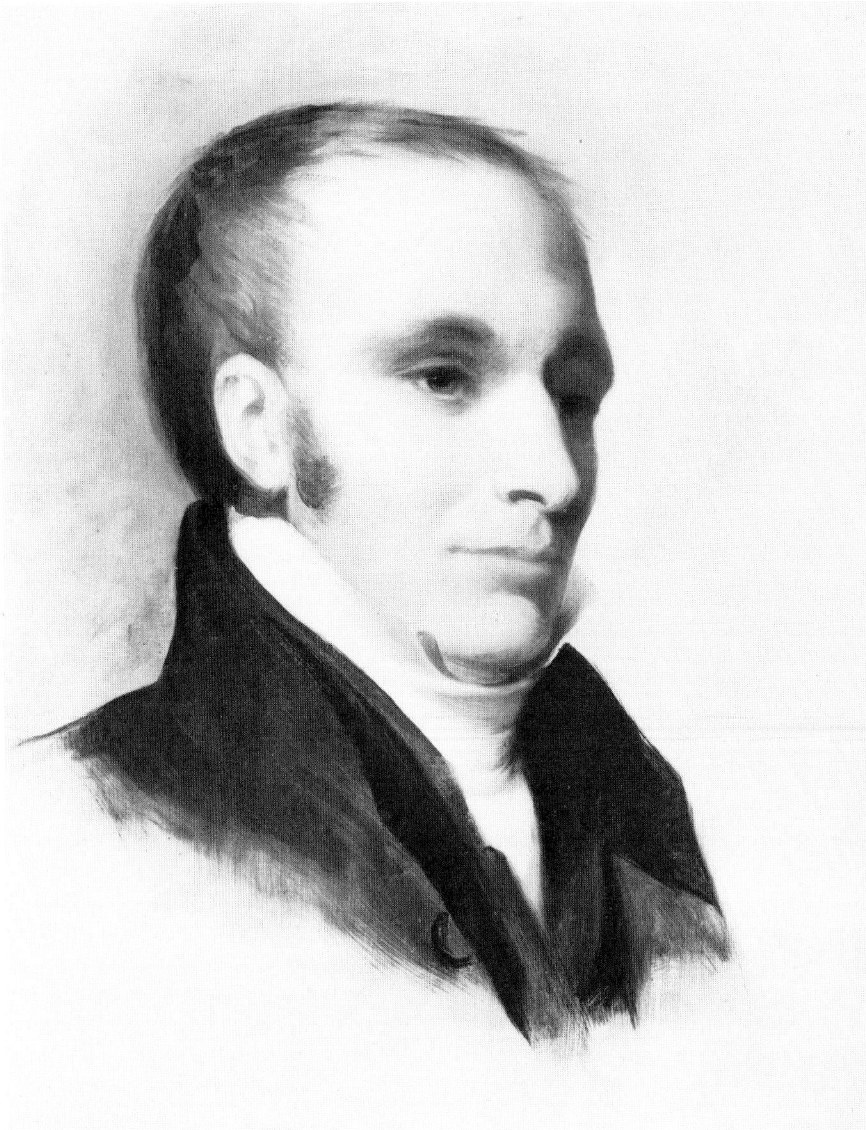

Samuel Emlen PA 112

then secretary to the Philadelphia Dispensary. He was a member of the Board of Guardians of the Poor and physician to the Magdalen Asylum, Orphan Asylum, and Friends Asylum for the Insane. In 1825 he was elected physician to the Pennsylvania Hospital and was secretary to the College of Physicians. As secretary to the Board of Health, he wrote a paper based on his observations of the yellow fever epidemic of 1820. He was co-editor of the *Journal of Foreign Medical Science and Literature* from 1821 to 1823. He was a founder of the Pennsylvania Society for Discouraging the Use of Ardent Spirits.

Artist: Thomas Sully (1783-1872)

For biography, see page 18.

Oil on board; 17 3/4 x 14 1/4. In Sully's Register of Portraits *this portrait is dated May 5–September 8, 1828, with the remark, "Deceased, from a cast Dr. Meigs." Since Dr. Emlen had died on April 17, 1828, this portrait was probably made after a death mask or sculpture cast either owned by or done by or for Dr. Meigs. The son of Dr. Charles Delucena Meigs said that his father was a capable amateur at both painting and modeling in clay and wax. Presented by Mr. John Thompson Emlen through the interest of Dr. William N. Bradley, 1945. PA 112*

Dr. Emlen's head is turned to the right and tilted slightly down. The background is a thin wash of tan, umber, and pale green above, with bare canvas below. The subject has sparse medium brown hair and long side-whiskers. His long, arched eyebrows surmount deepset blue eyes which look out in the direction of his head turn and tilt. The rounded face has thin lips and a slender nose with a small bump. The subject wears a white shirt with stand-up collar, a white stock, and a brown coat. The surface of the portrait has a thin coat of sketchy, rapidly painted, visible brush strokes. The features are soft and blurry. The romantic, dreamy expression, faraway look, and smooth skin are appropriate for a man who died in the prime of life.

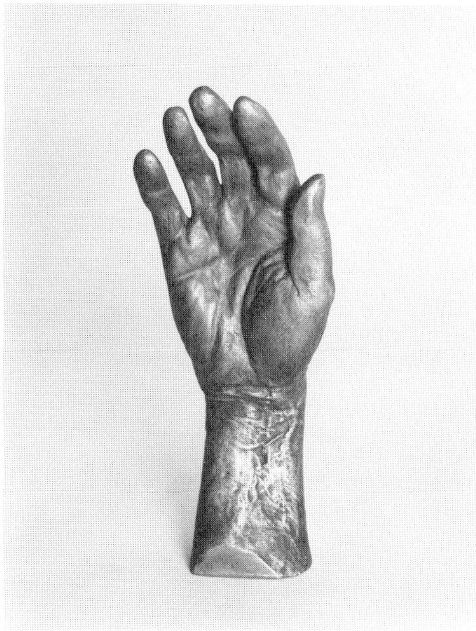

Hand of George Fetterholf ST 568

George Fetterolf (1869-1932)

The son of the president of Girard College, Fetterolf was born in Collegeville, Pennsylvania. He graduated from the University of Pennsylvania in 1887 and from its school of medicine in 1891. At the University he was appointed assistant demonstrator in anatomy and then assistant professor of anatomy. In 1924 he became the first professor of otolaryngology (previously the chairs of otology and laryngology had been separate). He was consulting laryngologist to the Henry Phipps Institute, Whitehaven Sanitarium, Eagleville Sanitarium, Eastern Pennsylvania Institute, Kensington Hospital, and Phoenixville Hospital. During World War I he served as a major in the Army Medical Corps. He belonged to many medical societies, including the American Laryngological Association, of which he was president in 1932. At the College of Physicians he was chairman of the section on otology and laryngology, a member of the Council, and chairman of the Mütter Museum committee. He was instrumental in obtaining the Chevalier Jackson, Cryer, and Fraser Collections for the Museum. He was the author of many articles on otolaryngology and served on the editorial boards of the *Annals of Otology, Rhinology and Laryngology*, and the *Archives of Otolaryngology*. He made important contributions to the etiology of pulmonary abscess, the treatment of laryngeal tuberculosis, the use of ephedrine, the study of vagotonia, and the relation of the upper respiratory tract to bronchial asthma. He received an honorary Sc.D. degree from Ursinus College in 1911.

Artist: Dr. and Mrs. Joseph Head

Bronze; 93/4 x 33/4 x 3; not signed or dated. According to a letter dated July 1, 1940, from Mrs. Albert Edward Kennedy to Dr. Bradley, "The work was done by Dr. and Mrs. Joseph Head, of Chestnut Hill, who have been for years expecially interested in the expression they find in hands." Presented by Mrs. George Fetterolf through Dr. Harry P. Schenck, 1967. ST 568

This bronze cast shows Dr. Fetterolf's right hand and wrist at rest. The long, curved fingers are close together, but not touching. The surface shows every detail of the skin texture. On the dorsal surface the vessels and tendons are very prominent. On the palmar side deep furrows in the hand and veins in the wrist attract the viewer's attention. Since there is no base, the sculpture can be displayed standing (as in this photograph) or lying horizontally on either side.

John Fothergill (1712-1780)

Born at Carr End, Wensleydale, Yorkshire, Fothergill was first apprenticed to an apothecary and then took the M.D. degree at the University of Edinburgh in 1736. He moved to London, where he worked and studied for two years at St. Thomas's Hospital, then opened a practice, and in 1744 became the first graduate of Edinburgh to be admitted as licentiate of the Royal College of Physicians. He was later elected a fellow of the Royal Society of Medicine in Paris and a fellow of the College in Edinburgh. His essay, "An Account of the Sore Throat Attended with Ulcers," was the first in English to give a clear description of diphtheria as a separate entity and to describe its treatment. It was translated into almost every European language. Other notable essays by Fothergill dealt with tic douloureux, migraine, and influenza. He had a vast collection of shells and insects, which passed into the Hunterian Museum, and a renowned collection of rare and valuable plants, excelling those in most royal gardens. A philanthropic Quaker, Fothergill founded the school for Quaker children at Ackworth. He contributed munificently to the library of the British Museum. Although he never went to America, he had family members there, and as late as 1774 he cooperated with Benjamin Franklin in drawing up a scheme for reconciliation between the two countries. He was a friend of the College of Philadelphia and adviser and patron in its early medical courses. He wrote a letter of recommendation to the trustees for Dr. William Shippen, Jr. (q.v.) and sent a present of anatomical plates, casts, and models to the Pennsylvania Hospital which he suggested should be used in lectures to be given at the College.

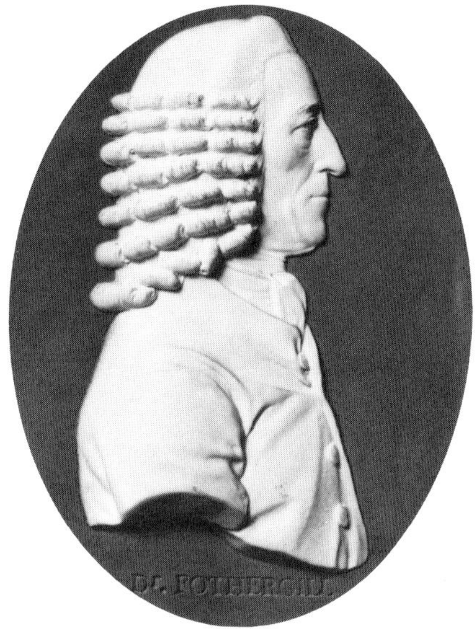

John Fothergill *PH 757*

Artist: Modelled by Patience Wright, produced by Josiah Wedgwood (1730–1795)

Wedgwood jasperware relief medallion; oval, 4 x 3. According to Henry Fertig, in "Josiah Wedgwood, Medallions and Physicians," Bulletin of the History of Medicine, *XXVIII, 8 (1954), this is one in a group of ten physicians in Class X, "Heads of Illustrious Moderns," in Wedgwood's sixth catalogue, and it is one of two separate medallions of Fothergill made prior to 1787, the other having been modelled by John Flaxman. Presented by Dr. D. Sergeant Pepper, from the collection of D. William Pepper, 1948.*
PH 757

Dr. Fothergill is shown bust length, with head and body in profile to the right. The figure is white, the background blue. An inscription, "Dr. Fothergill," appears below the figure. The wig has seven sets of horizontal curls extending in rows from eye level to shoulders. Under a delicate eyebrow, the eye, which has pupil and iris incised, looks straight ahead. Between high cheekbones, the tip of the long nose points down toward a wide mouth and pointed chin. Age lines appear at the eye, nose, and jaw. The subject wears a stock, a cravat, and a single-breasted, buttoned coat with no lapel. The head and body on this neoclassical medallion appear solid and three-dimensional, even though the carving is no more than 3/8 inch in depth. The surface is smooth with sharp contours and minute, crisply carved details of hair, face, and costume. The elongated face, tight mouth, and formal wig contribute to the serious demeanor, appropriate to the subject's inclusion in a group of "illustrious moderns."

John Foulke (1757–1796)

Descended from 17th century Welsh Quaker settlers in Gwynedd, Pennsylvania, Foulke was born in Philadelphia and received the M.B. degree from the University of Pennsylvania in 1780. After graduation he studied in Paris, where he was received cordially by Benjamin Franklin—then American Minister to France—and in Leipzig and Holland. On his return to Philadelphia he was physician to the Pennsylvania Hospital and a lecturer in anatomy there from 1784 to 1796. He also taught medicine privately at his own residence, giving Philadelphia its first systematic instruction in obstetrics. He was a junior founding fellow of the College of Physicians and secretary of the American Philosophical Society. While in France he became interested in aeronautics, the invention of the balloon just having been made public there. Soon after his return to Philadelphia he gave a "Lecture on Pneumatics" and exhibited the first balloon seen in this country to an audience at the University of Pennsylvania. In May, 1784, the same balloon was raised from the garden of the minister of France "twice or perhaps three Times the Height of the Houses, and then gently descended without Damage."

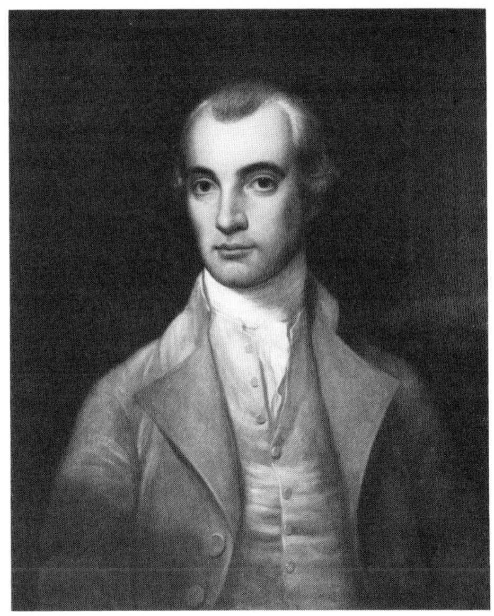

John Foulke *PA 6*

Artist: Attributed to Waugh

Samuel Bell Waugh (1814–1885)

Born in Mercer, Pennsylvania, Waugh studied art privately in Philadelphia, then removed to Canada, where he lived in Montreal and exhibited portraits with the Society of Artists and Amateurs in Toronto. He spent eight years abroad in Paris, in England, and especially in Italy, where he visited ancient ruins and studied old masters. After his return to America in 1843, most of his career was spent in Philadelphia. He became widely known for his "views" of Italy and for a panorama titled *Italia*; these were exhibited first in Philadelphia and were shown on a tour throughout the United States during which Waugh accompanied the paintings and charged admission. Waugh was widely sought after as a portraitist to society, the professions, and government leaders. Most of the paintings that he exhibited at Artists' Fund Society exhibitions and at annual exhibitions of the Pennsylvania Academy of the Fine Arts between 1843 and 1869 and intermittently at the National Academy of Design between 1842 and 1879 were portraits and figure studies. He was made an associate of the Pennsylvania Academy in 1847 and in 1860 and an honorary professional member of the National Academy of Design in 1848. He exhibited with the Artists Fund Society in the 1840s and served as a member of its council and board of control. The Samuel B. Waugh family included several other artists—his wife, Mary Eliza Young Waugh; his son, Frederick Judd Waugh (1861-1940); his daughter, Ida Waugh; and his nephew, Henry W. Waugh. The artist William Waugh is not a member of this family.

Ida Waugh (d. 1919)

Born in Philadelphia, Ida Waugh was the daughter of the portrait and landscape painter, Samuel Bell Waugh, and the miniaturist, Mary Eliza Young Waugh. She first studied at the Pennsylvania Academy of the Fine Arts in 1867 and was a member of its first women's life class in 1869. In Paris she studied at the Académie Julien under Julies Lefebvre and Jean Joseph Benjamin-Constant and at the Académie Delecluse under Paul Delance and Georges Callot; she exhibited at the Paris salons of 1889, 1890, and 1891. She was an associate at the Pennsylvania Academy, where her work appeared frequently in annual exhibitions between 1863 and 1905. She exhibited paintings and sculpture at the Philadelphia Centennial Exposition (1876) and at the Chicago Columbian Exposition (1893), where her work was included in the Gallery of Honor in the Woman's Building. She also showed work at the National Academy of Design, where she won the Dodge prize in 1896. She won a prize for a cover design of the *Ladies Home Journal* and was a well-known illustrator of books. Her painting, *Hagar and Ishmael in the Desert,* is in the collection of the Pennsylvania Academy.

Oil on canvas; 29 1/2 x 24 1/2; not signed or dated. There is no document at the College of Physicians to identify the artist, but the work is listed variously in several catalogues. In the record of the 1887 Centennial Celebration Loan Collection of Portraits, *it is stated that the work is owned by College of Physicians and the artist is "Waugh." The 1898-1915 Inventory says, "portrait artist Waugh (copy)." The 1940* Catalogue of College Collections *says, "copied by Waugh." The 1950* Catalog of Oil Portraits *states that the artist is "Ida Waugh after." The Bradley file suggests "S.B. Waugh (copy)." An Albert Rosenthal etching of Foulke, undated, says "from the painting in the possession of the College of Physicians." Presented by Mrs. Julia Powel Foulke (Mrs. William Parker Foulke, wife of Dr. Foulke's grandson) in 1869, according to College minutes of 1869. Although there is no known birth date for Ida Waugh, she was a student at the Academy in 1867 and 1869, so it seems unlikely that she would have received such a commission. However, more research would have to be done on the copy style of Samuel Waugh and on the identification of the original source to establish Samuel Waugh as the artist, without other positive documentation. PA 6*

Dr. Foulke is shown bust length, his body turned very slightly to the right, the head turned to the left and tilted slightly downward. The dark brownish-gray background includes the base and shaft of a fluted column on the right. Foulke's gray wig is brushed away from his face and has a formal curl at the ears. The eyebrows are dark. The large brown eyes gaze straight ahead in the direction of the head turn. The wide mouth is full-lipped. The subject wears a white stock and shirt frill, a yellow waistcoat with no collar or lapel, and a green single-breasted coat with wide lapels and a small stand-up collar. The surface of the portrait is smoothly painted, with no visible brush strokes. The head is moderately well constructed in three dimensions, and there is some sense of the body mass underlying the costume. The august symbolism of the column is contradicted by the youthful appearance of the sitter, his pink flesh tones, pastel-colored costume, and somewhat pouting facial expression.

Four Studies of the Progress of Fatigue in Athletes

Artist: Robert Tait McKenzie (1867-1938)

Dr. McKenzie was born in Ramsey, Ontario, to Scottish Canadian parents. While at high school in Almonte he received his only formal art training, drawing from casts and from life at night school. He received the A.B. degree from McGill University in 1889 and the M.D. in 1892. While a student, he earned tuition money as an assistant in the gymnasium and was active in competitive sports, especially gymnastics. This was a crucial experience in the formation of his three-pronged career in medicine, physical education, and sculpture. He established an orthopedic practice in Montreal and served as medical director of physical training and demonstrator of anatomy at McGill from 1895 to 1904. During this period he made anatomical models and masks to illustrate the process of fatigue for his students of anatomy; he also fashioned low relief plaques and medallions of heads and figures based on his thorough knowledge of anatomy. At the same time he accumulated anthropometric data on athletes' physiques and produced his first full-length sculptures of ideal modern athletes. He became known for his treatment of scoliosis. In 1904 McKenzie came to the University of Pennsylvania as the first professor of physical education. He became research professor in 1931 and emeritus professor in 1937. He was also appointed the first professor of physical therapy in the medical school. He expanded the department of physical education and its facilities, and he founded the School of

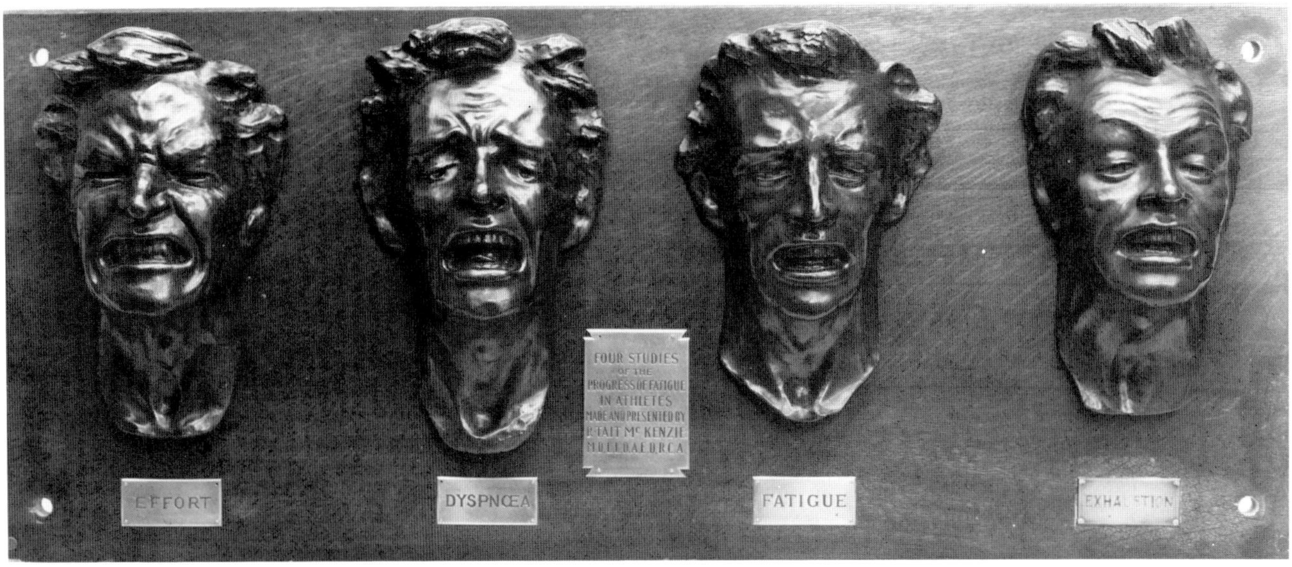

Four Studies of the Progress of Fatigue in Athletes ST 528

Public Health. During World War I he worked in rehabilitation and physical medicine as a member of the Royal Army Medical Corps. He was widely known for making facial masks for reconstructive plastic surgery. A leader in the field of physical education, he widened its horizons by emphasizing related psychological and social objectives as well as innovative corrective treatment. He served as president of the American Academy of Physical Medicine, the American Physical Education Association, and the Society of Directors of Physical Education in Colleges. He was a fellow of the College of Physicians and chairman of its section on medical history. He wrote a series of textbooks on physical education, including *Exercise in Education and Medicine* (1909) and *Reclaiming the Maimed in War* (1918). McKenzie was at least as well known as a sculptor. In addition to portrait plaques and medals, he made more than 200 statues of athletes in action and many famous war memorials, including those in Cambridge, London, Ottawa, Edinburgh, and Washington, D.C. His works of local interest include *The Boy Scout* at the Boy Scout Headquarters, *The Young Franklin* and portraits of the Reverend George Whitefield and Provost Edgar Fahs Smith at the University of Pennsylvania, and *Alma Mater* at Girard College. He was elected an honorary academician of the Royal Canadian Academy of Art and received honorary degrees from the University of Pennsylvania and St. Andrew's and McGill Universities. An early sculpture of a sprinter poised for action drew great praise at the Society of American Artists in New York (1902), the Royal Academy in London (1903), and the Paris Salon (1904). Sculptures of athletes were purchased by the Fitzwilliam Museum in Cambridge, the Ashmolean Museum in Oxford, and the Metropolitan Museum of Art. There were exhibitions of his work at the Heron Art Institute in Indianapolis (1908), the McClees Gallery in Philadelphia (1913), the Fine Arts Society in London (1920 and 1930), the Grand Central Galleries in New York (1934), and a retrospective exhibition at the University of Pennsylvania (1975), where the Lloyd P. Jones Gallery maintains at least sixty sculptures on permanent exhibition. His own career was a testimony to the motto, *mens fervida in corpore lacertoso* (the eager mind in the lithe body), for the Olympic shield that he designed.

Four bronze relief sculptures, their upper portions resting on wooden blocks, mounted on a wooden board, 17 5/8 x 42 x 1 1/8; "Effort," 12 1/2 x 8 x 5; "Dyspnoea," 13 3/8 x 8 x 5; "Fatigue," 12 x 8 x 5; "Exhaustion," 12 1/8 x 7 x 5; made in 1900. The brass plates reads, "Four Studies/of the/ Progress of Fatigue/ in Athletes/ Made and Presented by/ R.Tait McKenzie/ M.D., L.L.D., A.E.D., R.C.A." Presented in 1932. Shown in The Art of Philadelphia Medicine *exhibition, Philadelphia Museum of Art, 1965. Replicas at the Museum of the School of Anatomy, Cambridge University, and at the Lloyd P. Jones Gallery at the Gimbel Gymnasium, University of Pennsylvania.* ST 528

Although usually referred to as "masks," these studies were first modelled in clay from the observations of athletes in action and with the help of instantaneous photographs. The expressions on the faces are typical and not intended to be portraits of a single individual. They were used in McKenzie's anatomy classes and as illustrations in an article, "The Facial Expression of Violent Effort, Breathlessness and Fatigue" (*Journal of Anatomy and Physiology*, 1905, 40, 51), and in his book, *Exercise in Education and Medicine* (first published in 1909). The athletes were actual long-distance runners whom McKenzie studied not only during races but also during the recovery period. In his discussion of the physiological symptoms, the doctor relates the facial expressions to well known artistic and medical studies of emotion and to famous art works of athletes. "Effort" illustrates the extreme intensity of concentration shown in the frowning brows, closed eyes, distended nostrils, clenched teeth, and a facial expression close to rage. "Dyspnoea" shows the breathless state, in which the

Dr. Friebis is shown bust length, body and head turned slightly to the left. The background is dark brown. He has a high forehead, dark gray hair, a moustache and squared-off beard, and brown eyes which look up slightly. The nose is aquiline and the cheek-bones are high. The subject wears a white shirt with stand-up collar, a black necktie with tie pin, a black vest, and a black coat with wide lapels. The surface of the painting has been damaged, hence the style is difficult to assess. The details of the face are lightly indicated and there is paint loss throughout. The rendering was probably naturalistic, with a solidly constructed head and a flatter costume and body. The expression is serious, almost mournful.

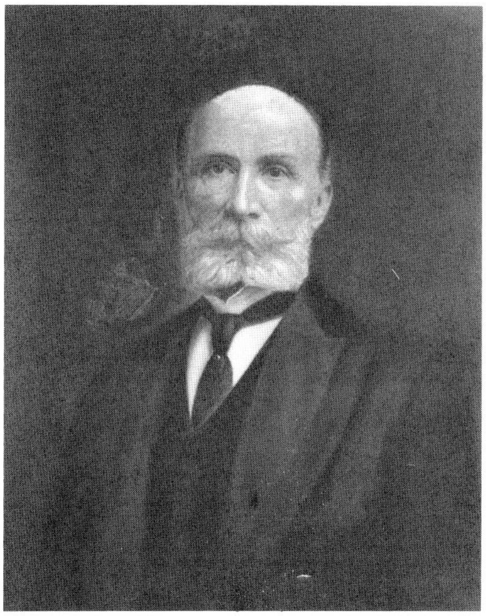

George Friebis *PA 93*

eyebrows are drawn up, the eyelids droop, the nostrils are dilated, the mouth gapes, and the expression resembles that of sorrow. "Fatigue" shows slightly frowning eyebrows, flaccid cheeks, half-open mouth, drooping jaw, and an expression of vacancy. "Exhaustion" shows the athlete fighting off collapse; there are doubly curved wrinkles in the forehead, drooping eyelids, lips drawn downward and outward, and an expression of surprise. All four heads are rendered in naturalistic anatomic detail, showing how all features change during each phase of exercise. The sculptor even included changes in the thick hair.

George Friebis (1846-1912)

Born at Edelsheim, Germany, Dr. Friebis also lived in France before his family moved to America. He was educated in Philadelphia and received the M.D. degree from Jefferson Medical College in 1879. At Jefferson he was appointed successively assistant to the professor of anatomy, William Pancoast (q.v.); demonstrator of anatomy; lecturer on diseases of the skin; assistant to the professor of otology and rhinolaryngology, Dr. Lawrence Turnbull; assistant to the professor of ophthalmology, Dr. William Thomson (q.v.); and from 1889 to 1895, clinical chief and lecturer on diseases of the eye. He contributed many articles on ophthalmology, especially to the *Medical Bulletin*, of which he was assistant editor.

Artist: Attributed to W. C. Hafner

Oil on canvas; 29 3/4 x 24 1/2; signed lower right, but signature indecipherable. In College of Physicians Inventory of 1898-1915, artist is listed as W. C. Hafner; presented by the subject's sisters in 1912, the year of his death. *PA 93*

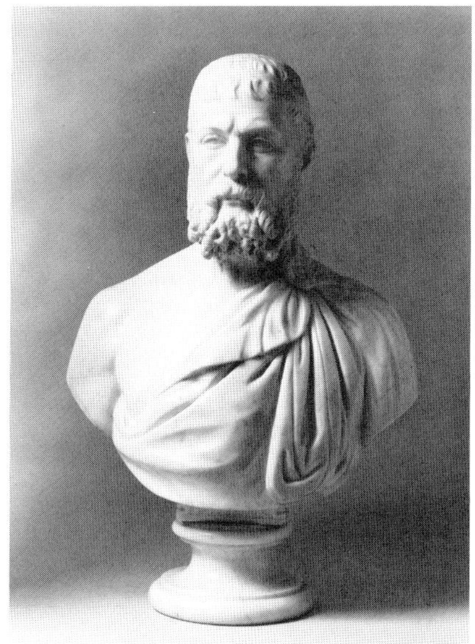

Galen *ST 502*

Galen (ca. 129-200 A.D.)

The most celebrated ancient physician after Hippocrates, Galen was born in Pergamon and was the son of an architect. In addition to medicine he studied mathematics, logic, and philosophy in many cities, including Pergamon, Smyrna, Corinth, and Alexandria. After his appointments as physician to gladiators in Pergamon and as a lecturer in Rome, he became official physician to the Emperor Marcus Aurelius. He wrote more than 500 treatises (100 extant) that exerted great influence on the development of medicine in late antiquity and the middle ages and that remained standard texts until superseded by the work of Vesalius (q.v.) in anatomy and Harvey (q.v.) in physiology. His greatest expertness was in anatomy and physiology, and he systematized and unified Greek knowledge and practice in those fields. By careful dissection of animals, including apes, he drew many conclusions about human anatomy. He gave an account of the fetal circulation and demonstrated that arteries carry blood, not air. He determined the mechanism of respiration and pulsation and analyzed the function of various glands, ducts, and cardiac structures. He believed that the mind is located in the brain, and he contributed to knowledge of the brain, spinal cord, and nerves. He also described and suggested treatment for fevers and for phthisis.

Artist: Unknown

Marble; 29 x 19 5/8 x 11 3/4; base, integral with sculpture, 1 1/4 in. high in front; resting on 4 3/4 in. high circular pedestal; inscription on center front of square base, "Gallienus." Presented by Dr. Richard H. Harte, 1912. In his presentation address, Dr. Harte stated that this is a bust of Galen, "a faithful copy of one now in a private collection in Rome." If the original sculpture could be located, it might answer the question of whether or not this bust is intended to represent Galen (as it has always been known at the College of Physicians) or Gallienus (the name of a Roman Emperor who reigned from 252 to 268), as the inscription says. The only extant ancient portrait of Galen is a 5th century manuscript in which the head is scarcely visible. This sculpture does not resemble any of the known portraits of Gallienus (for information and bibliographic references, see Elsbeth Dusenbery, "Sources and Development of Style in Portraits of Gallienus," Marsyas, *IV, 1945-47). Adding to the confusion is that the name "Galen" in other languages can be spelled "Galien," "Gallien," "Galeno," "Galenos," or "Galenus"—perhaps the artist misspelled the name. It is possible that the artist, probably a 19th century sculptor, merely intended to represent a general "philosopher" type. ST 502*

The subject is shown bust length, body frontal and head slightly to the left. The hair is combed in flat curls onto the forehead. Curly side-whiskers meet the downward curve of the thick moustache and square-cut beard, whose corkscrew curls are pierced. Below knitted brows, the deepset, narrow eyes are blank. The cheeks are hollow, the nose is wide-bridged, and the wide mouth has thin lips. The subject wears a narrow fillet and a toga fastened with a large round brooch on his left shoulder. The arrangement of vertical and diagonal folds leaves the right shoulder and upper torso bare. The surface of the marble is smooth, showing no tool marks. The piercing of the beard and the deeply set eyes and deep carving of the drapery folds cause a sharp contrast of light and shadow. The facial expression and costume convey a message of thoughtfulness, erudition, and dignity.

Joseph Louis Gay-Lussac (1778-1850)

The son of a lawyer, Gay-Lussac was born at St. Léonard, Haute-Vienne, France. He was graduated from the École Polytechnique in 1800 and then entered the school of civil engineering, the famous École National des Ponts et Chaussées. There he became the protégé of the chemist, Berthollet, who played an important role in his professional advancement. He held successive titles at the École Polytechnique and was made professor of chemistry in 1810. He was professor of physics at the Paris Faculty of Science at the Sorbonne from 1808 until 1832, when he resigned in order to become professor of chemistry at the Muséum d'Histoire Naturelle. He was made an academician in 1806. Although his career was devoted to science, he represented Haute-Vienne in the Chamber of Deputies in 1831 and was appointed to the Chamber of Peers by Louis Philippe in 1839. Gay-Lussac's early research was physical in character. He proved that equal volumes of gases expand equally with the same increase in temperature. By making ascents in a hydrogen balloon, he concluded that the magnetic intensity of the earth's surface is constant up to 4000 meters and that the proportion of oxygen in air was equal at 6000 meters to that on earth. With von Humboldt (q.v.), he devised a method for determining precisely the proportion of hydrogen and oxygen in water. He proved that the specific heat of gases is a function of their density. His most important discovery, still called Gay-Lussac's Law, is that when gases combine they do so in the simplest proportions by volume, and that the volume of any gaseous product formed bears a simple ratio to that of the constituents. Later he did research on the isolation and description of various substances and compounds and on improving the methods of organic analysis. He worked on the properties of potassium, sodium, boron, hydrofluoric acid, chlorine, oxymuriatic acid, sulfates, sulfides, salts, and prussic acid. Guy-Lussac's "principle" states that the weight of acids in salts is proportional to the oxygen in the corresponding oxide. He introduced the concept of permutation of the constitutent parts of salts. He contributed to the early history of isomerism and did vital work on volumetric analysis. He published almost 150 papers, in addition to his collaborative writings with von Humboldt, Berthollet, and Thenard.

Artist: Rembrant Peale (1778-1860)

For biography, see page 30.

Encaustic on canvas; 27 1/2 x 22 1/2; signed and dated lower right, "painted in wax by Rem.Peale/Paris 1810." Donor and date of donation are unrecorded. The portrait was located at Peale's Museum gallery until 1854, when it was sold to Charles S. Ogden at an auction of the museum's portraits (according to an annotated copy of the auction sale catalogue located at the Historical Society of Pennsylvania). It entered the collection of the College of Physicians between 1854 and 1887, when it was shown at the Centennial Celebration Loan Collection of Portraits *and listed as owned by the College. The painting was also shown at the* Loan Exhibition of Historical Portraits, *Pennsylvania Academy of the Fine Arts (1887-88), the* Exhibition of Portraits by Charles Willson Peale, James Peale and Rembrandt Peale, *Pennsylvania Academy (1923); and the* Rembrandt Peale Exhibition, *Municipal Museum of the City of Baltimore (1937). PA 37*

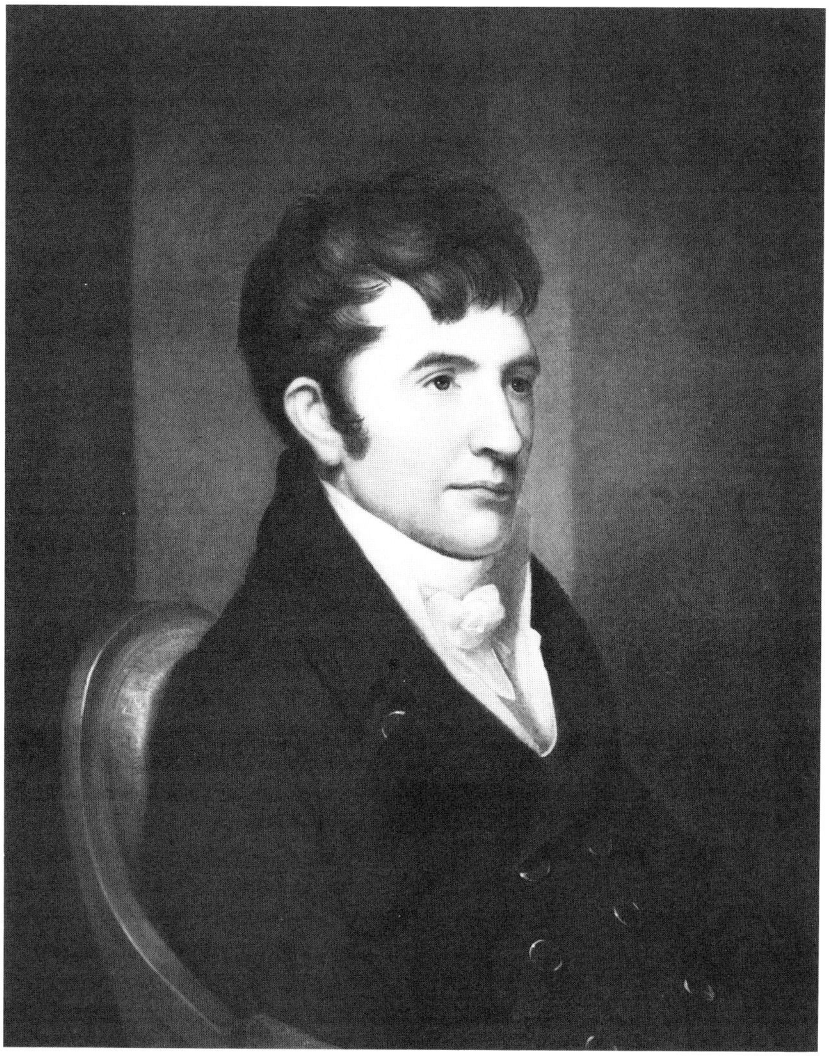

Joseph Louis Gay-Lussac PA 37

Gay-Lussac is shown bust length, body and head turned three-quarters to the right. He is shown seated, with both arms at his sides. The atmospheric background is divided into four vertical strips, giving a sense of architectural division of space. The strips are of uneven width and vary in color from dark brown on the left, medium brown on the right, and two lighter browns in the center behind the subject's head. The armchair has a rounded gold frame and red upholstered back and arm pads. The subject has dark brown wavy hair with soft, curly bangs on his forehead and temples; his brown eyes look straight out in the direction of the head turn. The rounded face has a straight nose, a wide mouth, and full lips. He wears a white stock, a white jabot, a white waistcoat with stand-up collar, and a black double-breasted coat with notched lapel and high collar. The paint style consists of smoothly brushed strokes and softly contoured forms; careful attention was paid to the highlights. The head is rendered solidly, with skillful gradation of planes giving a three-dimensional appearance. There is a sense of the bodily mass underlying the costume. The soft, curvilinear details in hair, eyebrows, shoulders, buttons, and chair back act as a foil against the rectangular shapes in the background. The subject's head and upper body are erect, but his lower torso is relaxed, almost slumping. The dreamy, poetic facial expression and posture and the romantic style of painting seem in opposition to the precise and demanding scientific research that Gay-Lussac had already accomplished by 1810.

William Wood Gerhard (1809–1872)

Born in Philadelphia of Moravian and Irish ancestry, Gerhard received the A.B. degree from Dickinson College in 1826 and the M.D. degree from the University of Pennsylvania in 1830. He spent the next two years in Paris, where he studied under Chomel, Andral, and Louis. He served as clinical lecturer at the Philadelphia Hospital, assistant professor of the institutes of medicine at the University of Pennsylvania, and visiting physician at the Pennsylvania Hospital. After his return to Philadelphia from Paris, he published papers on his European observations of the cholera epidemic of 1831–32, on the pathology of smallpox and tuberculous meningitis, and on pneumonia in children. His greatest contribution was the clinical and anatomical distinction between typhus and typhoid, based on his notes of the typhus epidemic of 1836 in Philadelphia. He was especially expert in diseases

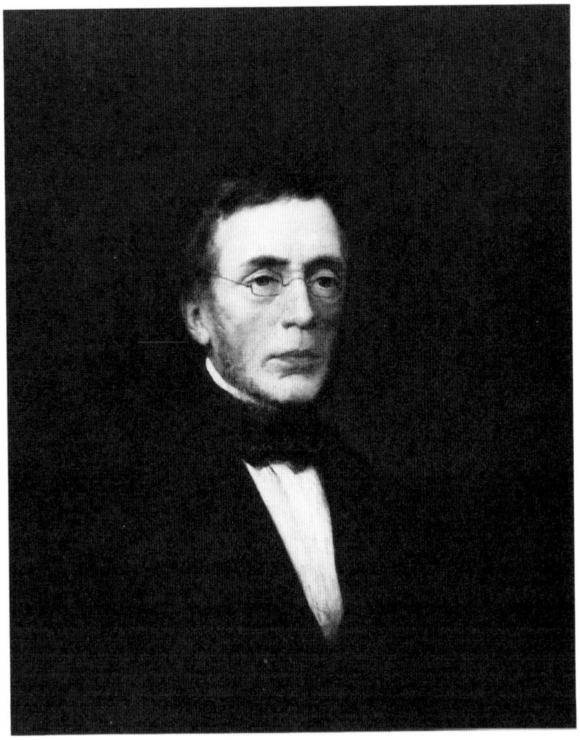

William Wood Gerhard *PA 63*

of the heart and lungs, as is shown by his book *Lectures on the Diagnosis, Pathology and Treatment of Diseases of the Chest* (1842). In addition to being a fellow of the College of Physicians of Philadelphia and member of the American Philosophical Society, Gerhard was president of the Pathological Society of Philadelphia.

Artist: Attributed to Robert Hinckley (1853-1941)

Born in Boston and descended from settlers of Plymouth Colony, Hinckley studied art in Paris, in the studio of Carolus-Duran and at the École des Beaux Arts. He spent 17 years abroad before returning to this country. He set up a studio in Washington, where he established a reputation for portraiture and taught portrait painting at the Corcoran Gallery School of Art for six years. He exhibited portraits at the National Academy of Design in 1877, 1883, and 1895-96. He spent the last thirty years of his life at Rehoboth Beach, Delaware. He is said to have painted 350 portraits of eminent Americans. Many are at Annapolis, West Point, and the United States Capitol Building.

Oil on canvas; 29 1/4 x 24 1/4; not signed or dated. Records of the College of Physicians attribute the painting to Hinckley but the College possesses no confirmatory evidence. There are two torn labels on the back of the painting, one from Washington (where Hinckley lived), the other from Philadelphia. If the painting was made by Hinckley, it would have to be a copy, as he returned to America after the death of Dr. Gerhard. The depiction resembles a portrait of Gerhard by Hannah Mae Horner, formerly located at Philadelphia General Hospital. Presented by the subject's family in 1897. *PA 63*

Gerhard is shown bust length, with head and body turned slightly to the right. The background is dark brown on the right, black on the left. The subject has short, dark brown hair, grayish side-whiskers, and a gray square-cut beard. His blue-gray eyes look straight ahead through metal-rimmed spectacles. There is a long gap between the short, straight nose and the full, pursed lips. The subject wears a white shirt, a wide black bow tie, a black vest, and a black coat. Although there is paint loss in the face and there is overpainting elsewhere, it can be inferred that the head was smoothly brushed and solidly constructed and that the costume was flat, with little sense of underlying body mass. Perhaps the damaged surface makes the facial expression more austere than the artist originally intended.

John Heysham Gibbon, Jr. (1903-1973)

A fifth-generation physician, Dr. Gibbon was born in Philadelphia. He was graduated from Princeton University and then from Jefferson Medical College in 1927. He served in the Army with the Pennsylvania Hospital Unit in the South Pacific and was chief of surgical services at the Mayo General Hospital in Galesburg, Illinois. Most of his career was spent at Jefferson Hospital, where he became professor of surgery and director of surgical research in 1946. He was Samuel D. Gross Professor of Surgery and chairman of the department of surgery from 1956 until 1967, when he became professor emeritus. He is widely known for his development of the artificial heart-lung apparatus, which permitted the development of open-heart surgery, including transplantation of the heart, valvular replacement, and coronary artery bypass. Dr. Gibbon was president of the College of Physicians of Philadelphia (1964-66), the Laennec Society, the Society of Vascular Surgery, the American Association for Thoracic Surgery, the Society of Clinical Surgery, and the American Surgical Association. In recognition of his pioneering medical research and leadership he received the honorary D.Sc. from Dickinson, Princeton, the University of Pennsylvania, Buffalo, and Duke and an LL.D. from Thomas Jefferson University. He was made an honorary fellow of the Royal College of Surgeons in England. He received the Strittmatter Award of the Philadelphia County Medical Society, the Distinguished Service Award of the International Society of Surgery, the Albert Lasker Award in Medical Science, the Dickson Prize in Medicine from the University of Pittsburgh School of Medicine, and the Philadelphia Award. He was the author of *Surgery of the Chest*, chairman of the editorial board of *Annals of Surgery*, and contributor of many chapters and articles to other publications.

Artist: Charles Sydney Hopkinson (1869-1962)

Born in Cambridge, Massachusetts, Hopkinson received the A.B. degree from Harvard in 1891 and

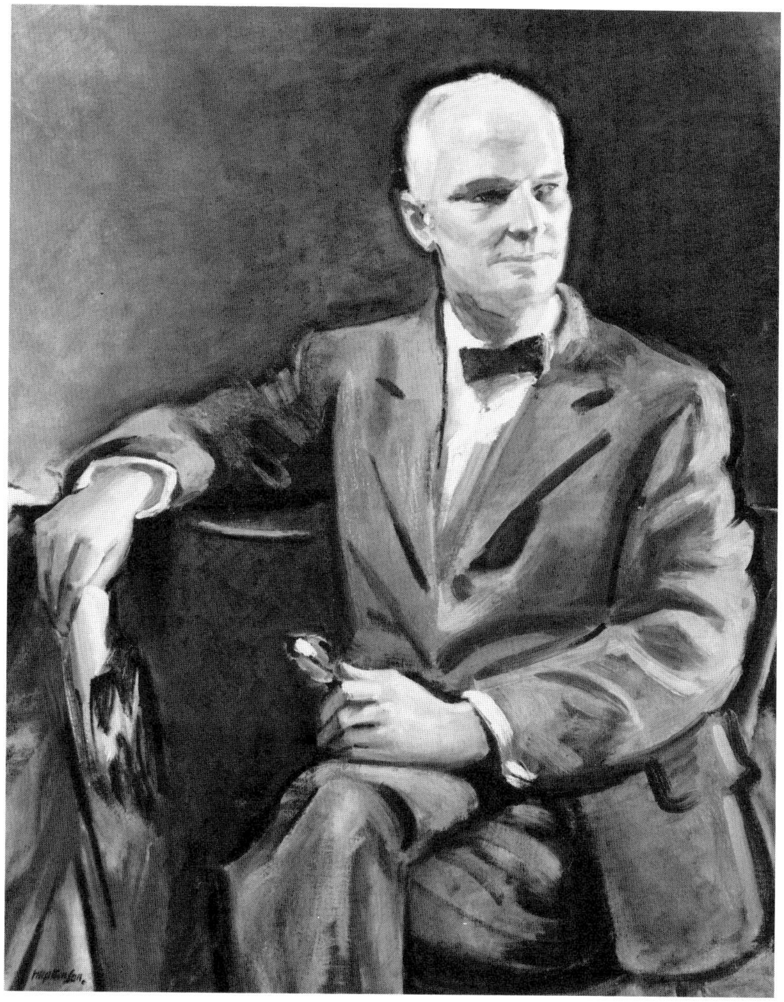

John Heysham Gibbon, Jr. *PA 130*

then studied art in Cambridge, at the Art Student's League in New York, and in Paris. He was a distinguished portrait painter and was made an academician of the National Academy of Design in 1929. He won awards at the Pan-American Exposition in Buffalo (1901), the Louisiana Purchase Exposition in St. Louis (1904), and the Beck gold medal at the Pennsylvania Academy of the Fine Arts (1915), the silver medal at the Panama-Pacific Exposition in San Francisco (1915), the silver medal at the Sesquicentennial Exposition in Philadelphia (1926), and the Logan medal of the Art Institute of Chicago (1926). In 1919 he was requested by the National Art Commission to paint portraits of war celebrities. His portraits can be found in many important collections, including those of The Rhode Island School of Design, the National Gallery of Art, the Brooklyn and Cleveland Museums, Radcliffe and Dartmouth Colleges,and Brown, Rochester, Harvard, and Virginia Universities.

Oil on canvas; 39 1/4 x 32 3/4; signed lower left, "C. Hopkinson"; date, 1953, documented by Mrs. John H. Gibbon, Jr., in her presentation of the portrait to the College of Physicians in 1973. Shown at the Pennsylvania Academy of the Fine Arts annual exhibition in 1954. *PA 130*

Dr. Gibbon is shown three-quarters length, seated, his head turned to the right and body slightly to the left. His right arm rests on a table and his right hand, which holds a paper, hangs over the edge of the table. His left arm rests on his lap and his left hand holds eyeglasses. His legs are crossed at the knees. The upper half of the background is light blue on the left and medium blue on the right. The lower half has a table with green printed fabric on the left and drapery on the right. The subject has a high forehead, white hair, and brownish-gray eyes which look to the right in the direction of the head turn. His square face has high cheekbones, a straight nose, and a wide mouth. He wears a white shirt, a maroon bow tie, a camel-colored single-breasted sport coat, and gray trousers. The painterly surface of the portrait has fluid strokes throughout, including broad outlines of facial features and costume. The dramatic shadows are green, violet, and blue. This animated surface produces a sketchy, somewhat flat dimensional quality. Although the chair is set at an angle of 45 degrees to the picture plane, the subject's head turns and his hips twist, suggesting high energy and action. This movement is enhanced by the bravura paint style and the strong contrast of light and shade. It is reinforced by the informal costume and by the alert, almost conversational facial expression. Almost all of Dr. Gibbon's biographers mention his warmth and charm, his ruggedly handsome physical appearance, and his wide interests, which include sports and art. He shared these interests with the artist, his father-in-law, who was 83 years old in 1953. Hopkinson successfully captured the essential characteristics of his subject, who was the toast of the medical world at this time.

William Gibson (1788-1868)

Dr. Gibson was born in Baltimore. After studying at St. John's College in Annapolis, he took the bachelor's degree at Princeton in 1806 and the medical degree in Edinburgh under John Bell in 1809. He stayed abroad for another year studying medicine with Sir Charles Bell and Sir Astley Cooper, in addition to studying art, music, botany, ornithology, and boxing. Returning to Baltimore, he helped establish the medical department of the University of Maryland, becoming professor of surgery at the age of 23. He was famous for two surgical procedures—ligation of the common iliac artery for aneurysm (1812) and a ligation of the left subclavian artery one day after its rupture (1828). Having observed and fought in the two battles of Corunna and Waterloo, he was expert in gunshot wounds and extracted a bullet from General Winfield Scott during the War of 1812. He was called to Philadelphia to succeed Dr. Philip Syng Physick (q.v.) in the chair of surgery at the University of Pennsylvania, a position he held from 1819 until 1854. When lecturing and demonstrating, he used his own enlarged wax and plaster models and magnified drawings and paintings in addition to dissection. He was considered one of the first to do clinical teaching by bringing a group of patients with similar diseases to the amphitheater for observation. His textbook, *The Institutes and Practice of Surgery*, went through eight editions. Gibson's most striking surgical success was the performance of Cesarean section twice on the same patient. This was before the days of asepsis and anesthesia.

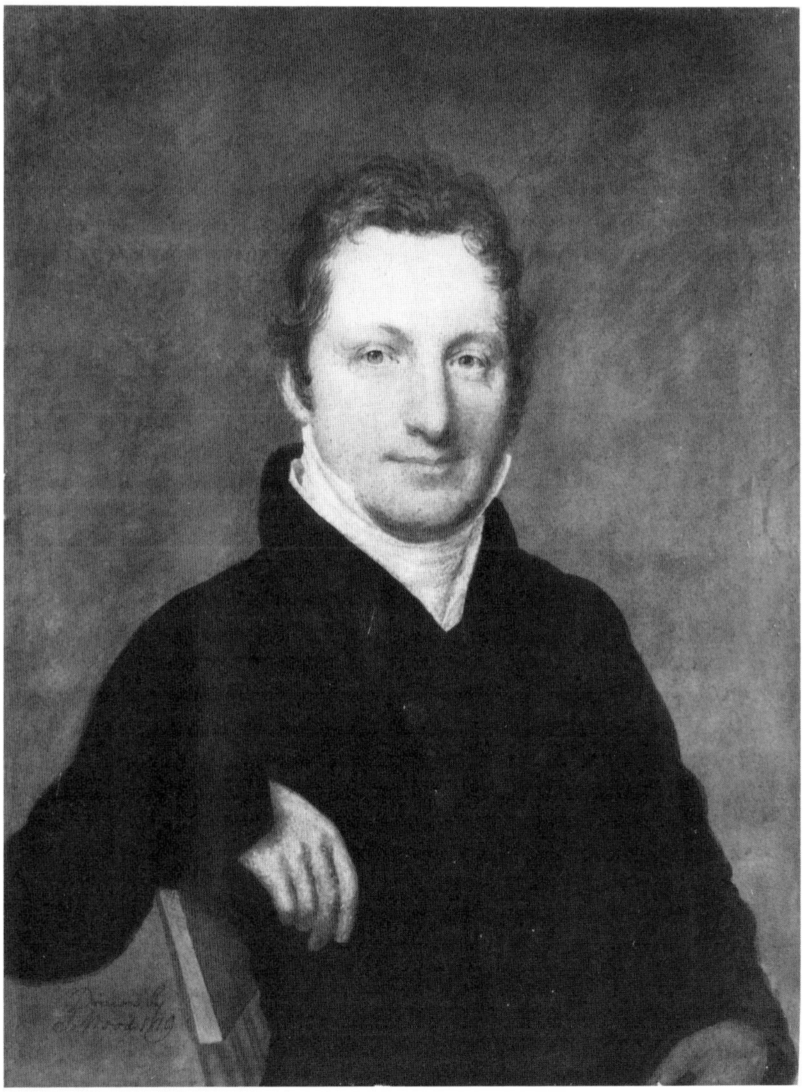

William Gibson *PA 54*

Artist: Joseph Wood (1778–1830)

Born in Clarkstown, New York, Wood was the son of a farmer and sheriff who was unalterably opposed to the boy's choice of career. Against his father's wishes, Wood went to New York City at the age of 15 and worked as a silversmith and violinist until he was able to support himself as an artist. His first professional venture was in 1804 as a partner in John Wesley Jarvis's studio of miniature painting. He received some instruction in miniature painting from Edmond G. Malbone. He became independent either in 1807 or 1811 and worked first in New York and then in Philadelphia, where he showed work in the annual exhibitions of the Pennsylvania Academy of the Fine Arts from 1811 to 1818 and later in Washington and Baltimore. Besides miniatures, Wood also painted cabinet-sized portraits of many of the political and professional notables of his day.

Oil on wood; 83/8 x 63/8; signed and dated lower left, "Drawn by/Jo: Wood 1819." Presented by Dr. Gibson's granddaughter, Anne L. Gibson, in 1923. PA 54

Dr. Gibson is shown half length, body and face turned slightly to the right. He is seated in a slat-back armchair. His right arm rests on the cresting rail, his right hand loosely bent at the wrist. His left arm is at his side, and his left hand is on his lap. The background is a warm greenish-brown. He has curly brown hair, pale blue eyes which look straight ahead towards the spectator, a full face with a long nose whose tip points down to a wide mouth, and a rounded chin. He wears a white shirt with standup collar high on his cheeks, a white stock, a white waistcoat, and a double-breasted black coat with low, pointed cuffs. The smoothly brushed surface of the painting shows anatomically solid and three-dimensional head and hands. Details, such as strands of hair and highlights on coat buttons, are rendered exquisitely. In order to face the spectator, Gibson has been turned in his chair, which is placed perpendicularly to the picture plane. This informal pose, in addition to the confident facial expression, portrays a subject at ease in his world.

Girl With Basin

Artist: Edward Fenno Hoffman III (b. 1916)

The son of an architect and painter, Hoffman was born in Philadelphia. After working in business and serving in World War II with the Philadelphia City Cavalry, he studied art at the Pennsylvania Academy of the Fine Arts from 1946 to 1950. At the Academy he won a Cresson traveling scholarship, the Stimson prize, and honorable mention for the Stewardson prize. In 1949 he won first prize in the annual competition of the American Academy Alumni in Rome. In 1951 he won a Tiffany Foundation grant and the Barnett prize at the National Academy of Design, and he spent six months as assistant to Paul Manship, the American

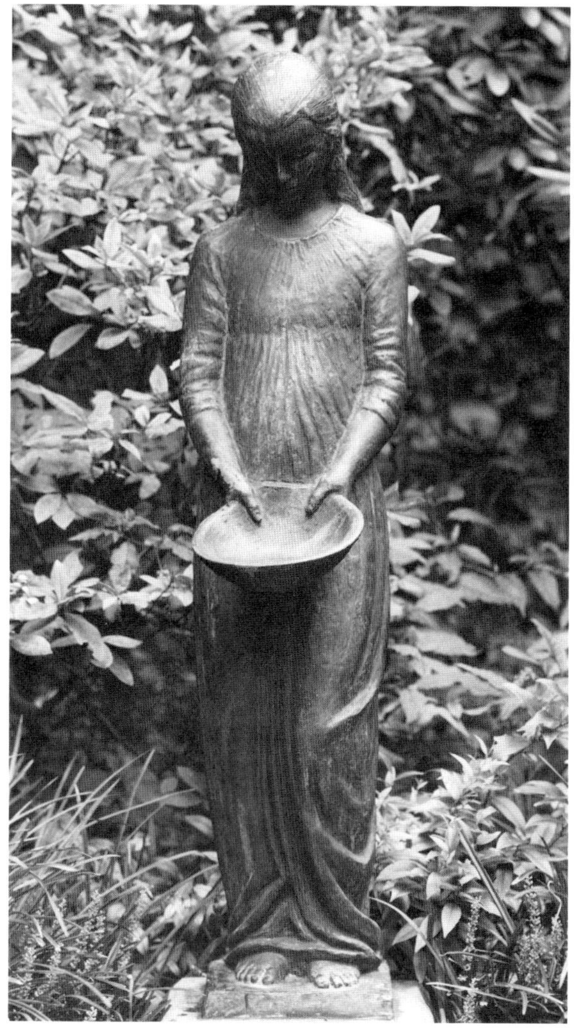

Girl With Basin *ST 579*

sculptor. From 1952 to 1955 he was sculptor-in-residence at the Henry Clews Memorial Art Foundation in La Napoule, France. Hoffman has been a consistent exhibitor and prize winner. He has had a solo exhibition in Cannes, the Philadelphia Art Alliance, Bryn Mawr Art Center, Grand Central Art Galleries in New York, Portland Museum of Art, Provident National Bank in Philadelphia, the Art Association of Newport, Rhode Island, and the Woodmere Art Gallery in Philadelphia. He won the Braverman sculpture prize at the Pennsylvania Academy, the best-in-show at the sculpture exhibition of the National Arts Club and National Sculpture Society, a silver medal at the American Artists' Professional League at the Smithsonian Institution, the gold medal of honor at the Allied Artists of America exhibition at the National Academy of Design, the Samuel F.B. Morse medal at the National Academy of Design, and the Huntington award of the American Artists' Professional League of New York. He is represented in the collections of the Philadelphia Museum of Art, the Pennsylvania Academy of Fine the Arts, Pennsylvania Hospital, Villanova University, and many other museums, universities, gardens, libraries, and churches.

Hoffman's sculptures are in bronze, stone, and marble. His subjects range from mythological and religious subjects to animals, portraits, and genre scenes.

Bronze; 41 3/4 x 11 1/2 x 16; bronze base integral with sculpture, 1 1/4 in. high; mounted on cement block, 14 in. high; signed and dated on top of bronze base on left side, "Edward F. Hoffman 1960/III." Presented by the Philadelphia Unit, Herb Society of America in 1958, replaced 1960.
ST 579

The full-length figure is shown with head and body frontal. The head is tilted downward. The arms are at the sides and hold a large basin. The subject's weight is on her right foot and her left leg is bent at the knee. Her long hair is brushed away from her face; her features are regular and idealized, and they have a benign expression. She wears a round-necked, high-waisted, ankle-length dress with three-quarter length sleeves. Delicate curving folds of drapery reveal her slender girlish body. She looks down toward the basin that is held in a position to catch rainwater for the birds. The attitude of the figure and the simplicity of the costume suggest a timeless, universal quality appropriate for this piece of garden sculpture.

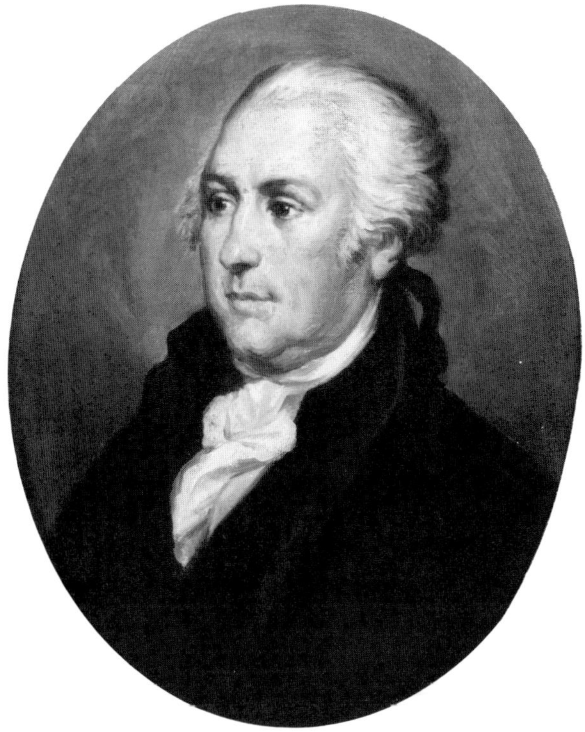

George Glentworth *PA 117*

George Glentworth (1735-1792)

Dr. Glentworth was born in Philadelphia and served an apprenticeship there with Dr. Peter Sonmans. Then he entered the British Army as a junior surgeon. From 1755 to 1758 he was in Europe. He is said to have received a medical degree from the University of Edinburgh. On his return to Philadelphia he became the partner of Dr. Sonmans. In addition to conducting a large practice, he was a founder of the Philadelphia Medical Society (1768); the entire membership of this organization was voted into the American Philosophical Society. He was an original member of the Society of Sons of St. George and one of the senior founding fellows of the College of Physicians of Philadelphia in 1787. During the Revolutionary War he served as regimental surgeon, senior surgeon of the general hospital, and director-general of the hospital in the Middle Department. It is said that after the battle of Brandywine he extracted a bullet from Lafayette's wound. After recovering from "hospital fever," which he contracted in 1780, he returned to private practice and joined the staffs of the Philadelphia Almshouse and the Humane Society.

Artist: Albert Rosenthal (1863-1939)

The son of the Russian immigrant artist Max Rosenthal, Albert Rosenthal was born in Philadelphia and studied painting and print-making first with his father and then at the Pennsylvania Academy of the Fine Arts. Later he went abroad and studied with Jean Léon Gérôme at the Académie des Beaux Arts and at the Munich Academy. After returning to Philadelphia he established a successful career as an etcher, engraver, and painter of portraits; many of these were reproductions of portraits of historic American subjects. He exhibited at the Pennsylvania Academy of the Fine Arts, the Chicago Art Institute, the Carnegie Institute, the Society of American Artists, and the Paris salon. Rosenthal was a prize winner at the Chicago Columbian Exposition (1893), the Buffalo Pan-American Exposition (1901), the St. Louis Louisiana Purchase Exposition (1904), and the San Francisco Panama-Pacific Exposition (1915). He belonged to art societies in many cities, and his work is to be found in museums in Philadelphia, Los Angeles, Youngstown, Kansas City, Brooklyn, Dallas, St. Louis, Providence, Newport, and Allentown.

Oil on canvas; oval, 23 3/4 x 18 1/2; not signed or dated. Copy after an original posthumous portrait painted by Charles Willson Peale, 1794, located at Independence National Historical Park. Proof that Albert Rosenthal is the copyist is contained in a document of the Bureau of City Property dated December 24, 1947, which says that in 1910 the city of Philadelphia acquired an oil of George Glentworth, painted by Albert Rosenthal, and that this Rosenthal copy had been kept in storage at Independence Hall until Miss Marguerite Glentworth, great-great-granddaughter of Dr. Glentworth, presented Peale's original portrait to the Independence Hall Historical Collection of Portraits in 1947, at which time an exchange was made. Miss Glentworth presented the Rosenthal portrait to the College of Physicians in 1948. *PA 117*

The subject is shown bust length, head and body turned three-quarters to the left. The greenish-gray atmospheric background is lighter around the face. The gray hair, brushed away from the forehead, is tied back in a black ribbon. The large and luminous brown eyes look straight ahead in the direction of the head turn. The face is wide, with a small mouth, a cleft chin, and heavy jowls. The figure wears a white stock, a white shirt frill, a brown waistcoat, and a brown open coat. The painterly surface has been brushed loosely with animated strokes, especially in the face, hair, and frill. In contrast to the well-formed head, the costume is flat and does not indicate the underlying body mass. The facial expression is bland and neutral. Comparison with Peale's original portrait of Glentworth shows that Rosenthal regularized the subject's facial features, animated the surface of the painting, changed the color of the eyes, costume, and background, and eliminated details of the setting. Peale's portrait is rectangular. On the right are drapery, a chair, and a table with medical books and cut pink roses; on the left is a window with a potted lily-of-the-valley plant. The flowers recall Dr. Glentworth's well-known interest in botany.

Plunket Fleeson Glentworth (1760–1833)

Dr. Glentworth was born in Philadelphia, the son of Dr. George Glentworth (q.v.). He received the M.D. from the University of Pennsylvania in 1790. He was secretary of the trustees of the College of Philadelphia in 1791, just before that institution merged with the University of the State of Pennsylvania to form the new University of Pennsylvania. He was elected a fellow of the College of Physicians of Philadelphia in 1792. He was a founder of the Pennsylvania Academy of the Fine Arts (1805), was its first treasurer (1806), and served on its board of directors (1807–19), its committee on correspondence (repeatedly between 1807 and 1818), and its committee on instruction (1813). According to letters, written in 1947–48 by his great-granddaughter, Marguerite Linton Glentworth, and preserved in the files of the College of Physicians, he was a friend and physician to both Joseph Bonaparte, King of Naples and Spain, and to George Washington. Miss Glentworth owned a letter from Washington to Glentworth "thanking him for coming down to Mount Vernon," and stating, "he was now in most excellent health." This is corroborated in a Commemorative Address in the Centennial Publication of the College of Physicians (1887), in which Dr. S. Weir Mitchell (q.v.) quotes a letter to John Lewis from Washington, who said about Glentworth, "No nobler man or more skillful physician ever lived," and called him his "estimable friend."

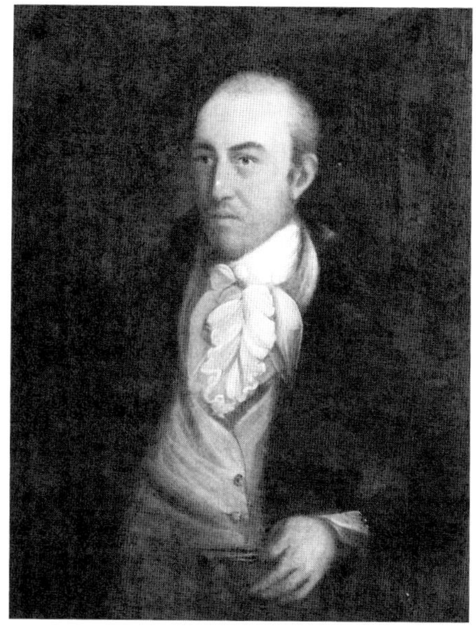

Plunkett Fleeson Glentworth *PA 116*

Artist: Unknown

Oil on canvas mounted on board; 30 x 23 1/2; not signed or dated. Presented by Henry R. Glentworth and Marguerite Linton Glentworth, great-grandchildren of Dr. Glentworth, in 1948. Correspondence dated 1947–48 in the files of the College of Physicians from Miss Glentworth indicates that the family originally believed this portrait to have been the work of Gilbert Stuart and that it was exhibited as a Stuart at the Columbian Exposition of 1893 in Chicago, the Pan-American Exposition of 1901 in Buffalo, and the College of Physicians' Centennial Celebration Loan Collection of Portraits *in 1887, when the painting was owned by Mrs. Caroline Glentworth, mother of Marguerite Glentworth. Many years later the family was informed by the Frick Art Reference Library that the painting was not a Stuart and could be a copy, but the artist could not be identified. For this reason additional research must be done on this work; contemporary experts still cannot establish the identity of the artist.* *PA 116*

Glentworth is shown half-length, the body frontal, the head turned to the right. He is standing with his right arm bent at the elbows. He is leaning on a table covered with green cloth. His right hand holds a small brown book and his index finger marks the place. His left arm extends sideways, cut off at mid-arm by the edge of the canvas. The crystalized varnish on the painting is so disfiguring that is is impossible to tell if any objects are present in the brownish background. Glentworth is depicted as having gray, close-cropped hair. His blue eyes look in the direction of the head turn. The tip of his straight nose points downward to a small mouth with thick lips and a pointed chin. He wears a white shirt with lace cuffs, a white stock (or a thick, white neckcloth), a white bow, a white jabot, a white double-breasted waistcoat, and a black jacket with a high, stand-up collar.

Because of the lamentable condition of the portrait, the style of the painting is difficult to judge, but one can assume that the head and hands were painted in solid, three-dimensional volumes while the costume, which appears flatter, was done with freer brush strokes. Although Glentworth has a somewhat ascetic appearance because of his small face and slender bone structure, his conventional, aristocratic posture is relaxed and his expression is confident.

Paul Beck Goddard (1811-1866)

Born in Baltimore, Dr. Goddard received the A.B. degree from Washington (now Trinity) College in Hartford, Connecticut, in 1828 and the M.D. degree from the medical school of the University of Pennsylvania in 1832. At the University he became an assistant to the professor of chemistry, Dr. Robert Hare (q.v.). Later he was preceptor under Dr. Joseph Leidy (q.v.), demonstrator of anatomy, and then professor of anatomy in the medical department. He was the author of many books, including *Plates of Cerebro-Spinal Nerves, with References for the Use of Medical Students* (1837), *Plates of the Arteries with References for the Use of Medical Students* (1839), and *The Anatomy, Physiology and Pathology of the Human Teeth with the Most Approved Methods of Treatment Including Operations and the Method of Making and Setting Artificial Teeth* (1844). He edited or revised books by Erasmus Wilson, T.B. Curling, F.J. Moreau, R. Rayer, and Samuel Ashwell. He was elected a member of the American Philosophical Society in 1840 in recognition of his pioneering work in photography. Dissatisfied with the slowness of Daguerre's process, he had discovered that by the use of bromine on the silvered plate, the printing could be accelerated. He also described a new method of making minute anatomical injections adapted for microscope, by means of vermilion in oil and sulphuric ether. He was elected a fellow of the College of Physicians in 1842.

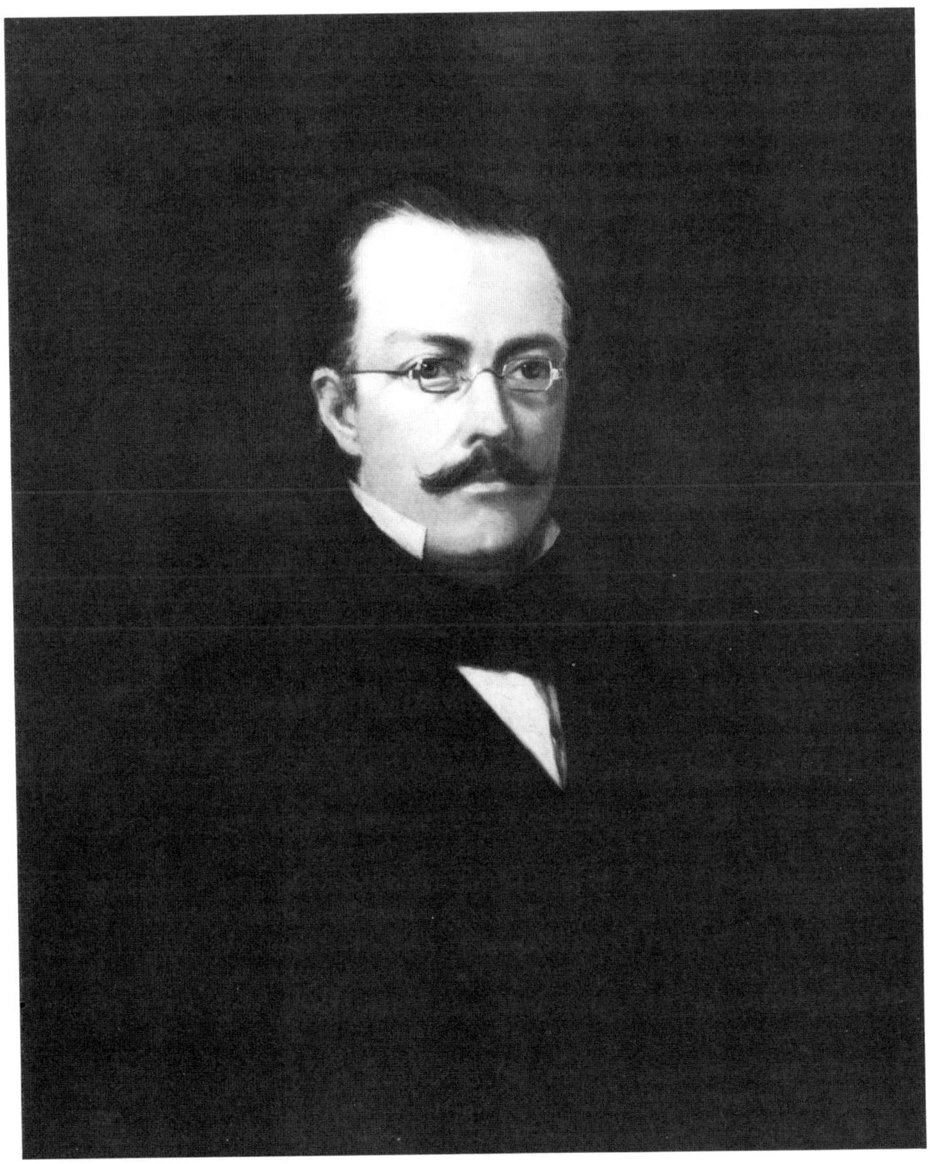

Paul Beck Goddard PA 52

Artist: Edward Bowers (b. ca. 1822, d. after 1870)

Bowers was a painter of portraits, genre paintings, and still-lifes in oils and crayons. He was born in Maryland. He worked in Baltimore (1850-52 and 1860-70), Philadelphia (1854-59), New York City (1859), and Detroit (1865). He exhibited work at the Maryland Historical Society, the Pennsylvania Academy of the Fine Arts, the National Academy of Design, and the Washington Art Association. He was elected an associate member of the National Academy and an associate of the Pennsylvania Academy, where he was nominated to be academician, but there is no record of his actual election to this dignity.

Oil on canvas; 29 x 24; not signed or dated. Since the portrait was shown in 1855 at the annual exhibition of the Pennsylvania Academy of Fine Arts (which listed it as the property of the artist Edward Bowers), it was probably painted either in 1854, when Bowers first came to Philadelphia, or in 1855. An engraving after this portrait reads, "engraving by John Sartain from a picture of E. Bowers." The painting was presented by Mrs. Louisa B. Goddard in 1901. *PA 52*

Goddard is shown bust length; the body and head are inclined slightly to the right. The atmospheric background is bluish-gray. The subject has collar-length, dark brown hair brushed away from his face and a brown moustache. His hazel eyes look straight ahead in the direction of the head turn, through metal-rimmed spectacles. His oval face has regular features and a dimpled chin. He wears a white shirt with stand-up collar, a wide black bow tie, a black vest, and a black coat. The painted surface is smooth and bears no visible brush strokes. The face has been constructed solidly. Skillful modeling of the planes produces a three-dimensional appearance. The costume is flatter, with little sense of underlying bodily forms. Although the expression is neutral and the gaze averted, the eyes are luminous and penetrating. This gives the impression of a thoughtful demeanor.

William Goodell (1829-1894)

Born in Malta, the son of a missionary, Dr. Goodell came to America to study at Williams College, where he graduated in 1851, and at Jefferson Medical College, where he received the M.D. degree in 1854. After some years both in Constantinople and in West Chester, Pennsylvania, he returned to Philadelphia and developed a distinguished career in obstetrics. In 1865 he was appointed physician-in-charge at the Preston Retreat, a gynecological hospital. At the University of Pennsylvania he was appointed lecturer in obstetrics and diseases of women in 1870. He served as clinical professor of the diseases of women and children from 1874 to 1894, when he was designated an honorary professor and also received an honorary LL.D. Jefferson Medical College awarded him an honorary LL.D. in 1893. He was a founder and president of the Philadelphia Obstetrical Society, president of the American Gynecological Society, honorary fellow of the Edinburgh Obstetrical Society, and fellow of the College of Physicians. Of his 113 published writings, the best known is *Lessons in Gynecology (1879).*

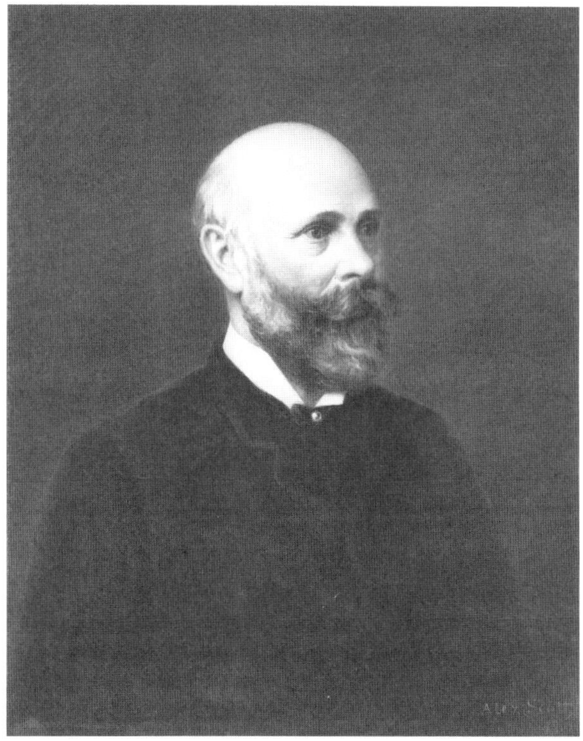

William Goodell *PA 81*

Artist: Alexander Scott

Alexander Scott is the son-in-law of Dr. Goodell.

Oil on canvas; 29 3/4 x 24 1/2; signed and dated lower right, "Alex: Scott/1910." Copy after a portrait by Robert Vonnoh (q.v.), University of Pennsylvania, 1895, which was painted after a photograph. Presented by the family of Dr. Goodell in 1911. *PA 81*

Goodell is shown bust length, with head and body turned to the right. The background is a medium-toned, gray-green. The head is bald, with a fringe of gray at the sides. Gray side-whiskers meet a full gray moustache and rounded beard. The light blue eyes look straight ahead in the direction of the head turn. The fair complexion is highlighted by pink cheeks. The subject wears a white shirt with stand-up collar, a black ascot with pearl pin, and a single breasted black coat with small lapels, buttoned high. Although the surface of the painting is in bad repair, a linear quality can be noted in the drawing of the head. In contrast to the sharp, clear details of the head, the costume is flat and vague, with no sense of underlying body mass. The subject's facial expression is dignified but neutral, and it is removed from any degree of animation, as might be expected in a copy of a painting which in itself was copied from a photograph.

Samuel Powel Griffitts (1759-1826)

The son of Philadelphia Quakers, Dr. Griffitts was educated at the College of Philadelphia. He began the study of medicine under Dr. Adam Kuhn (q.v.) and received the M.B. from the University of Pennsylvania in 1781. He then spent three years taking courses in Montpellier, in London, and in Edinburgh under Dr. William Cullen (q.v.). After returning to Philadelphia he developed a private practice and was active also in the establishment of several medical institutions, including the Philadelphia Dispensary (1786), the Southwark and Northern Liberties Dispensaries (1816), and the Friends Asylum (1811). He was a junior founding fellow of the College of Physicians of Philadelphia (1787) and served as its vice-president from 1817 to 1826. He was professor of materia medica at the University of Pennsylvania from 1792 to 1796. In 1795 he issued a revised edition of *Buchan's Domestic Medicine* and was active in helping to write pharmacopoeias for the United States and for the College of Physicians of Philadelphia. He was a member of the Humane Society, the Pennsylvania Society for Promoting the Abolition of Slavery, and the Society for Alleviating the Miseries of Public Prisons. He was a member of the American Philosophical Society and served on its council from 1791 until 1797.

Artist: Joseph Sansom (1767-1826)

For biography, see page 23.

Silhouette; black ink on buff paper; 4 3/4 x 3 5/8; written in black ink below the figure, "Dr. Samuel Powell [sic] Griffitts of Philad[a] / aged 31"; written in pencil, by another hand, below the name of the subject, "By Jos. Sansom—1789." This date is incorrect because Griffitts was 31 years old in 1790, and the silhouette is one of a group done during 1790-92; however, the identification of Sansom as the artist is correct, since although this silhouette is missing from Sansom's manuscript book of silhouettes at the Historical Society of Pennsylvania, it is listed in the table of contents with the information, "short, Philadelphia, 1759," i.e., Griffitts was of short stature and was born in Philadelphia in 1759. Presented by Hampton L. Carson in 1910.

PH 293

Griffitts is shown bust length, profile to the left, with a steep, concave curve in the torso which forms two sharp points, the one at the chest longer than that of the back. His hair is close-cropped along the flat top of his head and is worn in a shoulder-length queue. The hair and eyelashes are indicated by thin lines separated from the black mass. Individualistic features include a turned-up nose, protruding lips, and a round chin. The outlines of the silhouette are crisp and clear.

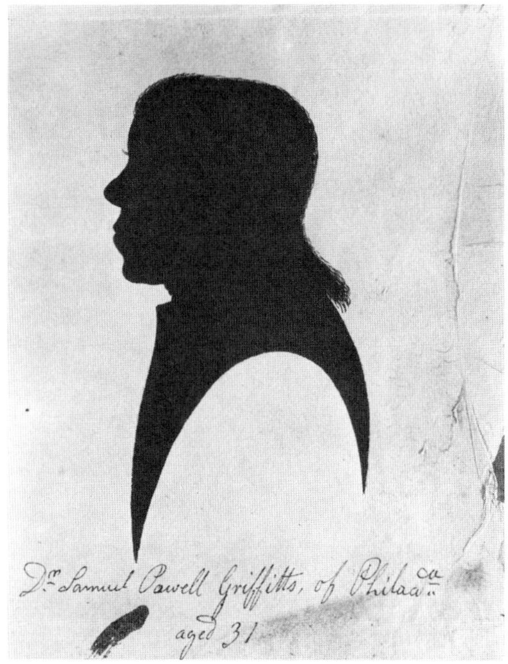

Samuel Powel Griffitts *PH 293*

Samuel David Gross (1805-1884)

Descended from 17th century Pennsylvania German farmers, Dr. Gross was born near Easton, Pennsylvania. He studied medicine first under a local preceptor and then at the Academy at Lawrenceville, New Jersey, in order to learn the classics. Thus prepared, he came to Philadelphia and enrolled with Dr. George McClellan as a private pupil. He then matriculated at the Jefferson Medical College, earning the M.D. degree in 1828. During the early years, when his practice in Philadelphia and Easton was slow, he occupied himself in translating French and German medical texts into English and by doing dissections and animal experiments. He gladly moved to Ohio when offered the position of demonstrator of anatomy in the Medical College of Ohio in 1833. In 1835, when the Cincinnati Medical College opened, he had the professorship of pathological anatomy. His great textbook, *Elements of Pathological Anatomy*, was published in 1839. In 1840 he became professor of surgery at the University of Louisville, where he remained until 1856 except for one year at the University of the City of New York. He returned once again to Philadelphia to become professor of surgery at Jefferson, where he remained until 1882. He was founder and president of the American Surgical Association, the Philadelphia Pathological Society, and the Philadelphia Academy of Surgery. He presided over the Inter-

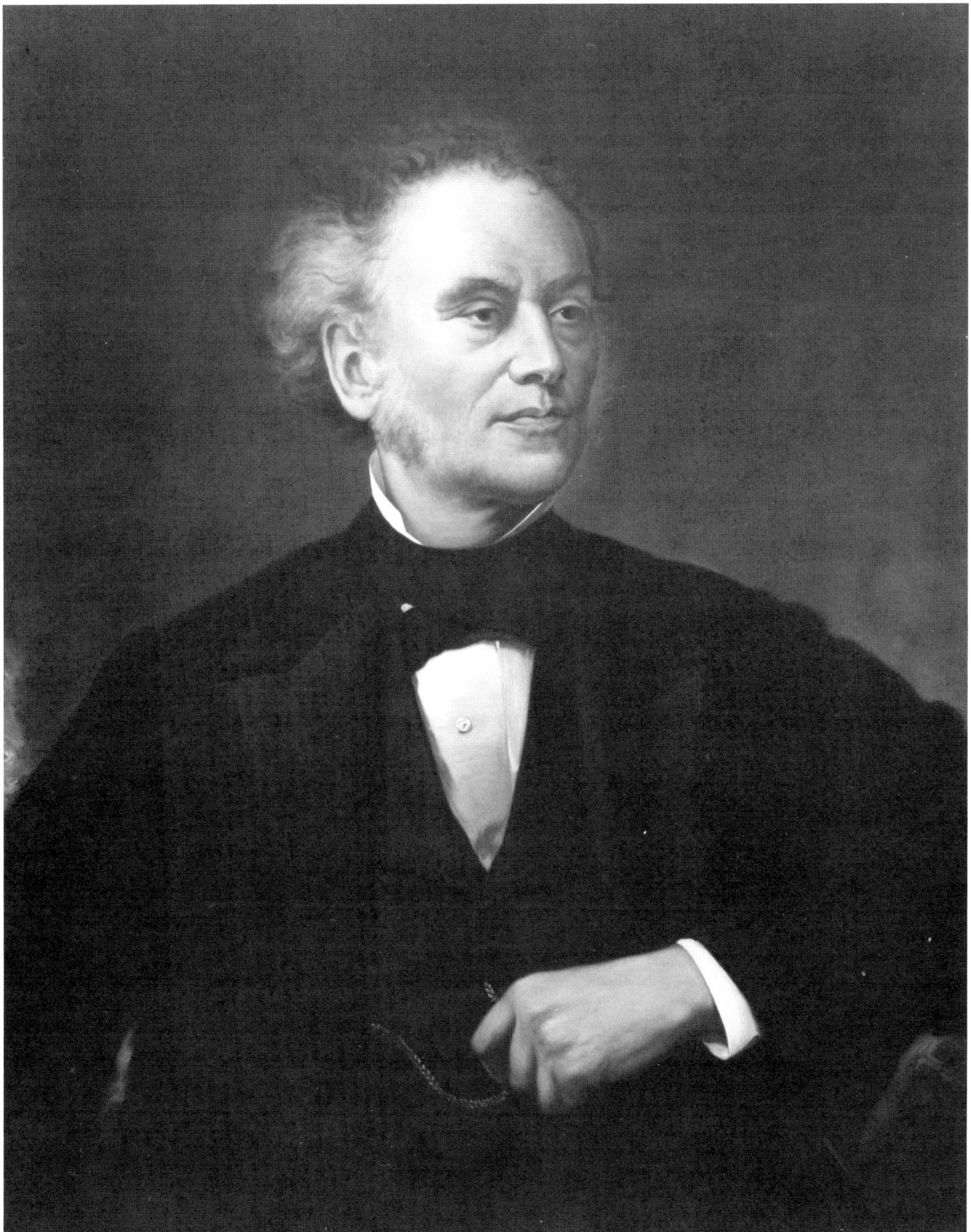

Samuel David Gross *PA 72*

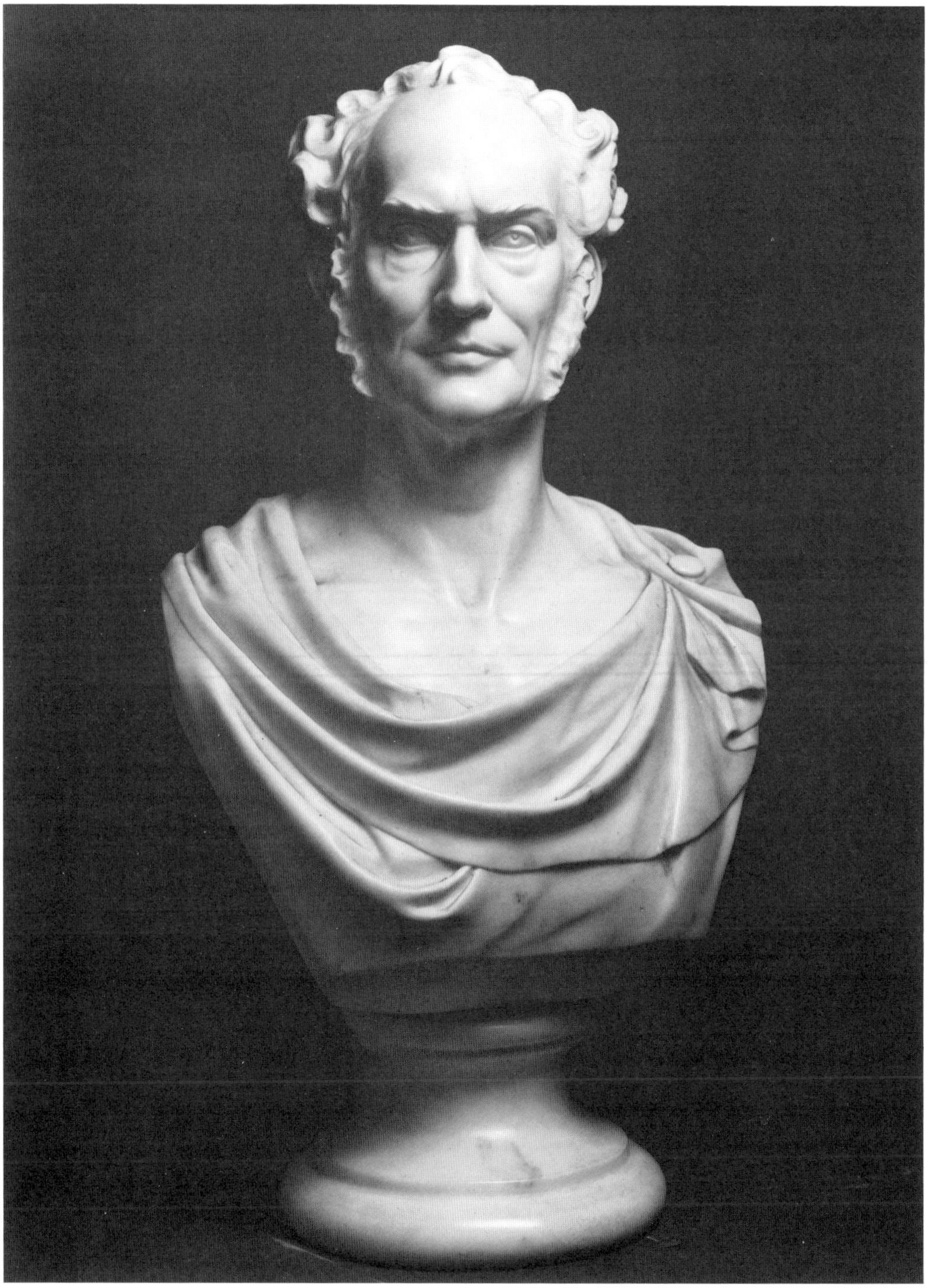

Samuel David Gross *ST 510*

national Congress of Surgeons (Philadelphia, 1876), the American Medical Association, the American Academy of Surgery, and the American Philosophical Society. He also made many contributions to medical literature, such as *A Practical Treatise on the Diseases and Injuries of the Urinary Bladder, the Prostate Gland and the Urethra* (1851), *A Practical Treatise on Foreign Bodies in the Air Passages* (1854), *A System of Surgery, Pathological, Diagnostic, Therapeutic and Operative* (1859), *Manual of Military Surgery* (1861), and *The Lives of Eminent American Physicians and Surgeons of the Nineteenth Century* (1861). He was editor of the *North American Medico-Chirurgical Review.* Dr. Gross also devised many surgical instruments and techniques. He left his extensive library of surgical and medical books to the Philadelphia Academy of Surgery with the proviso that it be housed at the College of Physicians of Philadelphia, where a special room was endowed by his children. He received many awards, including honorary LL.D. degrees from Edinburgh, Cambridge, and the University of Pennsylvania, the D.C.L. from Oxford, and innumerable honors from national and international societies. He was esteemed by colleagues, revered by patients, and admired by students, who appreciated the skill and clarity of his lectures, demonstrations, and textbooks.

Artist: T. Dimino

Oil on canvas; 35 1/4 x 28 1/4; signed and dated lower right, "T. Dimino/ Roma, 1909." Probably a copy of the portrait of Gross by Samuel Bell Waugh (for biography, see Foulke entry), located at Jefferson University and which was commissioned by Jefferson Alumni Executive Committee on April 16, 1874, and completed by February 8, 1875. Dimino's copy was presented by Dr. Gross's children, Maria Gross Horwitz and Albert Haller Gross, Esq., in 1909. A letter in the College of Physicians files from Albert Haller Gross states that he has two portraits of his father, but "neither does him justice, and my sister and I will take very great pleasure in having one painted for the College of Physicians." PA 72

Dr. Gross is shown half-length, with body frontal and head turned three-quarters to the right. His right arm is slightly akimbo. His left elbow leans on an unidentified piece of furniture covered with red cloth, while his left hand holds a gold watch chain. The background is grayish-umber, darker at the top. Gross's frizzy, long, gray-brown hair stands out from his head in all directions. He has a high forehead, knitted, thick gray eyebrows, and gray side-whiskers. His deepset brown eyes, which look in the direction of the head turn, are accentuated by heavy creases at the corners and deep pockets underneath. There are deep diagonal creases beneath the high cheekbones. The round face has a wide jaw and round chin. The subject wears a white shirt with stand-up collar and gold stud, a wide black bow tie, a black vest and gold watch chain, and a black double-breasted coat with wide lapels. The surface of the painting shows varied facture—painterly in the hair, moderately active in the face and hands, and smoothly brushed in the costume and background. The head is solidly constructed to produce a convincing three-dimensional appearance. The costume is flatter, the style is linear throughout. Details of the face and costume are insistently outlined. The individualistic face has a forthright, almost imperious expression. The expansiveness of the body, which fills the entire width of the lower half of the canvas, adds to the commanding presence. The copyist, Dimino, has been fairly faithful to Waugh's portrait in the subject's face, position, and costume. Interestingly, he has enlarged the original, adding the portion below the shirt front. Unfortunately, the trivial gesture, sharp white shirt cuff, and the confusing bit of furniture detract from the awesome impression of the head.

Artist: Joseph Obermeier

Marble; 25 1/4 x 17 x 12; resting on a marble base 6 1/4 in. high; signed on beveled edge below the subject's right shoulder, "Jos Obermeier." Presented by Albert Haller Gross, Esq., son of Dr. Gross, in 1884; resembles plaster busts of Gross by Obermeier, painted bronze color, at the Philadelphia County Medical Society and Jefferson Medical College. ST 510

Dr. Gross is shown bust length, with body frontal and head turned slightly to the left. His thick, wavy hair surmounts a high forehead and connects with heavy, chin-length whiskers. The long eyebrows curve sharply downward. The deepset narrow eyes, with irises and pupils incised, gaze upwards. The strong, aquiline nose points down to the wide, full mouth. The rectangular-shaped face has hollow cheeks and a square jaw. Indications of age include deep pockets under the eyes and asymmetrical creases next to the eyes and on the cheeks. The structure of the neck and chest is well described, especially the Adam's apple and the muscles of the neck. The subject wears a toga with U-shaped folds fastened with a simple brooch over the left shoulder. The marble surface of the sculpture is smooth. The planes have been sensitively carved to produce a solid, anatomically accurate rendering of the head and torso and of the deep folds in the drapery. The strong features and erect bearing express confidence and authority. In keeping with Obermeier's neoclassical conception, emphasized by the costume and upward glance, the subject's face and features, though recognizable, have been regularized and idealized, as is shown by comparison with portraits of Gross by Dimino, Waugh, and Thomas Eakins.

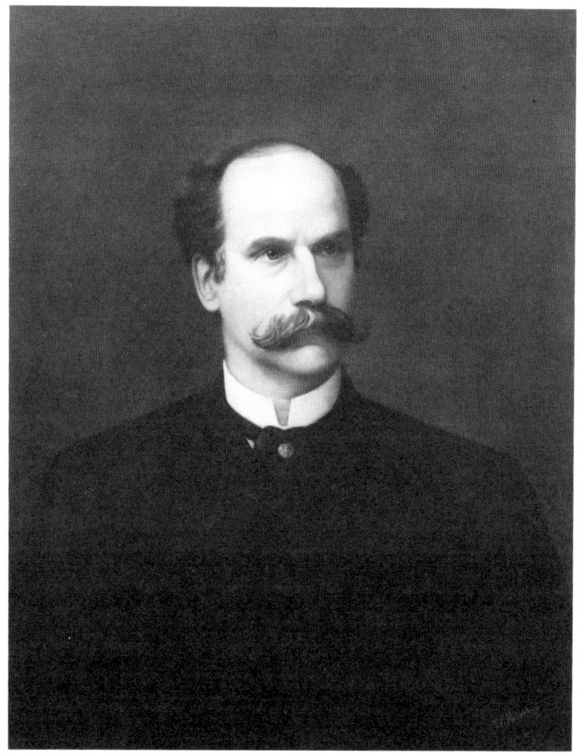

Samuel Weissel Gross PA 74

Samuel Weissel Gross (1837-1889)

Born in Cincinnati, the eldest son of Dr. Samuel David Gross (q.v.), Dr. Samuel W. Gross was graduated from Jefferson Medical College in 1857. For meritorious service as brigade surgeon during the Civil War, he was brevetted Lieutenant-Colonel. After the war he was lecturer on genito-urinary diseases at Jefferson Medical College and surgeon to the Howard, Philadelphia, and Jefferson Hospitals. On the retirement of his father from the chair of surgery at Jefferson, he was elected professor of principles of surgery and of clinical surgery. In addition to being a fellow of the College of Physicians of Philadelphia, Dr. Gross was a founder and vice-

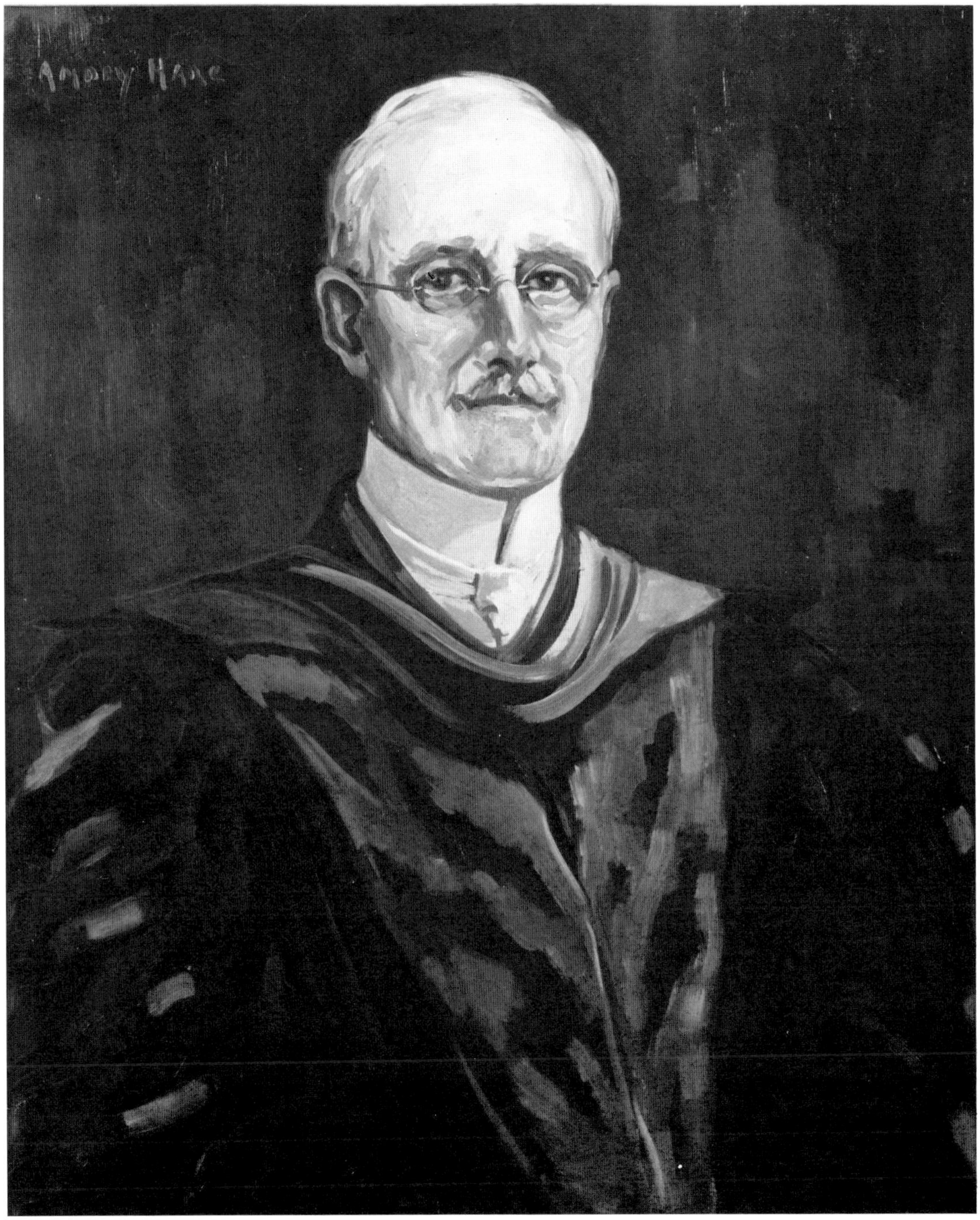

Hobart Amory Hare PA 23

president of the Academy of Surgery of Philadelphia, a founder of the American Genito-Urinary Association, and one of the original fellows of the American Surgical Association. He was one of the first to develop radical operations for cancer and one of the first surgeons in Philadelphia to employ antisepsis. His contributions to the medical literature include "Sarcoma of the Long Bones" (1879), *Tumors of the Mammary Gland* (1880), and *Practical Treatise on Impotence, Sterility and Disorders of the Male Sexual Organs* (1881). With his father he edited the *North American Medico-Chirurgical Review* and he aided his father in preparing various editions of the elder Gross's *System of Surgery.*

Artist: Mrs. Frances Van Horn Heberton (b. 1846)

Heberton studied at the Pennsylvania Academy of the Fine Arts, where she exhibited in 1891. She was a graduate of the School of Design for Women.

Oil on canvas; 26 1/2 x 21 1/2; signed lower right, "F.V. Heberton." Shown at the annual exhibition of the Pennsylvania Academy of Fine Arts in 1892. The painting resembles one of Gross by George W. Pettit, at Jefferson Medical College, done in 1890. Presented by Albert Haller Gross, Esq., and Mrs. S.W. Gross, 1890. PA 74

Dr. Gross is shown bust length, the body frontal, the head turned and tilted slightly to the right. The umber atmospheric background is darker on the left, lighter on the right. The high forehead has thick dark brown hair at the sides. The hazel eyes look straight ahead and slightly upward in the direction of the head turn. The nose has a pronounced bump at the bridge. The mouth is partly covered by a bushy, light brown moustache curled up at the ends. The subject wears a white shirt with stand-up collar, a black neckcloth with round gold pin, and a black, single-breasted coat with small lapels, buttoned high. The painted surface is very smooth, with no visible brush strokes except at the subject's sideburns and moustache, where individual thick hairs are differentiated. The well-constructed head appears solid and three-dimensional. In contrast, the flat costume conveys little sense of the underlying body mass. Although the subject's gaze is averted, his facial expression is alert. His body fills the entire lower width of the canvas; this gives an impression of commanding physical presence.

Hobart Amory Hare (1862-1931)

Dr. Hobart Amory Hare was born in Philadelphia. Included among his forbears who came to this country from England in 1773 were many distinguished ministers. He was educated at the University of Pennsylvania, where he received the M.D. degree in 1884. He then did physiological research in Leipzig, Berne, and London. After his return to Philadelphia he was appointed lecturer in physiology and, within a few years, clinical professor of diseases of children at the University of Pennsylvania. Between the years of these two appointments he won research awards from the Rhode Island Medical Society, the College of Physicians and Surgeons (New York), the Massachusetts General Hospital, the Royal Academy of Belgium, and Harvard University. He was the first non-English recipient of the Fothergillian gold medal of the Medical Society of London. This was awarded for his treatise, *Diseases of the Mediastinum.* Jefferson Medical College appointed him to the chair of therapeutics and materia medica in 1891, a post that he held until his death in 1931. He was secretary of the convention on the revision of the U.S. Pharmacopoeia (1890), a member of the Philadelphia Board of City Trusts (1912), recipient of an honorary LL.D. degree from the University of Pennsylvania (1921), and president of the College of Physicians (1925-28). He was a Naval Commander during World War I and served both in Washington and at various naval bases. In addition to teaching and research, he was founder and first editor of the *Medical Magazine* of the University of Pennsylvania and editor of *Medical News* and *Therapeutic Gazette.* He wrote *New and Altered Forms of Disease* (1886), *Epilepsy—Its Pathology and Treatment* (1889), *Fever—Its Pathology and Treatment* (1890), *Practical Therapeutics* (1890), *Practical Diagnosis* (1896), and *The Practice of Medicine* (1907).

Artist: Amory Hare (1885-1963)

Known professionally as Amory Hare, Mary Amory Hare (Mrs. James P. Hutchinson) was the daughter of Dr. Hobart Amory Hare. She was a painter of portraits, landscapes, and scenes of country life, especially hunting. She was even better known as an author. Her novels include *Deep Country* and *Gallant and Game.* Her books of verse, which won her the Browning Society's medal for poetry, include *Tossed Coins, Swept Hearth,* and *The Olympians.* She wrote two plays, *The Return of Hannibal* and *Private Enterprise,* as well as short stories published in *The Atlantic, Cosmopolitan,* and other magazines. She was a founder of the American National Theater and Academy (ANTA).

Oil on canvas; 29 1/2 x 24 1/2; signed upper left, "Amory Hare"; no date recorded. Presented by Mary Amory Hare in 1933. Resembles a portrait of Dr. Hare done in 1927 by William Thomson and held by Jefferson Medical College.
PA 23

Dr. Hare is shown bust length, with head and body turned slightly to the right. The background has geometric areas of warm umber, rust, and brown tones. The subject has gray hair. His grayish-blue eyes look out through metal-rimmed spectacles directly toward the viewer. He has a straight nose, a neat gray moustache, and a square jaw. He wears a white shirt with stand-up collar, a white neckcloth, and a black academic robe with green stripes on the sleeves, a triangular green panel at the front, and a thick curving red stripe on the mantle. The portrait has an all-over painterly surface consisting of loosely brushed, fluid strokes. The construction of the head is moderately three-dimensional; there is little sense of body underneath the expansive costume. The freedom of the paint style contributes to the immediacy of the subject's straightforward glance and pleasant expression. The cheerful red and green of the costume is reflected in the highlights and shadows of the face.

Robert Hare (1781-1858)

Dr. Robert Hare was born in Philadelphia, the son of an English immigrant. After working for a time at his father's brewery, where he invented a barrel capable of resisting the pressure of carbonic acid gas, he studied chemistry at the University of Pennsylvania. In 1818, after a few months as teacher at the College of William and Mary, he was appointed professor of chemistry at the University of Pennsylvania, a post he held for 30 years. As a teacher he excelled in the demonstration of principles, frequently with apparatus of his own invention. As early as 1801 he had devised an oxy-hydrogen blow-pipe, source of the highest degree of heat then known. He invented the calorimeter, a galvanic apparatus, and the deflagrator, a machine for generation of high electrical current. He introduced the use of the

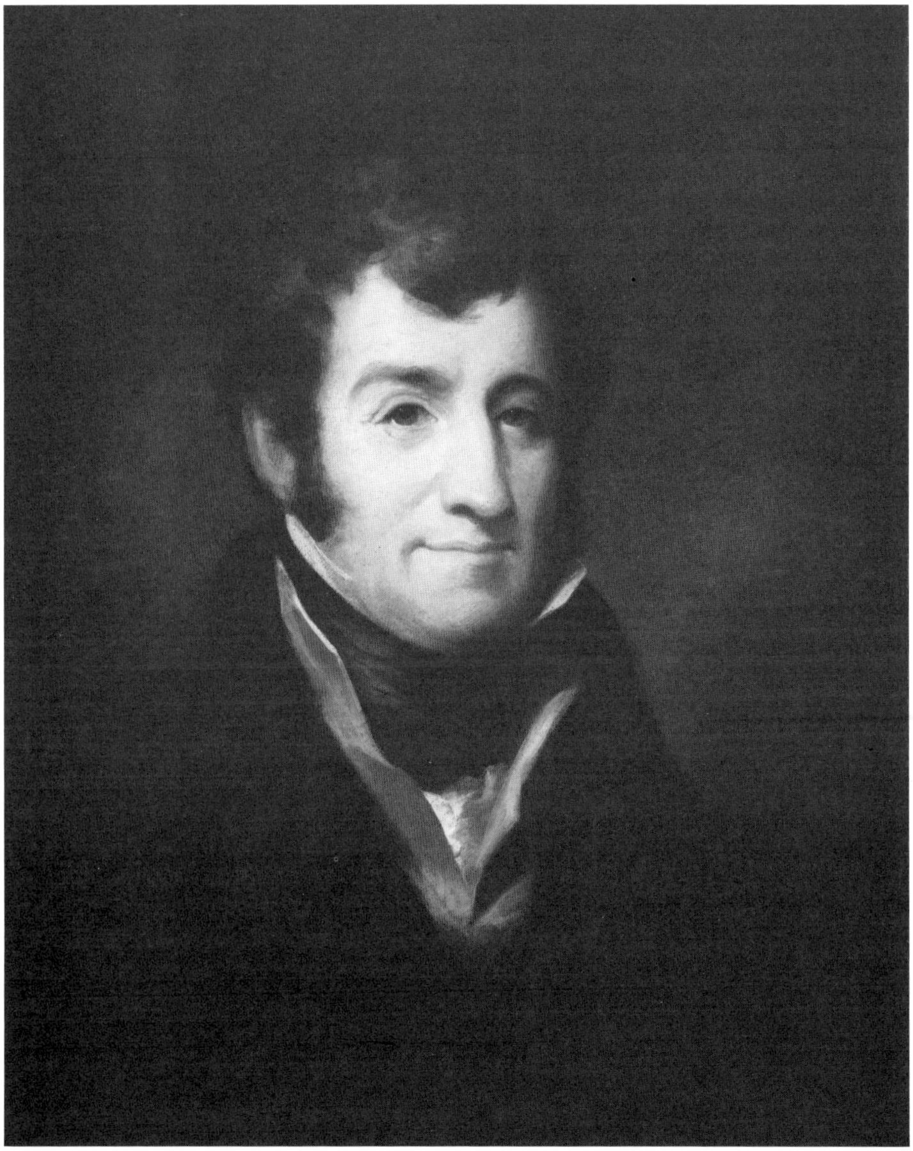

Robert Hare *PA 82*

mercury cathode in the electrolysis of aqueous solutions of metallic salts. He built an electric furnace in which he prepared phosphorus, calcium metal, calcium carbide, and artificial graphite from crude charcoal. When he retired from teaching, he gave his collection of apparatus to the Smithsonian Institution. In 1848 he was elected an honorary member of that organization. He received the honorary M.D. degree from Harvard and Yale Universities and received the Rumford medal of the American Academy of Arts and Sciences. He was a member of the American Philosophical Society. In addition to editing books on chemistry, he published his university lectures under the title, *A Compendium of the Course of Chemical Instruction* (1827). He wrote moral essays under a *nom de plume* for the *Portfolio* and lectured and wrote in support of spiritualism.

Artist: John Neagle (1796–1865)

For biography, see page 34.

Oil on canvas; 25 1/4 x 20 1/2; signed and dated lower left, "J.N. 1830." Presented by Charles Hare Hutchinson in 1892. Three letters in the files of the College trace the provenance of this portrait. The first, dated February 8, 1892, is from Garrett C. Neagle, the artist's son, to Charles Hare Hutchinson and reads, "The accompanying portrait which I take pleasure in sending to you and Miss Hutchinson to look at is an original painting from life, of Prof. Robert Hare, your great-uncle, I learn from my cousin Mr. L. Taylor Dickson. It was painted by my father John Neagle in 1830. See his initials in the lower left hand corner of the picture—'J.N. 1830.' This painting is a very fine example of my father's work— The flesh tints being exceptionally rich. . . . It is my intention to sell this portrait, my Dear Sir, and concluded that the descendants of Prof. Hare should first be notified. . . . The portrait will have a new gilt frame. Price for picture and frame—$150." The second letter, dated February 26, 1892, is from Charles Hare Hutchinson to Dr. S. Weir Mitchell, president of the College, and states that Dr. Hare's portrait will be delivered to the College by Garrett Neagle and should be presented in the name of Charles Hare Hutchinson, while the accompanying letter should be "placed on file as evidence of the authenticity of the *picture." The third letter, dated March 4, 1892, is from Garrett Neagle to Dr. Mitchell, the "accompanying letter" stating that the portrait was painted from life by Neagle in 1830, and that it is being presented to the College by its recent owner, Charles Hare Hutchinson.* *PA 82*

Dr. Hare is shown bust length, with body frontal and head turned slightly to the right. The grayish-brown atmospheric background is lighter around the face and darker above and below. His curly black hair is brushed toward his face and continues into long side-whiskers. The brown eyes look out of the corners toward the spectator. The tip of the long nose points down to a mouth whose thin lips give the hint of a smile. The oval face has a round chin. The subject wears a white shirt with stand-up collar, a wide black neckcloth, a white shirt with frill, an ivory-colored waistcoat with high, stand-up collar, and a dark brown coat, also with a high collar. The portrait has a painterly surface with visible brush strokes. The head has been constructed solidly with three-dimensional volumes; the flat costume does not indicate underlying bodily forms. The romantic portrayal gives soft edges to forms, particularly the curly hair, the facial features, and the shoulder line that melts into the background. The subject's head is large and his shoulders fill the width of the canvas. His physical presence not only commands the space of the canvas, but is so suffused with energy that it seems to penetrate the surface and to engage the viewer directly.

George Cuvier Harlan (1835-1909)

Son of the physician and naturalist, Dr. Richard Harlan, and named after his friend, the famous French naturalist Cuvier (q.v.), George Cuvier Harlan was born in Philadelphia. After receiving the B.A. and M.A. degrees from Delaware College, he was awarded the M.D. degree from the University of Pennsylvania in 1858. His professional affiliations were with Wills Eye Hospital, where he was surgeon from 1861 to 1901 and then consulting surgeon; St. Mary and Children's Hospitals, where he was attending surgeon; Pennsylvania Institution for Instruction of the Blind; eye and ear department of Pennsylvania Hospital; the Pennsylvania Institution for the Deaf and Dumb, where he was ophthalmologist; and the Polyclinic and School for Graduates in Medicine, where he occupied the first chair of ophthalmology. He was a member of numerous medical societies, including the College of Physicians, where he was an original member of the section on ophthalmology and chairman of the library committee. He was also president of the American Ophthalmological Society (1893) and chairman of the section on ophthalmology at the Universal Exposition in St. Louis (1904). His contributions to the medical literature include a book, *Eyesight and How to Care for It*, and the articles, "Diseases of the Eyelids" and "Operations Performed upon the Eyelids," in Norris and Oliver's *System of Diseases of the Eye*, as well as numerous articles in *Transactions* of the American Ophthalmological Society. He edited the journal *Ophthalmology*. During the Civil War he was assigned to the gunboat *Union* as an acting assistant surgeon. Then, desiring more active service, he was transferred to the Eleventh Regiment of the Pennsylvania Cavalry Volunteers as major and surgeon, and he attended wounded soldiers on the battlefield.

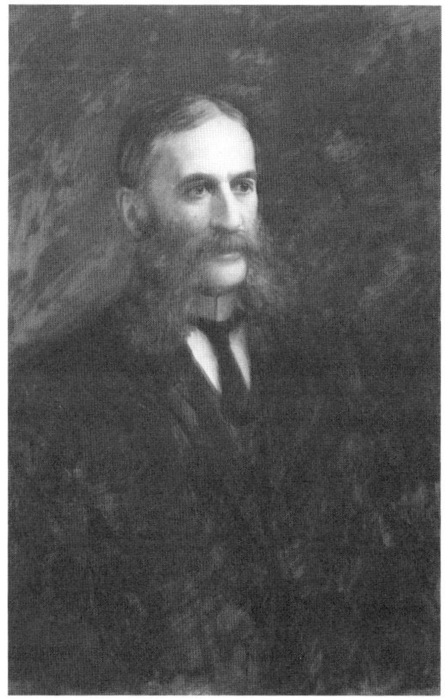

George Cuvier Harlan *PA 57*

Artist: William Wallace Gilchrist, Jr. (1879-1926)

Born in Philadelphia, Gilchrist studied at the Pennsylvania Academy of the Fine Arts, where he later became a member of its fellowship board of directors. He also studied in Munich, Paris, and London. He was an active member of the Philadelphia Art Club, the Philadelphia Water Color Club, and the Salmagundi Club. His awards include third prize at the National Academy of Design (1908), gold medal at the Washington Society of Artists (1914), gold medal at the Philadelphia Art Club, and silver medal at the Sesquicentennial Exposition in Philadelphia (1926). He maintained studios in Philadelphia, New York, and Boston, and he resided in Brunswick, Maine, at the time of his death.

Oil on canvas; 35 1/4 x 25 1/4; signed and dated on back of canvas, "W W Gilchrist Jr 1911/from photograph." Presented by Mrs. Henry Post Mitchell in 1911. Resembles portrait of Harlan by Adolphe Borie, 1910, Pennsylvania Hospital. *PA 57*

Harlan is shown half-length, with head and body turned to the right. The atmospheric background is gray. His grayish-brown hair joins side-whiskers that grow into an enormous muttonchop beard and moustache. His large blue eyes look in the direction of the head turn. He has an

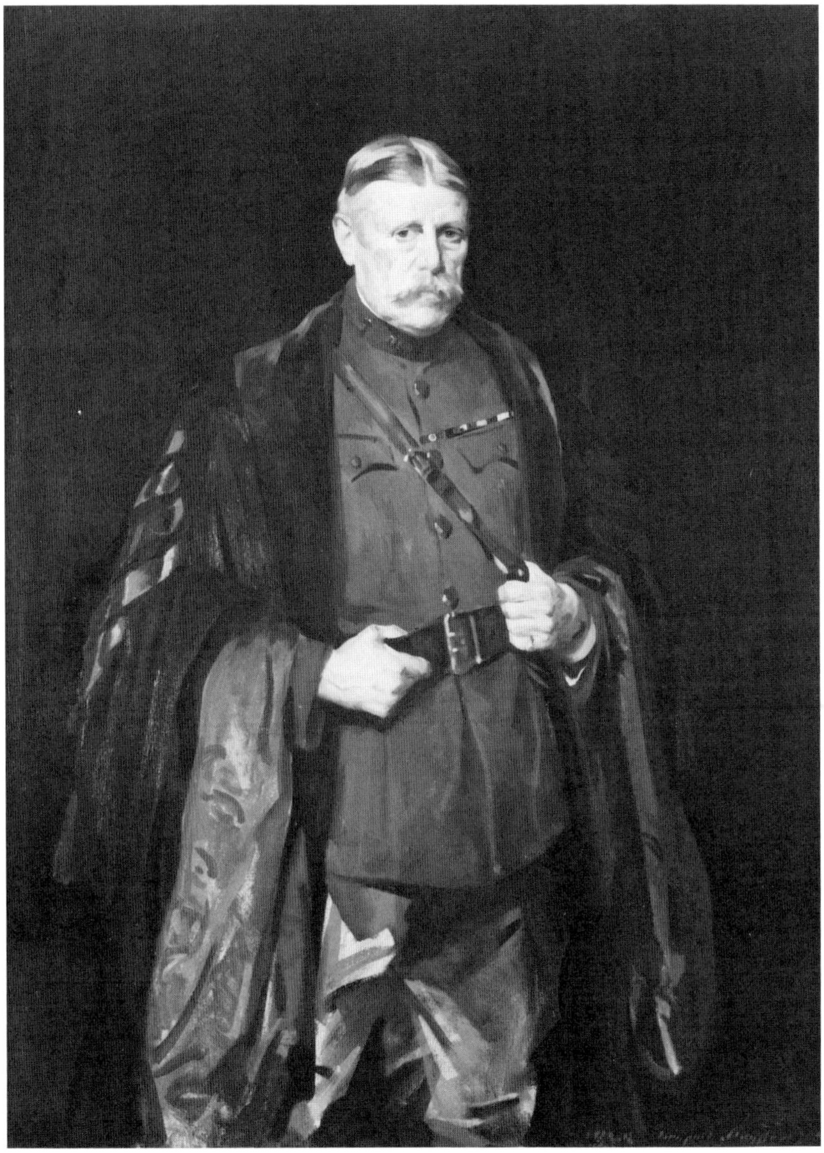

Richard Hickman Harte *PA 1*

oval face, a wide nose, and thin lips. He wears a white shirt with stand-up collar, and a black necktie, vest, and coat. Although the portrait is marred by varnish bloom and paint loss in the costume and background, the surface has a painterly quality, especially in the visible brush strokes that depict the beard. The face has been constructed very solidly with three-dimensional anatomical accuracy. The facial expression is neutral and bland, rather lacking in vitality.

Richard Hickman Harte (1855-1925)

Descendant of an Irish family, Harte was born in Little Rock, Illinois. His father, the owner and captain of a Mississippi River steamboat, died prematurely, leaving the family without financial resources. Through the aid of friends, Richard Harte was able to come to Philadelphia. He received the M.D. degree from the University of Pennsylvania in 1878. After studying in Europe for two years, he returned to Philadelphia. He was attending surgeon and then surgeon to the Pennsylvania Hospital; assistant to Dr. D. Hayes Agnew (q.v.) and Dr. John Ashhurst (q.v.); demonstrator of osteology and later associate professor of surgery at the University of Pennsylvania; surgeon to the Episcopal and Orthopaedic Hospitals; and consulting surgeon to St. Mary, St. Timothy's, Bryn Mawr, and Abington Hospitals. He contributed the section on surgery to Harrison Allen's (q.v.) *Handbook of Local Treatment*, and edited the *University Medical Magazine*. He served his country with great distinction during World War I. Before the United States entered the war he was surgeon at the American Ambulance Hospital at Neuilly, France. In 1917, in cooperation with the doctors, nurses, and managers of the Pennsylvania Hospital, he developed a military unit, designated as Pennsylvania Base Hospital No. 10, of which he became the commanding Officer in Le Tréport, France. Despite his age of 62 years, he also spent several weeks as head of an emergency surgery team on the Belgian front. In recognition of his wartime service, he was awarded the British Order of St. Michael and St. George, the Belgian Order of Leopold, and the American Distinguished Service Medal. He was elected a fellow of the Royal College of Surgeons of Ireland. He served as president of the College of Physicians (1916–18), the Philadelphia Academy of Surgery, and the American Surgical Association.

Artist: Leopold Gould Seyffert (1888–1956)

Seyffert was born in Missouri and studied at the Pennsylvania Academy of the Fine Arts from 1907 to 1912. He won two Cresson traveling scholarships for study in France and Spain. At the Academy he won the Fellowship prize (1913), the Beck gold medal (1918), the Temple gold medal (1921), the Stotesbury prize (1926), and the Lippincott prize (1929). He was made an associate in 1916 and an academician in 1925 at the National Academy of Design, where he won the Altman gold medal (1915), the first Hallgarten prize (1918), and the Proctor prize (1921). He won the Palmer, Logan, and Hearst prizes (1923–24) at the Art Institute of Chicago, a silver medal at the Panama-Pacific Exposition in San Francisco (1915), a gold medal at the Sesquicentennial Exposition in Philadelphia (1926), and the popular prize at the Carnegie International of 1930. His work can be found at the Metropolitan Museum of Art, Brooklyn Museum, Art Institute of Chicago, Corcoran Gallery, Carnegie Institute, Los Angeles County Museum, Detroit Art Institute, Pennsylvania Academy of the Fine Arts, and in many private and institutional collections.

Oil on canvas; 59 1/4 x 44 1/4; signed and dated, lower right, "19—[date indecipherable] Leopold Seyffert." Presented by members of the Harte family in 1920. Presumably painted in 1919 or 1920 after Dr. Harte's return from wartime duty in France in April, 1919; copied by Mr. Kenneth A. Smith-Brunet in 1968 for Pennsylvania Hospital on commission from Dr. Harte's children. *PA 1*

Dr. Harte is shown two-thirds length, the body turned to the right, the head to the right and tilted slightly down. He is depicted standing with legs spread apart. His hands hold onto a belt and diagonal strap across his chest. The background is dark blue-black and flat with no sense of atmospheric space. The subject has light grayish-brown hair and neat moustache. His blue eyes look straight out toward the viewer and slightly downward. The nose is straight, the jaw square. His extraordinary costume consists of both a United States Army colonel's uniform (khaki jodphurs and a khaki coat with high, round collar, brass buttons, wide brown belt and diagonal strap called a Sam Browne belt, and military decoration in red, blue, green, and yellow stripes) and also the presidential robe of the College of Physicians of Philadelphia (a black academic gown with green front panels and green stripes and lining of the voluminous sleeves). The paint style is fluid, with quickly brushed, broad strokes throughout. Although the head and hands are solidly constructed, there is little sense of bodily mass under the flowing drapery. The dramatic dark background also tends to flatten out the figure, as do the bare areas of canvas showing at the bottom. The bravado style of painting is in accord with the subject's swaggering stance and pugnacious facial expression.

Joseph Hartshorne (1779–1850)

Descended from English Quakers who came to America in 1669 and settled in what is now Sandy Hook, New Jersey, Dr. Hartshorne was born in Alexandria, Virginia. After working for a short time in his father's flour mill and warehouse, he started to read medicine and then entered the office of Dr. James Craik, physician and friend of George Washington. In 1801 he became resident apprentice and apothecary at the Pennsylvania Hospital. In 1805 he received the M.D. degree from the University of Pennsylvania. In the same year he published the first American edition of Alexis Boyer's *Treatise on Diseases of the Bones,* to which he added original notes and plates. In 1815, after two long voyages to India and a modest private practice supplemented by a brief partnership in an apothecary shop, he became surgeon to the Pennsylvania Hospital. He resigned this post in 1821, because a greatly enlarged practice now made increasing demands and his work came to include many consultations from other physicians, who admired his skill and his exactitude. He was elected a member of the Philadelphia Medical Society (1805), the American Philosophical Society (1815), and the College of Physicians of Philadelphia (1824). He served the College as treasurer and member of the committee to revise the pharmacopoeia.

Artist: George W. Pettit (1839–1910)

A native of England, Pettit resided in Philadelphia, where he exhibited portraits and figure studies at the Pennsylvania Academy of the Fine Arts intermittently between 1862 and 1887. He was made an associate of the Academy in 1863 and an academician in 1869. He also exhibited with the Art Club of Philadelphia in 1897 and 1899 and at the National Academy of Design in 1871.

Oil on canvas, mounted on wood; 35 1/2 x 28 1/4; signed and dated at lower right, "G.W. Pettit 1883." Presented by Edward Hartshorne in 1883. Shown in the College of Physicians Centennial Celebration Loan Collection of Portraits, *1887, with the annotation "G.W. Pettit (copy from photograph)." The source can now be identified as a daguerrotype by D.C. Collins. This was engraved by T.B. Welch in 1901.* *PA 76*

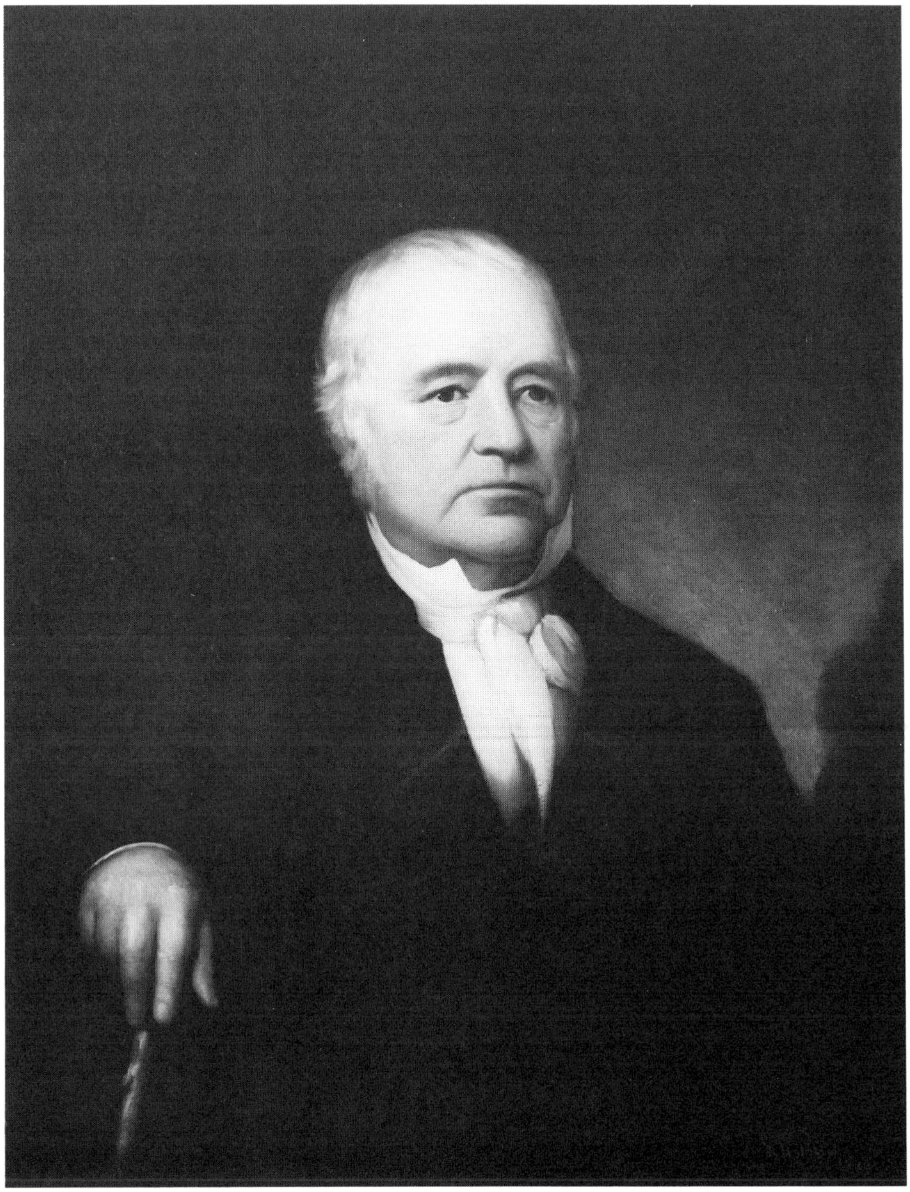

Joseph Hartshorne *PA 76*

Dr. Hartshorne is shown half-length, the body frontal, the head turned slightly to the right. His right arm is bent. His right hand rests on the handle of a bamboo cane; he had been lamed by smallpox in childhood. The dark brown atmospheric background becomes a lighter tan to the right of the head. The silvery-white hair is brushed onto the forehead and curled slightly over the ears. The blue eyes look straight ahead in the direction of the head turn. The face is round, the nose straight. The mouth is wide. The lips are thin and the cheeks and chin are rounded. The complexion is fair and the cheeks are pink. Prominent age lines are found in the lower lids and next to the nose and mouth. The subject wears a white shirt with stand-up collar, a white neckcloth tied in a bow, a black buttoned waistcoat with small standup collar, and a black opened coat with wide lapels. The portrait has been smoothly painted without visible brush strokes. The head and hand have been constructed solidly in three dimensions. Although the torso fills the width of the canvas, there is little sense of bodily mass underneath the costume. The facial expression is serious and dignified as the subject gazes thoughtfully into the distance.

William Harvey (1578-1657)

The great William Harvey, eldest son of a yeoman farmer and landowner, was born in Folkestone, Kent. He graduated from Caius College, Cambridge, in 1597 with a B.A. degree in arts and medicine. He completed his studies at the University of Padua in 1602 with an M.D. degree. His most outstanding teacher there was the anatomist, Girolamo Fabrici (Fabricius), discoverer of the valves in the veins. After his return to England Harvey was elected a fellow of the Royal College of Physicians in 1607 and served as Lumleian lecturer in surgery there from 1615 to 1656. Late in his life he endowed a museum and library at the College. In 1609 he was appointed physician to St. Bartholomew's Hospital, an office he held until 1643. He was named physician extraordinary to King James I and became senior physician ordinary to Charles I. He attended the King and the Earl of Arundel both in England

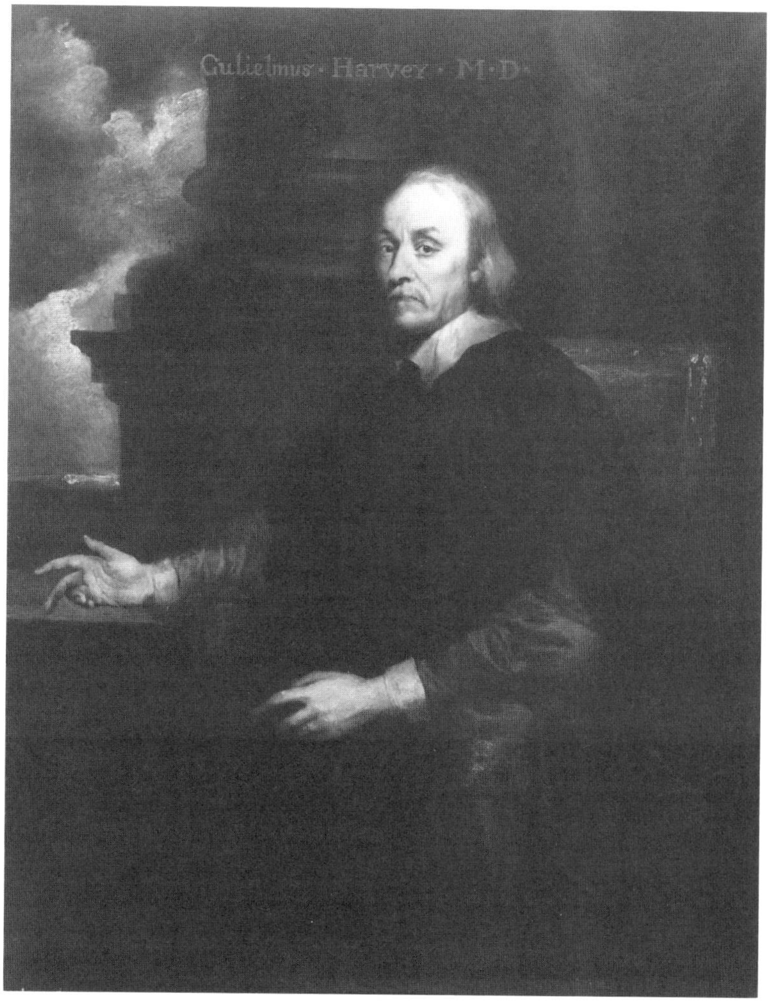

William Harvey *PA 36*

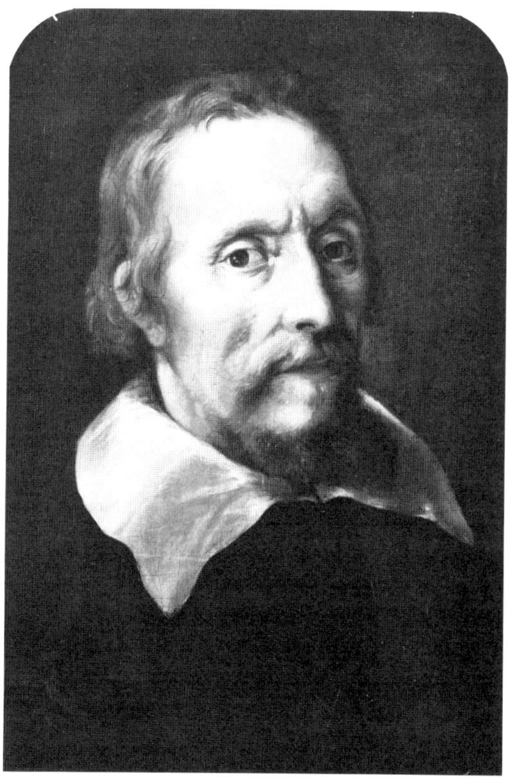

William Harvey *PA 61*

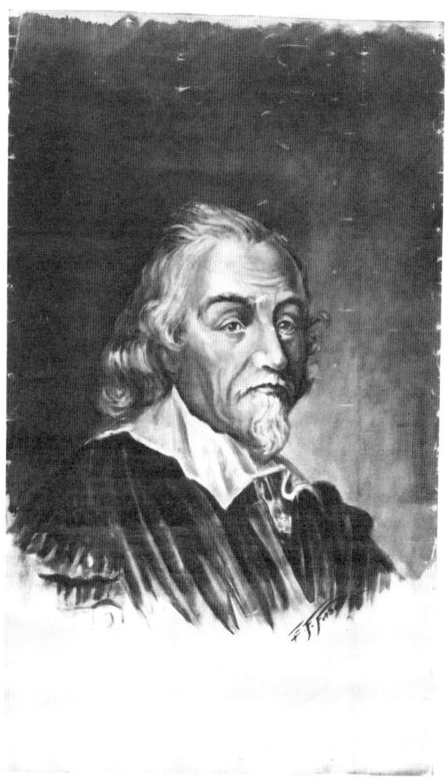

William Harvey *PA 96*

and on foreign trips and campaigns. The King consulted him on all issues in which medicine had even a remote bearing, and he encouraged and supported his research. From extant notes and published statements it is conjectured that Harvey contemplated a vast research program leading to the publication on such diverse subjects as motion of the heart, respiration, functions of the brain and spleen, animal locomotion and generation, and comparative and pathological anatomy. Although only his works on the heart and generation were published, his discovery of the circulation of the blood, announced in 1628 in *Exercitatio anatomica de motu cordis et sanguinis in animalibus,* was enough to ensure enduring fame. By direct experimental evidence and in contradiction to many of the esteemed ideas of Aristotle and Galen (q.v.), Harvey proved that the contraction of the heart coincides with the pulse, that the heart is the dynamic starting point of the blood, and that the blood is constantly recirculated. Harvey's *Exercitationes de generatione animalium,* published in 1651, is one of the foundations of modern embryology.

Artist: Anna Lea Merritt (Mrs. Henry Merritt) (1844–1930)

Anna Lea was born in Philadelphia, the eldest of six daughters of a prominent family whose forbears emigrated in the seventeenth century. Although her early classical education excluded art training, she went to exhibitions, studied reproductions, and read books on art theory. Before her family moved to Europe temporarily in 1865, she enrolled in a course in anatomy at the Woman's Medical College in Philadelphia. Since women were refused admittance in most European art academies, she studied privately with Stefano Ussi in Florence, Heinrich Hoffman in Dresden, and then with Henry Merritt in London. Henry Merritt was a conservator and art critic and was her teacher for seven years before they married in 1877. Although he died tragically just three months after their marriage, she was devoted to his memory and learned the art of etching to illustrate her late husband's writings, whose publication she oversaw. She became widely known as an etcher of portraits after painted or photographic originals. Although she was a consistent exhibitor and prize winner both in Europe and America, she was best known in England, where she associated with the English and American pre-Raphaelite painters, such as Whistler, Edward Burne-Jones, Sir Frederick Leighton, William Holman Hunt, Edward Austin Abbey, and others. In America she exhibited her work—portraits, allegorical and religious scenes, landscapes, and still lifes—at the Pennsylvania Academy of the Fine Arts (which purchased *Piping Shepherd* in 1895), the Avery Galleries in New York, and the National Academy of Design. She won a medal at the Centennial Exposition in Philadelphia for *The Patrician Mother* and *Saint Geneviève* (1876), two medals and a diploma at the Columbian Exposition in Chicago (1893), and a medal at the Pan-American Exposition in Buffalo (1901). In Europe she won honorable mention for *Camilla* at the Paris International Exposition of 1889. In London she exhibited frequently at the Royal Academy (between 1870 and 1906) and at the Royal Society of British Artists. She also showed her work in Liverpool and Manchester. Her best known work, *Love Locked Out,* was purchased by the Chantry Fund of the British National Collection for the Tate Gallery and was widely circulated through chromolithographic reproduction (she was the first woman so honored by the Fund). Her mural paintings include panels depicting women's occupations for the Women's Building at the Columbian Exposition in Chicago and religious subjects for St. Martin's Church, Chilworth, Surrey. She was an active member of the Royal Society of Painters and Etchers and wrote and illustrated two garden books. Portraiture was her primary source of income, and prominent sitters included Oliver Wendell Holmes, James Russell Lowell, Horace Furness, and Ellen Terry. For much of the above biographical information the author is indebted to Galina Gorokhoff, whose book, *Love Locked Out: The Memoirs of Anna Lea Merritt with a Checklist of Her Works,* was published in 1982 by the Museum of Fine Arts, Boston.

Oil on canvas; 52 1/2 x 41 1/2; not signed or dated. Presented as a bequest of Dr. S. Weir Mitchell in 1914. Shown in the College of Physicians' Centennial Celebration Loan Collection of Portraits, *1887. Label on back of portrait reads "Portrait of Wm. Harvey, M.D./copy by Anna Lea Merritt/ owned by Dr. S. Weir Mitchell/[stamped] May 20, 1902." Copied after portrait of Harvey at Royal College of Physicians, London. According to Geoffrey Keynes, (*The Portraiture of William Harvey, *London, 1949), the traditional attribution to Cornelius Janssen, also called Janson van Keulin, is "quite conjectural." Among other copies of the original portrait, Keynes mentions one "made for Dr. Weir Mitchell by Mrs. Merritt." In her* Memoirs, *the artist dates the work 1878 and says "For Dr. Weir Mitchell I copied at the College of Surgeons the portraits of Hunter and of Harvey by the great Sir Joshua Reynolds. These copies were to me a fine lesson and are now honored by a place in the College of Physicians of Philadelphia." Perhaps the portrait was attributed to Reynolds at the time of Merritt's copy.* *PA 36*

Harvey is shown three-quarter length, his body and head turned three-quarters to the left. He is seated in a red upholstered, square-backed armchair. His left arm rests on the chair arm and his left hand holds a black, round velvet hat between two fingers. His right arm also rests on the chair arm, and his awkwardly formed right hand is placed just above a stone parapet, in front of a column plinth placed in the middle ground. Mrs. Merritt has faithfully copied the awkward, open-handed gesture which in the original had been damaged and then repainted. It is conjectured that the hand might at one time have held a scroll. In addition to the stone column, the background contains sky and clouds on the upper left and red velvet drapery on the upper right. Harvey is depicted as having a high forehead and gray shoulder-length hair. Beneath knitted brows his brown eyes look out of the corners and directly toward the viewer. The face is angular with a long nose, tight mouth, narrow jaw, gray moustache, and a short beard. He wears a black gown which flows over the chair arm, a red velvet doublet, and a white shirt with pointed collar. Above his head is an inscription, "Gulielmus · Harvey · M.D." Mrs. Merritt did not attempt to reproduce the now almost indistinguishable coat of arms painted on the base of the column. Although this portrait has had extensive restoration, it maintains a painterly surface with visible brush strokes, especially in the head, hands, and collar. The anatomical structure of the head is depicted solidly; the body appears flat under the costume. The subject has a serious but lively and alert expression. His eyes appear to have moved just at this moment to regard the spectator.

Artist: Unknown

Oil on canvas; 21 x 14 1/2; not signed or dated. Presented by Mrs. Helen C. Jenks (Mrs. William F. Jenks), 1891. In The Portraiture of William Harvey *(London, 1949), Geoffrey Keynes includes this painting in a list of portraits formerly considered depictions of Harvey, but which he feels represent other persons. He adds, "an eighteenth century pastel drawing, possibly derived from this portrait, is in the Halford Collection at Wistow. Regarded by Dr. Weir Mitchell as 'undoubtedly of Harvey in middle life,' but the identification seems to me unacceptable." Elsewhere Keynes says, "This has a certain uncomfortable resemblance to Harvey, but not enough to be quite convincing."* *PA 61*

The subject is shown bust length, body to the right, head to the right and tilted. The medium-toned brown background is darker on the left. The subject has collar-length brown hair, round blue eyes which gaze out of their corners toward the observer, a long nose with a bump at the bridge, and a sparse, light brown moustache and wispy beard. His rectangular face has sunken cheeks and a square jaw. He wears a dark brown gown over a black doublet and a white shirt with a large pointed collar. The surface of the portrait is painterly, especially the highlights in head and collar. The well-constructed head is convincingly three-dimensional and solid. Lines in the forehead, under the eyes, and next to the nose give the subject a mature appearance and an expression of deep concentration. The gaze seems to stop short of the viewer.

Artist: Erwin Frank Faber (1866–1939)

For biography, see page 5.

Oil sketch on canvas; actual size, 40 1/4 x 24; signed below figure on right, "E.F. Faber"; dated 1878. Written in lower right corner in artist's hand, "Presented to the Coll of Physicians by the/artist on the occasion/of the Harvey/Tercentenary." Closely resembles the well-known engraving of Harvey by J. Houbraken, published in 1739, after the portrait by William Van Bemmel, now in the Hunterian Collection, University of Glasgow. *PA 96*

Harvey is shown bust length, body and head turned to the right. The background of this oil sketch is a thin wash of brown tones, darker on the left, lighter on the right; the bottom of the canvas has been left blank for 7 1/2 inches below the figure. Harvey is depicted as having a high forehead; wavy, gray, collar-length hair; brown eyes which look out in the direction of the head turn; high cheekbones and a narrow jaw; and a gray moustache and a short, narrow beard. He wears a white collar and dark brown robe. Although this is a rapidly done sketch with quickly executed brush strokes, the head is well constructed and seems quite three-dimensional. The paint is a thin wash in brown, tan, and gray tones, with the canvas showing through. The facial expression is one of dignity and serious purpose.

Isaac Hays (1796–1879)

Hays was born in Philadelphia, the son of a wealthy merchant. After receiving the A.B. degree from the University of Pennsylvania in 1816, he spent an unsatisfying year in business. He then began to study medicine under Dr. Nathaniel Chapman (q.v.); he earned the M.D. degree from the University in 1820. Specializing in surgery of the eye, he joined the staffs of the Wills Eye Hospital and Pennsylvania Infirmary for Eye Diseases. He recorded the first case of astigmatism in this country. Dr. Hays was an editor for fifty years. In addition to editing and translating books on medical and scientific subjects, he was the mainstay of a noted monthly journal. He

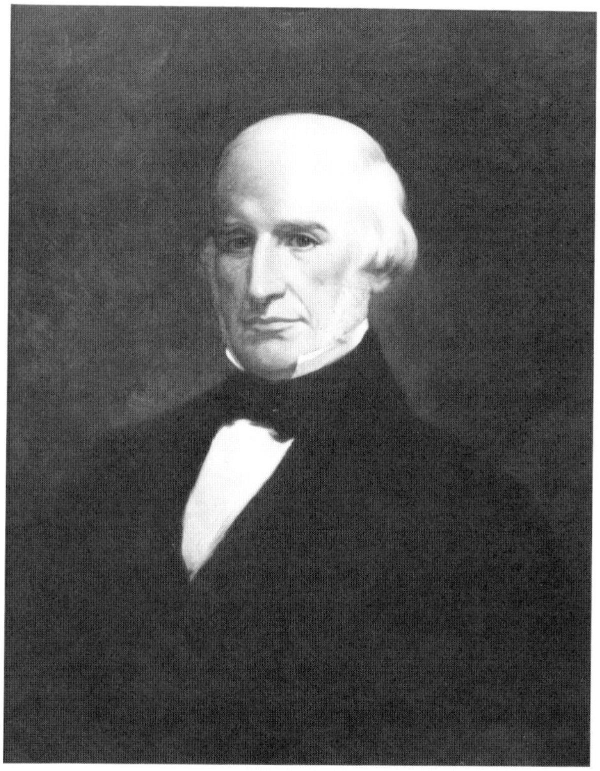

Isaac Hays *PA 64*

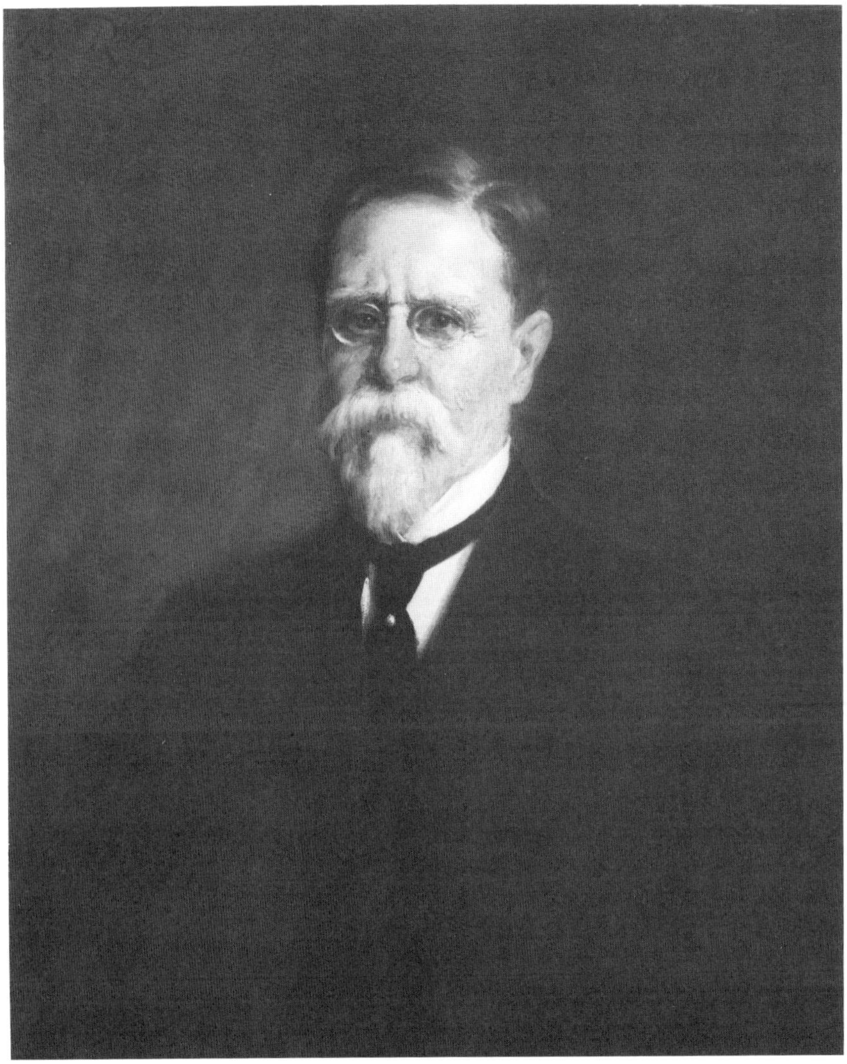

Frederick Porteous Henry *PA 51*

joined the editorial staff of the *Philadelphia Journal of Medical and Physical Sciences* in 1826 and in the next year became its sole editor. By changing its title to the *American Journal of Medical Sciences*, he was able to elicit contributions from the leading medical writers in the whole country. In 1869 he was joined by a co-editor, his son, Dr. Isaac Minis Hays. The original *Journal* gave rise to the weekly *Medical News* in 1843 and the monthly *Abstracts of Medical Science* in 1874. Dr. Hays was the first president of the Ophthalmological Society of Philadelphia and an honorary member of the American Ophthalmological Society. He was president of the Academy of Natural Sciences of Philadelphia from 1865 to 1869, a member of council of the American Philosophical Society, and a fellow of the College of Physicians.

Artist: Attributed to Ida Waugh (d. 1919)

For biography, see page 45.

Oil on canvas; 26 1/4 x 21 1/4; not signed or dated. Resembles a painting of Hays owned by the Academy of Natural Sciences and included in the College of Physicians' Centennial Celebration Loan Collection of Portraits in 1887, in which the designation is "copy, by Waugh," presumably S.B. Waugh. The Proceedings *of the Academy, vol. 32, 1880, contains a resolution thanking Mrs. Isaac Hays "for Waugh's excellent portrait of the late President, Isaac Hays." The College of Physicians' portrait is attributed to Ida Waugh, or "Miss Waugh" in most inventories, but there is no documentary evidence to substantiate this. Presented by Miss Henrietta M. Hays, daughter of Dr. Hays in 1912.* *PA 64*

Hays is shown bust length, body turned to the left, head turned to the left and tilted slightly downward. The scumbled, medium-toned brown background is darker on the right. The subject has ear-length white hair parted low and brushed across his forehead and frizzy white side-whiskers. Under straight brown eyebrows his hazel eyes look out of their corners toward the spectator. His long nose has a bump at the bridge, and its tip points down to the wide, full mouth. He wears a white shirt with stand-up collar, a wide, black bow tie, and a black vest and coat. The surface of the portrait is smoothly brushed. The head is moderately well constructed in three-dimensional volumes. The mass of the body is not indicated under the flat costume, whose shoulder line melts into the background. The neutral expression lacks vitality, probably because the portrait was not done from life.

Frederick Porteous Henry (1844-1919)

Henry's family home was in Mobile, Alabama, but he was born on his grandparents' farm in Middlesex County, New Jersey. After attending schools in Alabama, New Jersey, Dresden, and Tours and spending one-and-a-half years at Princeton University, Henry received the M.D. degree in 1868 from the College of Physicians and Surgeons in New York. He settled in Philadelphia and held staff positions at Episcopal, Philadelphia, and Jefferson Hospitals. He was professor of pathology and later of clinical medicine at the Philadelphia Polyclinic. At the Woman's Medical College of Pennsylvania he was professor of principles and practice of medicine from 1891 to 1917. He was one of the original 100 members of the Association of American Physicians. He was president of the Philadelphia County Medical Society and of the Pathological Society of Philadelphia. He was a corresponding member of the Royal Academy of Medicine in Rome and a fellow of the College of Physicians of Philadelphia, where he was honorary librarian for 29 years. He edited the seventh edition of Flint's *Practice of Medicine,* the *Standard History of Medicine in Philadelphia,* and the *Founders' Week Memorial Volume.* He was author of numerous articles, particularly on his pioneering work in blood studies, and on Addison's disease and Raynaud's disease. He was a winner of the Cartwright prize for his essay, "Observations with the Haemocytometer upon the Globular Composition of the Blood and Milk." He was awarded an honorary M.D. degree from Princeton University in 1891.

Artist: Lazar Raditz (1887-1958)

Born in Dvinsk, Russia, Raditz came to the United States in 1903. After working as assistant to a sign painter, he attended evening classes at the Graphic Sketch club, a free school for poor but talented art students. He also studied at the Pennsylvania Academy of the Fine Arts from 1903 to 1909 under Thomas Anshutz, Cecilia Beaux, Hugh Breckenridge, and William Merritt Chase. At the Academy he won Toppan prizes (1906, 1909) and Cresson traveling scholarships (1907, 1908). He studied at the Boston Museum School of Art (1909-10) under William Tarbell. He later returned to Philadelphia and taught at the Graphic Sketch Club for many years. A facile portrait painter, he captured likenesses that were pleasing to the public, and at the height of his career he was in great demand by Philadelphians prominent in government, the professions, and business. This is attested to by the number of public institutions in which his work is represented: the Pennsylvania Academy of the Fine Arts, the American Philosophical Society, the Academy of Natural Sciences, Dropsie College, the University of Pennsylvania, Jefferson Medical College, the Franklin Institute, the Free Library, Philadelphia City Hall, Temple University, Albert Einstein Medical Center, Girard College, the Germantown Friends School, the Convent of the Blessed Sacrament in Cornwells Heights, the Rabbinical Institute in New York, Rollins College, the State Capitol in Harrisburg, and Brown and Yale Universities. Raditz was awarded the bronze medal at the Panama-Pacific Exposition in San Francisco (1915) and the second Hallgarten Prize at the National Academy of Design (1918). He had one-man shows of his portraits at the Art Club of Philadelphia (1913) and at the McClees Galleries in Philadelphia (1935).

Oil on canvas; 29 1/2 x 24 1/2; signed upper left, "Lazar Raditz"; no date recorded. Presented by the subject's son, Dr. J. Norman Henry, on behalf of the family in 1919.
PA 51

Dr. Henry is shown bust length, his body turned slightly to the left, his head to the left and tilted slightly downward. The background is dark brown on the right and in the lower left corner, and reddish-brown on the left. He has dark brown hair and grayish-white eyebrows and side-whiskers. His large brown eyes look straight out in the direction of the head turn through metal-rimmed spectacles. His nose has a bulbous tip. His bushy white moustache and pointed beard almost conceal the lower part of his face. He wears a white shirt with stand-up collar, a black necktie with pearl pin, and a black vest and coat. The surface of the portrait is painterly, with animated brush strokes in the head and hair. The well-depicted head appears solidly three-dimensional. The costume is flat, giving no indications of underlying body volumes. The warmth of the yellowish-orange skin tones is accentuated by the reddish background. The knitted brows and large, luminous eyes give the subject a pensive, almost troubled expression.

Thomas Tickell Hewson (1773-1848)

A son of William Hewson, the celebrated English anatomist and physiologist, Thomas T. Hewson was born in London. A family friend was Benjamin Franklin, who resided in the Hewson household when he was a London agent of the colony of Pennsylvania. The widowed Mrs. Hewson took her family to Philadelphia in 1786. Thomas received the A.B. and A.M. degrees from the University of Pennsylvania in 1789 and then studied medicine for five years with Dr. John Foulke (q.v.). Between 1794 and 1800 he attended lectures at the University of Edinburgh and was a house-surgeon at St. Bartholomew's Hospital in London. After his return to Philadelphia he established a surgical and medical practice. He was physician to the Walnut Street Prison and the Orphan Asylum, surgeon to the Philadelphia Almshouse and the Pennsylvania Hospital, consulting surgeon to the Philadelphia Dispensary, and professor of comparative anatomy

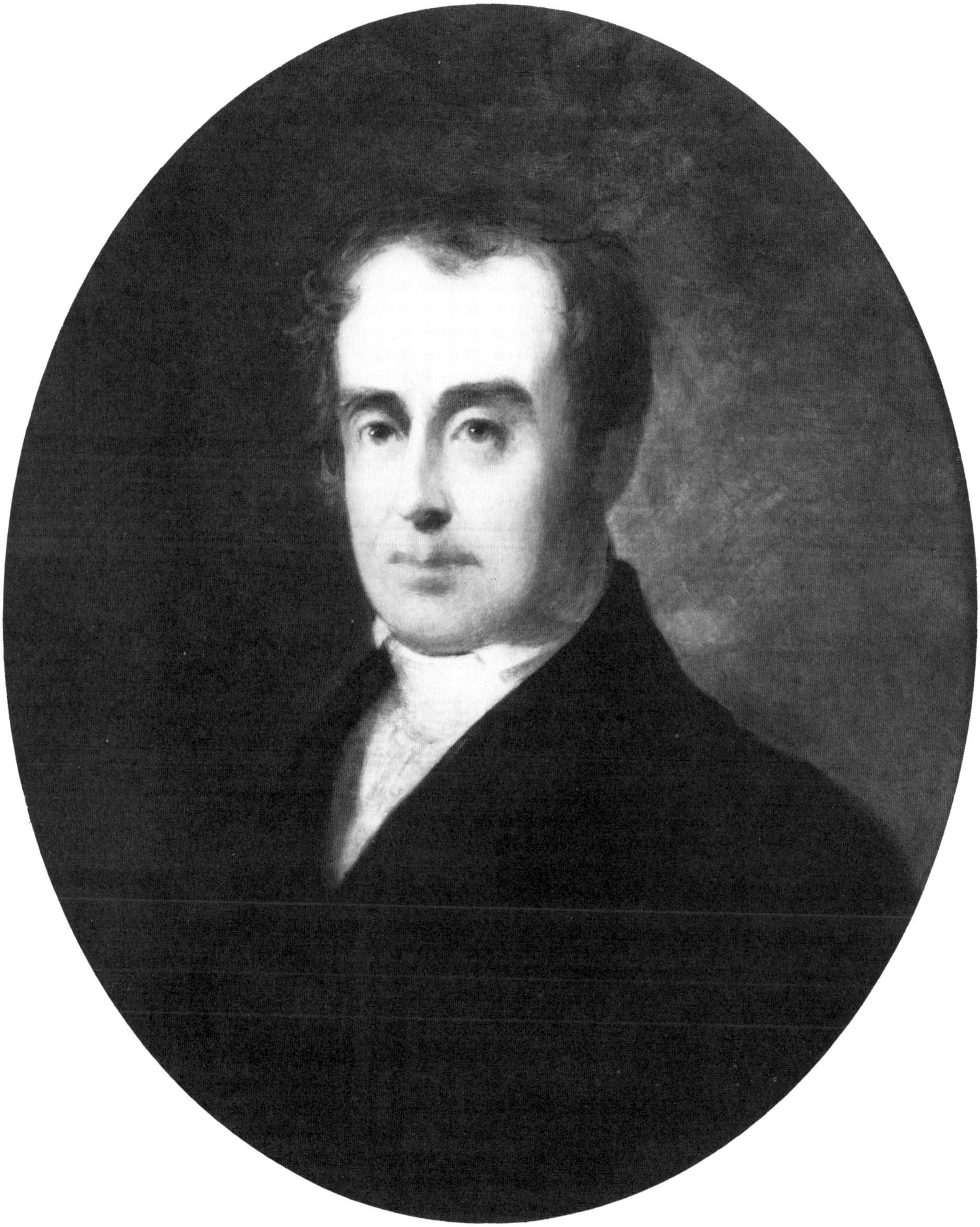

Thomas Tickell Hewson *PA 107*

at the University of Pennsylvania (1816–28). In 1822 he established a private medical school in which he taught anatomy. He was commended by the Board of Health for services rendered during the epidemics of yellow fever and typhus. He was a member of the American Philosophical Society, the American Linnaean Society, and the Edinburgh Medical Society. He received an honorary M.D. degree from Harvard University. He was an outstanding fellow of the College of Physicians, where he was successively secretary, censor, vice-president, and president (1835–48). The College appointed him a delegate to the regional and national conventions for formulating the National Pharmacopoeia. He served on the committee of publication and was chairman of the revision committee.

Artist: Thomas Sully (1783–1872)

For biography, see page 18.

Oil on canvas; 25 1/4 x 20 1/4; not signed or dated. Listed in Sully's Register of Portraits 1801–1871, *with the information that the subject was "deceased" and that the painting was painted in 1848. In* The Life and Works of Thomas Sully *(Charleston 1969), Edward Biddle and Mantle Fielding add that it was painted from a daguerrotype after the subject's death and that it was begun on February 25, 1848, and completed June 3, 1848. Exhibited at* the Memorial Exhibition of Portraits by Thomas Sully, *Pennsylvania Academy of the Fine Arts, 1922, and* The Art of Philadelphia Medicine, *Philadelphia Museum of Art, 1965. Presented by Dr. William Hewson, great-grandson of Dr. Thomas T. Hewson, on behalf of the children of Dr. Addinell Hewson, in 1941. PA 107*

Dr. Hewson is shown bust length, his face and body turned to the left. The atmospheric background is dark brown on the left, lighter umber on the right. Wispy brown hair curls around the high forehead. Under thick brown brows, the large gray eyes look out in the direction of the head turn and slightly upward. The face is oval, with pink cheeks, a straight nose, a wide mouth, and a round chin. The subject wears a white shirt with small collar turned down, a white stock, and a high-necked black coat. Although the portrait has undergone restoration, the painterly surface still shows visible brush strokes. The head is well-constructed in three-dimensional, solid volumes. The costume is flat, with no suggestion of the underlying body. The hair and details of features are soft-edged. The facial expression is dominated by the soft, luminous, unfocused eyes that give the subject a thoughtful, almost wistful expression.

Eugene T. Hinson (1873–1960)

Born in Philadelphia, Hinson traced his ancestry in Pennsylvania back 150 years. His grandfather owned the farmland upon which Lincoln University was built. In 1892 he graduated from the Institute

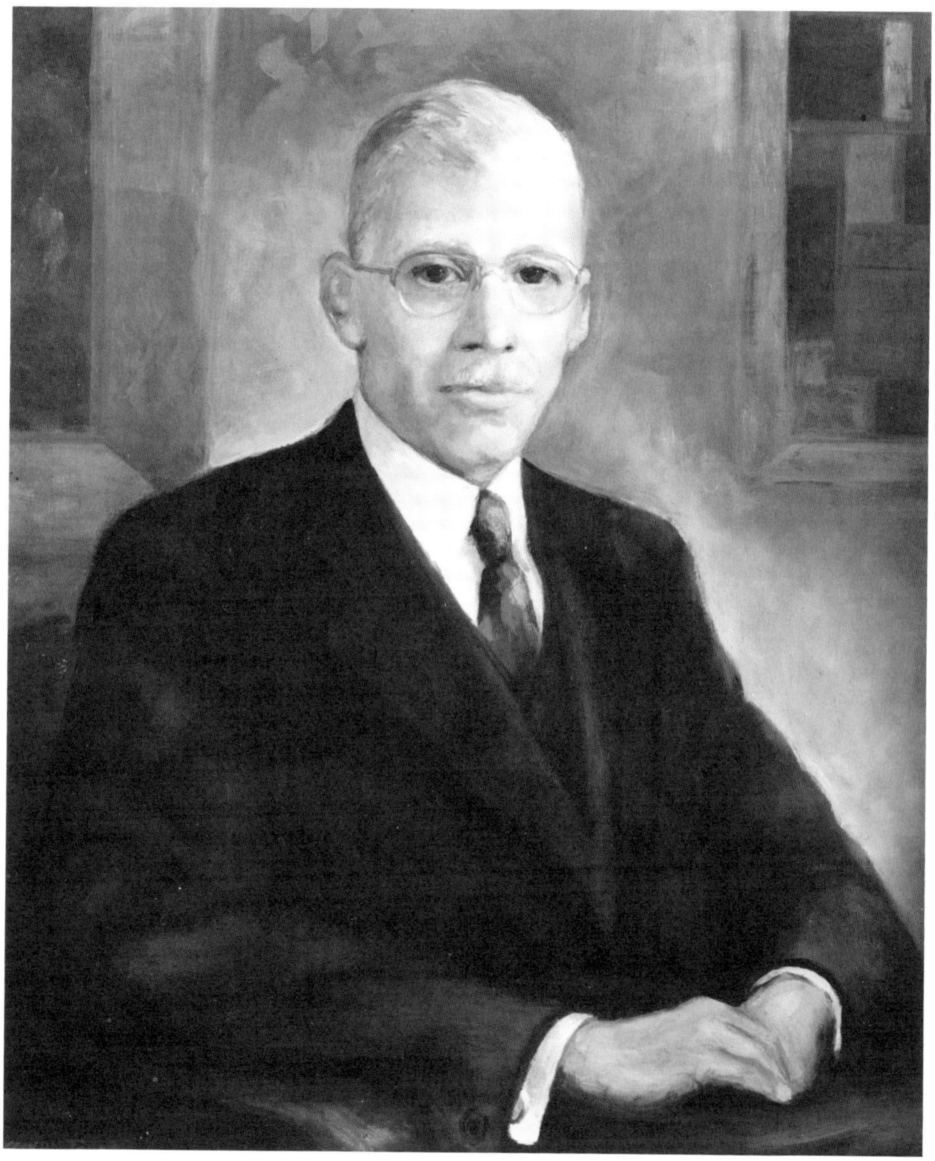

Eugene T. Hinson *PA 133*

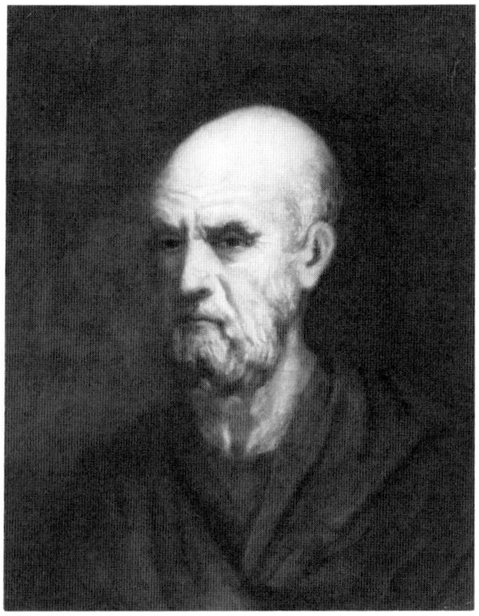

Hippocrates *PA 59*

for Colored Youth, a Quaker school. After teaching for two years at the Institute and in Gravity Hill, Maryland, he entered the medical school of the University of Pennsylvania and he graduated in 1898, an honor student and the second black graduate. After great difficulty in obtaining a hospital post he joined the staff of Frederick Douglass Hospital, then in operation only three years. Later, from 1900 to 1905, he was a member of its board of directors. He was a founder of the Mercy Hospital in 1907 and was chairman of its department of gynecology for 37 years. He continued in private practice until 1955. Hinson was a member of the American Medical Association and of the Philadelphia Academy of Medicine in Allied Sciences, an organization of black physicians, dentists, and pharmacists.

Artist: Henry Bozeman Jones (b. 1889)

Born in Philadelphia, Jones was a scholarship student at the Pennsylvania Academy of the Fine Arts from 1907 to 1910. His instructors included Cecilia Beaux, William Merritt Chase, Hugh Breckenridge, and Thomas Anshutz; he assisted in the latter's studio. As his career developed, Jones began to show his work at the Harmon Foundation's Exhibitions of Fine Arts, held at the Art Center in New York. This foundation, which gave awards for "distinguished achievements among Negroes," described Jones in its 1931 exhibition catalogue as a painter only in his spare time, "working as a bellboy, porter, cement worker, actor, printer and teacher. He is at present an instructor in physical education." The catalogue of 1933 stated that "he earns his living at both writing and painting." Sketchy biographical material adds that Jones exhibited at the Rumph Gallery, Warwick Galleries, A.C.A. Gallery, Reed Galleries, the Sketch Club, Print Club, Y.W.C.A., and the public schools, all in Philadelphia, and at the 135th Street branch of the New York Public Library.

Oil on canvas; 29¼ x 24¼; signed lower left, "Henry Jones." Originally commissioned by Sigma Pi Phi, a black medical fraternity, for Mercy-Douglass Hospital. Presented to the College of Physicians in 1974 by Mrs. Edith Longley, R.N., second cousin of Dr. Hinson. Shown at A Century of Black Presence at the University of Pennsylvania, 1879–1980, *an exhibition at the Van Pelt Library, University of Pennsylvania, 1980–81, and at* Three Hundred Years of Black History in the Commonwealth of Pennsylvania, *Afro-American Historical and Cultural Museum, 1981–82.* *PA 133*

Dr. Hinson is shown half-length, with body turned to the right and head very slightly to the right. He is seated in an armchair, with his right arm on the chair arm and his hands resting on his lap. The suggestion of an interior setting consists of a yellowish-orange background to the left and right of the head; on the wall are framed paintings in blue, green, red, orange, and yellow in geometric shapes on the right and more amorphous arrangements on the left. Hinson's hair and moustache are white, with cool green and gray shadows. His large brown eyes look straight ahead through gray plastic-framed glasses. He has a straight nose and a wide mouth with full lips. His tan skin tones have orange highlights. He wears a white shirt with cuff links, a blue necktie, and a dark blue three-piece suit. The surface of the portrait is very painterly, with loosely brushed, visible strokes in bright colors. The head and hands are moderately well constructed, but the costume is flatter, with little sense of underlying body forms. Hinson's posture is erect but relaxed. He gazes directly and confidently toward the viewer. A hint of a smile gives him a kind, compassionate, and pleasant facial expression.

Hippocrates (active 400 B.C.)

Though Hippocrates was the most famous of all ancient Greek physicians, little is known about his life. He is considered the founder of scientific medicine, and his fame has been recognized and venerated since the time of Plato. He has come to be the embodiment of an ideal physician. Soranus, a physician and biographer of the 2nd century A.D., said that Hippocrates was born on the island of Cos, off the coast of Asia Minor, where he was a member of the guild of Aesclepiadae (sons of Aesculepius, q.v.) and that he received his medical education at the famous temple of Aesculepius at Cos. He is said to have traveled widely and to have died at Larissa at an advanced age. The so-called Hippocratic Collection, books which deal with medicine, prognostics, dietetics, surgery, pharmacology, and health and diseases, show widely varying attitudes toward medicine. It is in dispute whether the Collection or

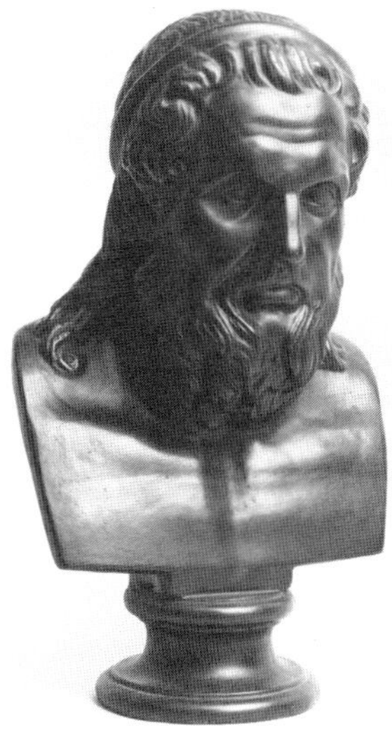

Hippocrates *ST 501*

even any fraction of it is truly an authentic work of Hippocrates. Probably it is the remnant of anonymous medical literature circulated in the 5th and 4th centuries B.C., brought together by the Alexandrian medical school soon after 300 B.C., and attributed to Hippocrates. It includes the famous Hippocratic Oath and the Aphorisms.

Artist: Fanny Darrach (Mrs. Hart Darrach)

For biography, see page 8.

Oil on canvas; 22 x 18; not signed or dated. Inscribed on back, "Hippocratic 1854." Shown at College of Physicians' Centennial Celebration Loan Collection of Portraits, *1887, the artist being listed as "Miss Darrach." In later inventories the artist is identified as Fanny Darrach and the work is said to have been presented by the artist. College minutes document the presentation date as 1869.* *PA 59*

Hippocrates is shown bust length, body frontal, head turned to the left and tilted down. The background is medium brown, darker on the right. The subject's head is bald, with fringes of gray hair and gray side-whiskers, short beard, and moustache. Under knitted brows his narrow gray eyes look down. His straight nose has a pointed tip, and his mouth is small. His long, thin face has deeply incised lines in the forehead and next to the nose. He wears a reddish-brown, round-necked robe of unknown type. The surface of the portrait is painterly, with visible brush strokes. The head is moderately well constructed with regard to anatomical accuracy. The long, thin face with its hollow cheeks and deeply incised lines and the exaggeratedly high dome of the head produce an ascetic appearance. The facial expression is thoughtful and rather disquieted. The gaze is unfocused, as though looking inward.

Artist: Unknown

Plaster, painted black; 24 1/2 x 14 1/2 x 12; 4 inch high round base, integral with sculpture; not signed or dated. Presented by Dr. Ludwig Loeb, in 1943, since which time the piece has been referred to as Hippocrates but with no documentation as to the identity or source. *ST 501*

When this sculpture is viewed frontally, both the body and head are frontal and the head is tilted down slightly. Its most distinguishing characteristics are the long, shoulder-length hair, bound by a rounded fillet, and the moustache, side-whiskers, and curly beard. The forehead has deeply incised horizontal lines. The deepset, large eyes are blank. The high cheekbones surmount hollow cheeks. The nose is straight with a flat bridge. The mouth has a full lower lip. The torso is cut off squarely, with just a hint of the structure of the chest. The surface of the sculpture is smooth, with no visible tool marks. Although the features of the face are idealized in what is probably a 19th century neoclassical conception, there is an intensity of facial expression. This is produced by the furrowed brow, the large round eyes, the protruding lower lip, and the disproportionately massive head that contrasts with the truncated body.

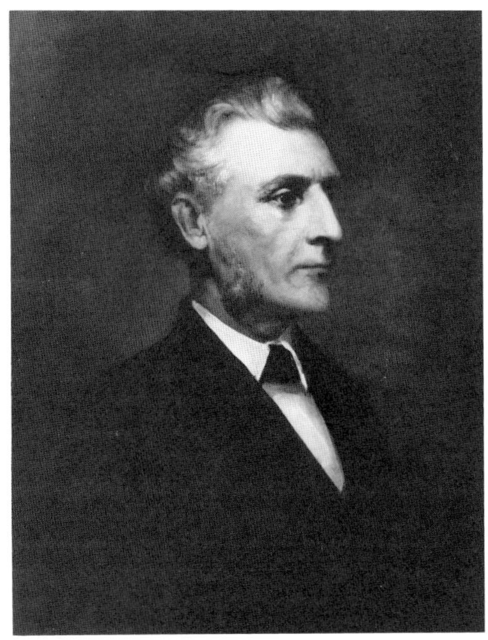

John Thompson Hodgen *PA 120*

John Thompson Hodgen (1826-1882)

Born in Hodgenville, Kentucky, Hodgen was graduated from Bethany College, West Virginia, and from McDowell's College of Medicine in St. Louis (now the University of the State of Missouri) in 1848. At his alma mater he was named demonstrator of anatomy and then professor of both anatomy and physiology. In 1862 he transferred to the St. Louis Medical College, where he filled respectively the chairs of physiology; anatomy; and surgical anatomy, fractures, and dislocation. In

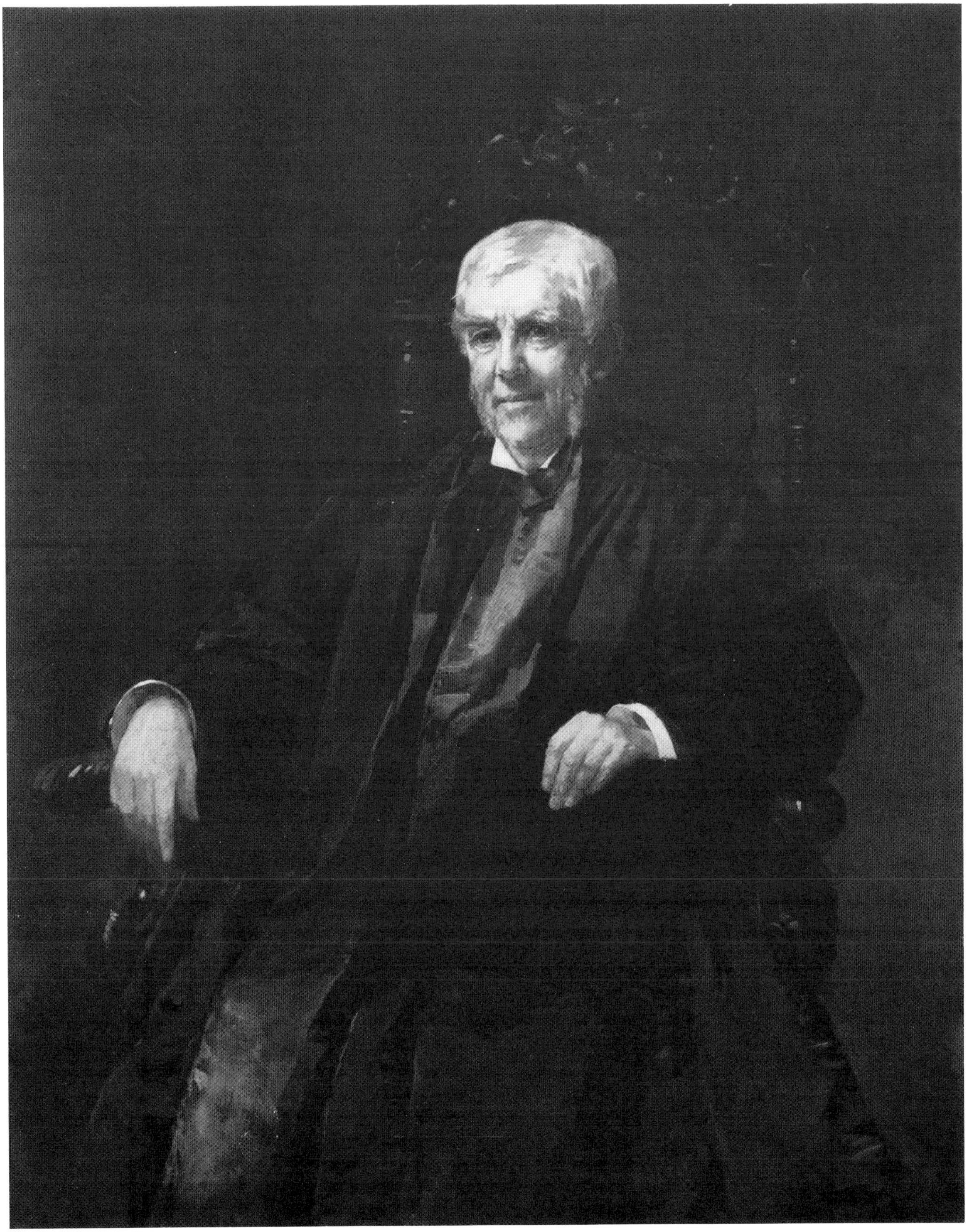

Oliver Wendell Holmes *PA 38*

1865 he was made dean of the faculty and held that position until his death in 1882. He taught surgery at the City Hospital of St. Louis from 1864 to 1882. During the Civil War he was surgeon-general of the Western Sanitary Commission, surgeon of the United States Volunteers, and surgeon-general of the State of Missouri. He was president of the St. Louis Medical Society, the Missouri State Medical Association, and the American Surgical Association. He had great mechanical aptitude and was the inventor of several medical devices, including the Hodgen splint, a wire suspension splint for fracture of the thigh. He also invented a suspension cord and pulleys permitting flexion, extension, and rotation of a fractured leg; a forceps dilator for removal of foreign bodies from air passages without tracheotomy; a cradle-splint for compound fracture of the thigh; a wire suspension splint for injury of the arm; a double-action syringe and stomach pump; and a hair-pin dilator for use in the trachea.

Artist: Unknown

Oil on canvas; 26 1/2 x 20 3/4; not signed or dated. Presented by Mr. Raoul Pantaleoni and Dr. Stuart Mudd in 1952.
PA 120

Dr. Hodgen is shown bust length, the body is turned three-quarters to the right, while the head is almost in profile to the right. The medium-toned gray background is lighter around the head. The subject has wavy gray hair and side-whiskers. His deep-set, dark brown eyes look straight out in the direction of the head turn. His angular face has a sharp nose, thin lips, and a pointed chin. He wears a white shirt with collar turned down, a thin black neckcloth, and a black coat. The surface of the portrait is painterly, with visible brush strokes in the head and hair. The head is moderately well constructed in terms of three-dimensional solidity. The costume is flat, with no indication of underlying bodily mass. The facial expression is dignified and sober, with slightly furrowed brows and tightly set lips.

Oliver Wendell Holmes (1809-1894)

The famed physician and author was born in Cambridge, Massachussetts. The son of a minister, he was descended from English settlers who came to Woodstock, Connecticut, in 1686. After graduating from Phillips Academy in Andover, Massachusetts, and from Harvard College in 1829, he spent one year in law school and then entered Harvard Medical School. He received the M.D. degree in 1836, after studying for an additional three years in Paris and Edinburgh. He was made physician to the Massachusetts General Hospital, and from 1838 to 1840 he was professor of anatomy at Dartmouth College in the summer months. He also taught at the Tremont Street Medical School, where courses supplementary to those of Harvard Medical School were given. Holmes was then elected to the newly established Parkman professorship of anatomy and physiology at Harvard, a position he held from 1847 to 1882. His popular lectures on anatomy were renowned for their erudition and wit. As a teacher he was foresighted in advocating the use of the microscope, which had just come into general use. In his medical writing he argued for what he considered good causes, rather than offering original discoveries. Examples of his essays are "Utility and Importance of Direct Exploration in Medical Science" (1837), an argument for more frequent use of the stethoscope; "Homeopathy and its Kindred Delusions" (1842), a scornful indictment against quackery of all kinds; "Currents and Counter-Currents in Medical Science" (1860), an insistence on scientifically tested therapeutic practices; and "Mechanism in Thought and Morals" (1871), an argument for the recognition of psychology in both morals and medicine. His most distinguished and most controversial essay was "The Contagiousness of Puerperal Fever" (1843), in which he contended that the disease was transmitted from patient to patient by the attending physician. Not unexpectedly, his article was opposed vigorously by America's leading obstetricians and he suffered personal abuse until his views were accepted. Holmes presented his personal library of 1000 volumes to the Boston Medical Library, of which he was president for 13 years. From his medical school days until the end of his life he published both verse and prose. He was a popular lecturer, whose "firecracker" wit exploded before delighted audiences. His essays and poems kept the newly founded *Atlantic Monthly* afloat in its early days. In 1886, he made a triumphant trip abroad, where he was the toast of the London season and received honorary degrees from Oxford, Cambridge, and Edinburgh Universities. He was elected an associate fellow of the College of Physicians of Philadelphia.

Artist: Sarah de St. Prix Wyman Whitman (Mrs. William Whitman) (1842-1904)

Sarah Whitman, born in Baltimore, studied art with William Morris Hunt in Boston and with Thomas Couture in Paris. A painter of portraits and landscapes, she was a frequent prize winner in major exhibitions. She won a bronze medal at the Columbian Exposition in Chicago (1893), gold and bronze medals at the Atlanta Exposition, and a diploma at the Pan American Exposition in Buffalo (1901). She was a member of the Society of American Artists in New York and of the Copley Society and the Water Color Club in Boston. In addition to having several works in the Boston Museum of Fine Arts, she is represented by glass windows in Memorial Hall, Cambridge, and in the Episcopal Church at Andover, Massachusetts.

Oil on canvas; 50 1/2 x 41 1/2; signed and dated upper left "MDCC SW [painter's initials in trefoil] CXII"; this is an error, since the correct equivalent for 1892 is MDCCCXCII. Presented by Dr. S. Weir Mitchell in 1892. The presentation of this portrait was accomplished under festive circumstances, arranged by Dr. Mitchell, then president of the College of Physicians and a lifelong friend of Dr. Holmes. Both were among the best-known physicians and men of letters of 19th century America. On April 30, 1892, a well-publicized gala dinner for 175 persons was held in the hall of the College to celebrate the presentation of portraits of Dr. Alfred Stillé (q.v.) and Dr. Holmes. After preliminary speeches and toasts, Dr. Mitchell presented the portrait of Dr. Holmes. His encomium in verse later appeared in a privately-printed booklet, in his Collected Poems *(1896), and in newspaper reports of the occasion. Although Dr. Holmes could not be present, he had forwarded his own "Lines," a gracious poetic response. The library of the College of Physicians owns the original manuscript of this poem, plus two separate four-page leaflet printings. The title of Dr. Mitchell's poem gave unusual tribute to the artist: "Verses Read on the Presentation by S. Weir Mitchell to the Philadelphia College of Physicians of Sarah W. Whitman's Portrait of Oliver Wendell Holmes, M.D."*
PA 38

Holmes is shown three-quarters length, seated in an armchair turned at an angle to the picture plane. He is turned slightly to the left; his head tilts down. His forearms rest on the chair arms, the right hand hangs loosely at the wrist, and the left hand holds a square black object, probably a mortarboard. The high-backed, William-and-Mary-style chair bears an elaborately pierced crest of a triple crown flanked by confronted horses; it has turned stiles and C-shaped volute arm supports. The subject has short, silver-white hair, and shaggy eyebrows and side-whiskers. His large hazel eyes look in the direction of the head turn. There are deep shadows under the brows and the lower eyelids are puffy. His round face has a straight nose, a full mouth with the hint of a smile, dimples, and pink round cheeks. He wears a white shirt with collar turned down, a black bow tie, and a black academic robe with red vertical panels in the center that are either a stole or the lining of the robe. The background of the portrait is painted smoothly. The deep folds of the costume have fluid, loosely brushed, visible strokes. The face and hands are solidly constructed with smaller strokes that render careful attention to the planes of anatomical detail. There is a sense of the bodily masses under the costume. The portrait radiates a sense of expansiveness. The large-scale figure and voluminous folds of the costume fill the canvas with a traditional pyramid shape. The subject's facial expression is outgoing and benign. The portrait embodies Dr. Mitchell's poetic allusion to the Apollo side of Dr. Holmes's nature:

> To wing the arrows of delightful mirth,
> To slay with jests the sadder things of earth.
> At his gay science melancholy dies,
> At his clear laugh each morbid fancy flies.

William Edmonds Horner (1793-1853)

Born in Warrenton, Virginia, of English forbears, Horner studied medicine first under Dr. John Spence and then at the University of Pennsylvania, where he received the M.D. degree in 1814. His studies had been interrupted by the War of 1812, in which he was commissioned surgeon's mate in the hospital department of the U.S. Army. His enthusiasm for the study of anatomy soon attracted the attention of Caspar Wistar (q.v.), professor of anatomy at the University of Pennsylvania, who hired him as dissector in 1816. Horner's career at the University was illustrious. He was made adjunct professor of anatomy and then professor (1831). He was dean of the medical school from 1822 to 1852 and dean of the faculty from 1835 to 1850. He was also surgeon to the Philadelphia Almshouse and a founder and first chief physician of St. Joseph's Catholic Hospital. In addition to his teaching and a large medical and surgical practice, Horner did research in pathology and was one of the first American physicians to make practical use of the microscope. He is credited with several anatomical discoveries. His writings include *Treatise on Special and General Anatomy,* the foremost American textbook of the period; *A Treatise on Pathological Anatomy; Lessons in Practical Anatomy for the Use of Dissectors*; and *Anatomical Atlas.* He bequeathed all his specimens, instruments, and apparatus to the medical department of the University of Pennsylvania. The collection, known then as the Wistar and Horner Museum, is housed today at the Wistar Institute of Anatomy.

Artist: Edward Dufrène (b. 1836)

A native of Belgium, Dufrène worked in Philadelphia in the years around 1850 to 1861. The city directories of 1860 and 1861 list him as a manufacturer of statuary and imitation marble.

Plaster, painted black; 26 3/4 x 17 3/8 x 11 3/4; base, integral with sculpture, 4 1/4 in. high; signed and dated, "Edward Dufrène Philad ÷," on beveled edge of shoulder, and "Sculp÷/1850," on rear of columnar base. Donor and date of donation are not recorded, but are prior to the Inventory of 1898-1915, in which it is included. *ST 524*

Horner is shown bust length, with body frontal and head turned slightly to the left. He has full, thick wavy hair, and curls around his forehead. The almond-shaped blank eyes have heavy upper lids. The long pointed nose has a bump at the bridge. The mouth is wide, the lips thin. The square face has high cheek bones and an angular jawline. The subject wears a toga with deeply carved, curving folds. The surface of the sculpture is smooth and shows no tool marks. The sense of anatomical structure is superficial; there is no sense of bodily forms underlying the costume. The sculpture combines a generalized neoclassical conception, emphasized by the blank eyes, costume, and dignified demeanor, with a certain individuality of features, especially the carefully differentiated strands of hair, prominent nose, high cheekbones, and wide mouth. Yet the impassive facial expression and smooth skin suggest a timeless, classical quality, belying the subject's age of fifty-seven years.

Friedrich Wilhelm Heinrich Alexander von Humboldt (1769-1859)

Humboldt was born in Berlin, the son of an ennobled Prussian officer. He studied at the Universities of Frankfurt and Göttingen and at the Academies of Commerce in Hamburg and of Mining in Freibert. His first employment was as an assessor and then director of mines in Franconia. A large inheritance allowed him to leave the civil service and to travel widely, and this provided the basis of his reputation as one of the founders of scientific geography. After careful exploration, he made one of the first sizable relief maps of Spain and as a result received permission to carry out a research tour through the Spanish colonies in South America. He spent the years from 1799 to 1804 making maps and amassing data in the fields of geomagnetism, meteorology, climatology, geology, mineralogy, oceanography, zoology, and ethnography. He observed and gathered more than 60,000 botanical specimens and he made historical and linguistic investigations. In 1804 he traveled to the United States, meeting with President Jefferson in Washington and stopping twice in Philadelphia, once to meet with the American Philosophical Society, which elected him to membership. His account of his American travels filled 35 volumes and was titled, *Voyage aux régions équinoxiales du Nouveau Continent.* Of all his scientific writings, the one that most seized the popular mind was the five-volume *Kosmos,* an attempt to describe physically the entire material world and to give the history of physical cosmography. Humboldt also established the fields of plant geography and

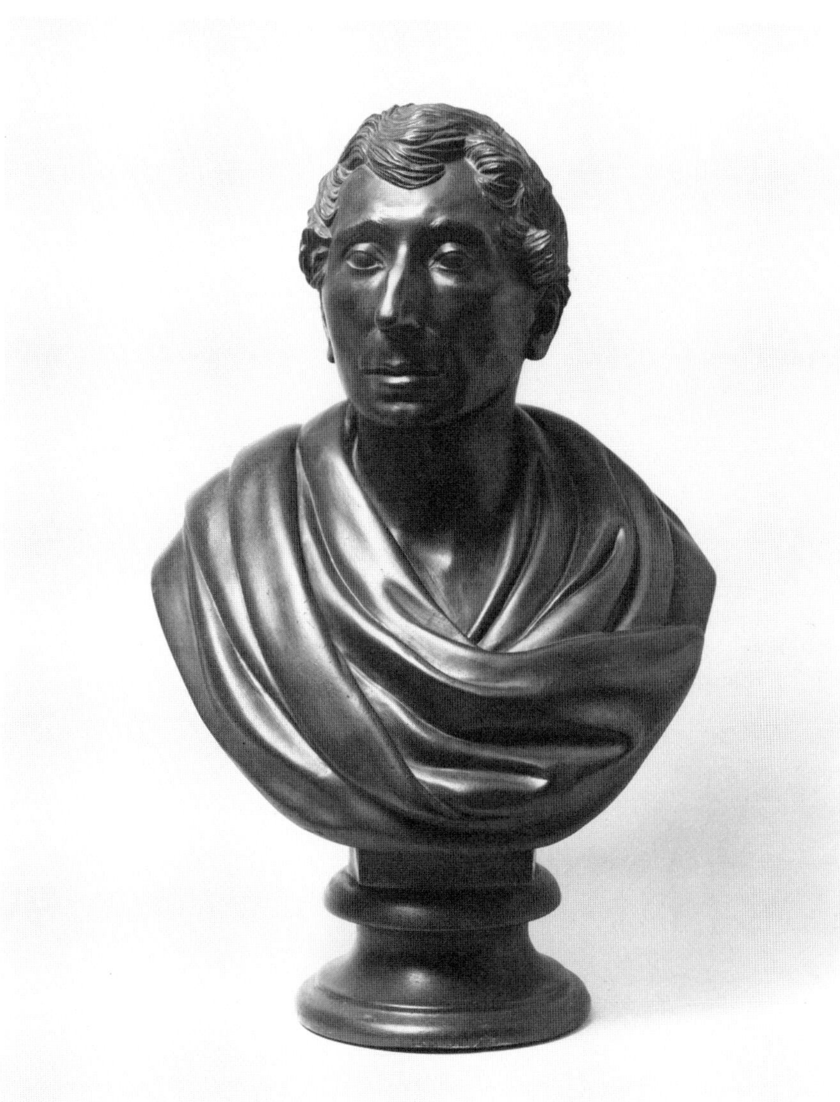

William Edmonds Horner *ST 524*

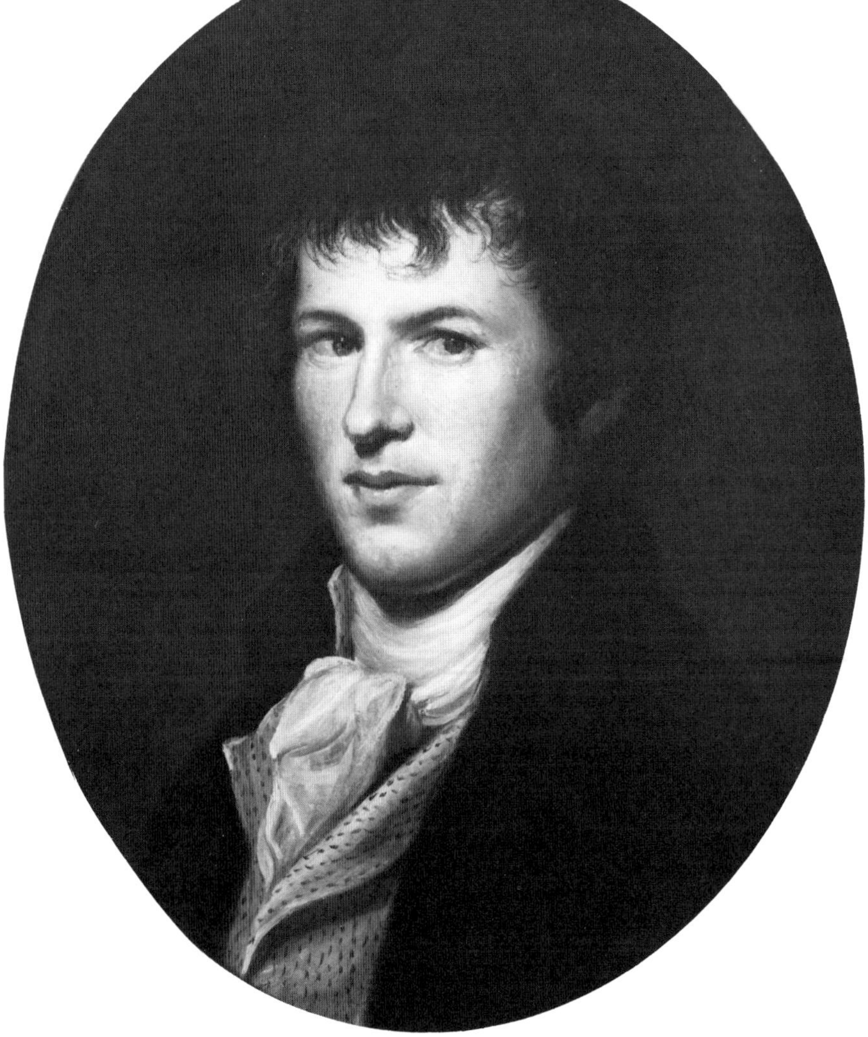

Friedrich Wilhelm Heinrich Alexander von Humbolt PA 47

orography, developed climatology as a separate science, formulated fissure theory of volcanology, and introduced the isotherm in meteorology. He was made a member of the Prussian Council of State, was sent on diplomatic missions, was made chancellor of the "Pour le Mérite" Order, was awarded six honorary degrees, and was elected to virtually all major international scientific societies. His scientific stature and social standing were so great that he received a state funeral.

Artist: Charles Willson Peale (1741-1827)

For biography, see page 26.

Oil on canvas; 21 x 17; not signed or dated. Inscription on back of relined canvas, "Baron Humboldt; the distinguished Traveling Writer/ an original portrait/ by Chas. Wilson [sic] Peale." Exact date of portrait and Peale's attitude toward the subject and the painting are revealed in letters at the American Philosophical Society, written after Peale had made the arrangements for Humboldt to meet President Jefferson and had accompanied him on the trip to Washington. On June 21, 1804, he wrote to his sons Rembrandt and Raphaelle expressing doubt that Humboldt would sit for a portrait. On June 23 he told his sons that Baron Humboldt would sit the next day. On June 27 in a letter to John de Peyster, he said, "I had this morning finished a portrait of him for the Museum. . . . I told the Baron that I had not painted for 6 years past and probably I should make a daub of it, yet it should be a likeness, and to my surprise it was a better painting than any I had painted for the Museum before." He said of Humboldt, "I have been richly rewarded for the trouble and expense of a journey. . . . He is the fountain of knowledge which flows in copious streams—to drop this metaphor and take another, he is a great luminary diffusing light on every branch of science. . . . His company is courted by the learned wherever he goes." No donor or date of donation is recorded. The portrait was located at Peale's Philadelphia Museum gallery from 1804 until 1854, when it was sold to "Nagle" at an auction of the gallery's portraits (according to an annotated copy of the auction sale catalogue located at the Historical Society of Pennsylvania). It entered the College of Physicians' collection between 1854 and 1887, when it was shown at the College's

Centennial Celebration Loan Collection of Portraits, *listed as owned by the College. It was also shown at two exhibitions at the Pennsylvania Academy of the Fine Arts: the* Loan Exhibition of Historical Portraits, *1887–88; and the* Exhibition of Portraits by Charles Willson, James and Rembrandt Peale, *1923.* *PA 47*

Humboldt is shown bust length, body to the left, head turned slightly to the left. The atmospheric background is a medium gray-brown. The subject has dark brown, collar-length hair brushed in wavy strands onto his forehead. His blue eyes gaze out of their corners to the right. His oval face has a straight nose, full lips, and a ruddy complexion. He wears a white stock and neckcloth, a white waistcoat with tan dotted stripes, and a black coat with a high collar. The surface of the portrait has been painted smoothly except for details in the hair and costume. The head is constructed in solid, three-dimensional volumes. The edges of forms are soft and there is no sense of bodily forms underlying the costume. Humboldt is portrayed as a youthful, self-confident man at the height of his powers. His facial expression is affable, yet determined. His glance adds to the effect of animation and energy.

William Hunt (1825–1896)

Dr. Hunt, born in Philadelphia, was descended from Scottish Quakers who settled in the years around 1680 in the areas that are now New Jersey and Pennsylvania. After a brief stay in his father's publishing house, he began to study medicine with Dr. George B. Wood (q.v.) and received the M.D. degree from the University of Pennsylvania in 1849. At the University he became assistant demonstrator of anatomy under Dr. Joseph Leidy (q.v.) and then demonstrator. During this time he was also on the surgical staffs of the Episcopal and Wills Eye Hospitals. He resigned the last two positions to become surgeon at the Pennsylvania Hospital, where he remained from 1863 to 1893. He was a fellow in the College of Physicians, which he served as chairman of the Mütter Museum Committee. He was president of the Philadelphia Academy of Surgery, an honorary member of the American Surgical Association, a trustee of the University of Pennsylvania, and a director of the Philadelphia Contributionship. He was one of the original members of the microscopical and biological section of the Academy of Natural Sciences and the Biological Club. During the Civil War he was acting assistant surgeon in the U.S. Army and a special investigator of the general hospitals of the Army. He was an editor of the *Annual of the Universal Medical Sciences*, a contributor to the *American Journal of the Medical Sciences*, and author, with Dr. Thomas G. Morton (q.v.), of *History of Surgery in the Pennsylvania Hospital* (1880).

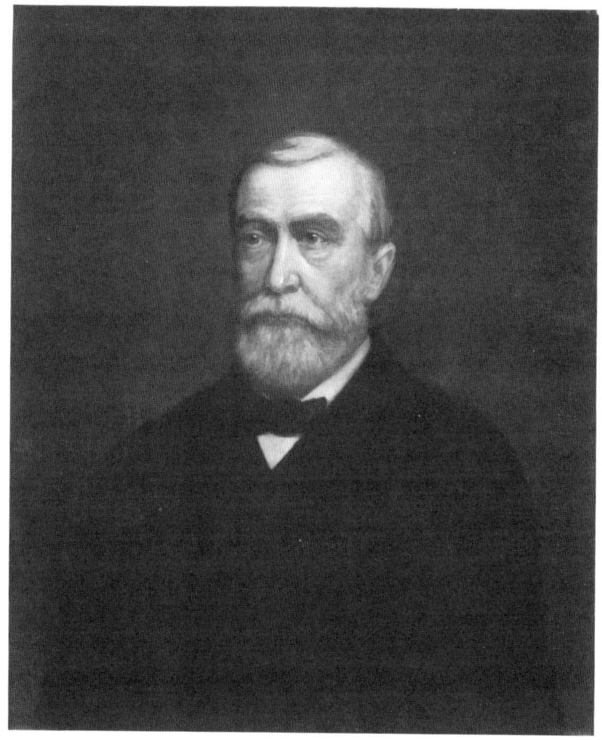

William Hunt *PA 62*

Artist: Louis Hasselbusch (1863–1938)

Born in Philadelphia, Hasselbusch studied at the Pennsylvania Academy of the Fine Arts, at the Académie Julien in Paris under Jean Joseph Benjamin-Constant and Jules Joseph Lefebvre, and at the Royal Academy in Munich. He specialized in portraits, and his works are represented in private collections, libraries, universities, and other institutions. His obituary in the *Philadelphia Evening Bulletin* mentioned that he left three paintings to the Melita Lodge, No. 295, Masonic Home of Pennsylvania, and "the balance of his pictures, sketches, and the equipment of his studio going to the Philadelphia Sketch Club for use there, or for worthy students." He also bequeathed $500 to the Club for refreshments at yearly meetings, "in the memory of old and deceased Members." He was a member of and exhibitor with the Art Club of Philadelphia and a member of the fellowship and an exhibitor at the Pennsylvania Academy of the Fine Arts.

Oil on canvas; 29 1/4 x 24 1/4; signed and dated on the back, "Wm. Hunt.M.D. / Louis Hasselbusch / pnx /MDCCCXCVII / apres photo." According to College minutes of 1897, presented by "subscribers," presumably fellows of the College of Physicians. *PA 62*

Dr. Hunt is shown bust length, with head and body turned slightly to the left. The atmospheric background is reddish-brown. He has gray hair, side-whiskers, a moustache, and a short beard. His blue eyes look straight out in the direction of the head turn. There are age lines on his forehead, under his eyes, and next to his nose. His

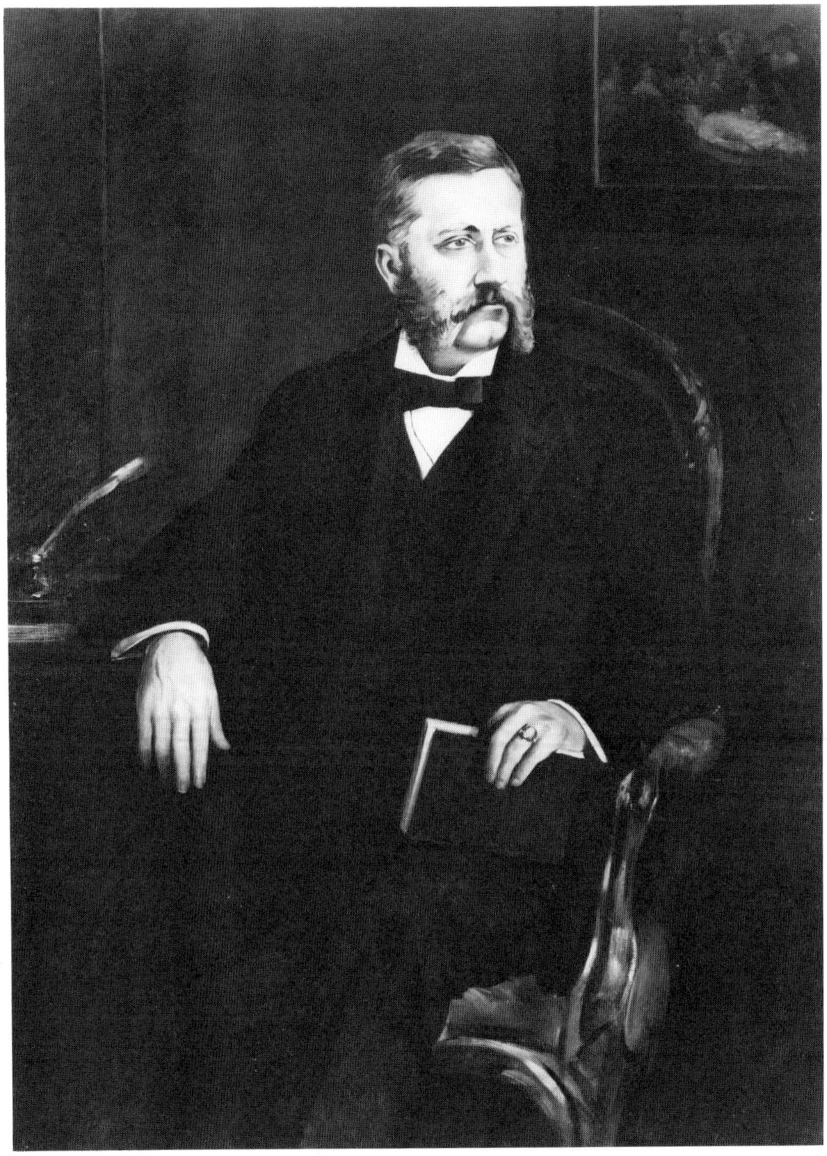

Charles Thomas Hunter *PA 91*

rectangular face has a straight nose and a wide mouth with thin lips. He wears a white shirt, a black bow tie, and a double-breasted black coat. The paint style is smooth on the background and costume and painterly in the head, which is well constructed in solid, three-dimensional volumes. The costume is flat with no suggestion of underlying bodily masses. The paint is thin in some areas, revealing pencil marks that outline features. The subject's bearing is erect and dignified, and his facial expression is rather somber.

Charles Thomas Hunter (1843-1884)

Born in New Bloomfield, Ohio, Hunter received the M.D. degree from the University of Pennsylvania in 1868. After serving as resident physician at the Pennsylvania Hospital, he was appointed chief of clinic and private assistant to Dr. D. Hayes Agnew (q.v.). He was demonstrator of surgery and demonstrator of anatomy at the University of Pennsylvania, assistant surgeon at the University Hospital, and surgeon to the out-patient department of Pennsylvania Hospital and the Episcopal Hospital. He was a fellow of the College of Physicians. During the summer of 1881 he sustained a wound of his left thumb while operating. No treatment could correct the ensuing infection that resulted in his death three years later. A colleague said, "There is to his many friends a peculiar sadness in his death at a time when his professional success was assured, at a time when the fruits of his diligence and faithfulness were within his grasp."

Artist: Henry R. Rittenberg (1879-1969)

Born in Libau, Russia, Rittenberg was brought to the United States in 1885. He studied art at the Pennsylvania Academy of the Fine Arts under William Merritt Chase from 1897 to 1900 and at the Munich Academy in 1902. He maintained his home and studio in New York City and taught at the Art Students' League and Beaux Arts Institute of Design.

He was in charge of special portrait classes at the National Academy of Design and was elected an academician in 1927. He was a frequent exhibitor and won several awards, including the Cresson traveling scholarship of the Pennsylvania Academy (1904), honorable mention at the Art Club of Philadelphia (1906), the Maynard portrait prize of the National Academy of Design (1920), the Harris prize at the Art Institute of Chicago (1925), and the Proctor portrait prize at the National Academy of Design (1926). He was a member of numerous art societies and clubs in New York, Washington, and Philadelphia. He was an officer in the Allied Artists of America and the National Commission to Advance American Art, and he was a member of the council of the National Academy of Design. His works are represented in museums, universities, libraries, hospitals, corporations, government buildings, cultural organizations, and private collections throughout the East Coast.

Oil on canvas; 51 3/4 x 38 3/4; signed lower right, but indecipherable. All inventories and a bronze plaque at the College of Physicians list Henry Rittenberg as the painter of this portrait. Disparity in dating shows that the portrait could not have been done from life. The pose and costume in the oil painting resemble those in a bust-length engraving of 1911, formerly owned by Dr. William N. Bradley. Presented by Mrs. Elizabeth R. Moulton, sister of Dr. Hunter, in 1913. *PA 91*

Hunter is shown three-quarter length, the body turned to the left and the head to the right. He is seated in a French-style upholstered armchair. His left arm rests on the chair arm and the left hand holds a blue book; his index finger marks the place. His right arm rests on the top of a desk, and the right hand hangs loosely over the edge. The interior architectural setting includes moldings on the dark brown wall, a framed reproduction of Rembrandt's *Anatomy Lesson of Dr. Tulp* in the upper right corner, a desk top with two green bound books, and a brass writing stand with quill pen. The subject's hair, side-whiskers, and moustache are brown, flecked with gray. He has long, narrow, blue eyes which look straight out in the direction of the head turn. The nostrils are flaring, the cleft chin is square. The subject wears a white shirt with turned down collar, a black bow tie, a black vest and suit, and a jewelled ring. In spite of paint loss and retouching, it can be seen that the surface of the portrait has fluid, painterly brush strokes. The head and hands are moderately well constructed in three-dimensional volumes and there is a suggestion of the body masses under the costume. The expression is dignified and it is appropriate to the somewhat pretentious setting. Even though the turn of the head and the marking of the book denote action, the figure is not convincingly lively and energetic. This is probably due to the fact that it was not painted from life.

John Hunter (1728-1793)

The youngest of ten children of a Scottish farmer, Hunter was born in Long Calderwood, Lanarkshire. With little formal education and three years of apprenticeship to a cabinetmaker in Glasgow, he visited his older brother, William, the London anatomist, hoping to become his assistant. John showed such promise that he soon attended surgical classes at St. George's and St. Bartholomew's Hospitals and became a pupil of William Cheselden and Percival Pott. Although considered ill-spoken and uncouth, at this early stage in his career he made his first anatomical discovery, the *gubernaculum testis.* In 1760 he joined the army as a staff surgeon during the Seven Years' War, gaining the battlefield experience that he later incorporated into his great work, *Treatise on the Blood, Inflammation and Gun-Shot Wounds* (1794). In 1767, on the basis of his anatomical and physiological investigations, he was elected a fellow of the Royal Society. Although impeded by his lack of formal credentials, at the age of 40 he was a successful candidate for the diploma of the Company of Surgeons, and in that same year he was appointed surgeon at St. George's. He opened his own school of anatomy. There his lectures on applied and comparative anatomy and on surgery attracted such illustrious students as Astley Cooper, Edward Jenner (q.v.), John Abernethy, and the Americans John Jones (q.v.), John Morgan (q.v.), Philip Syng Physick (q.v.), and William Shippen, Jr. (q.v.). In 1788, at the urging of Benjamin Franklin, Hunter was elected an honorary member of the American Philosophical Society. During these years he published his treatise, *The Natural History of the Human Teeth,* his *Treatise on Venereal Disease,* and *An Account of Mr. Hunter's Method of Performing the Operation for the Cure of Popliteal Aneurism* as described by Everard Home, his assistant. As Hunter's clinical practice flourished, he bought two adjacent houses which were later connected by a lecture hall, picture gallery, and natural history museum. Hunter was well acquainted with many artists, notably Sir Joshua Reynolds, Thomas Gainsborough, Angelica Kauffmann, Thomas Rowlandson, and Johann Zoffany. In later years he was accorded many honors, including the Copley Medal of the Royal Society; appointments as surgeon-extraordinary to King George III, surgeon-general to the army, and inspector-general of hospitals; and member of the Académie Royale de Chirurgie de Paris. He was widely regarded as the founder of scientific surgery. His museum was transferred to the Royal College of Surgeons in 1800, with the proviso that 24 lectures on comparative anatomy be delivered annually.

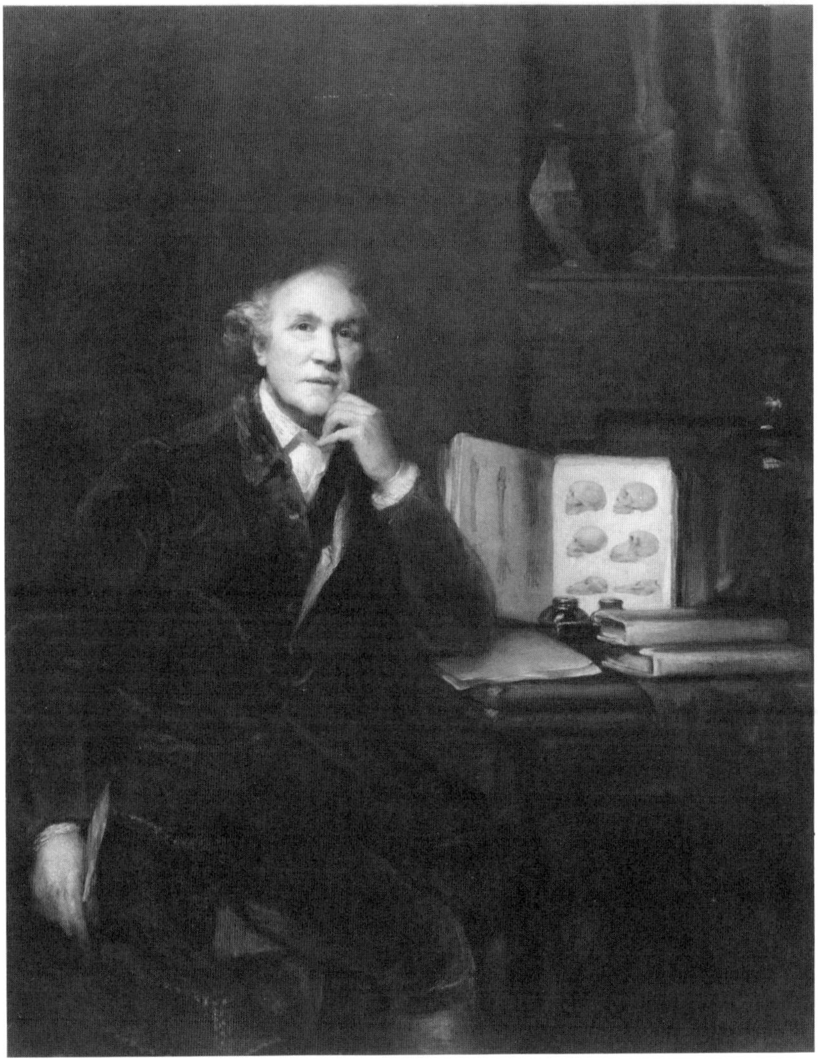

John Hunter *PA 33*

Artist: Anna Lea Merritt (Mrs. Henry Merritt) (1844–1930)

For biography, see page 70.

Oil on canvas; 55 3/4 x 44 3/4; not signed or dated. Label on back reads, "Portrait/copy by Anna Lea Merritt/owned by S. Weir Mitchell." Painted after the original by Sir Joshua Reynolds, ca. 1785–86, Royal College of Surgeons, London. In her Memoirs, *the artist dates the work 1878 and says, "For Dr. Weir Mitchell I copied at the College of Surgeons the portraits of Hunter and of Harvey by the great Sir Joshua Reynolds. These copies were to me a fine lesson and are now honoured by a place in the College of Physicians in Philadelphia" (see Galina Gorokhoff,* Love Locked Out: The Memoirs of Anna Lea Merritt, *Boston 1982). Reynolds, who was a friend of Hunter, used his great prestige to support the doctor's candidacy for the post of surgeon at St. George's Hospital. Hunter was Reynolds's physician and attended Reynolds during his final illness, assisted at the autopsy, and participated in the elaborate funeral services. It is said that the portrait was painted at the behest of the engraver William Sharp, a friend of both men, who wanted to gain fame by engraving the portrait. There are many tales, perhaps apocryphal, about the painter's frustrations at his failure to secure a satisfactory pose. It is said that Hunter became fatigued and fell into a train of thought, and that the artist quickly captured his subject's instinctive posture of reflection (see Jane M. Oppenheimer, "John and William Hunter and Some Contemporaries in Literature and Art,"* Bulletin of the History of Medicine, *XXIII, 1949). Presented by bequest of Dr. S. Weir Mitchell in 1914. Shown at the College of Physicians* Centennial Celebration Loan Collection of Portraits, *1887, while owned by Mitchell.* *PA 33*

Hunter is shown three-quarter length, seated. The lower trunk is turned to the right, the head and upper torso slightly to the right. His right arm hangs down at his side, and his right hand holds a quill. His left arm, bent at the elbow, rests on a table, and his left hand supports his chin. The architectural setting is an office or library in which Hunter sits in a green leather-upholstered chair in front of a table covered with green cloth. The objects on the table include a white paper (which in the original shows drawings of arterial branches), two closed books (which in the original are identified as *Natural History of Vegetables* and *Natural History of Fossils*), a bell jar with a specimen (which in the original is clearly a case with an injected bronchial tree), and an open folio of anatomical drawings of skulls and hands. On the right wall is a niche that shows the legs of O'Brien, the famous Irish giant.

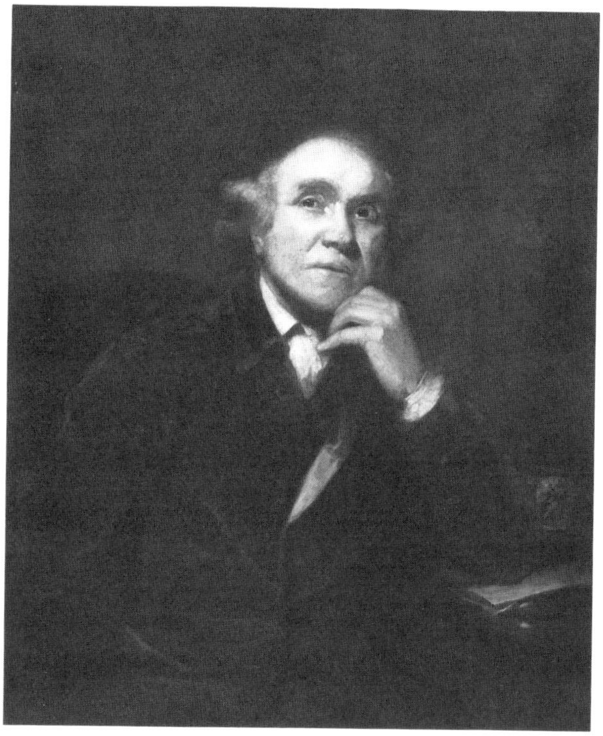

John Hunter PA 80

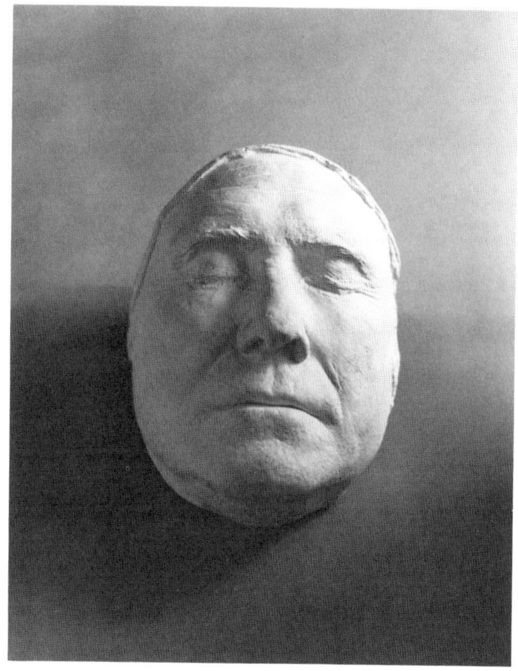

John Hunter ST 13055

Next to the giant's right foot is the open metacarpal bone of an ass, injected to show the finer arteries. (For a thorough study of Reynolds's original portrait, see Lord Brock, "Background Details in Reynolds' Portrait of John Hunter," *Annals of the Royal College of Surgeons of England,* 48, 1971). Hunter has collar-length, reddish-blond hair, full at the sides. His hazel eyes look upward. His round face has a ruddy complexion, his lips are slightly parted. He wears a white shirt with white frill and a maroon velvet coat and breeches. The portrait has a painterly surface with lively brush strokes throughout, especially in the dark shadows and bright highlights. The head and hands are well constructed in solid, three-dimensional forms. There is a sense of bodily volumes underneath the costume. The subject's mood is reflective, as though he were pausing for a moment to seek respite from his efforts or inspiration to continue his work. Despite the indicated momentary relaxation, the gesture, posture, and gaze show a figure full of energy and intense thought. The objects surrounding Hunter were chosen to demonstrate his versatility as a naturalist, botanist, geologist, pathologist, anatomist, experimental surgeon, and collector.

Artist: Attributed to Charles Robert Leslie (1794–1859)

Born of American parents in London, Leslie's father, a clockmaker, brought the family back to Philadelphia in 1799; there Leslie was apprenticed to the firm of Bradford and Inskeep, publishers. When Mr. Bradford, a director of the Pennsylvania Academy of the Fine Arts, recognized the skill of Leslie's early drawings and watercolors, he convinced the directors of the youth's "promise of great celebrity" and obtained permission for him to enter the Academy. Leslie, however, was encouraged by Thomas Sully, who gave him a few lessons; he was determined to study in London. Therefore, the Academy and a group of prominent merchants subscribed funds for the trip. In London he enrolled at the Royal Academy and received instruction from Benjamin West and Washington Allston. Letters of introduction and his own charm and grace soon put him in touch with some of the artistic and literary luminaries of the day, including Samuel Taylor Coleridge, John Constable, Sir Walter Scott, Sir Edwin Landseer, and the Americans Samuel F. B. Morse (a fellow student), Charles Bird King, and Washington Irving. He was elected to the Royal Academy in 1826, was professor of painting there from 1847 to 1852, and exhibited frequently there between 1813 and 1839. The subjects of his paintings included scenes from history and the Bible. He drew illustrations for writings of Shakespeare, Cervantes, Sterne, Addison, Goldsmith, Moliére, and Scott. His humorous genre scenes from literature endeared him to the public. The subjects of his portraits included the Queen, the nobility, and contemporary theatrical personalities. Except for six months as a teacher of drawing at the United States Military Academy at West Point, Leslie passed his entire career in London. However, he exhibited in America at the Pennsylvania Academy of the Fine Arts from 1811 to 1865, and he was made an honorary member and was nominated to be an academician. The Academy possesses several of his paintings. He also was an honorary member of the National Academy of Design, where he exhibited between 1827 and 1854. His writings include *Handbook for Young Painters* (1855), *The*

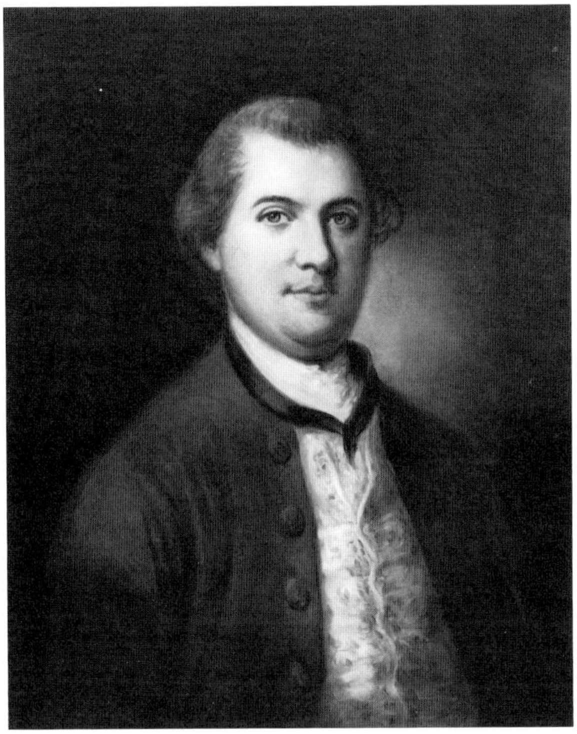

James Hutchinson *PA 22*

Life of Constable (1843), *Autobiographical Recollections* (1860), and *The Life of Reynolds* (1865). A collection of 30 works by Leslie was shown at the Royal Academy in 1870. A number of his best paintings can be found at the National Gallery, South Kensington Museum, the National Portrait Gallery, and Buckingham Palace.

Oil on canvas; 29 x 24 1/2; not signed or dated. Although confirmatory evidence is lacking, all inventories at the College of Physicians list this portrait as the work of Leslie. The painting is a copy of an original by Sir Joshua Reynolds, 1785-86, at the Royal College of Surgeons, London (for details, see entry above). A bronze plaque at the College says that the portrait was presented by Dr. Alfred Stillé, 1901, and is a copy by Leslie of the Reynolds portrait of Hunter. However, Dr. Stillé died in 1900.
PA 80

By copying only a portion of Reynolds's portrait of Hunter (see description above), Leslie has changed the interpretation. By eliminating architectural space in the room, he closes in on the subject. By eliminating most of the scientific objects on the table and on the wall and by eliminating the lower half of the figure, he emphasizes the subject's head and hand. Compared with the portrait by Merritt, here the tilted head is supported more convincingly by the hand. He has added one feature, the thick volume at Hunter's elbow. The result is that the painting is no longer a *portrait d'apparat,* but that of the traditional philosopher, with the head resting on the hand and the eyes upraised. Leslie has been faithful in the coloring and in the details of face and costume. This painting, too, has a lively, animated surface, and the figure is convincingly solid and three dimensional.

Artist: Unknown

Plaster, painted white; 8 1/8 x 6 1/4 x 4 1/2; cast of the original life mask, 1788, at the Hunterian Museum, Royal College of Surgeons, London. Received from the curator of the Royal College of Surgeons by William Williams Keen (q.v.), who presented one copy to the College of Physicians in 1900 and a second copy (ST 17832.73) in 1925. *ST 13055*

The original was made when Hunter was 60 years old, about two years after Reynolds's portrait (see above). It shows the subject's face in almost surrealistic anatomical detail—including the pores of the skin and the wrinkles in the forehead, corners of the eyes, and next to the nose. It accords with the general configuration of the face portrayed in the paintings, with the obvious difference that the eyes and mouth are closed and that the hair does not show. Although the corners of the mouth turn down, the face has a serene expression.

James Hutchinson (1752-1793)

The son of a Quaker farmer, Hutchinson was born in Wakefield, Bucks County, Pennsylvania. After his father's death he lived with his uncle, Israel Pemberton, in Philadelphia, where he served as apprentice to an apothecary and then received a bachelor's degree with first honors from the College of Philadelphia. He studied medicine first under Dr. Cadwalader Evans and then at the College of Philadelphia, from which he received the Bachelor of Medicine degree with a gold medal for proficiency in chemistry in 1774. In that year he went to London to study with Dr. John Fothergill (q.v.) and, at St. Bartholomew's Hospital, with Percival Pott, John Hunter (q.v.), William Hunter, and others. Because of political events, he decided to return home by way of France in 1777 and brought with him important dispatches from Benjamin Franklin, then foreign minister in France. When his ship was attacked by the British, he left under fire in an open boat in order to save the dispatches. At home he immediately joined the American army, serving as surgeon general of Pennsylvania from 1778 to 1781. After the war he established a medical practice in Philadelphia and was appointed professor of materia medica at the University of the State of Pennsylvania. In 1791, when that institution merged with the College of Philadelphia, he became professor of chemistry. He was also physician to the Pennsylvania Hospital and physician of the port of Philadelphia. He was a senior founder of the College of Physicians and its first secretary, and he was a member of the American Philosophical Society; he also served on the Committee of Safety. His death was caused by yellow fever, which he contracted while fighting the disease in the epidemic of 1793.

Artist: Attributed to M. Louise Wood (Mrs. John Wright) (b. 1875)

Born in Philadelphia, Wood studied at the Pennsylvania Academy of the Fine Arts in 1885, 1888-89, and again in 1895-96. She studied in Paris at the Académie Julien and with James McNeill Whistler; in London she studied with F.W. Jackson. She was a member of the fellowship at the Pennsylvania Academy, exhibited at annual exhibitions there in 1889, 1895, and 1902-05, and won the Toppan prize. She exhibited at the Paris Salons of 1900-02 and widely in Philadelphia, New York, Boston, Chicago, Washington, and St. Louis. She belonged to and exhibited with the Philadelphia and New York Water Color Clubs; she was a vice-president of the Pennsylvania Society of Miniature Painters, with whom she exhibited (1903-04). She exhibited with the Art Club of Philadelphia (1891-94, 1899, and 1904). In 1904 she won a bronze medal at the Louisiana Purchase Exposition in St. Louis.

*Oil on canvas; 29½ x 24½; not signed or dated; written on back of canvas before relining in 1980, "copied 1897 by Louise Wood after Healy" [G.P.A. Healy, 1813-1894]. There is a similar portrait of Hutchinson by Louise Wood at the Pennsylvania Hospital. Another similar portrait of Hutchinson, possibly the original Healy, is at the University of Pennsylvania. At the College of Physicians there is a mezzotint of an engraving by Samuel Sartain, made after the Healy painting. According to Charles Coleman Sellers (*Portraits and Miniatures by Charles Willson Peale*, Philadelphia, American Philosophical Society, 1952) Healy's portrait was painted after a miniature, now lost, by Charles Willson Peale that was made at Valley Forge in May, 1778. Presented by Pemberton S. Hutchinson, Margaretta Hutchinson, and Emlen Hutchinson in 1897. Most inventories at the College of Physicians list the artist as unknown. PA 22*

Dr. Hutchinson is shown bust length, with body turned to the right and head slightly to the right. The atmospheric background is dark brownish-black except for pale grayish-green to the right of the head. The gray hair is brushed away from the face and probably was tied in the back. Under dark eyebrows the round, luminous gray eyes look straight out toward the viewer. The face is round, the nose is straight. The red lips are full and there is a double chin. The subject wears a white stock, a white shirt with a black solitaire tucked into the shirt front, a white waistcoat with an orange-brown design, and a single-breasted, blue coat worn open. The painterly surface is loosely brushed. The head and body are moderately well constructed in three-dimensional volumes. Dr. Hutchinson's portly figure fills the canvas with a sense of his roundness and girth. His facial expression is pleasant and his gaze is direct.

James Howell Hutchinson (1834-1889)

A grandson of James Hutchinson (q.v.), James Howell Hutchinson was born in Cintra, Portugal, where his father was engaged in business. Hutchinson was educated in this country and graduated from the University of Pennsylvania (where he was elected to Phi Beta Kappa) in 1854 and from the medical department of the University in 1858. After studying in Paris and Vienna, he returned to Philadelphia and set up a medical practice. He became physician to the Children's Hospital, Pennsylvania Hospital, and the Hospital of the Protestant Episcopal Church. During the Civil War he was acting assistant surgeon in the United States Army. He was president of the Pathological Society of Philadelphia, vice-president of the College of Physicians (1889), and a member of the American Philosophical Society. He was also a director of the Library Company of Philadelphia, a trustee of the University of Pennsylvania, manager of the University Hospital, and a director of the National Bank of Commerce. He was editor of two editions of Bristowe's *Practice of Medicine*, editor of the *Philadelphia Medical Times*, and a contributor to Pepper and Starr's *System of Medicine*.

Artist: Unknown

Oil on canvas; 29½ x 24½; not signed or dated. Presented by friends in 1890. Closely resembles a three-quarter-length portrait of Hutchinson by Carl Newman at the Pennsylvania Hospital. PA 25

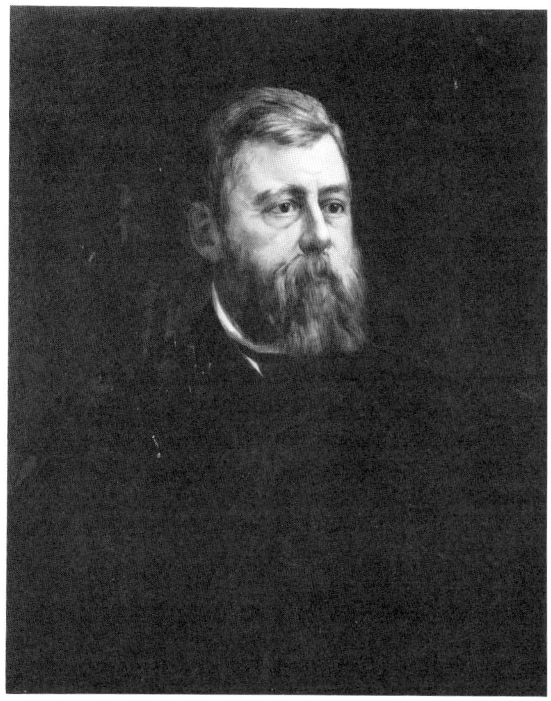

James Howell Hutchinson PA 25

Dr. Hutchinson is shown half length, with body frontal and head turned to the right. The background is dark brown. The most prominent features are the luxuriant grayish-brown hair, side-whiskers, shaggy moustache, and short, square beard. The blue eyes look straight ahead in the direction of the head turn. The brows are knitted, the lower lids are puffy. There are wrinkles at the corners of the eyes and next to the nose. The subject wears a white shirt with a small stand-up collar, a maroon necktie, and a black, single-breasted coat buttoned up to the small notched lapel. In spite of damage and paint loss, the surface of the painting is smoothly brushed, except for visible touches in the hair. The naturalistic rendering of the head is solid and three-dimensional. The costume is flat, with no indication of underlying bodily forms. The stocky upper body of the subject fills the width of the canvas, giving the observer a sense of the subject's immediate physical presence. His facial expression is very serious, almost mournful.

Samuel Jackson (1787-1872)

The son of a physician, Jackson was born in Philadelphia. While working at his father's apothecary shop, he attended the University of Pennsylvania and received the M.D. degree in 1808. During the War of 1812 he served with the First Troop Philadelphia City Cavalry. After the war he established a medical practice. By 1820 he was chairman of the Board of Health and organized the efforts against the yellow fever epidemic of that year. He was a founder of the Philadelphia College of Pharmacy and was its first professor of materia medica (1821). His association with Dr. Nathaniel Chapman (q.v.) started that same year when he became a lecturer at Chapman's summer school, the Medical Institute of Philadelphia. In 1827 he became an assistant to Dr. Chapman at the University of Pennsylvania and lectured on institutes of medicine (physiology). He was professor of this subject from 1835 to 1863. His lectures in the wards of the Philadelphia Hospital attracted many students. He was one of the physicians who fought the cholera epidemic of 1832 most actively. His medical writings include many articles on yellow fever, cholera, and pulmonary diseases. His best known work is *Principles of Medicine, Founded on the Structure and Functions of the Animal Organisms* (1832). Jackson was a member of the College of Physicians, the American Philosophical Society, and other learned societies.

Artist: Daniel Huntington (1816-1906)

Born in New York City, Huntington studied at Yale and at Hamilton College, where he met a portrait painter, Charles Loring Elliott, who encouraged him to become an artist. In 1836 he went to New York and studied with Samuel F. B. Morse and Henry Inman. He studied abroad in 1839, traveled to Rome (1842-45), and worked in England (1851-58,

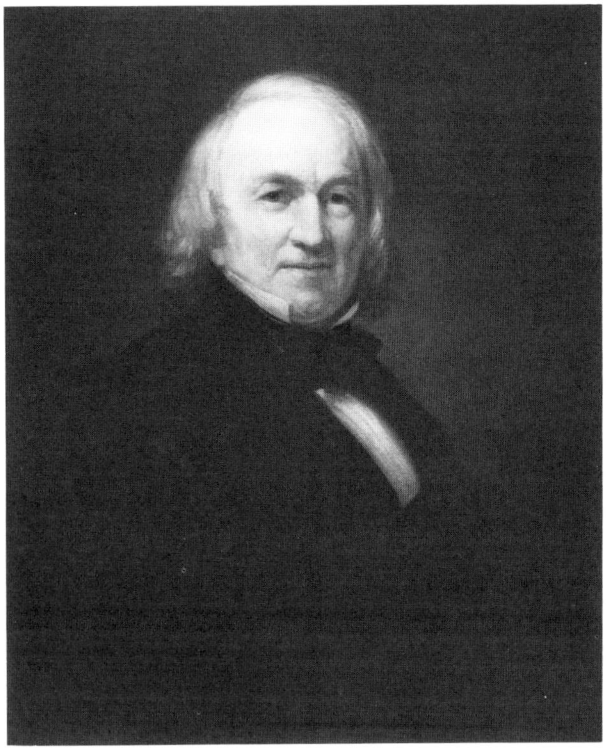

Samuel Jackson *PA 65*

1882). Huntington produced more than 1000 portraits, in addition to landscapes, genre paintings, religious works, and illustrations from literature. Although his style of portraiture changed from one of liveliness and animation to a dry and stiff manner, he was sought after by persons prominent in business, professional life, and social affairs, and he is said to have become wealthy. In Philadelphia he exhibited at the Pennsylvania Academy of the Fine Arts with the Artists' Fund Society from 1842 to 1845 and at the Academy annuals frequently between 1843 and 1868. He was made an honorary member of the Academy in 1854. He exhibited at the National Academy of Design annuals every year from 1836 to 1900, always represented by at least two works, and once by fourteen. He was elected an associate member in 1840 and a member in 1841, and he served the organization as its president from 1862 to 1870 and 1877 to 1890. He was also a vice-president of the Metropolitan Museum of Art from 1870 to 1903.

Oil on canvas mounted on board; 29 1/2 x 24 1/2; initials in lower right corner almost indecipherable [D.H.?]. Presented by Mrs. M.M. Jackson, date unrecorded but prior to 1887, when the portrait appeared in the College of Physicians' Centennial Celebration Loan Collection of Portraits *and was owned by the College then.* *PA 65*

Dr. Jackson is shown bust length, with body turned to the right and head almost frontal, turned slightly to the right. The atmospheric background is mostly dark greenish-brown but is lighter grayish-green around the head. The straight, collar-length hair is whitish-blond. The brown eyes look straight ahead. The nose has a bump on its bridge. The lips are slightly parted. The oval face has a cleft chin and there is a deep dimple in the left cheek. The subject wears a white shirt with stand-up collar, a black neckcloth tied in a bow, a black waistcoat, and a black coat. The style of painting is smooth in the background and costume, with more visible brush strokes in the face and hair. There is no sense of bodily forms under the flat costume. In spite of repeated restoration, the facial expression retains a pleasant, direct, almost conversational quality. It cannot be known whether the artist ever fully accorded to his subject the vivacious personality and sparkling eyes mentioned by biographers.

Thomas Chalkley James (1766–1835)

Descended from English Quakers, James was born in Philadelphia, the son of a leading merchant. He studied medicine under Dr. Adam Kuhn (q.v.) and then at the University of the State of Pennsylvania, where he received the Bachelor of Medicine degree in 1787 and the Doctor of Medicine degree in 1811. Heeding the advice of Philip Syng Physick (q.v.) to study abroad, James went to London in 1792 and became a pupil of John Hunter (q.v.) at St. George's Hospital. He studied obstetrics at Story Street Lying-in Hospital and continued his studies in Edinburgh in 1792–93. After his return to Philadelphia he established a practice and began his first course of lectures in obstetrics in 1802. The lectures were continued at the University of Pennsylvania starting in 1810, the first time such a course had ever been offered there. In 1807 Dr. James was appointed physician to the Pennsylvania Hospital. In 1810, at his own request, he was transferred to the post of obstetrician. He was also physician to the Philadelphia Dispensary. He was president of the Philadelphia College of Surgeons and a member of the American Philosophical Society. He served the College of Physicians as treasurer, secretary, vice-president, and president (1835). In 1810 he read a paper about the first successful artificial induction of premature labor in a case of contracted pelvis. He was an editor of the *Eclectic Repertory*, a journal of abstracts from foreign medical journals. He commanded a knowledge of classical and modern languages and published anonymous verses and essays.

Artist: Attributed to Waugh

For biographies, see page 44.

Oil on canvas; 35 1/2 x 28 1/2; not signed or dated. Presented by Dr. George B. Wood in 1866. Shown in the College of Physicians' Centennial Celebration Loan Collection of Portraits, *1887, with the designation, "Artist. Waugh. Copy of small painting by Wood [presumably Joseph Wood, the Miniaturist, 1778–1830] Owner, College of Physicians." Later inventories and catalogues list the artist as Ida Waugh or Samuel B. Waugh, but no document yet uncovered substantiates either attribution. The College of Physicians owns two engravings of James by John Neagle after Wood, one published by S.C. Atkinson for the* Casket, *the other published by Joseph Delaplaine and printed by Harrison and Porter; the painting resembles a portrait of James at the University of Pennsylvania in which his right arm is not shown.* *PA 16*

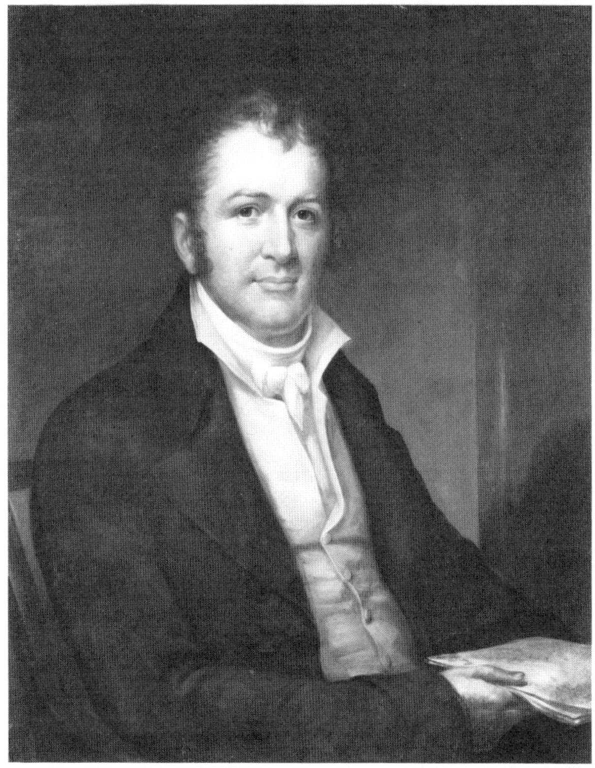

Thomas Chalkley James *PA 16*

Dr. James is shown half-length, the body turned to the right, the head almost frontal, slightly to the right. He is seated in a red upholstered, low-backed, Empire-style chair. His right arm, which rests on the chair arm, sweeps across his body; his right hand holds a sheaf of papers. The vaguely architectural background is maroonish-brown on the left and lighter buff color on the right, with a curving dark maroon shadow on the lower right. The subject has brown hair, falling in wisps on his high forehead, and long side-whiskers. His blue eyes look straight ahead toward the viewer. His face is round, the nose is straight. The lips are full and the complexion florid. He wears a white shirt, a white neckcloth tied in a bow (slightly askew), a yellow waistcoat with a high stand-up collar, and a dark green double-breasted coat with M-notched lapels and wide cuffs. The surface of the portrait is smoothly brushed. The head is well constructed in a solid, three-dimensional way and there is suggestion of the body mass underlying the costume. Dr. James's pleasant expression and direct gaze produce an aura of well-being and confidence.

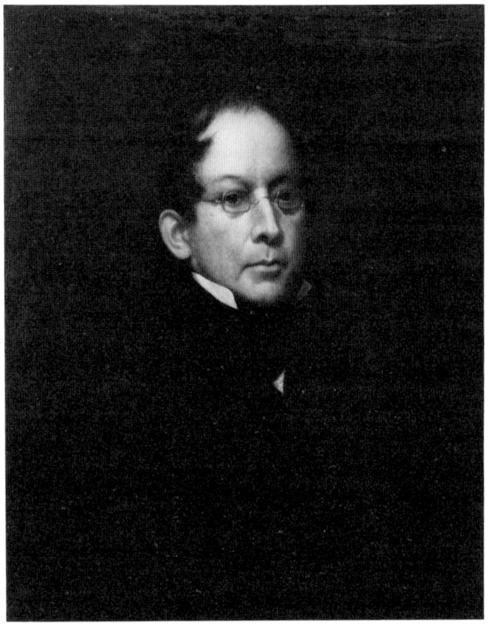

Benjamin Say Janney *PA 95*

Benjamin Say Janney (1790 or 1799–1859)

Descended from English Quakers who came to Pennsylvania in 1683, Janney was born in Lower Merion, Pennsylvania. After graduating from the Jesuits College in Baltimore, he came to Philadelphia. He entered the Pennsylvania Hospital as an apprentice and studied at the University of Pennsylvania under Benjamin Rush (q.v.). He received the M.D. degree in 1813. After a few disheartening attempts in several locales, he succeeded in establishing in Philadelphia a large medical practice, which lasted for almost half a century until the very day of his death. He was a fellow of the College of Physicians of Philadelphia, a vice president of the Philadelphia County Medical Association, and a delegate in 1859 to the Medical Society of the State of Pennsylvania. He was a founder and president of the Northern Medical Association, the organization which founded the Episcopal Hospital to serve the northern section of Philadelphia, and he was a manager of the Episcopal Hospital.

Artist: Unknown

Oil on canvas, backed with wood; 26 1/4 x 21 1/4; not signed or dated. Presented by Mrs. Gertrude Bolles in 1934.
PA 95

Dr. Janney is shown bust length, with head and body turned slightly to the right. The background is dark brown. The hair is thin and dark brown with two eccentrically placed clumps brushed onto the forehead. The light brown eyes look straight out through metal-rimmed spectacles in the direction of the head turn. The nose is straight, the mouth is full, and the chin is square. The subject wears a white shirt with stand-up collar, a black neckcloth, and a black coat. Because of damage and subsequent overpainting, the original quality of the surface is difficult to assess. At present the portrait appears smoothly painted throughout. The head is solid and three-dimensional, although features and some contours are blurred. The costume is so flat and dark that it is scarcely distinguishable from the background. The facial expression is neutral and remote. The blurred, somewhat hazy surface and the veiled expression could be due to the fact that this portrait was not painted from life. In fact, it closely resembles a work in the collection of the College of Physicians, an engraving signed by A.B. Walters (1820–1875), after a daguerreotype by Richards.

Edward Jenner (1749–1823)

Born in Berkeley, Gloucestershire, Jenner was the son of a country vicar. He began his medical education as apprentice to a surgeon in Sodbury. Coming to London to study at St. George's Hospital, he was a house pupil of John Hunter (q.v.), who became his devoted friend and who directed his zoological experiments that won him election to the Royal Society in 1789. He received the M.D. from St. Andrew's University in 1792. While establishing a medical practice in Berkeley, Jenner started to investigate smallpox, a disease constantly prevalent in England. Jenner discovered that persons who had had cowpox could not be inoculated successfully for smallpox, and he surmised that cowpox should give complete and permanent immunity to smallpox. In 1796 he inoculated an eight-year-old boy with

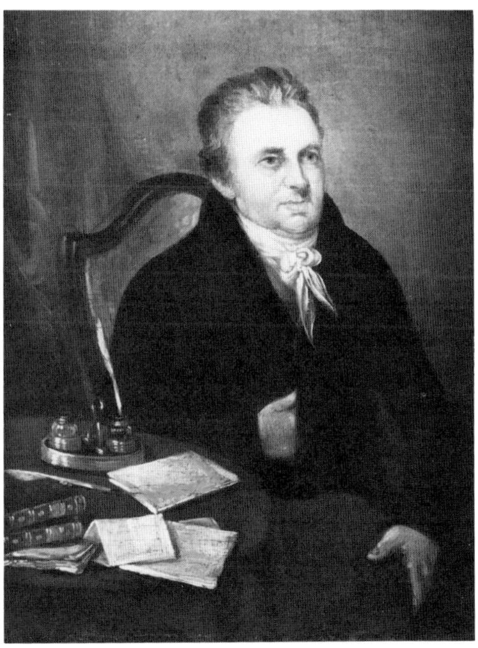

Edward Jenner *PA 101*

matter from a cowpox lesion taken from a dairymaid's hand. Two months later the boy was inoculated with smallpox, but the disease did not follow. In 1797 he offered a short treatise on his work to the Royal College of Surgeons, but the paper was refused. He published his results privately in 1798, under the title *An Inquiry into the Causes and Effects of the Variolae Vaccinae a disease discovered in some of the Western Counties of England particularly Gloucestershire, and known by the name of the Cow Pox.* Although controversial at first, by 1800 the concept was accepted in England and spread throughout Europe and the Americas. He received two grants of £10,000 from Parliament to compensate for time spent away from his practice in experimentation, inoculation, and subsequent voluminous correspondence. In 1803 the Royal Jennerian Society was founded, later to be replaced by the National Vaccine Establishment. In the garden of the vicarage where he lived in Berkeley, Jenner built a "Temple of Vaccinia," which he used as a surgery for vaccinating the poor. He received an honorary degree from Oxford University in 1813.

Artist: Unknown

Oil on canvas; 9 3/4 x 7 1/2; not signed or dated. Presented by heirs of Mrs. Louisa Webb in 1912. Shown in College of Physicians' Centennial Celebration Loan Collection of Portraits, *1887; the owner was Dr. William H. Webb.*
PA 101

Jenner is shown two-thirds length, seated, with body and head turned to the right. His right hand reaches under one flap of his coat. His left hand appears to be resting on an object which is unidentifiable because of paint loss; it could be the knee of a crossed leg. The complex setting includes red drapery on the upper left side of this small painting, a Hepplewhite-style shield-back armchair upholstered in red, a round table covered in green cloth, and objects on the table, including a silver and glass writing stand, two quills, two books, and four sheaves of paper. The subject has brown hair brushed away from his face, gray eyes which look straight out in the direction of the head turn, a straight nose, a full lower lip, and prominent jowls. He wears a white shirt, a white neckcloth tied in a bow, a red waistcoat, and a black coat with shawl collar. Although there has been much loss of paint and much repainting, the surface of the portrait appears smoothly brushed. The head is only moderately well constructed. The hands are awkwardly placed and partly hidden. The costume is flat, with no indication of the underlying body. The subject's expression is neutral and his gestures conventional, as he turns away from the table. The objects on the table, which suggest the writing of his important treatise, are treated in such detail that they detract attention from the figure.

John Jones (1729–1791)

The son, grandson, and great-grandson of Welsh Quaker physicians, Jones was born in Jamaica, Long Island. After studying medicine with his cousin, Dr. Thomas Cadwalader (q.v.) of Philadelphia, he spent three years abroad. He studied in London with William Cheselden, Percival Pott, and William Hunter; he also studied in Paris, Leyden, and Edinburgh. He received the M.D. degree from the University of Rheims in 1751. After returning to New York he began a surgical practice and was appointed army surgeon in the colonial campaign against the French. He was the first professor of surgery at the newly opened medical department of King's College (1767) and was a co-founder of New York Hospital. It is said that he was the first surgeon in New York to perform a lithotomy. The first book on surgery written in the United States was his treatise, *Plain Remarks upon Wounds and Fractures designed for the Use of Young Military Surgeons of America,* published in 1775. He organized the medical department of the revolutionary army in 1777–78 and was transferred to Philadelphia, where he remained after the war. He was made physician to Pennsylvania Hospital, first president of the Humane Society, and consulting physician to the Philadelphia Dispensary. He was a member of the American Philosophical Society and a founding senior fellow and vice president of the College of Physicians. He was an intimate friend and physician of Benjamin Franklin and was the physician of George Washington when the government was situated in Philadelphia.

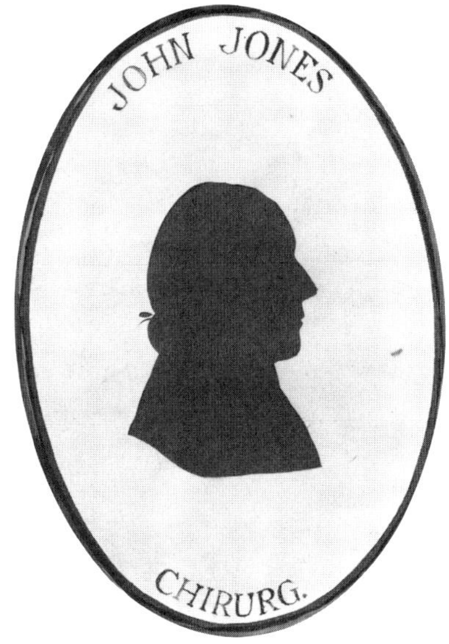

John Jones *PH 577*

Artist: Unknown

Silhouette, negative image cut out of white paper, pasted onto gray paper so that the figure is dark; oval, 6 x 4; not signed or dated. Presented by Dr. Samuel X. Radbill in 1946.
PH 577

Dr. Jones is shown bust length, with profile to the right. The once-white paper background is now grayish. Inscriptions printed in black ink are, "JOHN JONES" above the figure and "CHIRURG." below the figure. There are smooth contours to his hair, which is tied at the nape of his neck in a bow. The features are regular and not strongly individualized. No details of costume are indicated. The lower edge of the silhouette is pointed at the ends, with a wide V-shaped curve in the center.

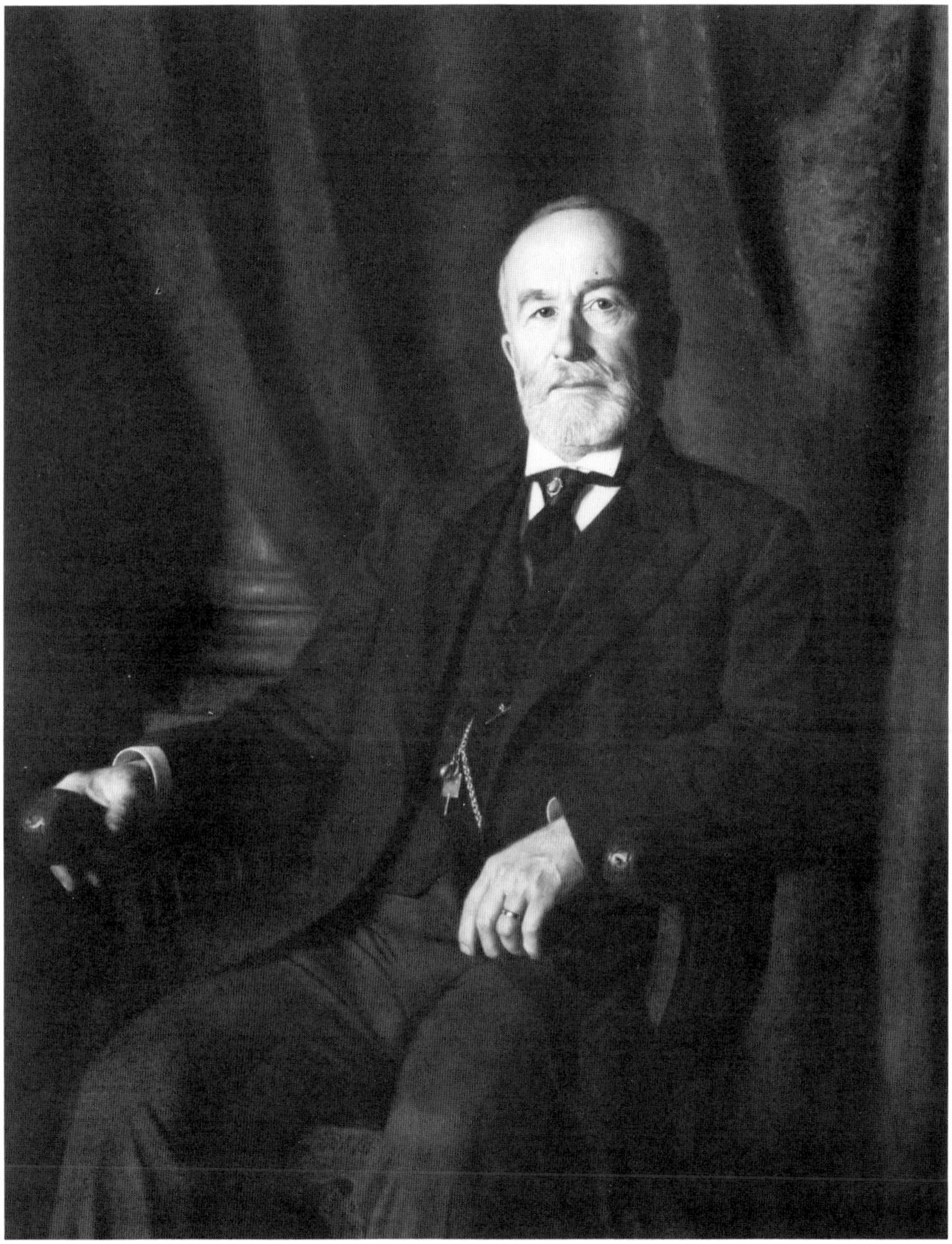

William Williams Keen *PA 75*

William Williams Keen (1837-1932)

Descended from Swedish settlers who came to Fort Christina on the Delaware in 1643, Keen was born in Philadelphia. He was graduated from Brown University in 1859 and entered Jefferson Medical College in 1860. His medical studies were interrupted when he was asked to serve as surgeon to the Fifth Massachusetts Regiment in the Civil War. Following his discharge after the Battle of Bull Run, he returned to Jefferson and received his M.D. in 1862. Two months later he was commissioned as acting assistant surgeon in the U.S. Army and was in charge of hospitals in Washington, D.C., and Maryland before being assigned to Satterlee Hospital in Philadelphia. From there he was transferred to the Christian Street Hospital, where he worked with S. Weir Mitchell (q.v.) and George R. Morehouse on studies of nerve injuries and co-authored with them the classic monograph, "Gunshot Wounds and Other Injuries of Nerves" (1864). Keen next spent two years abroad doing postgraduate work in Paris and with Virchow in Berlin. Returning to Philadelphia in 1866, he lectured on surgical pathology at Jefferson. Soon after, he became head of the Philadelphia School of Anatomy until it dissolved in 1875. He taught artistic as well as descriptive and surgical anatomy, and later he became professor of artistic anatomy at the Pennsylvania Academy of the Fine Arts. He was professor of surgery at the Woman's Medical College in 1884 and at Jefferson from 1889 until 1907, when he became emeritus professor. Keen was not only an excellent lecturer and popular teacher, but was also a bold and

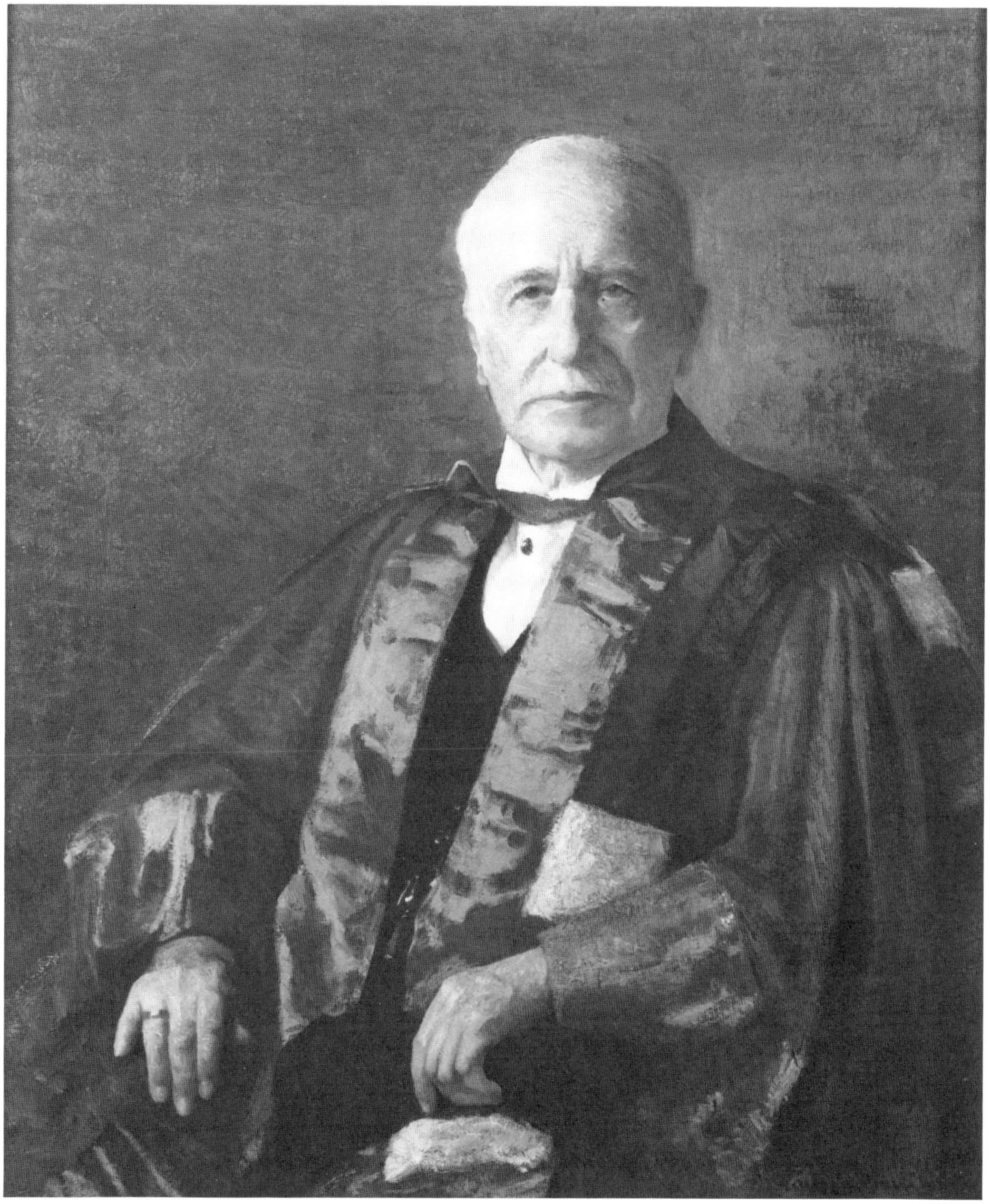

William Williams Keen *PA 29*

innovative surgeon. He was the first in Philadelphia to use Lister's methods of antiseptic surgery, introducing it at St. Mary's Hospital. At St. Mary's in 1887 he performed the first successful operation in the United States for removal of a brain tumor. His efforts to improve the techniques of brain surgery led him to use the osteoplastic flap rather than the simple incision, to use electrical stimulation of the cerebral cortex to aid in localization of the tumor, and to use bone chips to fill the skull defect. Other contributions to neurosurgery included performing cerebral surgery for focal epilepsy, treating tic douloureux by removing the Gasserian ganglion, devising an operation for spasmodic torticollis, tapping the cerebral ventricles, suturing nerves, surgically treating brain abscesses, and performing the first operation in America to correct microcephaly. In general surgery he was noted for his work in hepatic tumors and was one of the first four surgeons to do cholecystotomy. In 1893 he assisted Dr. Joseph Bryant in the successful removal of a cancerous tumor from the jaw of President Grover Cleveland, the operation being conducted in utmost secrecy aboard a private yacht in Long Island Sound. Recognized as a leader in surgery both in this country and abroad, he served as president of the American Surgical Association, the American Medical Association, the Philadelphia Academy of Surgery, the American Philosophical Society, the International Society of Surgery, and the College of Physicians (1900–01). In addition, he had honorary fellowships in many foreign surgical societies and received honorary degrees from major universities in the United States, Canada, Great

Britain, and Europe. He was the first recipient of the Colver-Rosenberger Medal of Honor awarded by Brown University (of which he was a trustee), and he also received the Bigelow Medal of the Boston Surgical Society. His literary output was great and spanned a period of 65 years. He wrote works on religion, medical history, and education; he wrote for the popular media as well as for the scholarly press. Works for the latter included editing two editions of *Gray's Anatomy,* an edition with J.W. White of *An American Text-book of Surgery* (1892), and an edition with John Chalmers da Costa of volumes IV and V of the eight-volume work, *Surgery, Its Principles and Practice* (1906–21).

Artist: James Longacre Wood (1867–1938)

Descended from a distinguished medical family, James L. Wood was born in Philadelphia, the son of Dr. Horatio C Wood (q.v.). He was the grandson of James Barton Longacre (1794–1869), who served as chief engraver of the U.S. Mint and engraver (after original portraits) for John Sanderson's *Biographies of the Signers of the Declaration of Independence* (1820–27). He collaborated with James Herring in *The National Portrait Gallery of Distinguished Americans* (1833). Records at the Pennsylvania Academy of the Fine Arts reveal that James L. Wood studied in the antique class in 1881 and 1883 and in the life class in 1885. The circular of the Committee on Instruction of 1882–83 instituted a new regulation that students had to be at least sixteen years of age, and Wood was ineligible in 1882. He attended a summer session at the University of Pennsylvania in 1884. Later he continued his studies in Paris. He was a student of Gustave Boulanger and Jules Joseph Lefebvre at the Académie Julien when he matriculated at the École des Beaux Arts in February, 1888. He was then enrolled in the atelier of Jean Léon Gérôme in March, 1888, and he remained there at least until July 11, 1890, when he won an honorable mention for studio work. According to information obtained through correspondence with Professor H. Barbara Weinberg of Queens College, New, York, and from her article, "Nineteenth Century American Painters at the École des Beaux Arts" (*American Art Journal,* Autumn, 1981), he may still have been a matriculate at the École in February, 1891. Wood returned to Philadelphia and was appointed to the art department of Drexel University, which was inaugurated in 1891 or 1892 and lasted until 1905. At Drexel he taught drawing from the antique from 1892 on, artistic anatomy from 1896 on, and art history from 1899 on, and he is known to have been one of several faculty members who gave free public lectures on the history of art in the late 1890s. Starting in 1893, Wood is listed in the Gopsill's *Philadelphia City Directory* as "artist," with separate addresses for his home and work. He exhibited work at the Pennsylvania Academy annuals in 1893, 1896–97, and 1899 and at the Art Club of Philadelphia almost yearly from 1892 to 1904. Although he painted some landscapes and genre scenes, he is best known as a portrait painter in the naturalistic tradition of his Parisian teachers and of Thomas Eakins, with whom he probably studied at the Academy. He also studied with Eakins at the Art Students' League after the latter's dismissal from the Academy in 1866. Lloyd Goodrich adds that Eakins painted Wood's portrait about 1890, but that it has since "disappeared" (*Thomas Eakins: His Life and Work,* 1933). In addition to the portraits at the College of Physicians are portraits of Doctors Harrison Allen, Horatio C Wood, John Ashhurst, and Joseph Leidy at the University of Pennsylvania, additional portraits of Leidy at the Historical Society of Pennsylvania and the American Philosophical Society, and a portrait of D. Hayes Agnew at Mercersberg Academy. None of these portraits is dated later than 1905. Although additional genre scenes and landscapes are extant and perhaps other portraits are included in family collections, Wood's public career seems to have ended abruptly at this time. Family members say that his deafness had increased steadily and that in spite of loving attention from his wife and daughter, he became more reclusive in later years. His wife died in 1923 in Milford, Pennsylvania, an area in which Wood is known to have owned a working farm and where he served as a part-time lay minister in a Methodist church.

Oil on canvas; 46 1/2 x 36 1/2; signed and dated lower right, "J.L. Wood 1901." Presented by fellows of the College, 1902. *PA 75*

Dr. Keen is shown three-quarters length, the body turned to the left, the head almost frontal and tilted to the right. He is seated in a low-backed, Renaissance revival-style armchair, with both his arms resting on the chair arms, the right hand grasping the hand hold, and the left hand hanging loosely from the wrist. His legs are spread apart. The interior setting includes a maroon drapery which falls in curving folds behind the figure from upper left to lower right and the base of a reddish column whose shaft is largely hidden by the curtain. The atmospheric space on the left is dark reddish-brown. The subject has sparse, dark gray hair and lighter gray, neatly trimmed side-whiskers, a moustache, and a short beard. His small gray eyes look out in the direction of the head turn and slightly upward. His face is oval. His nose has a pronounced bump. His mouth is wide. He is dressed impeccably in a white shirt with wing collar, a black necktie, a black vest, black trousers, and a black double-breasted cutaway coat with wide lapels; he wears a jeweled tie pin, a gold ring, and a gold watch chain with two gold ornaments, which perhaps are medals. The smooth paint style of the portrait shows meticulous brush strokes. The solid volumes of head, hands, and body underlying the costume gives the illusion of being three-dimensional. The planes of each shape are carefully modeled in light and shadow. The composition is tightly knit, with the diagonals of the drapery countered by the opposing diagonal of the figure. Keen's posture is erect, somewhat tense, and full of energy. His eyes do not engage the viewer but gaze past him. It is the viewer who regards the subject, not vice versa. The high-fashioned chair, column, and drapery, combined with the subject's posture and elegant attire, suggest his education, high status, and professional accomplishments.

Artist: Robert William Vonnoh (1858–1933)

For biography, see page 31.

Oil on canvas; 35 1/2 x 29 1/2; signed and dated lower right, "Vonnoh Phila. 1925." Presented by the daughters of Dr. Keen in 1925. On the back of the painting are four labels, two which do not mention an exhibiting institution. The other two are from the Art Alliance of Philadelphia (no date), and the Pennsylvania Academy of the Fine Arts Annual Exhibition *of 1926.* *PA 29*

Dr. Keen is shown two-thirds length, seated, with body turned to the left and head almost frontal. His left hand holds a black academic hat, while his right hand rests on his thigh. The mottled background is a dusky warm pink underneath, covered by a thick, green layer above. The subject has a high forehead, sparse white hair on head and eyebrows, and a trim moustache. His small, hooded brown eyes look straight ahead. His long nose has a bump at the bridge. The mouth is wide. The rectangular face has deep lines between the eyes and next to the nose. The subject wears a white shirt with wing collar, a black vest with ornamented gold watch chain, a white necktie with red tie tack, a gold ring, and the brilliant red academic robe of the University of St. Andrew with red-orange highlights and bands of blue and white trim. The bands of white fur are the "epitoga" of the *doctor honoris causa* of the University of Paris. The painterly, almost impressionistic surface of the portrait is composed of broad strokes throughout. The head and hands are moderately well constructed in three-dimensional solidity. The warmth and mottled strokes of the background bring it forward and do not suggest atmospheric space. The brilliant color, voluminous folds, wide base, deep shadows, and bright highlights of the costume project it forward and attract the viewer's attention at the expense of the subject. The all-over use of green, both in the background and as shadows in the face, hands, and shirt collar, also serve to unite the background and the figure on very close planes of depth. Keen's posture is erect. His knitted brows and tight lips give him a serious, tense expression. The head turn allows him to gaze directly at the viewer in a way that is almost challenging.

Artist: Samuel Aloysius Murray (1870–1941)

For biography, see page 3.

Plaster, painted grayish-bronze color; 15 3/8 x 8 1/2 x 9 1/4; square base 1 1/2 in. high, integral with sculpture; mounted on pedestal 11 1/4 in. high, with inscription, "W.W.KEEN./ SVRGEON"; signed and dated on rear of head, "S. Murray/ 1920." Presented by Mrs. Samuel Murray, through Dr. William N. Bradley in 1942. *ST 554*

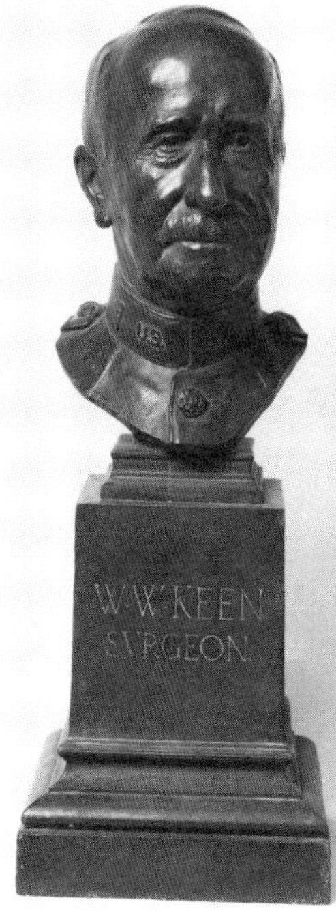

William Williams Keen *ST 554*

Keen is shown head-and-neck length, with head turned slightly to the right. He has a receding hairline, with thin hair and a trim moustache. His small eyes, which have carved irises and pupils and deeply lined corners and lower lids, look straight ahead to the viewer. The ears are long and narrow. The nose has a pronounced bump in the center and is slightly out of alignment. The wide mouth has a thin upper lip. The face is narrow, the chin is square, and there are deeply set lines next to the nose and mouth. The abbreviated shoulder and chest area, which slightly overhangs the base, was included to show the subject's military uniform with its high round collar decorated with the initials *U.S.*, the caduceus, and eagle-emblazoned buttons. The surface of the sculpture is smooth in the head, textured in the uniform. Subtly modeled planes define the shape of the solid, anatomically convincing head. The naturalistic style emphasizes Keen's strongly individualistic features. His expression is serious, yet full of energy and vitality.

Artist: Robert Tait McKenzie (1867–1938)

For biography, see page 45.

Plaster of Paris death mask, white; 10 x 7 x 6 3/4; signed and dated on rear, "Dr. William Williams Keen Aet. 95/Taken 12 hrs. P.M./ By R. Tait McKenzie June 28, 1932." Presented in 1964 by Dr. Samuel Sturgis (q.v.), to whom it was given by Mrs. William Williams Keen, with the written stipulation that it be given to the College of Physicians "not earlier than 1960." *ST 566*

This death mask shows Keen at the age of 95 with very sparse hair on his head, eyebrows, and moustache. There are deep hollows under the closed eyes. The hook of the nose forces it out of alignment and is even more

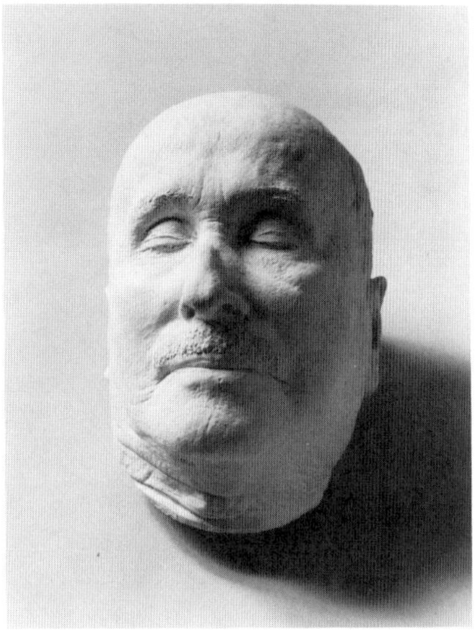

William Williams Keen *ST 566*

pronounced than in the Murray bust or the Wood and Vonnoh paintings. The mouth is wide, the chin is square, and the neck is deeply lined. The surface of the mask has a very even, grainy, uniform texture except for the areas with hair. Even though every detail is paradigmatically specific and unique to this subject, somehow the stark, white color and relaxation of the features give the image a timeless quality.

Richard Arminius Kern (1891-1982)

Dr. Kern was born in Columbia, Pennsylvania, the son of a minister. He received the A.B. degree at the University of Pennsylvania in 1910 and the M.D. in 1914. At the university he was successively instructor in medicine, associate, assistant professor, and professor of clinical medicine (1934–46). He was physician to the Hospital of the University of Pennsylvania and chief of the medical outpatient department and allergy section there; he organized its first allergy clinic in 1920. He was also professor of clinical medicine at the Graduate School of Medicine of the University of Pennsylvania. After World War II, he transferred to Temple University School of Medicine and Hospital where he was professor of medicine and head of the department of medicine from 1946 to 1956. He became professor emeritus in 1956. Dr. Kern also had a distinguished military career. During World War I he served with the navy medical corps on the U.S. hospital ship, *Solace*. In 1935 he organized a group of University of Pennsylvania colleagues into the Medical Specialists Unit Number 31 of the navy reserve. It was called to active duty in 1942. Kern was made the chief of medical service aboard the *Solace*, which both evacuated and treated patients in battle zones in the South Pacific. In 1943 Kern was promoted to commodore and assigned as medical consultant to the staff of Admiral William Halsey, who wrote a letter of commendation in his honor. He also received a Distinguished Public Service Medal from the Department of Defense. After the war he served as consultant with the Surgeons General of the Army and Navy, the Armed Forces Institute of Pathology, the Department of Defense Science Board, the Office of Emergency Preparedness, and the Committee on Naval Medical Research of the National Research Council. He received letters of commendation from Secretary Thomas for his work with the Naval Reserve and from Secretary Forrestal for rehabilitation work at the Philadelphia Naval Hospital. Dr. Kern was chairman of the Joint Committee on Accreditation of Hospitals and president of the Board of Health of the City of Philadelphia, the Philadelphia County Medical Society, the Pennsylvania Medical Society, the Association of Military Surgeons, the American College of Physicians, the International Society of Internal Medicine, the Association for the Study of Allergy, the Society for the Study of Asthma and Allied Conditions, and the College of Physicians of Philadelphia (1952–54). In addition to contributing articles to numerous journals, he served as editor of the *American Journal of Medical Sciences* and *Military Medicine*. He received the Mastership and the Alfred Stengel awards of the American College of Physicians. He was co-winner of the Casselbery award of the American Laryngological Association. He received the Strittmatter award of the Philadelphia County Medical Society and honorary degrees from Temple University, Bucknell University, Franklin and Marshall College, and Lebanon Valley College.

Artist: Harry S. Moskovitz (1894–1956)

Moskovitz was born in Philadelphia and studied at the Graphic Sketch Club and the School of Industrial Art. He continued his training abroad at the Beaune Art School in France and at the Hilde School in Germany. During World War I he served in the 54th Pioneer Infantry with the American Expeditionary Force in the Meuse-Argonne offensive. After the war he was an instructor in art in the Third Army Troop Education Center in Coblentz. For this work he received official commendation. He was portrait painter to many distinguished citizens, including Presidents Franklin Delano Roosevelt and Harry S. Truman, Justice H. Edgar Barnes, Cardinal Dougherty, Samuel S. Fleisher, the Honorable James Putnam Goodrich, Ellis Gimbel, Henry Kaiser, Frederick H. Ecker, A. Lawrence Lowell, Jay Chapman Root, Justice Nelson Sharpe, Samuel Price Wetherill, Peter A. B. Widener, James M. Willcox, and Admiral David Taylor. His works can be found in many government and corporate buildings and in private collections.

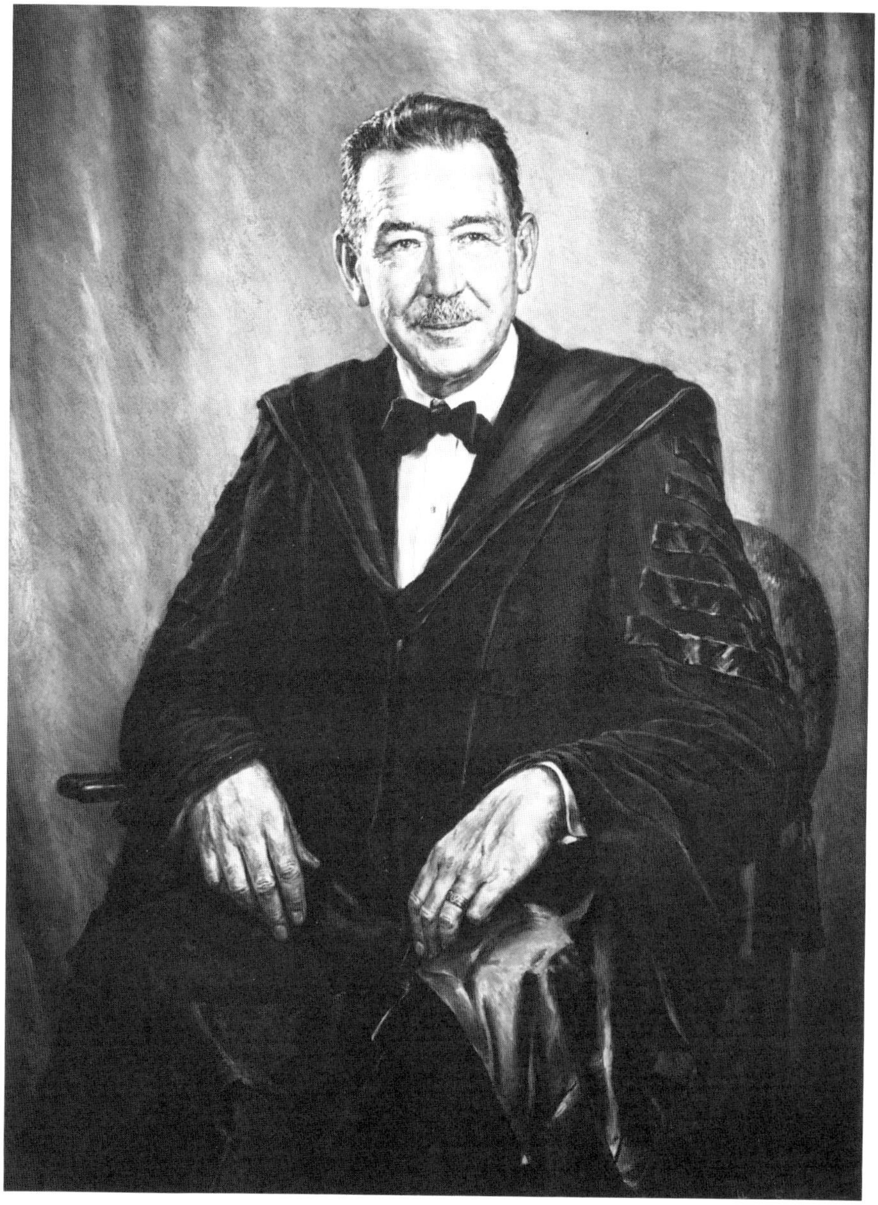

Richard Arminius Kern PA 121

Oil on canvas; 47 1/4 x 35 1/4; signed and dated lower right, "Harry S. Moskovitz.1953." Label on back of canvas gives artist's name, his Philadelphia address, and information that he does "portrait painting and portrait etching." Presented by Dr. Richard A. Kern in 1953. *PA 121*

Dr. Kern is shown three-quarters length, with body turned slightly to the left and head almost frontal and tilted to the right. He is seated in an upholstered armchair with the green tassel of his mortarboard hanging over the rounded chair back. His arms rest on the chair arms; the hands bend loosely at the wrists. The yellow-green background is non-specific but is suggestive of drapery. The subject has wavy brown hair and a brush moustache. His small brown eyes look in the direction of the head turn. His nose is broad. His thin lips form a pleasant smile. Details include wavy horizontal lines in his forehead, wrinkles around his eyes, deep furrows next to his nose, and dimples in his cheeks. He wears a white shirt, a black bow tie, a gold ring, and a black academic robe whose wide sleeves are lined in bright green and have five green horizontal stripes on the upper half and green vertical panels in the front. The V-shaped hood has alternating red and green sections. The surface of the painting uses both smooth and painterly brushwork. The head and hands are rendered in solid, three-dimensional volumes, and there is a sense of bodily forms underlying the costume. The anatomy of the head and hands are treated in ultra-linear detail, not surprising for a painter who was also an etcher. The amount of detail, combined with the conventional studio pose and expression and the bright light source from front and left—there are two highlights in each eye—give the portrait a photographic quality.

Thomas Story Kirkbride (1809-1883)

Descended from English Quakers who came to America with William Penn, Dr. Kirkbride was born on a farm near Morrisville, Pennsylvania. He graduated with honors from the medical department

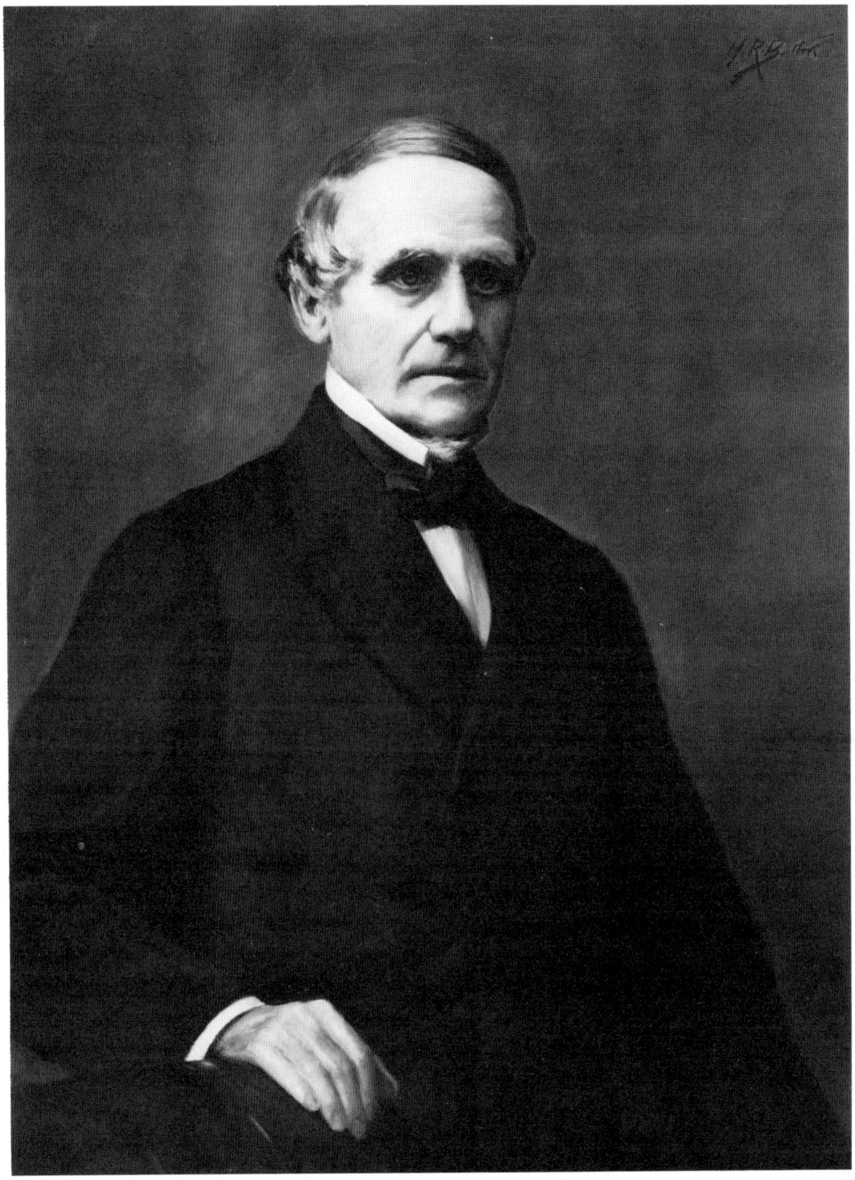

Thomas Story Kirkbride *PA 79*

of the University of Pennsylvania in 1832. He was appointed resident physician to the Friends Asylum for the Insane and to the Pennsylvania Hospital, where he directed the treatment of the mentally ill. When he left the Pennsylvania Hospital in 1835 to set up a medical practice, he already had a large reputation in the treatment of insanity. He was named physician to the House of Refuge, the Magdalen Hospital, and the Institute for the Blind. In 1840, when the new building of the Pennsylvania Hospital for the Insane was erected, Kirkbride was elected physician-in-chief and superintendent; he held these posts until his death. He was a founder of the Association of Medical Superintendents of American Institutions for the Insane, its first secretary and treasurer, and later its president. In addition to being a fellow of the College of Physicians, he was a member of the American Philosophical Society and an honorary member of the British Medico-Psychological Association. He contributed many articles to the medical literature, including *The Construction, Organization and General Arrangement of Hospitals for the Insane* (1856), which made the "Kirkbride Plan" the standard authority for the construction of mental hospitals. He was admired for his executive ability, his devotion to patients, his pedagogic skill, and his advanced ideas regarding insanity as a disease that should be treated in a hospital, not an asylum.

Artist: Howard Russell Butler (1856–1934)

Born in New York, Butler graduated from Princeton University in 1876 and from the Columbia Law School in 1882. He had obtained wide-ranging scientific, commercial, and legal experience before he resolved to pursue an artistic career. He began his studies of art with the landscape painter, Frederick Church, in Mexico. Then he enrolled in the Art Students' League in New York. He spent the next two years studying landscape and figure painting in France, Italy, England, and Holland. After returning to New York in 1887, he became a member of the Society of American Artists and was elected to the Architectural League of New York. He became an associate of the National Academy of Design in 1898 and a full member in 1902; he served as its president from 1916 to 1921. He was a founder of the American Fine Arts Society in 1889 and its president until 1906, and he was the president of the Carnegie Music Hall Association from 1896 to 1905. He moved easily in society, and many of his contacts in art and business developed as a result of his friendship with Andrew Carnegie, whose portrait he painted at least 13 times. He also supervised the building of Carnegie's New York residence. A consistent prize winner at important expositions, he won honorable mention at the Paris salon (1886) and silver medals at the Pennsylvania Academy of Fine Arts (1888), Universal Exposition in Paris (1889), Columbian Exposition in Chicago (1893), Atlanta Exposition (1895), Pan-American Exposition (Buffalo, 1901), and Panama-Pacific Exposition (San Francisco, 1915). He won a bronze medal at the St. Louis Exposition (1904) and the Carnegie prize at the National Academy of Design (1916). Butler painted solar eclipses on three occasions and was appointed supervisor of astronomical exhibits at the American Museum of Natural History in 1925. He was elected a member of the American Astronomical Society. Although he was much in demand as a portraitist, Butler derived the most satisfaction from his seascapes, especially those done from his summer house in East Hampton, Long Island, and those done in California, where he lived for many years.

Oil on canvas; 34 1/2 x 26 1/2; signed upper right, "H.R. Butler." Presented by the family of Dr. Kirkbride in 1898. Must be a copy of an earlier portrait or photograph, since the artist did not begin his studies of art until the year after the subject's death. The face, costume, and pose resemble those in a photograph in the collection of the College of Physicians of Philadelphia. *PA 79*

Dr. Kirkbride is shown half-length with head and body turned to the right. He is depicted standing with his right hand resting on the back of a chair. The atmospheric background is medium-toned umber. His gray hair is brushed across his head and curled forward at the ears. His thick gray eyebrows overhang the deepset, large, grayish-hazel eyes which look in the direction of the head turn. His nose has a broad tip. The lips of the wide mouth are slightly parted. The square face has deep lines in the forehead and next to the nose and mouth. He wears a white shirt with stand-up collar, a black bow tie, and a single-breasted black coat with notched lapels. The surface of the portrait is smoothly brushed. The planes of the head are well modeled in light and shade, making solid and three-dimensional forms. There is a suggestion of the body under the costume. Kirkbride's posture is erect and his expression is dignified and earnest, his lips parted as though he were about to speak.

Edward Bell Krumbhaar (1882-1966)

Descended from a family whose English forbears arrived in America in 1633, Dr. Krumbhaar was born in Philadelphia. He received the A.B. degree from Harvard University (1904) and the M.D. (1908) and the Ph.D. (1916) from the University of Pennsylvania. While a resident physician at the Pennsylvania Hospital, he came under the guiding influence of Warfield T. Longcope, who introduced him to the fields in which he ultimately became famous—physiology and pathology of the heart, and diseases of the blood, spleen, and bone marrow. Krumbhaar was the first in Philadelphia to use the string galvanometer in diagnosing cardiac pathology. He was appointed director of the pathology laboratory at Philadelphia General Hospital and associate professor of pathology at The Graduate School of Medicine of the University of Pennsylvania; he held both positions from 1920 to 1927. He was professor of pathology at the University of Pennsylvania from 1927 to 1948 and became professor emeritus in 1948. During World War I he served in the Medical Corps as major with the Pennsylvania Hospital Unit (U.S. Base Hospital No. 10) at Le Tréport, France, from 1917 to 1919. In addition to his teaching and research, Krumbhaar was editor of the *Journal of the Medical Sciences* (1925-50) and of *Clio Medica*, a series of concise texts on the history of medicine. He served on the editorial boards of *Folio Haematologica*, the *Journal of Clinical Investigation*, and *Annals of Medical History*. He also translated into English several important German and Italian works, notably Arturo Castiglioni's *A History of Medicine*. Krumbhaar was noted also for his contributions to the field of medical history. In 1905, when the College of Physicians founded its section on medical history, he served as chairman. In June, 1924, he organized a meeting at the College to found the American Association of the History of Medicine, which he served as secretary-treasurer and, for two terms, as president. He was a steady contributor of papers and articles on medical history, especially to the *Annals of Medical History*, and he was a frequent delegate to the International Society of the History of Medicine. He was president of the American Association of Pathologists and Bacteriologists, the American Society of Experimental Pathology, the American Association for Cancer Research, the American Heart Association, the Pathological Society of Philadelphia, and the Physiological Society of Philadelphia. He was an honorary fellow of the Royal Society of London and corresponding member of medical societies in Mexico, France, Italy, Spain, and Rumania. Special mention should be made of his contributions to the College of Physicians. In addition to serving on the history of medicine committee, the council, and the library committee, he was president of the College from 1940 to

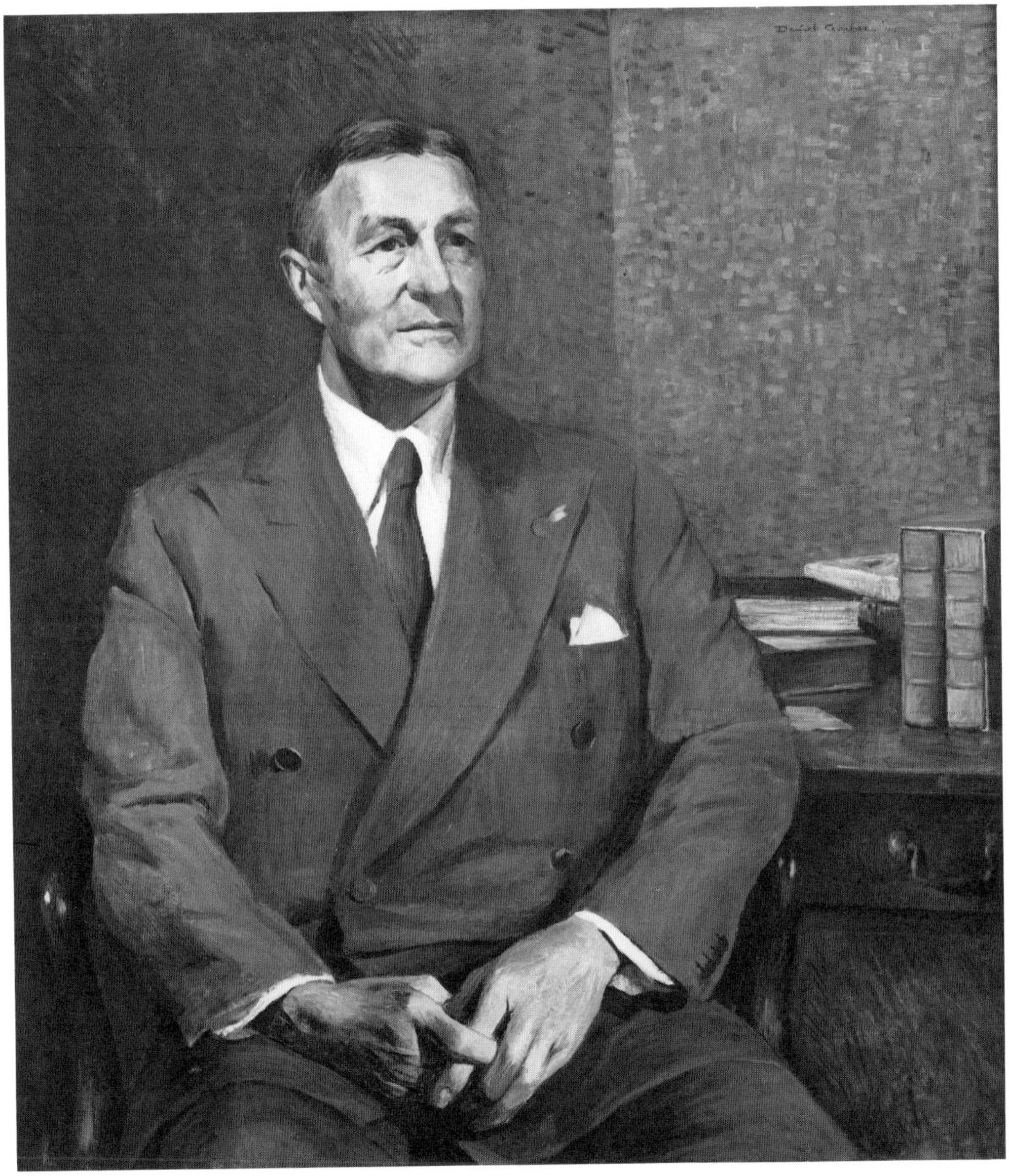

Edward Bell Krumbhaar *PA 114*

1943. His magnanimous donations include rare books, medals, medical instruments, casts, prints, and archival material. In recognition of his contributions, the section on medical history created the Krumbhaar prize in 1957, to be awarded annually to a medical student for accomplishment in the history of medicine.

Artist: Daniel Garber (1880–1958)

For biography, see page 16.

Oil on canvas; 39 1/2 x 35 1/2; signed and dated upper right, "Daniel Garber '45." Presented by Mrs. Edward B. Krumbhaar, 1946. *PA 114*

Krumbhaar is shown two-thirds length, body frontal and head turned slightly to the right. He is seated squarely in a low-backed Queen Anne-style armchair, arms loosely at his sides, hands on his lap with thumbs and index fingers overlapping. The interior setting includes a period table with two orange-bound books standing in a box and four other books lying horizontally. The background suggests the corner of a room—on the left and lower right are dark brown and rust-colored diagonal linear strokes; on the right is an under layer of light brown, covered with multicolored geometric strokes of blue, violet, purple, rust, and tan. The subject has brown hair, blue eyes which look out in direction of the head turn, and a square-shaped face with high cheekbones, straight nose, wide mouth, and a prominent jaw line. He wears a white shirt, reddish-brown necktie, white pocket handkerchief, double-breasted light brown suit, and a lapel pin with an orange ornament. The impressionistic surface of this portrait is covered throughout with varying kinds of brush strokes. The head and hands are solidly constructed and there is a sense of the underlying bodily forms. The high-keyed colors in the head and hands include vivid oranges with light blue highlights and dark blue shadows; these colors are also included in the background and books, so that all elements in the painting are related by color. The strength of the color is in accord with the subject's robust physical presence, confident posture, and eager facial expression—he looks relaxed but full of energy, as though pausing before an imminent action.

Artist: A. Zellr

Although the portrait of Krumbhaar is clearly signed "A. Zellr," no information about an artist of that name has been found. There was a sculptor named August Zeller listed as a student at the Pennsylvania Academy of the Fine Arts and who showed work at the Academy's annual exhibitions of 1885 and 1907. According to the *American Art Annual* of 1918, Zeller was a sculptor and teacher who was born in Bordentown, New Jersey, in 1863. He studied at the Franklin Institute and Pennsylvania Academy of the Fine Arts; in Paris he studied at the École des Beaux Arts under Thomas and with Rodin. He taught architectural sculpture at the Carnegie Technical Schools in Pittsburgh and was the custodian of architectural sculpture at the Carnegie Institute. His work includes a *Last Supper* at the Episcopal Church, Fox Chase, Pennsylvania, and a Schuylkill County military monument in Pottsville, Pennsylvania. He died in 1918. Further research is necessary to attribute the Krumbhaar portrait to Zeller and to establish whether "Zeller" could be a variant or misspelling of the name "Zellr."

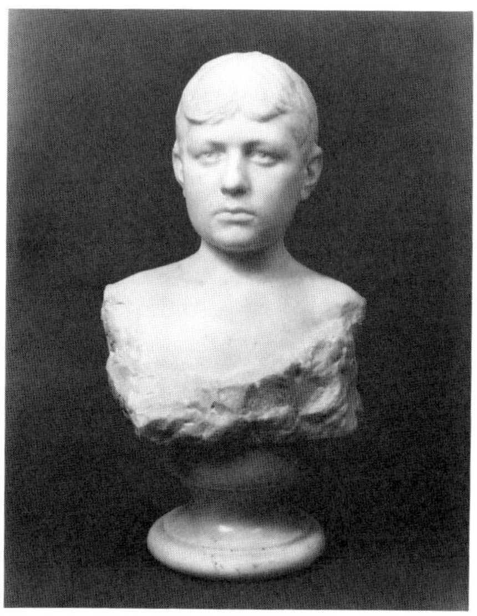

Edward Bell Krumbhaar *ST 572*

Marble; 16 3/4 x 12 3/4 x 9 3/4; no base; rests on a round marble pedestal 5 5/8 in. high; signed and dated lower left corner, rear, "A. Zellr/1897." Presented by Peter D. Krumbhaar, son of Dr. E.B. Krumbhaar, in 1969. If the sculpture had been done from life, the subject would be 15 years old, but according to the College of Physicians files, he was 12 or 13 and he looks even younger than this. More work must be done to trace the source of this sculpture and to find information about the sculptor. *ST 572*

The young Krumbhaar is shown bust length, with body frontal and head turned very slightly to the left. His smooth hair is parted in the center, with curving wings to each side. Delicately formed eyebrows overhang narrow eyes that look straight ahead with carved irises and pupils. The round face has a straight nose, round cheeks, and a full mouth. The neck and chest are described anatomically above and terminated in rough, unfinished marble on the sides and below. The face and chest of the romantically expressive sculpture have been finished smoothly with delicate gradations of planes. This is in sharp contrast to the irregular, unpolished texture below. There is additional contrast between the softness of hair and eyes and the more linear carving of ears, nose, and mouth. The boy's expression is quiet and dreamy.

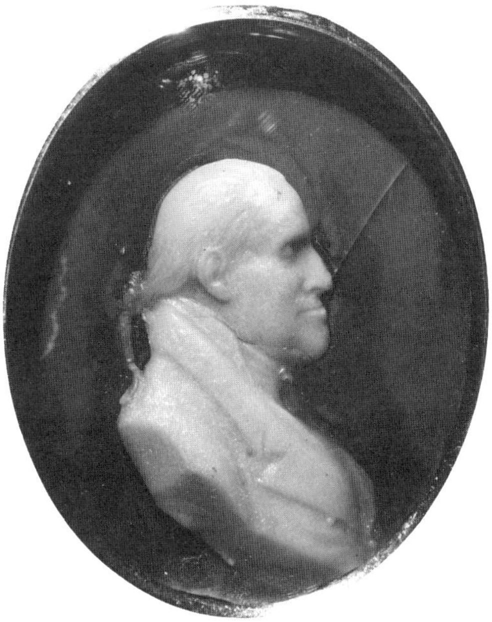

Adam Kuhn *MISC 989*

Adam Kuhn (1741-1817)

Born in Philadelphia of Swabian immigrant parents, Kuhn studied medicine first with his father. In 1761 he went abroad to study medicine and botany at the University of Upsala. There the botanist Linnaeus was so impressed with his aptitude that he named an American plant after Kuhn. After residing in London for a year, he went to Edinburgh, where he received the M.D. degree in 1767 and dedicated his thesis to Linnaeus. He returned to Philadelphia in 1768 and established a medical practice. In the same year he was appointed professor of materia medica and botany in the College of Philadelphia. He was physician to the Pennsylvania Hospital from 1775 to 1798 and consulting physician to the Philadelphia Dispensary. He was a senior founding fellow of the College of Physicians of Philadelphia and its president from 1808 to 1817. He was also a member of the American Philosophical Society. He was professor of the theory and practice of medicine at the University of Pennsylvania from 1789 to 1797. In 1773, during a severe epidemic of smallpox, he joined a society of doctors who inoculated the poor against this disease. He was also active in treating victims of yellow fever in the epidemics of 1793 and 1794.

Artist: George M. Miller (d. 1818 or 1819)

A native of Scotland, Miller came to America in the late 1790s. He is thought to have modeled a wax portrait of George Washington in Philadelphia in 1798. He was in Baltimore from 1810 to 1812 and in Philadelphia again by 1813. He exhibited wax sculptures at the Pennsylvania Academy of the Fine Arts from 1813 to 1815. Works by Miller were also shown posthumously in 1821 and 1852. He is known to have made busts of Thomas Jefferson, Bishop William White, Charles Willson Peale, Mrs. James Madison, Albert Gallatin, and other notables. He was a member of the Pennsylvania Academy of the Fine Arts and the Columbian Society of Arts.

White wax relief sculpture; 21/2 x 13/4 x 1/2; mounted on glass with black paper on verso, on an oval backing; not signed or dated. Authenticated as a work by Miller by Ethel Stanwood Bolton, in Wax Portraits and Silhouettes *(Boston, 1914). Bolton adds, "eyes closed and from expression evidently taken after death" (i.e., 1817). Presented by Mrs. C. Hartman Kuhn, date unrecorded, but prior to 1887, when it was shown at the College of Physicians'* Centennial Celebration Loan Collection of Portraits *with owner listed as College of Physicians.* *MISC 989*

Kuhn is shown bust length with profile to the right. His wig is pulled back in a long queue. His forehead recedes, his eye is closed, his large nose has a bump on its bridge, the lower lip protrudes, and the chin juts out. The subject wears a stock, a waistcoat with high collar, and a coat with high collar and M-notched lapel. The surface is smoothly modeled and has an even grain to its texture. Delicate lines describe the hair and folds of the stock. The prognathous profile and distorted chest may have have resulted from cracking or melting of the sculpture.

Artist: Louis Hasselbusch (1863-1938)

For biography, see page 83.

Oil on canvas; 291/2 x 241/2; signed lower left, "L. Hasselbusch"; written on new lining on back of canvas, "Adam Kuhn M.D. 1741-1817/Louis Hasselbusch/copy." Probably copied after the wax relief sculpture by George Miller (see above). Closely resembles a painting of Kuhn by Hasselbusch at the University of Pennsylvania. Presented by C. Hartman Kuhn in 1910. *PA 26*

Kuhn is shown half-length, the head in profile to the right, the body almost in profile. Part of the left arm is visible. The background is a dark, neutral color consisting of green, brown, and gray. Kuhn wears a grayish-white wig tied into a queue in the back, ending in a shoulder-

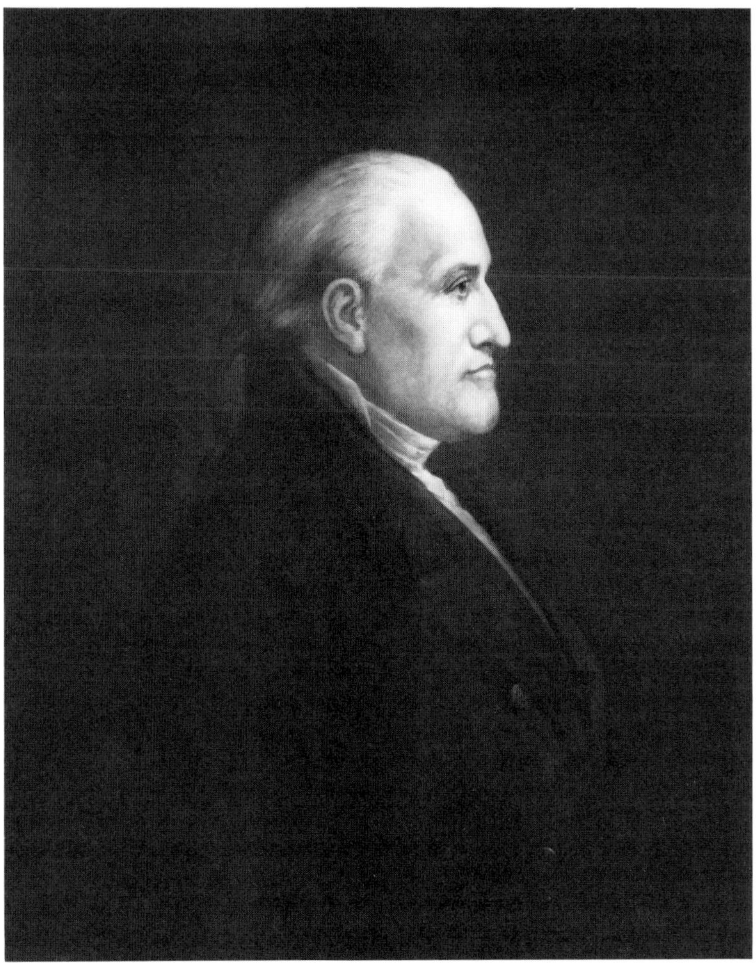

Adam Kuhn *PA 26*

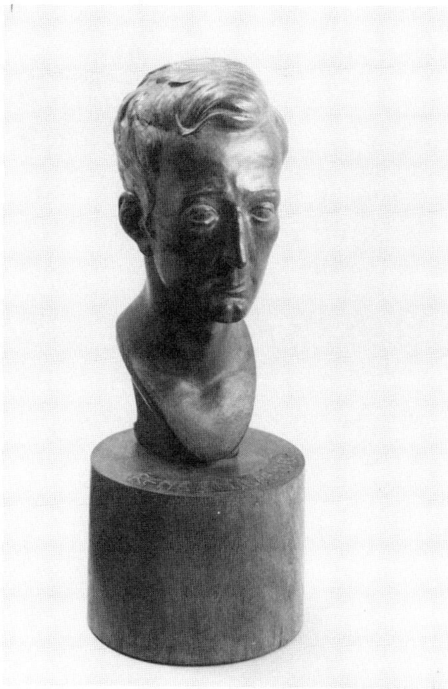

René Théophile-Hyacinthe Laënnec ST 570

length curl. His brown eye looks straight ahead. The tip of his long nose points down toward a tightly closed mouth and a jutting chin. He wears a white stock, a white waistcoat with stand-up collar, and a maroon double-breasted coat with M-notched lapels and brass buttons. The surface of this portrait shows visible brush strokes, especially in the highlights and shadows. The head is well constructed in three-dimensional solidity. The costume is painted flatly, but is rounded over the abdomen. The subject looks stiff and wooden, without any expression or trace of animation. The portrait is a modification of the original wax source (or at least of its present condition).

René Théophile-Hyacinthe Laënnec (1781-1826)

Born in Brittany, Laënnec studied medicine first with an uncle at the University of Nantes who had been a student of John Hunter (q.v.). After serving as a regimental surgeon in the French army, he received the M.D. degree from the Hôpital de Charité in Paris in 1804; his teachers included Corvisart, Bichat, Bayle, and Dupuytren (q.v.). Laënnec succeeded Bayle as head of the Hôpital Necker in 1816. It was here that Laënnec invented the stethoscope and where three years later he wrote his famous work, *Traité de l'auscultation médiate.* Laënnec's early stethoscope was made of a foot-length wooden cylinder with a hollow center. Although his treatise was received with indifference initially, it revolutionized the study of clinical pathology of the thorax and abdomen, and the descriptions of cardiac and respiratory diseases added technical terms that are still in use today. Laënnec correlated the breath and heart sounds with the changes made by diseases. His fame spread within a few years. He was appointed professor at the Collège de France in 1822 and physician to the Charité the following year. Just after having completed a second edition of his book, he died of tuberculosis, a disease he had helped to elucidate.

Artist: Charlotte Geffken

Plaster, painted bronze color; 12 3/4 x 5 1/2 x 7 1/4; rests on a circular base 5 1/8 in. high, with an inscription on a copper plaque, "RENE TH LAENNEC"; signed and dated on rear of bust, "C. Geffken/1936." Presented by Miss Charlotte Geffken in 1968. *ST 570*

Laënnec is shown head-and-neck length, the head frontal. He has thick hair, knitted brows, diagonally set blank eyes, a very long, thin nose, a small mouth, and a cleft chin. The chest area below the neck is abbreviated. The surface of the sculpture is smooth. The features are superficial without convincing anatomical depth. The dour facial expression, added to the elongated features and shape of the face, give the subject an ascetic appearance.

René La Roche (1795-1872)

The son of a French physician who practiced in San Domingo until an insurrection forced him to flee, La Roche was born in Philadelphia, where his father cared for French families residing there. Before receiving his M.D. from the University of Pennsylvania in 1820, he served as captain in the War of 1812 and engaged in business. Although he had a successful medical practice for more than 50 years, he was best known for his active participation in medical societies and for his literary work. He

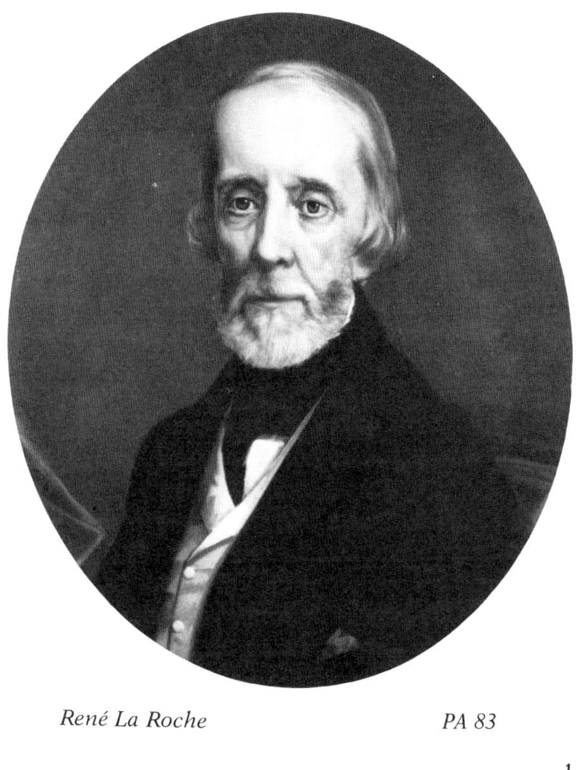

René La Roche *PA 83*

belonged to the Kappa Lambda Association of the United States, which sponsored the *North American Medical and Surgical Journal,* of which he was an editor. This society was succeeded by the Monday Evening Club, said to be the first medical club in the United States. La Roche was also a founder and president of the Pathological Society of Philadelphia, a trustee of the University of Pennsylvania, president of the medical society of the State of Pennsylvania, a fellow of the College of Physicians, and a member of the American Philosophical Society. His chief work, which became a medical classic, was *Yellow Fever Considered in Its Historical, Pathological, Etiological and Therapeutic Relations* (1855). A portion of his own vast collection of books on yellow fever has come to the College of Physicians. He also had a large and valuable collection of books on music.

Artist: Unknown

Oil on canvas mounted on board, oval, 24 1/4 x 19 3/4; not signed or dated. Presented in 1915 by a grandson of Dr. La Roche, J. Percy Keating. He had received it from the doctor's daughter, who commissioned the work, possibly while living in Brussels. *PA 83*

Dr. La Roche is shown bust length, with body turned to the left and head turned slightly to the left. He sits in a straight-backed, upholstered armchair. The atmospheric background is a warm greenish-gray. The subject has thinning, gray-white, ear-length hair, a moustache and short beard, a very high and straight forehead, heavy-lidded blue eyes which look out in the direction of the head turn, a long rectangular face with a prominent nose, a thin mouth, sunken cheeks, deep circles under his eyes, and broad lines next to his nose. He wears a black neckcloth, a white vest, and a black coat with a white pocket handkerchief. The surface of the portrait has been painted smoothly. The head is constructed in three-dimensional volumes; there is a suggestion of the body under the costume. Details of facial features and costume are delineated crisply. The subject is of slender build, advanced age, and serious demeanor. Nonetheless, he radiates a feeling of energy, zest for life, and strength.

Michael Leib (1760-1822)

The son of a native of Strasaelbourg who came to America in 1753, Leib was born in Philadelphia. He studied medicine under Dr. Benjamin Rush (q.v) and then was surgeon to the Philadelphia militia. After the war he was active in medical affairs for fifteen years, as attending physician to the Philadelphia Dispensary, the Philadelphia Almshouse and Hospital, and the Bush Hill Hospital. He was a fellow of the College of Physicians and a member of the Pennsylvania Prison Society. Activities in the Democratic Society, the German Republican Society, and the Assembly launched him into a political career which precluded the practice of

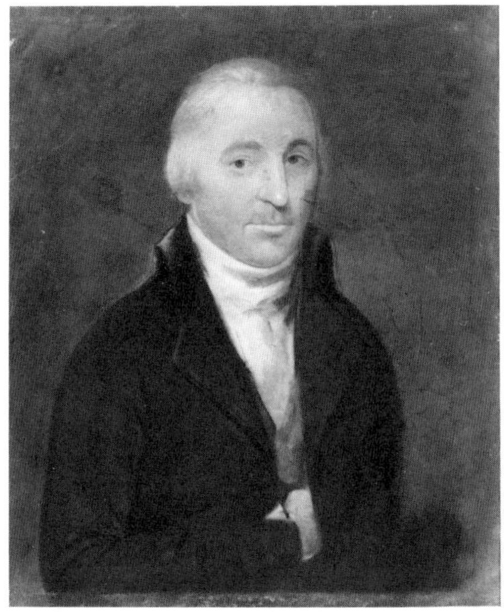

Michael Leib *PA 79*

medicine. He served in the Pennsylvania House of Representatives (1797-98), the United States House of Representatives (1799-1806), and the United States Senate (1809-14). He was a Democratic presidential-elector (1808), brigadier-general of militia (1807-11), and postmaster of Philadelphia (1814-15). Hostility to his political views forced him from the latter post, and he returned to the Assembly (1817-18) and the State Senate (1818-21). In 1822 he was prothonotary of the United States District Court at Philadelphia.

Artist: Unknown

Pastel on paper; 25 x 21. Presented by Thomas Skelton Harrison, 1920. *PA 79*

Dr. Leib is shown half-length with head and body slightly to the right. His right arm is bent at the elbow, the hand tucked under the coat. The subject has smooth white hair, brown eyes which look out of their corners toward the viewer, a long nose with tip pointed down, and a wide mouth with full bottom lip. His round face has smooth skin with pink highlights and gray shadows. He wears a white shirt and stock, a gray waistcoat, and a black coat with a high folded collar. The surface of this portrait is much damaged and the smoothly applied color is worn through, so that underlying outlines of some details are visible. There is little sense of anatomical structure in the head or body. The expression is bland.

Joseph Leidy (1823-1891)

Descended from German immigrants who came to America in 1719, Leidy was born in Philadelphia, the son of a hatmaker. As a child he showed talent for drawing and intense interest in natural history. He studied medicine at the University of Pennsylvania under Dr. Paul Goddard (q.v.) and Dr. William

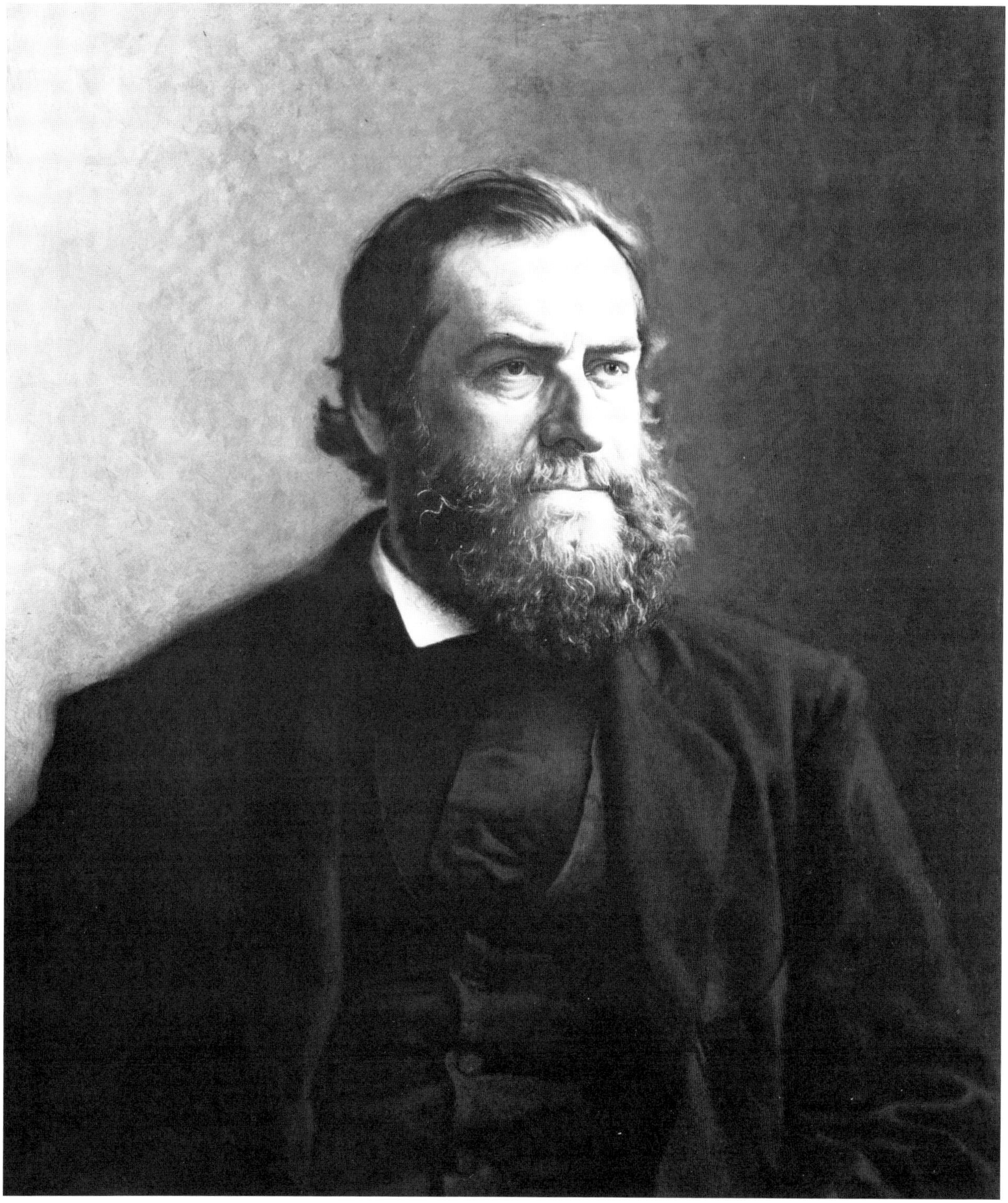

Joseph Leidy PA 39

Horner (q.v.), receiving the M.D. degree in 1844. In 1845 he was appointed prosector to Dr. Horner and in 1847 he delivered lectures on human anatomy to Horner's students. The following year the two men traveled to Europe, visiting hospitals and anatomical museums. In 1850 he accepted the offer of Dr. George B. Wood (q.v.) to accompany him to Europe to collect models, casts, and preparations for teaching material. On their return Leidy lectured on physiology at the Medical Institute of Philadelphia. On the death of Dr. Horner in 1853, Leidy was elected professor of anatomy at the University of Pennsylvania. He filled that chair for 38 years, in addition to the chairs of zoology and comparative anatomy. He was also professor of natural history at Swarthmore College. He was regarded as the foremost American anatomist of his time, and his *Elementary Treatise on Human Anatomy* (1861) remains a classic. He served as acting assistant surgeon with the U.S. Army during the Civil War. In addition to his accomplishments in anatomy, his nearly 600 publications extend into the fields of

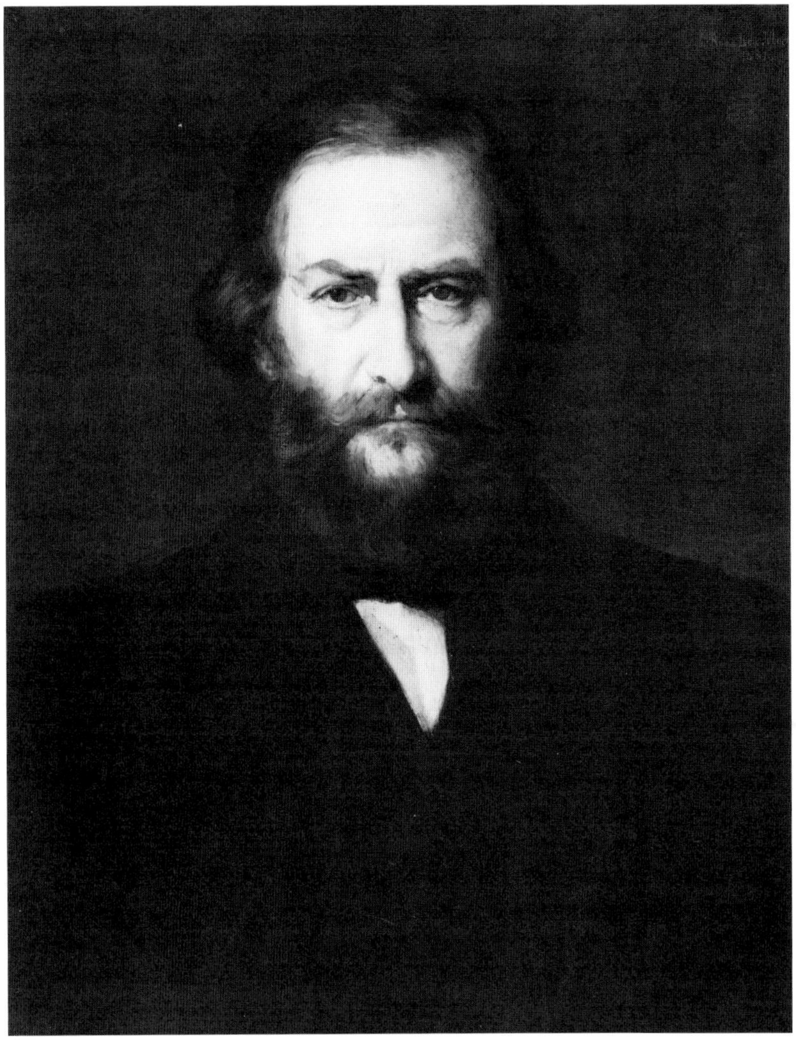

Joseph Leidy PA 85

botany, minerology, paleontology, zoology, and anthropology; many are illustrated with his own drawings. His work with animal parasites, particularly *Trichinella spiralis* and intestinal worms, is noteworthy. His treatise, *Flora and Fauna within Living Animals* (1853) has been called "epoch-making." He identified more than 100 new species of entozoa. His monograph, *Extinct Mammalian Fauna of Nebraska and Dakota* (1869), is considered one of the most important contributions to vertebrate paleontology. He was elected to the Boston Society of Natural History and the Academy of Natural Sciences of Philadelphia, which he served as President from 1882 to 1891. He was elected a member of the National Academy of Science in 1863, president of the Wagner Free Institute of Science in 1885, and president of the Association of American Anatomists in 1889. He was a fellow of the College of Physicians and an honorary member of more than forty American and European learned societies. He received an honorary LL.D. from Harvard University and medals and prizes from the Boston Society of Natural History, the Royal Microscopical Society, the Geological Society of London, and the Paris Academy of Science.

Artist: James Longacre Wood (1867-1938)

For biography, see page 96.

Oil on canvas; 29 1/2 x 25 1/2; signed and dated lower right, "from photo/James L. Wood/1901." Presented by Mrs. Joseph Leidy, Jr., in 1901. Other portraits of Leidy by Wood are at the American Philosophical Society (ca. 1900), the Historical Society of Pennsylvania (1900), and the University of Pennsylvania (1892). PA 39

Dr. Leidy is shown bust length, with body frontal and head turned to the right. The atmospheric background is warm, light yellowish-brown on the left and darker brown in the right. His brown hair has a few loose strands on top and turns up at the collar. Under knitted brows his blue eyes gaze straight ahead in the direction of the head turn. His prominent nose has a bump on the bridge and a tip that points down to a wide mouth whose lower lip protrudes beyond the thin upper lip, giving a slightly pouting look. The side-whiskers, moustache, and beard are rendered in precise linear detail. He wears a white shirt with a wing collar, a black plastron, a buttoned black vest which spans his girth, and a rumpled black coat worn informally open. The surface of the portrait is smoothly brushed. The head and body are constructed in solid, three-dimensional volumes, modeled

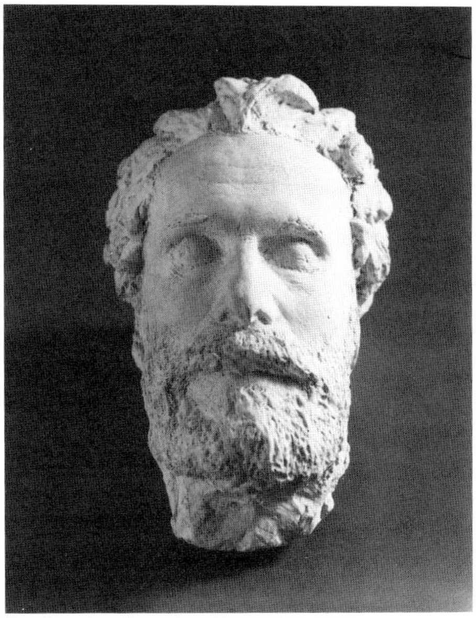

Joseph Leidy *ST 13056*

in light and shade in such a way as to give a sculptural quality. Another feature that is characteristic of this artist is the emphasis on detail, such as the puffy eyelids, individual hairs, and wrinkles in the costume. This gives the portrait a vivid, photographic quality. The horizontal expanse of the body and the forceful facial expression depict an assertive, energetic personality, but it is not intimidating to the viewer because the subject looks off into the distance.

Artist: Anna Lea Merritt (Mrs. Henry Merritt) (1844-1930)

For biography, see page 70.

Oil on canvas; 261/2 x 211/2; signed and dated upper right, "Anna Lea Merritt/1881." Given by Mrs. Anna Lea Merritt in 1881. *PA 85*

Dr. Leidy is shown bust length with head and body frontal. The background is a thin layer of green over an umber undercoat which shows through. The smooth brown hair, flecked with gray around the face, is worn full at the ears. The side-whiskers, moustache, and rounded beard are also brown with gray. The grayish-green eyes look straight ahead toward the observer. The long nose has a bump at the bridge and a long tip which points down toward the thin-lipped mouth. There are creases in the forehead, the corners of the eyes, and next to the nose. The subject wears a white shirt, a black bow tie, a black vest with shawl collar, and a black coat. The surface of the portrait has visible brush strokes. The head has been rendered solidly. The costume is flat with little suggestion of underlying bodily forms. The direct stare, knitted brows, and tight lips give a solemn expression which challenges the viewer to respond. The massive head and breadth of shoulders produce an air of physical strength and authority, emphasized by the dramatic contrast of light and shade on the face.

Artist: Attributed to Samuel Aloysius Murray (1870-1941)

For biography, see page 3.

Plaster of Paris death mask, white; 113/4 x 81/4 x 6; 1891; there is no base; not signed. Presented by Dr. Joseph Leidy, Jr., in 1902. Replicas at the American Philosophical Society and the Historical Society of Pennsylvania. The Bradley File attributes this work to Murray, although there is no additional documentary evidence to corroborate this. However, Bradley knew Murray in later life and had a portrait bust made by him. *ST 13056*

Dr. Leidy has very thick hair brushed away from his face. He has scanty eyebrows, closed eyes, a prominent nose with the tip pointing down and a bump at the bridge, a moustache, a short beard, and a mouth whose lower lip is recessed behind the upper lip. The irregular surface texture shows details of skin and the rough thickness of hair and beard.

Charles Lester Leonard (1861-1913)

Descended from English ancestors who settled in Massachusetts in 1632, Leonard was born in Easthampton, Massachusetts. He received A.B. degrees from the University of Pennsylvania in 1885 and Harvard in 1886, an M.D. degree in 1889, and an A.M. degree in 1892, both from the University of Pennsylvania. After studying abroad from 1889 to 1892 and then working on photomicrography at the Pepper Laboratory, he became interested in the new field of roentgenology; he devoted the remainder of his career to X-ray techniques and diagnosis. He became director of the roentgen laboratories at the University of Pennsylvania and the Methodist Episcopal Hospital and professor of roentgenology at the Philadelphia Polyclinic. He was a fellow of the College of Physicians, founder and secretary of the Philadelphia Roentgen Ray Society, president of the American Roentgen Ray Society, and fellow of the British and German Roentgen Ray Societies. He was a delegate to many international congresses of radiology. He was an associate editor of the *Archives of the Roentgen Ray, Zeitschrift für Röntgenkunde,* and the *Journal de Radiologie.* Leonard is regarded as a pioneer in this new specialty, which had just been discovered and announced in 1895. He was one of the first physicians in America to demonstrate the presence of stones in the urinary tract by means of X-rays; he wrote 44 papers on the diagnostic use of X-rays and their application in the treatment of cancer. As a result of excessive exposure to X-rays, he developed chronic skin ulcers on his hands. After suffering amputations, he died of cancer induced by radiation.

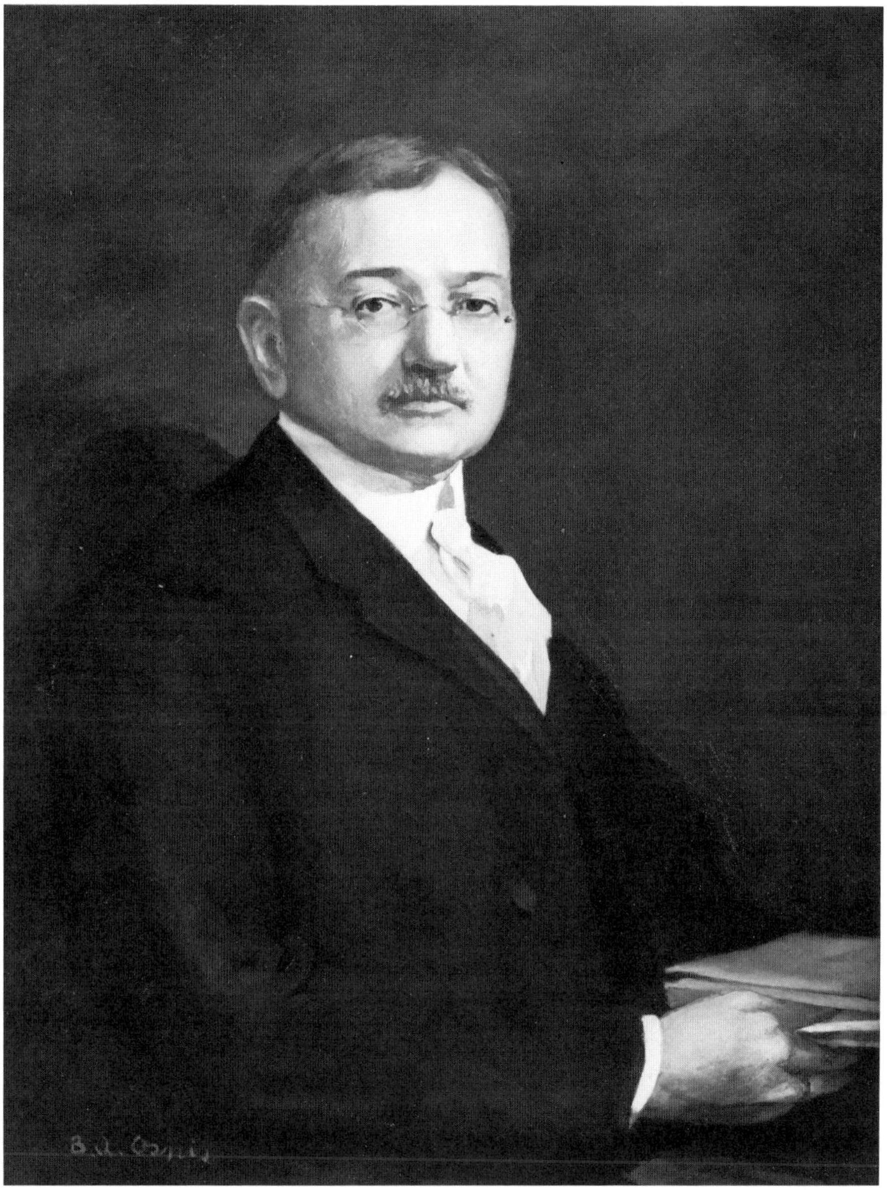

Charles Lester Leonard *PA 98*

Artist: Benedict Anton Osnis (1872–1941)

Born in Russia, Osnis came to the United States in 1886 and studied art at the Pennsylvania Academy of the Fine Arts (1895–1906) under William Merritt Chase. He was a well-known portrait painter whose subjects included President Calvin Coolidge, Dennis Cardinal Dougherty, General John H. Pershing, Mayor Harry Mackey, General Charles P. Summerall, and many other leaders. His work and that of his wife, Daisy Hartman Osnis, were exhibited jointly at the Art Club Gallery in 1936. A copy of his portrait of Benjamin Franklin is located at the office of the postmaster general in Washington. Osnis was also well known for portrait sketches in charcoal, twenty-six of which were exhibited at West Point.

Oil on canvas; 35 1/2 x 27 1/2; signed lower left, "B.A. Osnis." Commissioned by the Philadelphia Roentgen Ray Society in 1937 and presented by the Society to the College of Physicians in 1937. *PA 98*

Dr. Leonard is shown half-length, with body turned three-quarters to the right and head rotated slightly to the right. His right arm rests on the arm of a red upholstered chair. His right hand holds and marks a book with a bright pinkish-orange cover. The background is purplish-gray in the upper left, greenish-gray on the right. Leonard has short, light brown hair and hazel eyes which gaze at the viewer through rimless glasses. His face is square. The nose and jaw are wide. A gray brush moustache extends over a full mouth. The complexion is high keyed, with several shades of bright pink. He wears a white shirt, a white necktie with pastel design, and a dark blue-black vest and coat. The surface of the portrait is painterly throughout, with fluid brush strokes. The head is well-constructed in solid forms, and there is a suggestion of ample body masses under the clothing. The subject sits erect and turns his head to regard the viewer with a benign expression. Even though the painting was not made during Dr. Leonard's lifetime, the artist has conveyed an expression of energy and vitality.

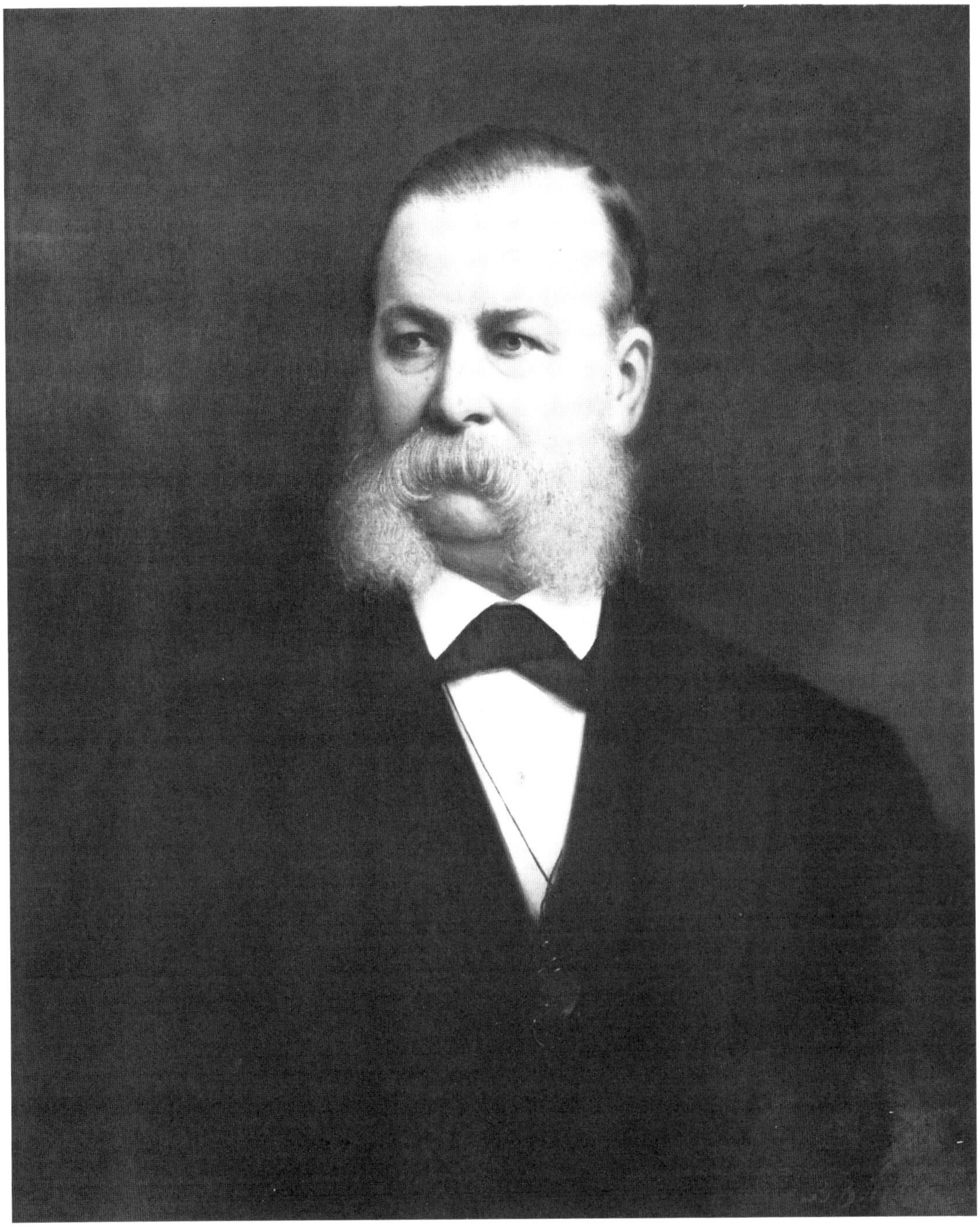

Samuel Lewis *PA 11*

Samuel Lewis (1813–1890)

Born in Barbados, West Indies, Lewis came to Philadelphia with his guardian uncle and studied medicine for one year at the University of Pennsylvania. He completed his medical education at the Universities of Dublin, London, and Edinburgh. From the last-named he received the M.D. degree in 1840. He was elected a member of the Royal Medical Society and of the Royal Physical Society of Edinburgh. He returned to Philadelphia in 1840 and established an office practice which he had to abandon after a few years because his health was bad. He was an editor of the *Medical Examiner,* an original member of the Philadelphia Pathological Society, a censor of the Philadelphia County Medical Society, and a founder of the Children's Hospital. His overriding interest was in the collection of medical books and in service to the College of Physicians, of which he was a fellow for 42 years. He was a member of its library committee and publication committee, a censor, and, in 1844, its president. In 1864 he presented his medical library of 2500 volumes to the College. During the following years his donation increased to more than 10,000 volumes, including many from the library of Dr. La Roche (q.v.). that he had bought at auction.

Artist: Samuel Bell Waugh (1814-1885)

For biography, see page 44.

Oil on canvas mounted on board; 29 1/4 x 24 1/4; signed and dated lower right, "S.B. Waugh, 1873." Presented by fellows of the College of Physicians in 1873. *PA 11*

Dr. Lewis is shown bust length, with body frontal and head turned slightly to the left. The atmospheric background is gray. The subject has smooth brown hair, grayish-blue eyes which look toward the left and slightly down, and very fair skin. There are lines below his eyes and next to the straight nose. He has muttonchop whiskers and a luxuriantly full moustache that conceals his mouth. He wears a white shirt and a black bow tie, a black vest with shawl collar, a black coat, and a pince-nez that hangs from a black cord around his neck. The paint style of this portrait is smooth and slick. The head has been modeled meticulously in solid, three-dimensional forms. The costume is flat with no sense of underlying bodily forms. The gaze is directed away from the viewer, as though the subject were lost in thought.

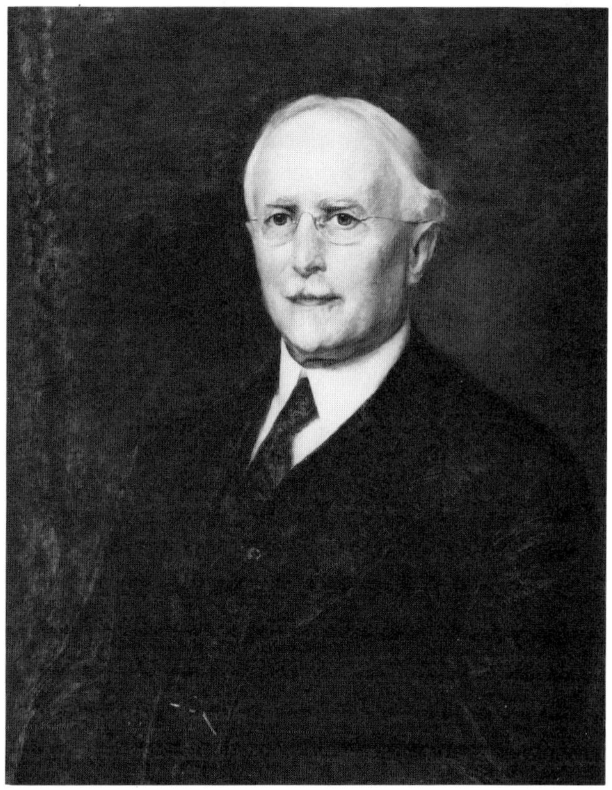

Ludwig Loeb *PA 144*

Ludwig Loeb (1866-1957)

Born in Palatinate, Germany, Loeb received a certificate from the Teachers' Seminary in Kaiserlautern in 1885. He received the M.D. degree from Jefferson Medical College in 1890 and continued his education with post-doctoral work at the graduate school of the University of Pennsylvania and then in Berlin. He was appointed instructor of surgery at the graduate school of the University of Pennsylvania and chief obstetrician and medical director of the Jewish Maternity Hospital (1892-1924). He was attending physician and medical chief of the Jewish Hospital of Philadelphia (now the Albert Einstein Medical Center, Northern Division) from 1894 to 1934; he served thereafter as consultant. He was co-founder of the American Hospital for Diseases of the Stomach (1905); co-founder, medical director, and chief physician of the National Stomach Hospital (1914-31); and consulting physician to the Mt. Sinai Hospital (now Albert Einstein Medical Center, Southern Division) from 1930 to 1932. His most outstanding contributions to the medical literature were in the field of gastrointestinal diseases.

Artist: Julius Thiengen Bloch (1888-1966)

Born in Kehl, Germany, Bloch came to America in 1893 and spent the remainder of his life in Philadelphia. He studied at the Pennsylvania Museum School of Industrial Art from 1905 to 1908 and at the Pennsylvania Academy of the Fine Arts from 1908 to 1912, where he won two Cresson fellowships and a Toppan prize (1911, 1912). He was an instructor in painting at the Academy from 1948 to 1962 and received the Percy M. Owens Memorial Prize from its fellowship in 1962. He served in the United States Army during World War I. He was well known as a portrait painter of friends and colleagues, as well as of members of society and the professions. During the 1930s and 1940s he developed a special following in the black community for his pictures of American Negroes which expressed social protest and for his portraits of distinguished black leaders and artists. His paintings also showed sympathy to problems of the American worker. He contributed regularly to annual exhibitions of the Pyramid Club, a Philadelphia black professional society which honored him with a one-man show. He exhibited widely in annual national exhibitions at the Pennsylvania Academy of the Fine Arts, the Whitney Museum of American Art, the Museum of Modern Art, the Metropolitan Museum of Art, the Print Club of Philadelphia, the Corcoran Gallery, the Art Institute of Chicago, and at international expositions in San Francisco and New York in 1939. He was active in the Works Projects Administration projects in Philadelphia. He had one-man shows at the Little Theater (1929), Edward Side Gallery (1930), Little Gallery of Woodstock, N.Y. (1931), Philadelphia Art Alliance (1938), the Pennsylvania Academy of the Fine Arts (1948), Robert Carlen Gallery (1950), Woodmere Art Gallery (1954), Jewish Community Art Center (Wilkes-Barre, 1956), Newman Gallery (1959), and memorial exhibitions at the Art Alliance and Little Gallery of Contemporary Art (1967). He received awards from the Worcester Art Museum (1933), the Wanamaker Gallery of Art (1934), and the Yarnall Abbott Prize from the Art

Alliance (1939). His work is represented in many major museums and colleges, including the Philadelphia Museum of Art, which owns a large collection of his prints and drawings; they held an exhibition of his work in 1983 and devoted its *Bulletin* of Summer, 1983, (essay by Patricia Likos) to a biography of the artist.

Oil on canvas; 27 1/4 x 21 1/4; signed upper left, "Julius Bloch"; dated 1945 on the back. Presented by the subject's children, Sophie Loeb Siegel (Mrs. Adrian Siegel) and Daniel Stern Loeb, 1981. *PA 144*

Dr. Loeb is shown bust length, with body turned to the left and head slightly to the left. He is seated in a red-backed chair. The background is blue over an umber undercoat, lighter on the right and darker on the left side, which has a vertical stripe, perhaps a fold of drapery. The subject has white hair, a brush moustache, and a small, pointed beard. He has large brown eyes which look toward the viewer through rimless spectacles. He has a long aquiline nose, generous red lips, and a ruddy complexion. He wears a white shirt, a maroon necktie, a brown vest, a brown coat, and a gold watch chain. The surface of the naturalistic portrait is painterly, with an all-over mottled look, except for the face, which has more deliberate, small strokes, painstakingly brushed to render solid and three-dimensional forms. There is a sense of the body underlying the costume. Loeb, at the age of 79, has an erect and dignified bearing. His luminous eyes, warm skin tones, and pleasant facial expression give him a kindly and vital appearance.

Willis Fastnacht Manges (1876–1936)

Born in Luthersburg, Clearfield County, Pennsylvania, Manges was the son of a Lutheran minister. After studying at Gettysburg College, he received the M.D. degree from Jefferson Medical College in 1903. He remained at Jefferson for 32 years and was appointed roentgenologist (1904), clinical professor (1925), and professor of roentgenology (1929). He was also physician to the Philadelphia General and Bryn Mawr Hospitals. With Dr. Charles Lester Leonard (q.v.) he was a founder of the Philadelphia Roentgen Ray Society, which he later served as president. He served the American Roentgen Ray Society as secretary, then as president (1918). He was a member of the American Board of Radiology and a fellow of the College of Physicians. In 1918 he enlisted in the U.S. Medical Corps and organized the Camp Greenleaf School of Roentgenology at Fort Oglethorpe, Georgia. Manges was an ingenious practitioner of medical radiology and wrote many articles on his innovations, such as exact measurement of the female pelvis, introduction of pyeloscopy, and application of the biplane roentgenoscope (with Dr. Chevalier Jackson) for localizing and removing foreign bodies from the respiratory and digestive channels and from the eye. He also

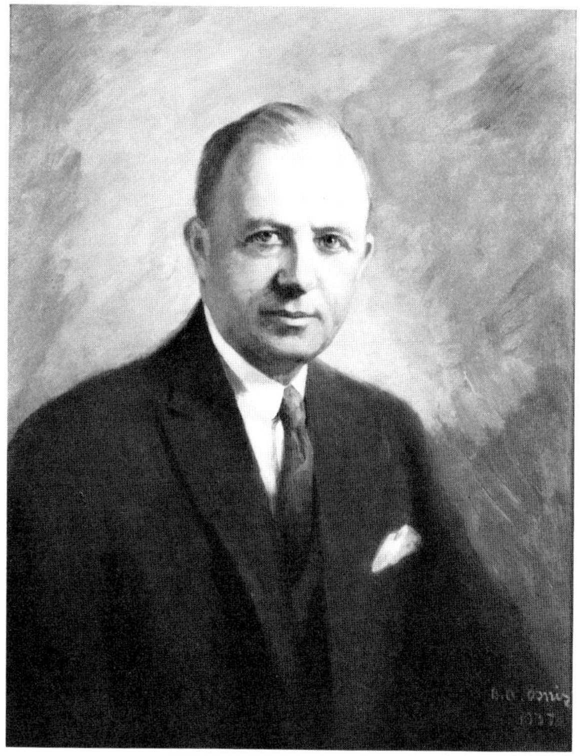

Willis Fastnacht Manges *PA 97*

wrote on the use of roentgen therapy for infections, the association of sinus disease with chronic chest conditions, and the description of the mechanism and diagnostic significance of obstructive emphysema and atelectasis in connection with radiolucent foreign bodies and endobronchial lesions.

Artist: Benedict Anton Osnis (1872–1941)

For biography, see page 110.

Oil on canvas; 29 x 23; signed and dated lower right, "B.A. Osnis, 1937." Commissioned by the Philadelphia Roentgen Ray Society in 1937 and presented by that society to the College of Physicians in 1937. Similar to a portrait of Manges at Jefferson Medical Hospital, painted by Osnis in 1936. *PA 97*

Manges is shown bust length, with body and head turned slightly to the right and head tilted slightly down. The background is composed of warm-toned yellow, green, and umber patches of paint, lightest around the head. The light brown hair is brushed away from the face. The light bluish-green eyes look straight ahead toward the viewer. The face is oval, the nose is straight, the lips are full, and the chin is round. The complexion is vividly colored, with bright pink highlights on the cheeks and red lips. The subject wears a white shirt and white pocket handkerchief, a brown tie, and a brown vest and coat. The surface of the portrait is painterly, with large visible strokes throughout. The head has been constructed in three-dimensional and solid forms. The coloring is unusually high-keyed, especially in the face and background. The costume is flatter, with little detail and with no sense of underlying bodily forms. The facial expression is pleasant, with the hint of a smile. Although not painted from life, the subject seems to emit a sense of energy and liveliness.

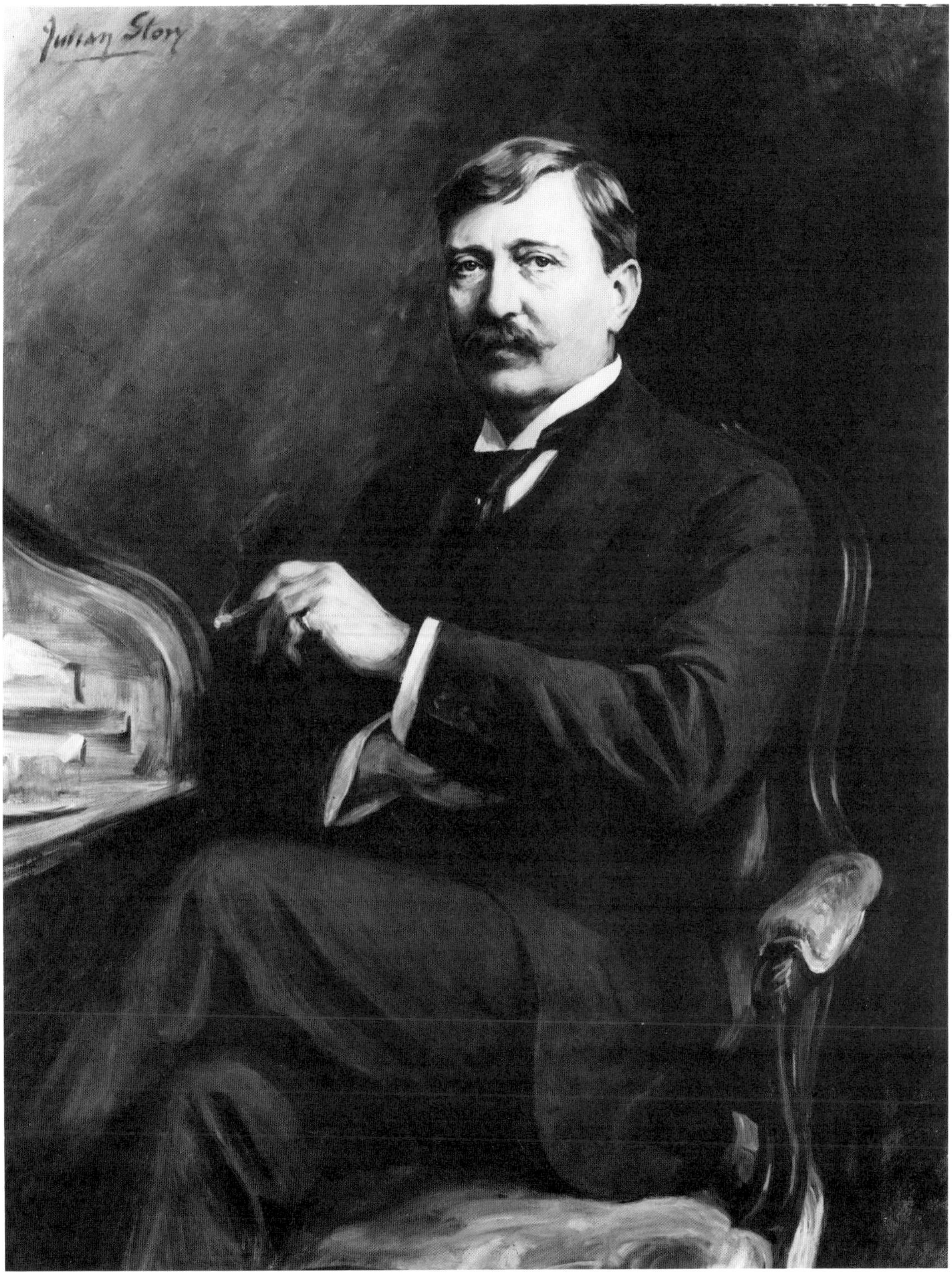

George McClellan *PA 88*

George McClellan (1849–1913)

McClellan was descended from a long line of distinguished Scottish forbears who supported the house of Stuart and came to America in the early 1700s. His grandfather, for whom he was named, was the founder of Jefferson Medical College and his father, John H. B. McClellan, was a surgeon and an anatomist. Dr. George McClellan was born in Philadelphia and studied art for three years at the University of Pennsylvania. He then went to Jefferson, receiving an M.D. degree in 1870. He completed his medical education in Vienna under the master anatomist, Hyrtl, who was celebrated for the beauty of his anatomical specimens. On his return to Philadelphia in 1873 he established a surgical practice and became surgeon to the Philadelphia and Howard Hospitals. In 1881 he founded the Pennsylvania School of Anatomy and Surgery. This private school attracted throngs of medical students, one of whom said that the beauty of his dissections, clarity of his demonstrations, and speed, accuracy, and dexterity of the pictures he drew on the board were of such high quality that "his anatomy was art. He dissected a body as a great sculptor would carve a statue." In 1890 he was elected professor of artistic anatomy at the Pennsylvania Academy of the Fine Arts. He was finally recognized by his alma mater by being made professor of applied anatomy at Jefferson in 1906. His monumental works, *Regional Anatomy* (1891-92) and *Anatomy in Relation to Art* (1900), were illustrated with original photographs of drawings of dissections. He was a fellow of the College of Physicians.

Artist: Julian Story (1857-1919)

For biography, see page 34.

Oil on canvas; 44 x 34; signed upper left, "Julian Story." Presented by Mrs. George McClellan in 1914. *PA 88*

Dr. McClellan is shown three-quarter length, the body being turned three-quarters to the left, the head slightly to the left. He is seated in a French-style upholstered armchair with his legs crossed, arms folded across his body, and his left hand holding a smoking cigar. The chair is turned away from the desk so that it is parallel to the picture plane, and the subject sits at an angle in the chair. The atmospheric background is dark brown on the right, lighter tan on the left. McClellan has light brown hair and moustache, blue eyes which gaze directly at the viewer, a straight nose, full lower lip, and square jaw. He wears a white shirt with wing collar, a dark blue necktie with jeweled tie pin, a dark gray three-piece suit, and a jeweled ring. The head is rendered in solid, three-dimensional volumes, and there is a suggestion of underlying bodily forms beneath the costume. The elegant furniture, the fashionable attire, the cigar, and the absence of books or writing materials on the desk (other than a few papers) present the subject in an attitude that is unusual in portraits of physicians. He is shown at a moment of ease, appearing to have just turned away from his desk to address the viewer. His posture is relaxed but energetic. His alert expression and direct gaze invite the viewer's admiration and response.

Robert Tait McKenzie (1867-1938)

For biography, see page 45.

Artist: Violet Oakley (1874-1961)

Born in Bergen Heights, New Jersey, to a family of artists, Miss Oakley studied at the Art Students' League in New York with Carroll Beckwith, in Rye, England, and at the Académie Montparnasse in Paris. Upon her return to America she studied at the Pennsylvania Academy of the Fine Arts with Joseph de Camp (q.v.) and Cecilia Beaux and at Drexel Institute with the illustrator, Howard Pyle. At Drexel she befriended two students, Jessie Willcox Smith and Elizabeth Shippen Green, with whom she later shared a series of studios. Pyle arranged for Oakley and Willcox to collaborate on illustrations for Longfellow's poem, *Evangeline*. Afterwards Oakley received numerous commissions to illustrate books and magazines. For this work she was awarded a gold medal for illustration at the St. Louis Exposition (1904). At about this time her ambition for a career in mural painting and large-scale decorative ensembles was beginning to be realized. Her first major decorative commission (1900) was for five lancet windows, two large murals, and a mosaic altarpiece for All Angels Church in New York, for which she won a silver medal at St. Louis. Two years later she became the first woman to be entrusted with the mural decoration of a major government building; she painted 13 murals for the Pennsylvania state capitol buildings in Harrisburg (between 1902 and 1927). The first series of murals won her a gold medal at the 100th anniversary celebration of the Pennsylvania Academy (1905). Her windows for the Collier House near New York won a medal at the Panama-Pacific International Exposition in San Francisco in 1915. She also did murals and stained glass decorations for the Yarnall house, St. Peter's Church, Chestnut Hill Academy, Fleisher Art Memorial, Philadelphia Naval Base, and First Presbyterian Church (all in Philadelphia) and the Gibson house (Wynnewood, Pennsylvania), Westtown School (Westtown, Pennsylvania), Cuyahoga County Courthouse (Cleveland), and the Vassar College Alumnae House. She was also a noted portrait painter and produced hundreds of portraits in crayon, pastel, and oil. She exhibited at the Pennsylvania Academy from 1896 through the 1940s and taught a class there in mural decoration from 1913 to 1917. She won the Academy gold medal (1905) and the Pennell Memorial (1932), Lippincott (1940), Emily Drayton Taylor (1941), and Mary Smith (1948) prizes there. She was a founding member of the Plastic Club, the Philadelphia Water Color Club, and the Philadelphia Art Alliance. She was an academician of the National Academy of Design. There was a one-man show of her work at the Philadelphia Museum of Art in 1979. As she prospered, her studio and estate at Cogslea, in Mt. Airy, attracted the attention of the press and women's magazines, and for a time it became a school as well as a salon and gathering place for writers, artists, dancers, and musicians. Today it houses the Violet Oakley Memorial Foundation. A very socially conscious and pacifistic Quaker, she attended meetings at the League of Nations and was an active member of the Women's International League for Peace and Freedom. Her art work is mystical and esoteric, with frequent spiritual and allegorical references, and it often includes powerful female images clad in medieval costume.

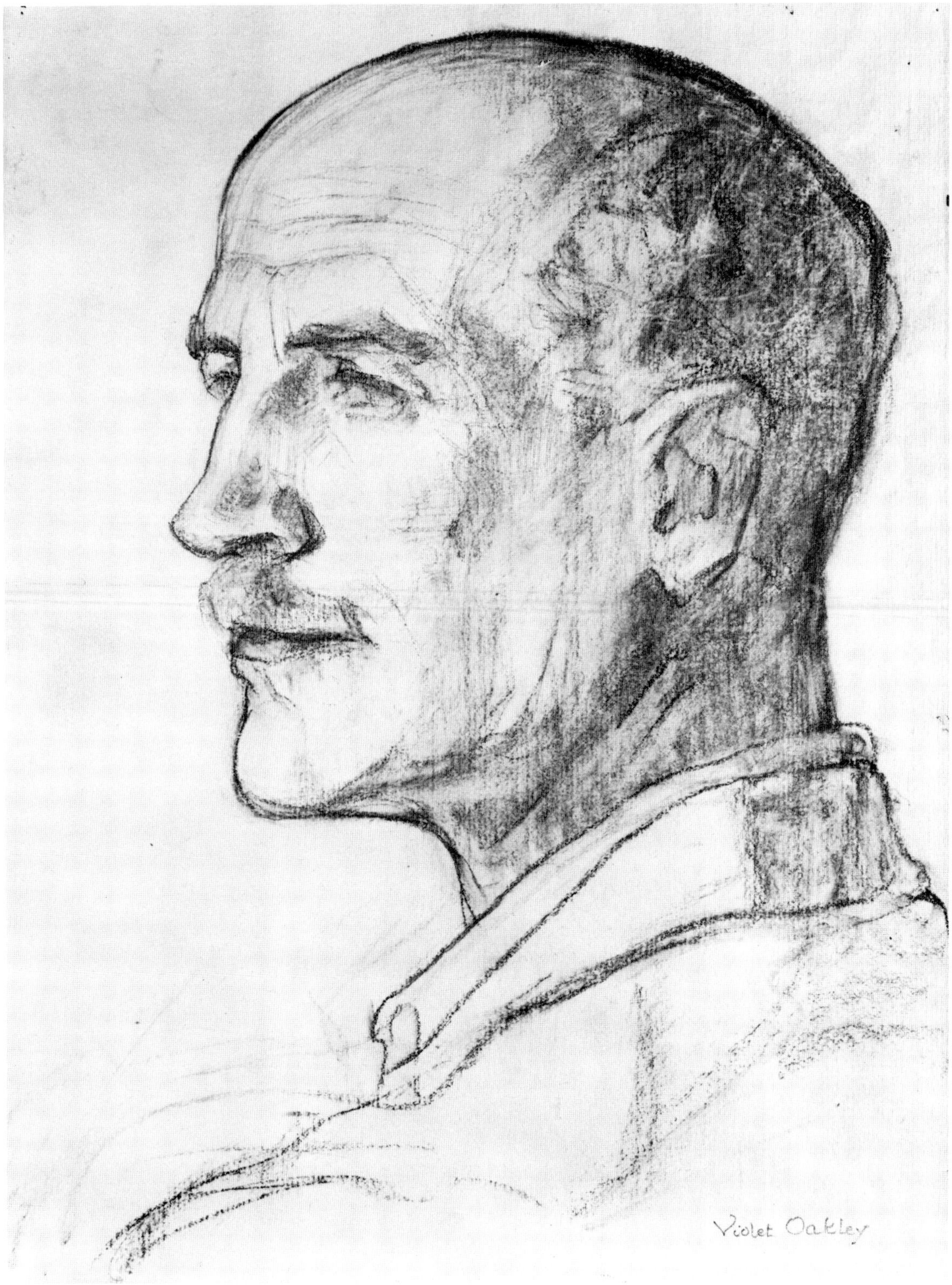

Robert Tait McKenzie *PH 581*

Burnt sienna pastel on buff paper; actual size 14 1/2 x 11; signed lower right, "Violet Oakley." Presented by Dr. James Monroe Thorington in 1953. *PH 581*

Dr. McKenzie is shown head-and-neck length, almost totally in profile, facing left. His high forehead is faintly wrinkled. His hair is close-cropped at the back and sides. His eyes look straight forward in the direction of the head turn. His nose has a bump at the bridge and a pointed tip; a neat brush moustache covers his upper lip. His costume consists of a shirt collar and coat collar. The strong style of drawing uses heavy contours around the features and delicately shaded recessed areas; the paper becomes the areas of light. The anatomical structure of the head is rendered solidly. The subject has the appearance of athletic strength, with his thick neck, chiseled features, and erect bearing.

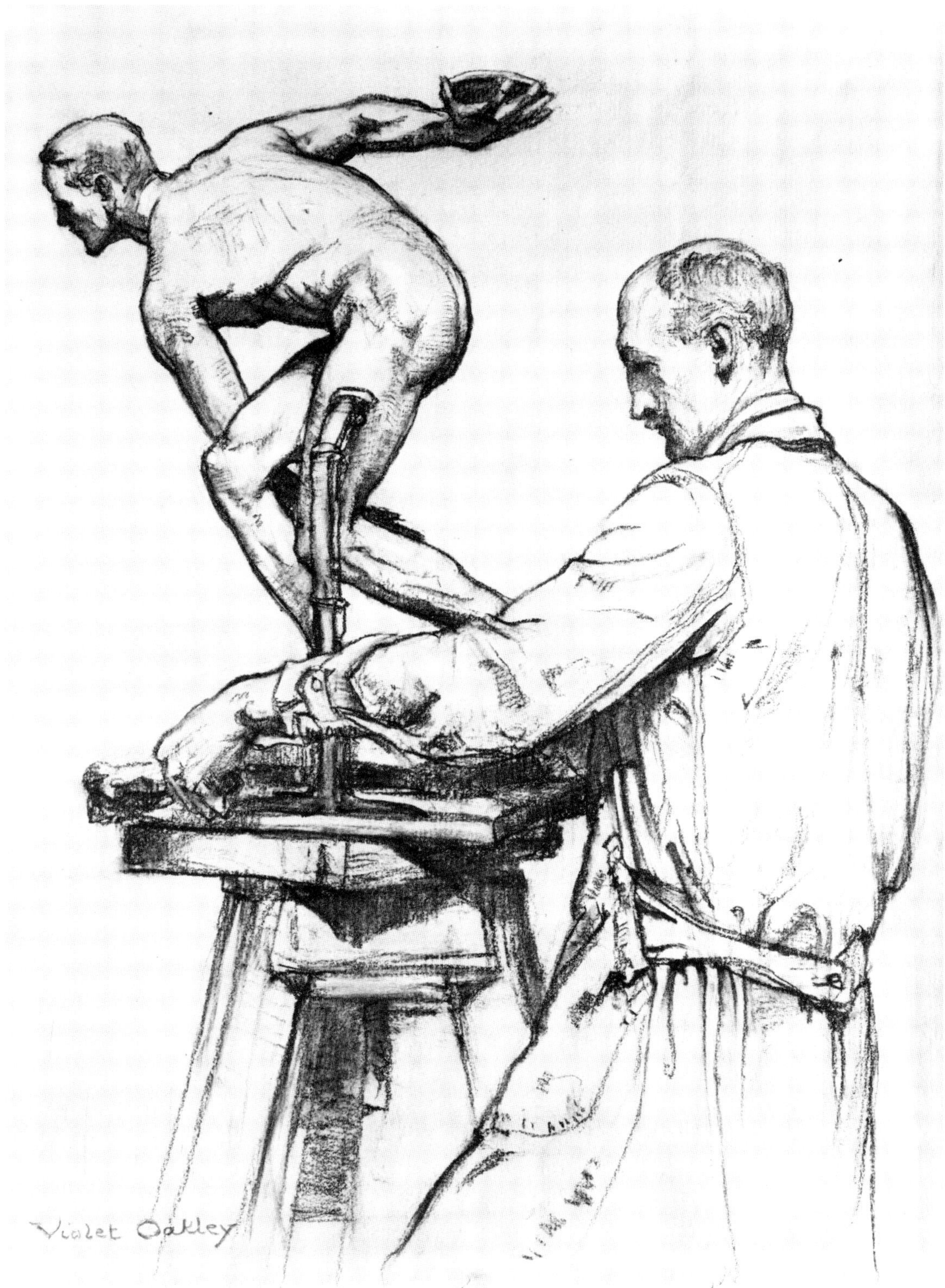

Robert Tait McKenzie *PH 579*

Burnt sienna pastel on buff paper; actual size 147/8 x 11; signed lower left, "Violet Oakley." Presented by Dr. James Monroe Thorington in 1952. *PH 579*

McKenzie is shown two-thirds length, with head in profile and body in two-thirds view from the back. His left arm is stretched out over a workstool, on which are several wood blocks and perhaps a drawing board, and a vertical post that braces a sculpture of a discus thrower in action. McKenzie's head is tilted down toward the stool. He wears a shirt and a long-sleeved work coat, belted in back. The drawing is done in calligraphic style with a variety of lines ranging from heavy contours to hatching and heavy shading. The composition is dramatic—the artist's large figure is on the right side, and the forearm of his disproportionately long limb is at the focal point of the picture, where he is making adjustments to the work. Significantly, the flung-back right arm of the discus thrower parallels the arm of the sculptor, and their profiles are strikingly similar.

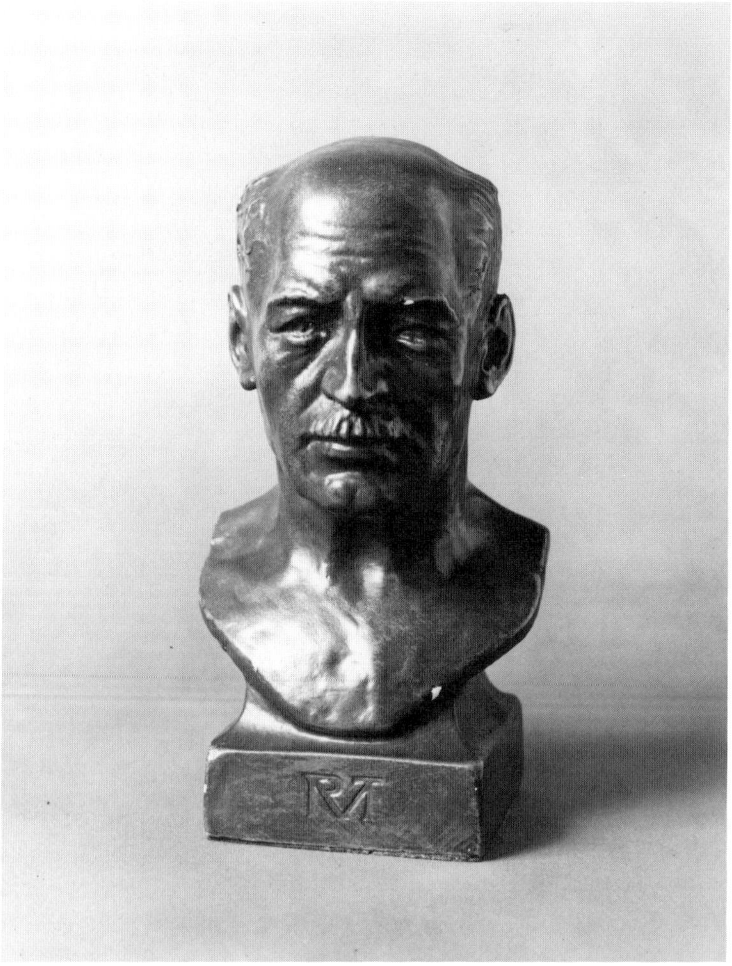

Robert Tait McKenzie *ST 563*

Artist: Joseph Brown (b. 1909)

Brown was born in Philadelphia and received a B.S. in Education from Temple University. He was an apprentice and studio assistant to Robert Tait McKenzie (q.v.) from 1931 to 1938 and shared his mentor's interest in athletics. Brown was a professional boxer and then a boxing coach at Princeton University. He was a resident sculptor and member of the faculty there from 1939 on. He became professor in 1962 and professor emeritus in 1977. His naturalistic portraits and sculptures of athletes were exhibited at the Pennsylvania Academy of the Fine Arts (1932–42), the National Academy of Design (1933–78), the Art Institute of Chicago, the Philadelphia Museum of Art, the New York World's Fair (1965), Expo '67 in Montreal, and the Architectural League of New York. He has had one-man shows at the National Academy of Arts and Letters, the National Education Association, the 1968 Olympic Games in Mexico City, galleries in New York and Philadelphia, and at Yale, Johns Hopkins, Bucknell, Virginia, Colgate, and Princeton Universities. He is an associate of the National Academy of Design and recipient of its Barnett prize (1944), fellow of the National Sculpture Society, winner of the Creative Award from the American Academy of Physical Education (1968), and winner of a distinguished service citation from the American Association of Health, Physical Education, and Recreation of the National Education Association (1967). His work, represented in many museums and universities, includes heroic bronze sculptures of a discus thrower and a runner at Johns Hopkins, a monument of a swimmer at Yale, bronze gymnasts at Temple University, and four monumental bronze athletes at Veterans' Stadium in Philadelphia.

Plaster, painted bronze color; 9 1/4 x 5 x 5 3/8; base 1 1/4 high, integral with sculpture, with stylized monogram, "RTM," on the front edge; signed and dated on right side above base, "Joe Brown '38." Presented by Dr. Douglas Macfarlan in 1959. *ST 563*

Dr. McKenzie is shown head-and-neck length, the head and body frontal. His head is bald except for a fringe of hair at the sides. His brows are knitted. His narrow eyes, with carved irises and pupils, look straight ahead. His thin nose has a bump at the bridge. A brush moustache surmounts a full mouth. There are wrinkles in the forehead and lower lids. The cheekbones are high, the jaw is square, and the chin is cleft. The surface of this naturalistic portrait is irregular and lively. The head is modeled with understanding of the anatomical structure. The facial expression is somber but retains a sense of energy and vitality.

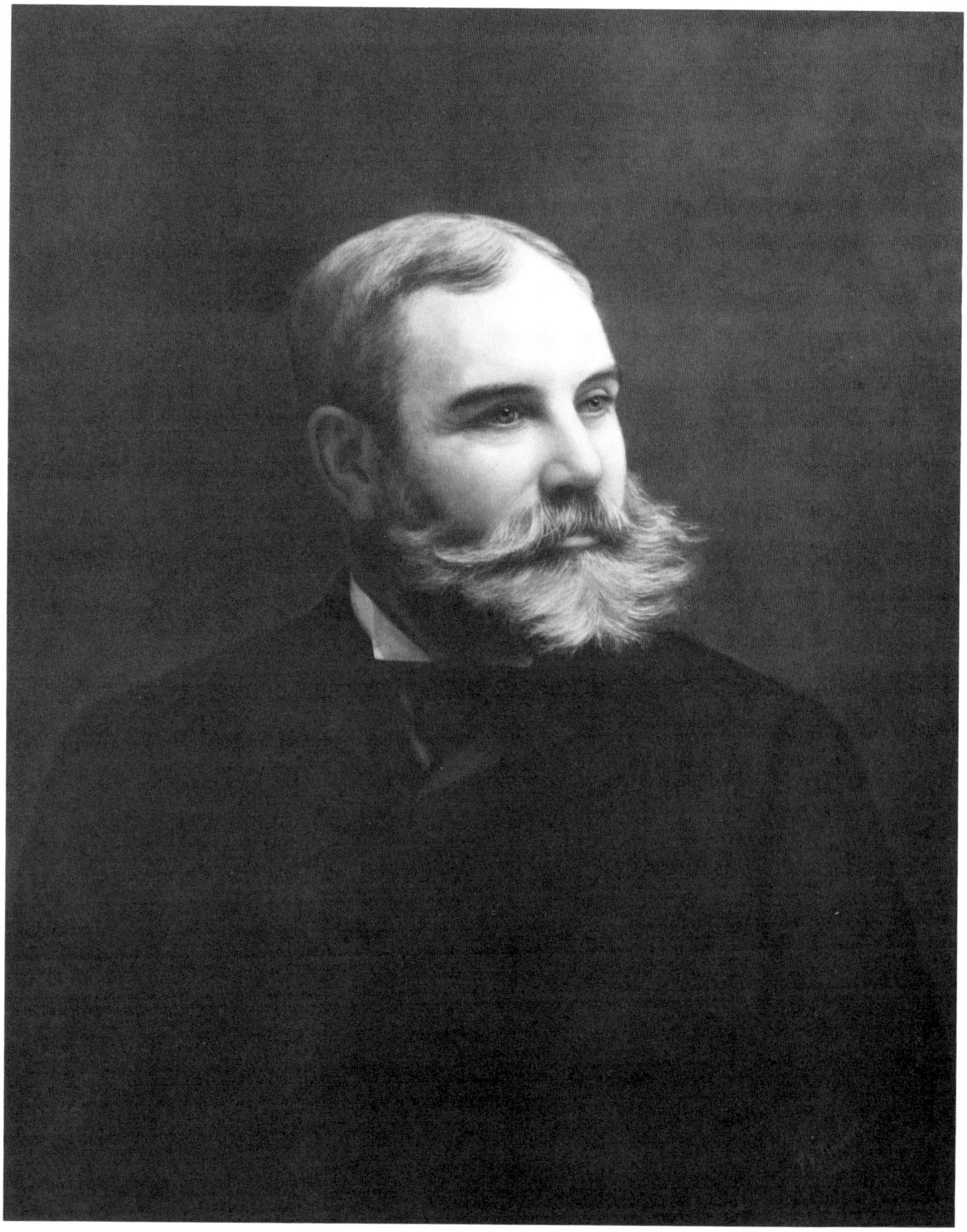

James Ewing Mears *PA 73*

James Ewing Mears (1838-1919)

Born in Indianapolis, the son of a physician, Mears was graduated with A.B. and B.S. degrees from Trinity College, Hartford, in 1858. During the Civil War he was a captain in the Quartermaster's Corps of the Indiana Volunteers and served in a military hospital. He received the M.D. degree from Jefferson Medical College in 1865. He became an assistant in the ovarian clinic of Dr. Washington L. Atlee (q.v.) and helped in the publication of his case reports. He also was associated with the Jefferson Surgical Clinic and was one of those who formed a quiz class to prepare students for their examinations. He was a charter member of the American Surgical Association and its president in 1893. He was a fellow of the College of Physicians, which he served as recorder, as editor of the *Transactions*, and as chairman of the hall committee. He contributed liberally to the building and book funds. He was professor of anatomy at the Philadelphia College of Dental Surgery, demonstrator of surgery at Jefferson Medical College, lecturer and gynecologist at Jefferson Medical College Hospital, and surgeon to St. Mary and St. Agnes Hospitals. In addition, for many years he performed abdominal and gynecological operations at his private hospital. He was author of *Practical Surgery* (1878) and *Surgery of the Abdomen* (1888), and he wrote on ankylosis of the jaw. Deeply interested in eugenics, he published a book, *The Problem of Race Betterment,* in which he advocated surgical procedures to sterilize mental defectives and criminals, and he left $100,000 to Harvard University to establish a course in eugenics. He left a large medical library to the State of Indiana Medical Society, established a scholarship at Jefferson Medical College, and left $10,000 to the Harvard Cancer Commission.

Artist: Mrs. Francis Van Horn Heberton (b. 1846)

For biography, see page 62.

Oil on canvas; 26 3/4 x 21 3/4; signed lower right, "F.V. Heberton/ Philad." Donor and date are unrecorded, but the painting is included in the College of Physicians 1898–1915 inventory. *PA 73*

Dr. Mears is shown bust length, with body frontal and head turned sharply to the right. The atmospheric background is greenish-gray, darker on the left, lighter on the right. He has short gray hair, parted in the center, as are his long moustache and forked, full beard. His deepset, light blue eyes look out in the direction of the head turn. The straight nose is thick at the bridge. The lower lip juts out and the upper lip is concealed by the moustache. He wears a white shirt with wing collar, a black necktie, and a black double-breasted coat, buttoned high. The paint style of this portrait is very smooth and slick without visible brush strokes, except in the luxuriant moustache and beard, in which animated strokes describe individual strands. The head is rendered in solid and three-dimensional anatomical forms. The costume is flat, without indication of underlying bodily forms. The subject's head is turned stiffly away from the viewer and has a neutral expression. Though depicted flat, the body almost fills the width of the canvas and is presented frontally, giving a sense of physical strength and power.

Arthur Vincent Meigs (1850-1912)

Dr. Meigs was born in Philadelphia of English forbears who came to America before 1640. He was the son and grandson of the physicians, J. Forsyth Meigs and Charles D. Meigs (q.v.). After studying at the University of Pennsylvania for two years, he entered its medical school, receiving the M.D. degree in 1871. He spent the next two years in Vienna. Upon his return to Philadelphia, he established a medical practice which he continued until his death. He was attending physician at the Children's Hospital, Pennsylvania Hospital, and the Sheltering Arms (a home for foundlings) and consulting physician at the Eastern Penitentiary and the Pennsylvania Institute for the Instruction of the Blind. He was a fellow of the College of Physicians and its president from 1904 to 1907. He was president of the Philadelphia Pathological Society, a trustee of the University of Pennsylvania and of the Wistar Institute, and a member of the American Philosophical Society. His scientific work on the comparative chemistry of the milk of humans and cows was begun in the 1880s, when he published a treatise, *Milk Analysis and Infant Feeding,* and was continued until about 1908, when he worked in the Hare Laboratory of the University of Pennsylvania. During the research for two other books, *The Origin of Disease* and *Human Bloodvessels in Health and Disease,* he discovered that the capillaries of the heart actually enter the myocardial fibers.

Artist: William Merritt Chase (1849–1916)

Born in Williamsburg, Indiana, Chase studied art at the school of the National Academy of Design from 1869 to 1871 and then at the Royal Academy in Munich, where he came under the influence of the realist, Wilhelm Leibl, and acquired the contemporary admiration for dark colors and bravura brushwork of the 17th century Dutch and Spanish painters. He returned to New York in 1878, where his exotically appointed studio in the Tenth Street Studio Building served as a salon for his friends and fellow artists. He travelled to Europe frequently throughout his career, often staying for extended periods. Chase was an activist in professional art organizations. He participated in the first exhibition of the Society of American Artists and was its president from 1885 to 1895. Although this organization was formed in protest against the excessively conservative policies of the National Academy of Design, Chase accepted election as an academician in 1890. He was a founding member of the Society of Painters in Pastel in 1884 and joined the Ten American Painters in 1910. He was an influential teacher at some of America's finest art schools, including the Art Students' League (1878–96, 1907–12), the Brooklyn Art School, the Chicago Art Institute, the Pennsylvania Academy of the Fine Arts (1897–1909), and his own Chase school, founded in 1896 (later the New York School of Art, and then Parsons School). He gave summer classes in Shinnecock, Long Island. He was a virtuoso painter of representational portraits, landscapes, still lifes, and interior scenes in an eclectic variety of techniques and in many media. He executed a large number of commissioned portraits. He was one of only a few Americans who was asked to paint a self-portrait for the collection at the Uffizi Gallery in Florence. His work is represented in most of America's major museums, and he received many honors and awards, including three gold medals in 1901 alone. His admiring students include many of America's most important modernists.

Oil on canvas; 35 1/4 x 28 1/2; signed lower right, "Wm M Chase." Presented by friends of Dr. Meigs in 1910. *PA 3*

Dr. Meigs is shown two-thirds length, with body turned to the left and head slightly to the left. He is seated in an armchair, his left forearm placed diagonally across his body, while the right arm rests on the chair arm and the right hand holds a soft-covered book, his index finger

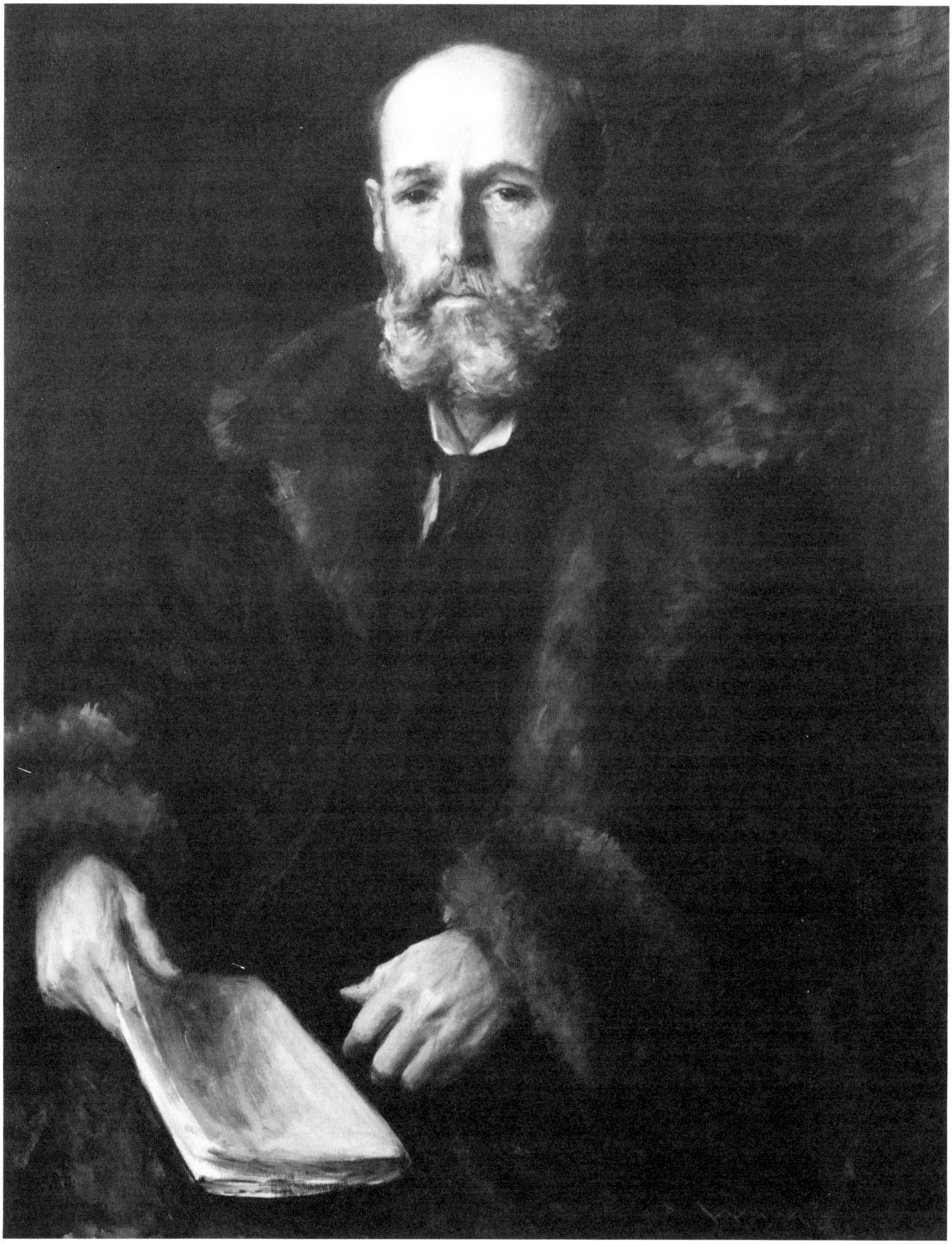

Arthur Vincent Meigs PA 3

marking the place. The background consists of large, dark brown diagonal strokes. Meigs is depicted as almost totally bald, with a little dark brown hair at the sides of his head. His brown eyes stare straight ahead. His nose has a bump at the bridge. His mouth is just visible amid the long gray hairs of his moustache. He has side-whiskers and a short, forked beard. He wears a white shirt with wing collar, a maroon necktie, a black vest, and a black overcoat with fur-trimmed collar, lapels, and wide cuffs. The surface of the portrait consists of loosely brushed, animated strokes. The head and hands are well constructed in three-dimensional volumes but the body is enveloped by the costume. This is a conventional pose in which the subject is supposed to have just looked away from his reading for a moment to regard the viewer. In this case, however, the figure seems curiously unanimated, with a somber, almost mournful expression, in direct opposition to the artist's assertive tour-de-force brushwork.

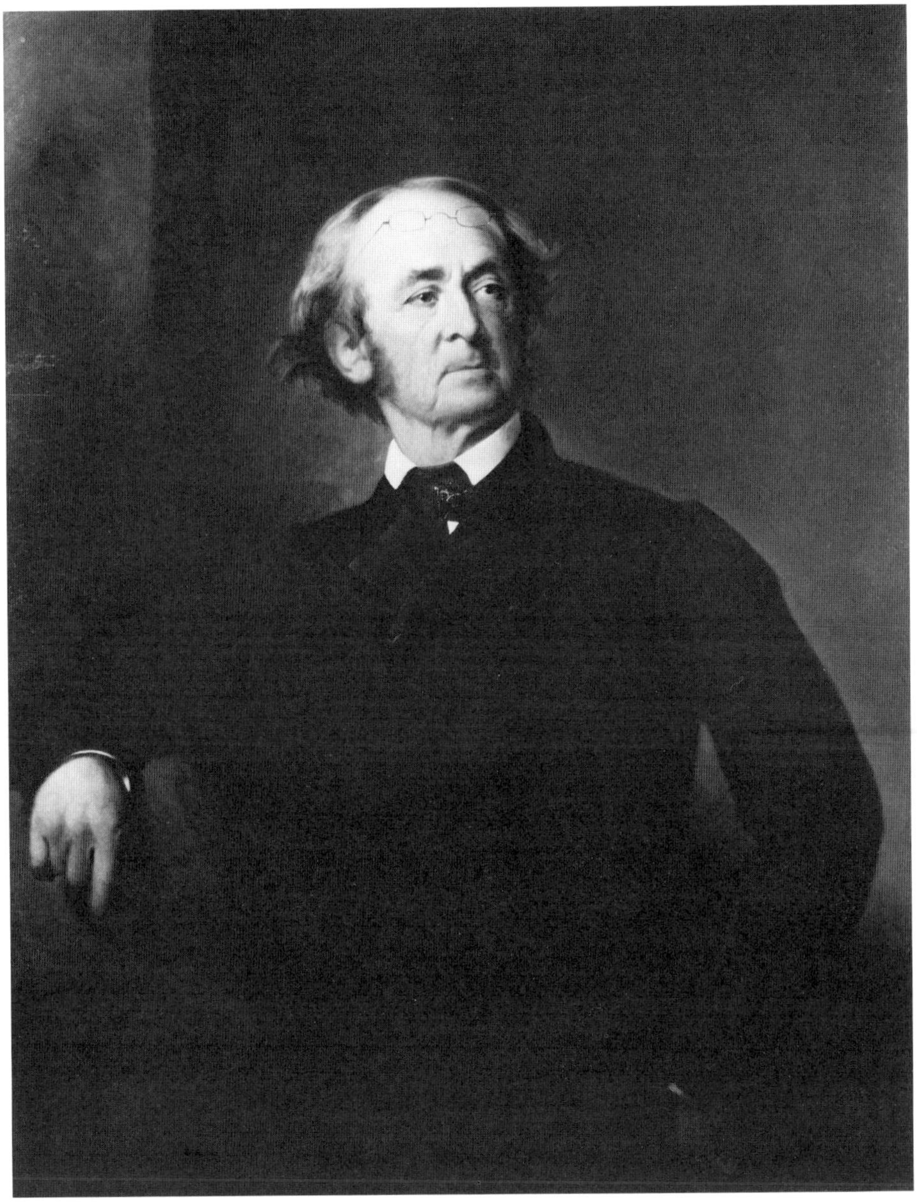

Charles Delucena Meigs *PA 113*

Charles Delucena Meigs (1792-1869)

Born in St. George, Bermuda, Meigs was a lineal descendant of Vincent Meigs, who emigrated from Dorset, England, to Connecticut before 1640. Dr. Meigs graduated in 1809 from the University of Georgia, of which his father was president, and received the M.D. degree from the University of Pennsylvania in 1817. He set up practice in Philadelphia and in 1826 became one of the first editors of the *North American Medical and Surgical Journal.* As his practice began to concentrate on obstetrics, he lectured on midwifery at William Gibson's private school of medicine and he translated from the French Velpeau's monograph, *Elementary Treatise on Midwifery* (1831). At the College of Physicians, which he served as vice president from 1848 to 1855, he was appointed a member of the committee which founded the Preston Retreat. He was elected professor of obstetrics and diseases of women and children at Jefferson Medical College in 1841, a post he filled for twenty years, and where he was known as an eloquent speaker and an advocate of elevating the standards of medical education. He was physician to the Pennsylvania Hospital and a member of the American Philosophical Society. He made significant contributions to the obstetrical literature, including *Woman, Her Diseases and Remedies* (1847), *Obstetrics, the Science and Art* (1849), *Treatise on Acute and Chronic Diseases of the Neck of the Uterus* (1850), and *On the Nature and Treatment of Childbed Fevers* (1854). He is sometimes best remembered, unfairly, for his strenuous opposition to the belief that puerperal fever is an infectious disease. It is not often remembered that he made an important contribution by identifying coronary thrombosis (and not syncope) as a cause of sudden death in childbirth.

Artist: Samuel Bell Waugh (1814-1885)

For biography, see page 44.

Oil on canvas; 35 1/2 x 44 1/2; signed and dated lower left, "S.B. Waugh, 186[?, last digit undecipherable]." Shown at the Pennsylvania Academy of the Fine Arts Loan Collection of Historical Portraits *(1887-88) and at the College of Physicians'* Centennial Celebration Loan Collection of Portraits *(1887) when it was owned by Arthur V. Meigs (q.v.). Presented by Dr. John Wister Meigs, the great-great-grandson of C.D. Meigs, in 1975. The portrait was commissioned and given to the subject as a token of esteem by either the graduating class of 1856 or the class of 1861, depending on whether one reads a letter from the donor in the files of the College of Physicians, a presentation speech in the* Transactions and Studies of the College of Physicians of Philadelphia *(vol. 43, 1975-76), or two notes in the* College and Clinical Record *of Jefferson College (Jan. 15, Feb 1, 1880), which offer conflicting statements. This portrait remained with the Meigs family until its presentation to the College of Physicians. In 1872, Samuel Bell Waugh made a bust-length copy which is at Jefferson Medical College. The College of Physicians portrait was briefly lent to the Solis-Cohen amphitheater of Thomas Jefferson University in 1982.* *PA 113*

Dr. Meigs is shown half-length, with body frontal and head turned to the right. He is standing with his left arm akimbo, while his right arm rests on a red, cloth-covered piece of furniture (perhaps a lectern) and his right hand is pendent. The atmospheric background is dark greenish-brown. There is a suggestion of a frame or window in the upper left corner. Meigs's wire-rimmed spectacles rest on his high forehead. His long gray hair projects from the sides of his head. Under thick eyebrows his brown eyes look out in the direction of the head turn; he has a thin upper lip, a jutting lower lip, and a square chin. There are age lines in the knitted brows and lower lids and next to the nose and mouth. He wears a white shirt, a wide black bow tie with a tie pin, and a black double-breasted coat buttoned high. The paint style of this portrait is very smooth, without visible brush strokes. The head and hands are well constructed in convincingly solid and three-dimensional volumes, and there is a sense of the bodily forms underlying the costume. The aristocratic posture, averted gaze, and serious facial expression give the subject a commanding, authoritative presence—he might be in the process of delivering an eloquent lecture on midwifery to an unseen audience. The use of dramatically lighted background and brilliant white of the shirt collar and cuffs focus attention on the subject's head and hands.

Russel F. Miller (1901-1980)

Reared in Nesquehoning, Pennsylvania, Miller received the B.S. degree from Pennsylvania State University in 1922 and the M.D. degree from the University of Pennsylvania in 1926. After studying pathology and serving as chief of pathology at Pottsville Hospital (1927-29), he moved to Philadelphia and completed a residency in radiology at Philadelphia General Hospital (1932). He was chief of the diagnostic radiology division there for 41 years and was greatly respected as a teacher and clinician. He was associate professor of radiology in the graduate school of medicine at the University of Pennsylvania and was director of radiology at the Women's Hospital. During World War II he had the rank of lieutenant colonel. He was a fellow of the College of Physicians.

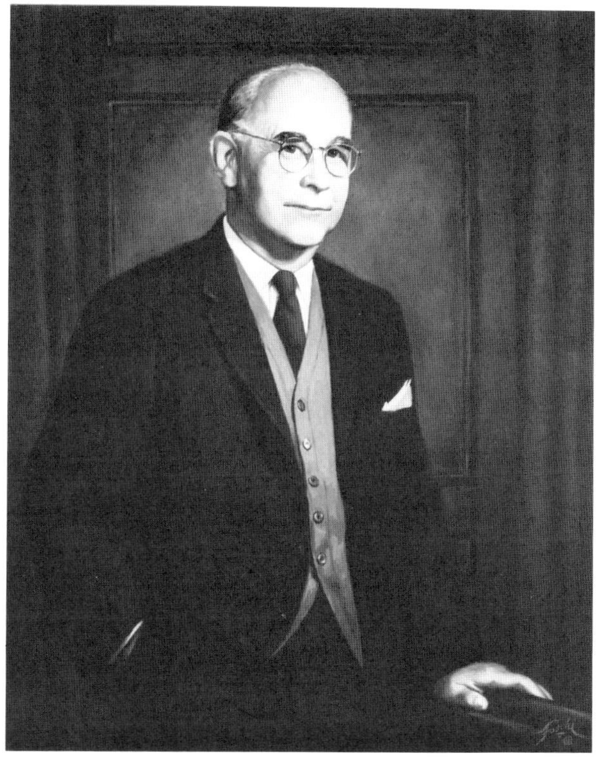

Russel F. Miller *PA 139*

Artist: Foschi Portrait Studio

Oil on canvas; 35 1/2 x 29 1/4; signed lower right, "Foschi"; painted from photographs in a collaborative portrait studio. Originally commissioned by the Blockley Radiological Society, the portrait was presented to the radiology department of Philadelphia General Hospital and then to the city of Philadelphia, which in turn presented it on permanent loan to the College of Physicians in 1977. *PA 139*

Dr. Miller is shown half-length, with body turned slightly to the right and head to the right and tilted down. He is standing with his right hand in his trouser pocket and his left hand resting on the back of a green chair. The geometric background is composed of square wooden paneling flanked by maroon draperies with regular, vertical folds. The subject has a high forehead with short gray hair. Under black eyebrows his blue eyes look out past the viewer through gold-rimmed spectacles. He has a small, straight nose and a wide, thin-lipped mouth. A grin makes his cheeks puff out. He wears a white shirt, a maroon tie, a gray cardigan sweater or vest, and a blue single-breasted suit with a white pocket handkerchief.

The surface of the portrait is smoothly brushed in the figure, more painterly in the background. The head and hand have been constructed solidly. The costume is flatter, with some sense of the underlying bodily forms. The pose, facial expression, and choice of costume are unusually informal. Because of the team effort involved in the manufacture of this type of portrait, the subject has an artificial, lifeless look, even though the likeness is probably accurate. In addition, there is no feeling of real space between the subject and the studio background.

Thomas Grier Miller (1886-1981)

Born in Statesville, North Carolina, Miller graduated from the University of North Carolina in 1906 and from the University of Pennsylvania School of Medicine in 1911. He spent the rest of his illustrious medical career at the University, where he was appointed successively instructor (1913), assistant professor (1928), professor of clinical medicine (1934), professor of medicine (1947), and emeritus professor (1952). At the beginning of his career he was offered the first fellowship in medicine established at the University, and at the end of that year he became the associate of Dr. Alfred Stengel (q.v.). At the University he founded the gastrointestinal section of the department of medicine in 1926 and established a subsection of the gastrointestinal department in psychiatry, which later evolved into the department of psychiatry, in 1949. In 1930, with Dr. Alfred Newton Richards, he made an extensive study at the request of the newly-installed president, Thomas S. Gates, of university medical schools to prepare a guide for recommendations for development of the University of Pennsylvania Medical School. Miller was well known as the developer, with Dr. William Osler Abbott, of the long double-lumen intestinal tube, which became an important device in the study and treatment of intestinal disorders. He was president of the American Gastroenterological Association, the American College of Physicians, the American Clinical and Climatological Association, the Philadelphia County Medical Society, the Interurban Clinical Club, the medical board of the Hospital of the University of Pennsylvania, and the College of Physicians of Philadelphia (1949-51). Among his awards are an honorary LL.D. from the University of North Carolina and the Friedenwald Medal of the American Gastroenterological Association (1957). At the University of Pennsylvania he was honored by the building of the T. Grier Miller Plaza adjacent to the medical education building and by the creation of the T. Grier Miller Chair in Medicine (1977). He wrote more than 100 articles in journals and textbooks, including the chapter on bronchitis, bronchiectasis, and foreign bodies in the lung in Cecil's *Textbook on Medicine* (editions of 1933, 1940, and 1943). He was an early investigator of miner's silicosis (formerly thought to be tuberculosis), the intranasal use of ephedrine, and the synthetic preparations of it that were subsequently developed.

Artist: Charles Baskerville (b. 1896)

Born in Raleigh, North Carolina, the son of a professor of chemistry at the University of North Carolina, Baskerville graduated from Cornell University in 1919. He studied at the Art Students' League in New York and at the Académie Julien in Paris. He has had an adventurous life, both in the military and artistic spheres. During World War I he was a lieutenant of infantry in the Rainbow Division. He received the silver cross for gallantry in action, a purple heart with oak leaf clusters, and the conspicuous service cross. As lieutenant-colonel during World War II he was official portraitist of the U.S. Army Air Forces and was decorated with the legion of merit for his depiction of 72 heroes and officers, a collection which is now on permanent display at the Pentagon. In 1945 he organized an exhibition of "Significant War Scenes" for the Chrysler Corporation, a collection now installed in its corporate headquarters after a two-year tour with the American Federation of Arts. He has traveled around the world four times in search of exotic subject matter and has painted portraits of such eastern dignitaries as the king and the prime minister maharajah of Nepal, Prime Minister Nehru of India, and the family of the Maharajah of Jaipur. The subjects of his portraits include an international list of diplomats, corporate leaders, actors, members of society, and professional leaders, such as Helen Hayes, the Duchess of Windsor, Bernard Baruch, and members of the Whitney, Mellon, Payson, Paley, duPont, Kellogg, Ingersoll, Hearst, Vanderbilt, Rockefeller, and Auchincloss families. Baskerville is also well known as a muralist and was president of the National Society of Murals Painters from 1957 to 1959. He has created murals for the S.S. *America*, three ships of the Grace Line, the Wall Street Club, Princeton University, the conference room of the Joint Committee on Military Affairs of the U.S. House of Representatives and Senate, and the homes of Mrs. Marjorie Merriweather Post, Gene Tunney, Harcourt Amory, the Viscount de Sibour, and many others. He has had thirteen one-man shows, including a command exhibition at the Viceroy's Palace in New Delhi. He has also exhibited at the National Gallery of Art, the Metropolitan Museum, the Whitney Museum, the Architectural League, the Carnegie Institute, the Chicago Art Institute, the Four Arts Society in Palm Beach, the Art Association of Newport, and Cornell University. In addition to being in private collections, his work is represented in many museums, corporate headquarters, and universities.

Oil on canvas; 47 1/2 x 35 1/2; signed and dated lower left, "Charles Baskerville-1952." Presented by Dr. T. Grier Miller in 1952. *PA 119*

Miller is shown three-quarters length, with body turned to the right and head frontal. He is seated in an upholstered chair, with his legs crossed at the knees. His right arm and hand rests on the chair arm, his left hand holds a book which rests on his knee, and his index finger marks the place. The background consists of a maroon curtain with vertical folds on the left and a warm greenish-gray wall behind, divided by a molding. The subject has an oval face with brown hair, blue eyes which look straight ahead through horn-rimmed glasses, a broad nose, a wide mouth with thin lips, a wide lower jaw, and a cleft chin. He wears a white shirt, a black bow tie, black trousers, and a black academic robe whose full sleeves have five green stripes and a green lining. There are green panels down the center front and a mantle with alternating red and green trim. The surface of the portrait is painterly throughout, but the head and hands are painted with tighter, more meticulous strokes to emphasize the three-dimensional solidity of the forms. The costume is more loosely brushed, but there is still a sense of the underlying bodily forms, in particular the foreshortened thigh and the dramatic highlight on the projecting knee. Although the chair is turned at a angle of 45 degrees to the picture plane, the subject's lower body twists around and his head is turned to gaze intently at the viewer, as though he had just been interrupted in his reading to respond to an unseen visitor.

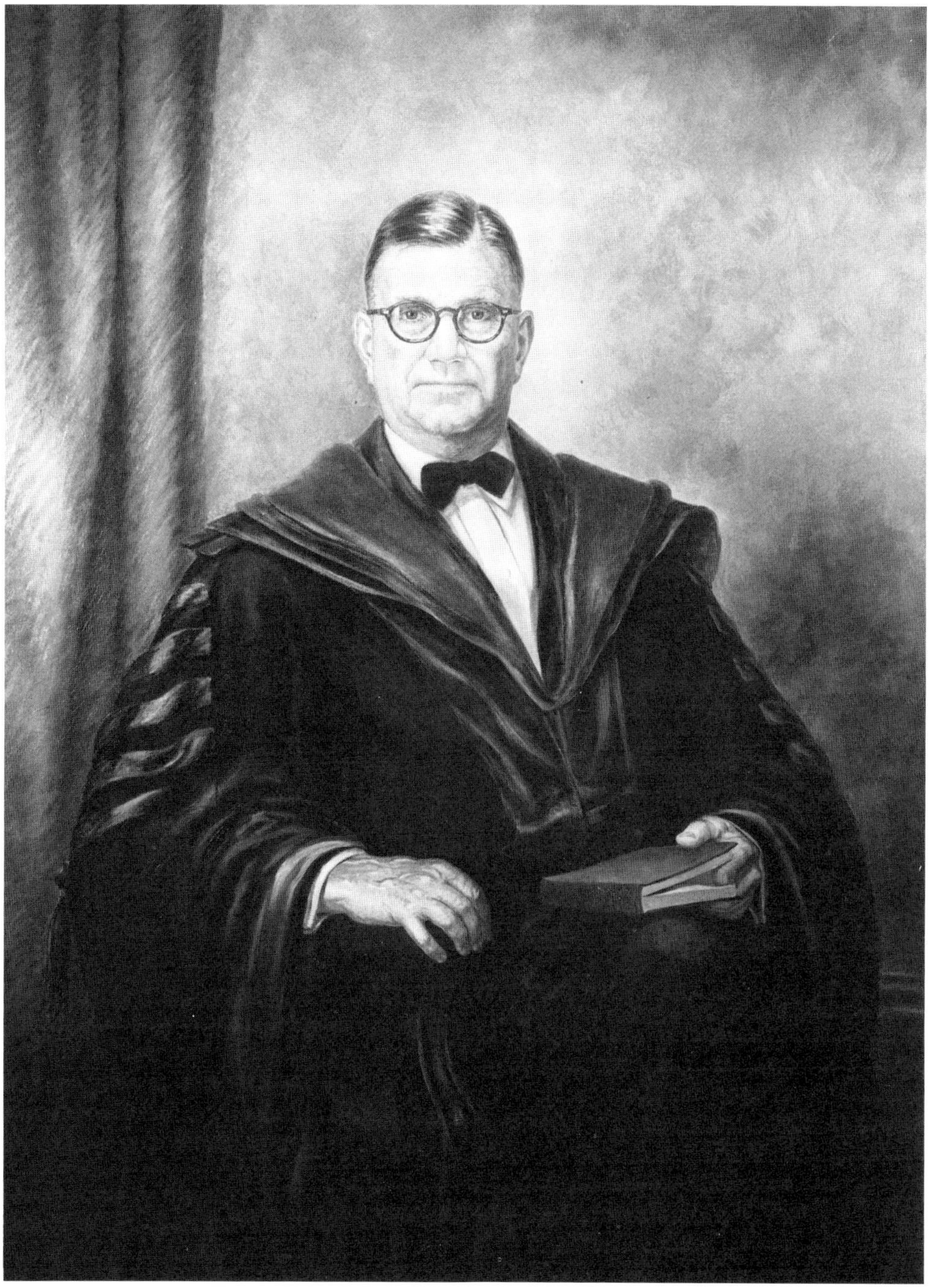

Thomas Grier Miller *PA 119*

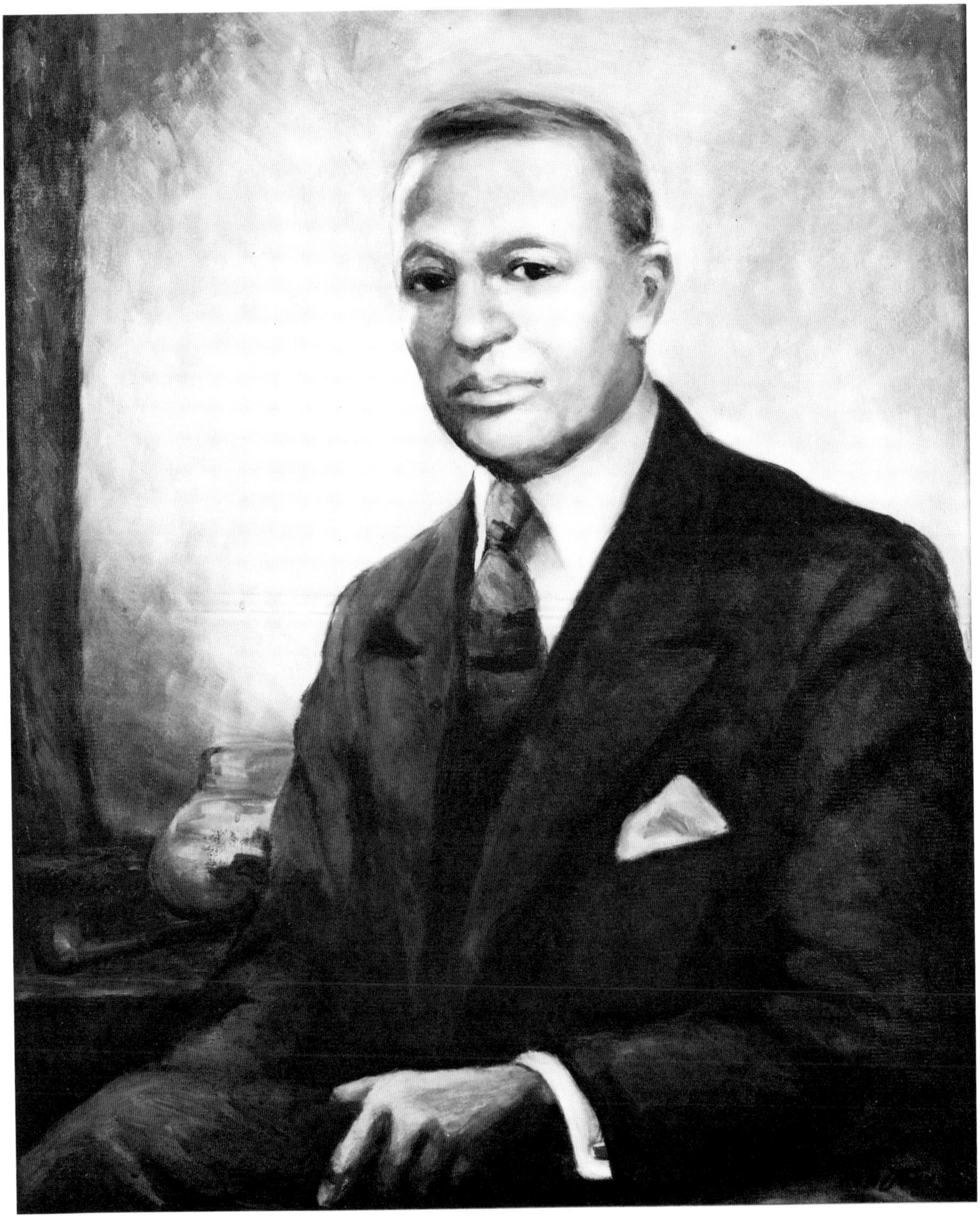

Henry McKee Minton *PA 134*

Henry McKee Minton (1870–1946)

Minton was born in Columbia, South Carolina. He was a grandson of Henry Minton, a well-known Philadelphia caterer who was devoted to elevating the social and economic status of black residents of his city. After attending the Washington, D.C., public schools and the Academy of Howard University, Minton entered Phillips Exeter Academy in New Hampshire, where he proved to be an outstanding scholar, athlete, debater, editor, and commencement orator. After one year at the University of Pennsylvania Law School, he recognized that science and medicine were his dominant interests. He transferred to the Philadelphia College of Pharmacy, where he earned the Ph.G. degree in 1895. He became the proprietor of the first black-owned pharmacy in Philadelphia, but after seven years in this business he decided to become a physician and earned the M.D. degree at Jefferson Medical College in 1906. He joined the staff of the first black hospital in Philadelphia, Douglass Hospital, as its pharmacist; he was later made secretary of its board of directors. In 1920 he joined the Mercy

Hospital, where his father, an attorney, served on the board. Minton was superintendent and director of Mercy Hospital for 24 years and was on the staff of the Henry Phipps Institute from 1915 to 1946. He was the founder of the Sigma Pi Phi medical fraternity and was a member of the American Medical Association, the Laennec Society, and the Philadelphia County and the Pennsylvania Medical Societies. He wrote three monographs, *The Early History of Negroes in Business in Philadelphia, Some of the Problems of Hospital Administration,* and *Early Diagnosis of Tuberculosis.*

Artist: Henry Bozeman Jones (b. 1889)

For biography, see page 76.

Oil on canvas; 29 1/4 x 24 1/2; signed lower right, "Hen Jones." Commissioned by the Olde Philadelphia Club and hung at Mercy-Douglass Hospital until presented to the College of Physicians by Dr. Russell F. Minton, nephew of the subject, in 1976. Shown at A Century of Black Presence at the University of Pennsylvania, 1879–1980, *at the Van Pelt Library, University of Pennsylvania, 1980–81.*

PA 134

Dr. Minton is shown half-length, with body and head turned to the left. He is seated, with legs crossed and with his left arm and hand rested on his left leg. In the left background there is a table with a pipe and a glass bowl upon it and bluish-purple drapery. The color behind the subject ranges from a warm yellow to green. Minton's face is square. He has a high forehead, brownish-gray hair, dark brown eyes which gaze out of their corners toward the viewer, a wide nose, full lips, and a firm chin. The skin tones are of a medium hue. He wears a white shirt and a white pocket handkerchief, a necktie striped in blue, green, and red, a dark brown three-piece suit, and cuff links. The surface of the portrait is painterly throughout. The head and hand are moderately solid. There is some feeling for the bodily forms underlying the costume. The contours of features and costume are outlined. The green, blue, and purple of the background are mixed with the local color of the suit. His posture is energetic and his gaze is riveted on the spectator, as though the subject were about to converse.

Silas Weir Mitchell (1829–1914)

The famed neurologist, novelist, and poet was born in Philadelphia, the son and grandson of physicians. He attended the University of Pennsylvania and received the M.D. degree from Jefferson Medical College in 1850. He continued his education in Paris, studying physiology and microscopy. At his father's urging he also took courses in surgery, but he felt unsuited for that specialty. Upon his return to Philadelphia, he established a medical practice that he continued for the rest of his career, but he was always more inclined toward scientific investigation. As early as 1853 he was elected a member of the Academy of Natural Sciences. He wrote a monograph on the venom of the rattlesnake (1860) and other papers in natural science. He was a founder of the Pathological Society of Philadelphia and presented a paper at its first meeting in 1857. He was elected a member of the American Philosophical Society in 1862. One of his earliest teaching positions was as lecturer in physiology for the Philadelphia Association for Medical Instruction, an organization for extramural medical teaching. He was disappointed never to have been named professor at Jefferson or at the University of Pennsylvania, although later in his career he was elected professor at the Philadelphia Polyclinic and College for Graduates in Medicine and was regarded as a skillful and inspiring teacher. He was also physician to the Southern Hospital, St. Joseph's Hospital, the Pennsylvania Institute for the Instruction of the Blind, Presbyterian Hospital, the Orthopaedic Hospital and Infirmary for Nervous Diseases, State Lying-in Hospital and Infirmary, and the Insane Department of Philadelphia Hospital. During the Civil War he was appointed an acting assistant surgeon, and the wards of two large military hospitals in Philadelphia were set aside for him and his two colleagues, W.W. Keen (q.v.) and G.R. Morehouse, to study and treat injuries of the peripheral nerves and of the central nervous system. The observations made there were used for the books, *Gunshot Wounds and Other Injuries of Nerves* (1864) and *Injuries to Nerves and Their Consequences* (1872). Mitchell did pioneering work in the description and treatment of various nervous disorders, including causalgia, reflex paralysis, erythromelalgia, diseases of the cerebellum, neuralgia, locomotor ataxia, headache, facial tic, spastic paralysis, trophic disorders, and physical and mental manifestations that result from amputation. In the popular mind his reputation is based on the rest cure, known as the Weir Mitchell treatment, in which he advocated a cure by means of repose, isolation, massage, and a milk diet. Some colleagues attacked him as a charlatan and a "fashionable doctor," and the "cure" was abused by other physicians for inappropriate application, but it is agreed today that he showed great insight into the role of emotions in illness in general and in neuroses in particular and that he tried to influence the mind of his patients. He is credited with pioneering insights into psychosomatic medicine. He was an active trustee at the University of Pennsylvania for 35 years and he was a successful fund-raiser and force behind the school of biology and the building of new laboratories. He served the College of Physicians for two terms as president (1886–88, 1892–94). He was a generous benefactor to the Mütter Museum, the College Collections, the library, and to the library and entertainment funds. The S. Weir Mitchell Oration, an annual lectureship, was named in his honor. He received honorary degrees from Harvard, Princeton,

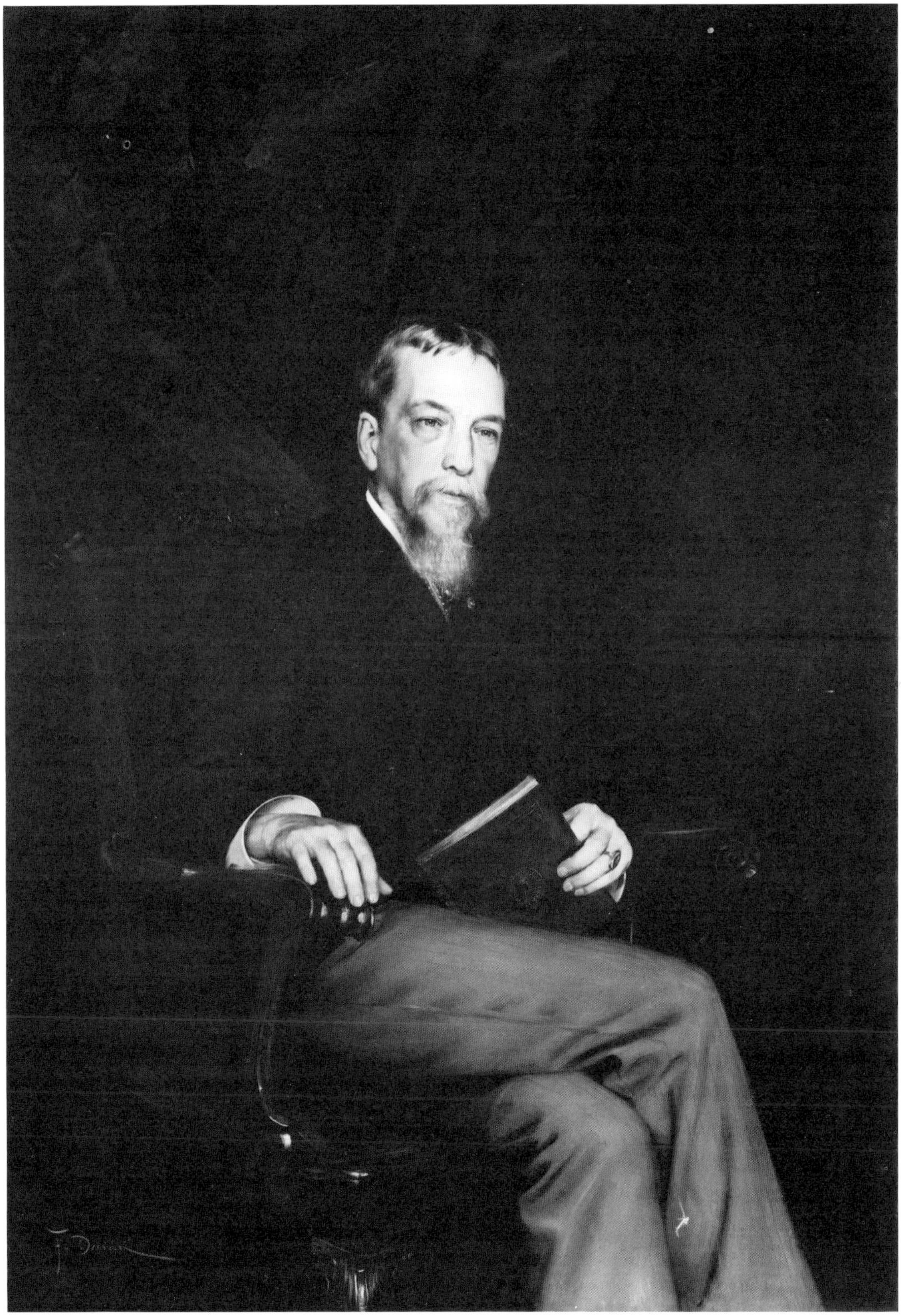

Silas Weir Mitchell *PA 87*

Jefferson, Toronto, Bologna, and Edinburgh Universities and was an honorary member of many foreign scientific societies. Because of his literary fame, he is often compared to his Boston counterpart, Oliver Wendell Holmes (q.v.). Mitchell's first novels appeared when he had already achieved an international reputation as a neurologist and they continued well into his 80s. Some of the better known titles are *In Wartime; When All the Woods are Green; Hugh Wynne, Free Quaker; The Adventures of Francois; Constance Truscot; The Red City; John Sherwood, Iron Master;* and *Westaways.* He also published short stories and books of poetry. His last poem, "Vesperal," was written the year of his death and begins with the lines:

> I know the night is near at hand,
> The mists lie low on hill and bay,
> The autumn sheaves are dewless, dry;
> But I have had the day.

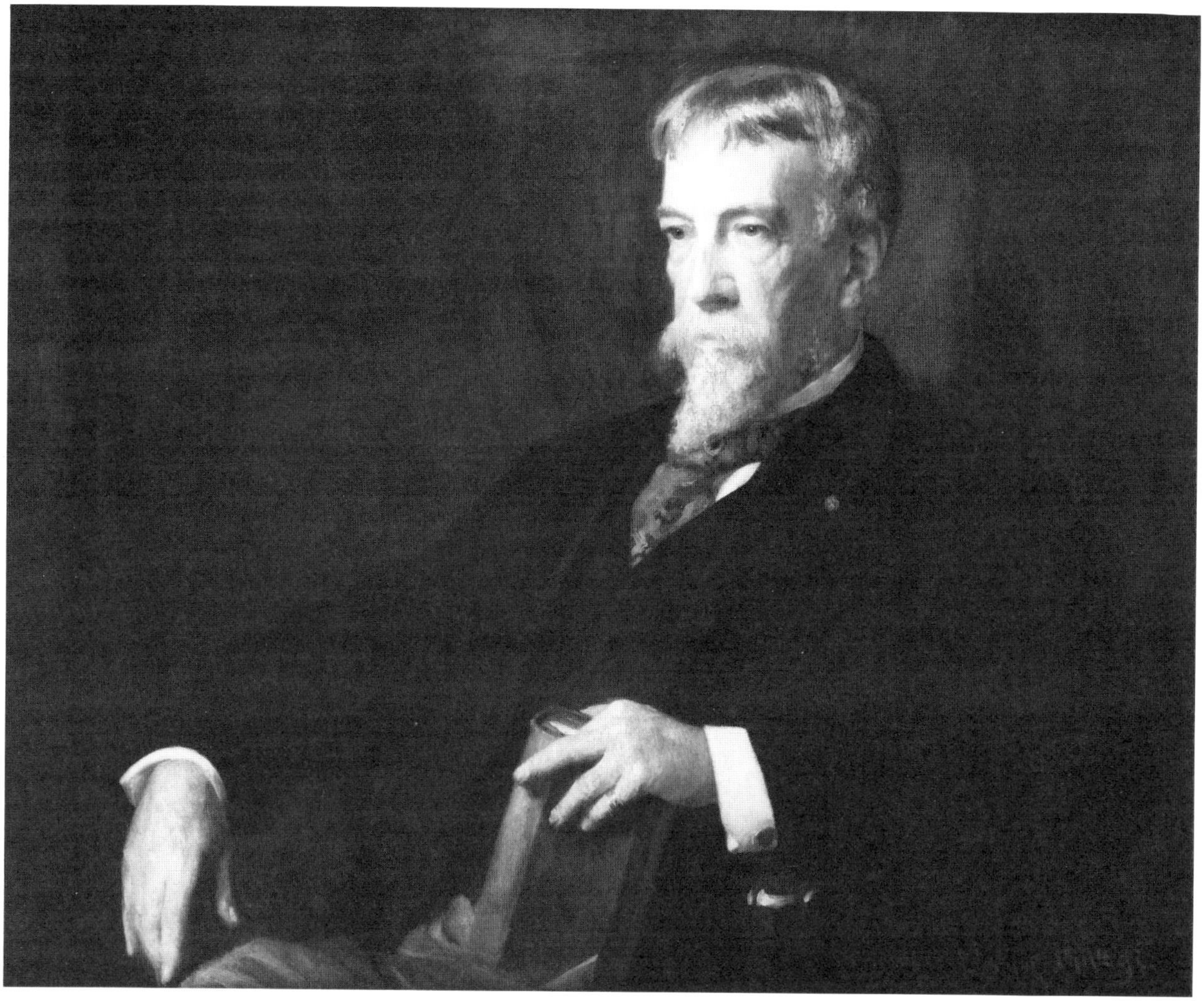

Silas Weir Mitchell

PA 24

Artist: Franz Dvorak (b. 1862)

Born in Prelouc, Bohemia, Dvorak was trained at the Academy in Vienna and then under W. Lindenschmit and O.V.R. Seitein in Munich. He showed his earliest work at exhibitions in Berlin and Vienna, starting in 1886. After a short stay in Paris he was in America from 1890 to 1895 and was in great demand as a portrait painter in Philadelphia, New York, and Chicago. He returned to Europe and was a constant exhibitor of portraits, figure studies, and religious paintings in Paris salons and expositions and at the Royal Academy in London.

Oil on canvas, backed with wood; 56 1/2 x 39 1/2; signed lower left, "F. Dvorak." Probably painted during the artist's stay in America between 1890 and 1895. Presented by friends at a special dinner in 1890. *PA 87*

Dr. Mitchell is shown three-quarters length, with body turned to the right and head turned to the right and tilted down. He is seated in a chair turned at an angle of 45 degrees to the picture plane, with his legs crossed at the knees and with his right arm and hand resting on the chair arm. His left hand holds a book whose place is marked by his index finger. The book has a red cover imprinted with the seal of the College of Physicians. The elegant interior setting is a library containing book shelves lined with books on the right and gray drapery that falls in diagonal folds from the upper left to the lower right corner. Mitchell sits on an elegant Chippendale-style chair with a maroon padded seat, an urn splat back, a cupid's-bow cresting rail with volute ears and a carved shell in the center, volute hands holds, and an acanthus-leaf carving on the knees. Mitchell has gray hair with a center part and carefully arranged bangs, a long gray moustache, side-whiskers, and a small triangular patch of beard on his chin with a narrow beard extending from the base of his chin. His blue eyes look down in the direction of the head turn. His face is elongated. The nose has a bump at the bridge. He has a small mouth, hollow cheeks, and shadows under the eyes. The subject is dressed immaculately in a white shirt, blue and white polka-dotted necktie or cloth, a black vest, a black high-buttoned cutaway coat, and gray trousers. He wears a jeweled tie pin, cuff links, a lapel pin, and a ring. The surface of the portrait has been painted very smoothly throughout, with meticulous, tight brush strokes. The head and hands are illusionistically, almost sculpturally, solid and three-dimensional. The tailoring and folds of the costume are rendered in precise detail and give a feeling for the underlying bodily forms. There are sparking highlights on the figure, costume, and furniture. The posture of the subject is very active. He leans back into the upper right corner of the chair and his hips twist around from the left to the right, so that his legs project

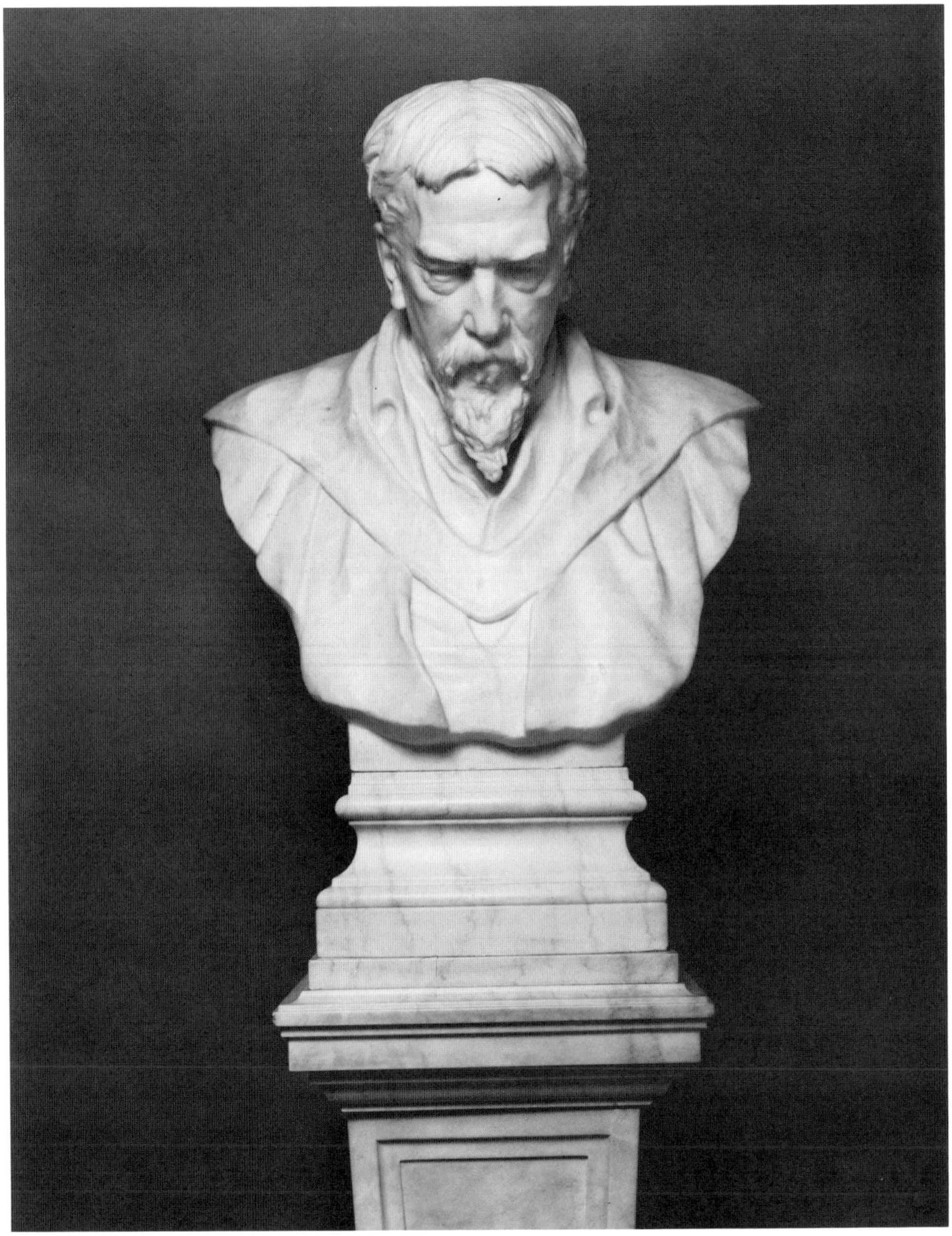

Silas Weir Mitchell ST 527

into space and set up a barrier between him and the viewer. His expression is actively thoughtful, with a gaze directed away from the viewer. His posture and expression, added to the elegant interior and fashionable costume, present a figure to be admired from a distance.

Artist: Robert William Vonnoh (1858–1933)

For biography, see page 31.

Oil on canvas; 28 1/2 x 35 1/2; signed lower right, "Vonnoh Phila—97." Presented by Mary Cadwalader Mitchell in 1900. Shown at an exhibition of the Society of American Artists, New York; at the annual exhibition of the Pennsylvania Academy of the Fine Arts in 1908; and at the Portraits of Yesterday and Today *exhibition at Portraits, Inc., New York, in 1968.* PA 24

Dr. Mitchell is shown half-length, with body turned to the left and head turned to the left and tilted down. He is seated in an armchair, with both arms resting on the chair arms, his right hand pendent, and his left hand holding a book whose place is marked with his index finger. The atmospheric background is green, darker on the right, lighter on the left. His silver-gray hair has a center part and carefully arranged bangs. His narrow blue eyes look down in the direction of the head turn. His nose has a broad bump at the bridge. The gray side-whiskers, moustache, and pointed beard are sparse. He has puffy lower lids and age lines on his hollow cheeks. The subject wears a white shirt, a bright red-patterned necktie, a black vest, a black coat, gray trousers, a lapel pin, cuff links, and a gold ring. The surface of the portrait is painterly throughout. The head and hands have been constructed solidly, with quick, impressionistic strokes.

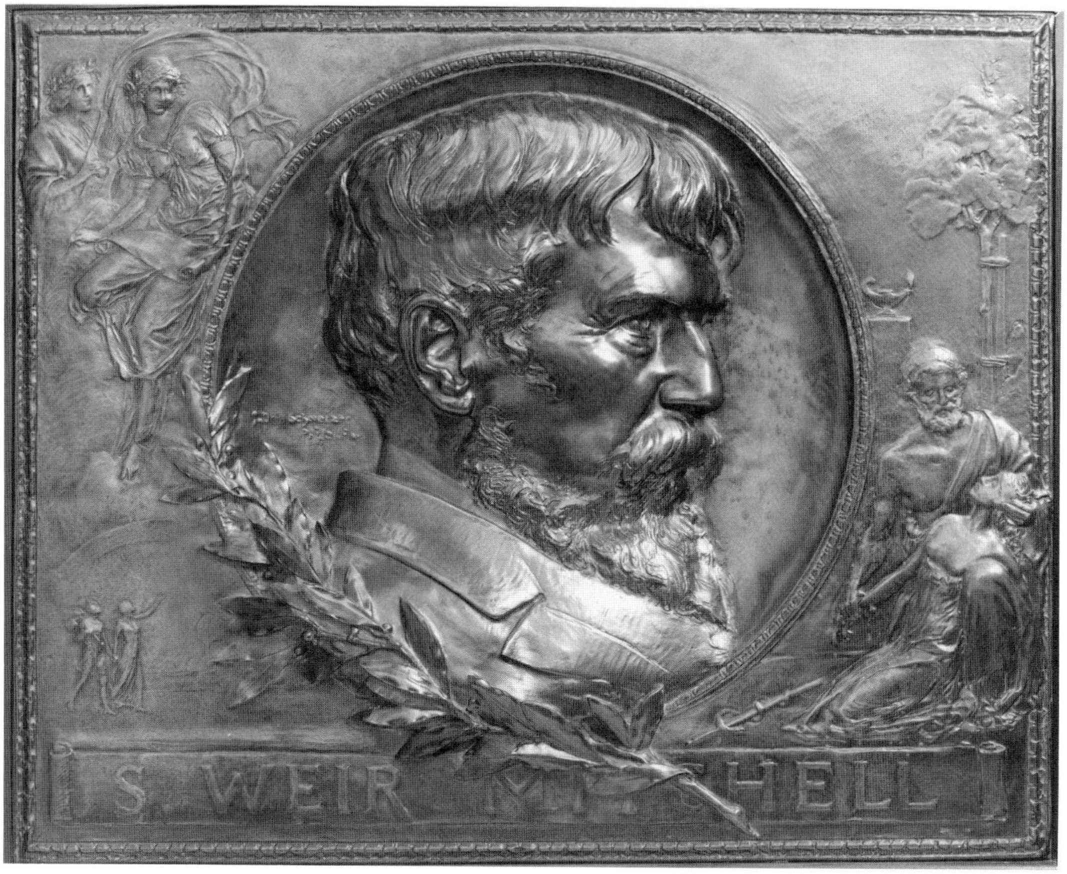

Silas Weir Mitchell *M 1048*

The costume and background are more fluidly painted. There is a suggestion of the bodily forms underlying the costume. The subject leans back in his chair, which is placed at an angle of 45 degrees to the picture plane. Although his expression is meditative, almost brooding, there is a sense of immediacy with the subject because of his placement on the canvas. Compared with Dvorak's portrait of Mitchell (see above) in which the figure is three-quarters length in a large, object-filled environment, here the subject is half-length, seen close-up, and without the distractions of an elaborate setting. Therefore, the viewer concentrates on the head and hands, feels a sense of empathy with the subject, and responds to his mournful expression.

Artist: William Ordway Partridge (1861–1930)

An American born in Paris, Partridge was the son of a wealthy agent for a New York merchant. He was educated first at private military academies and then at Columbia University. He studied sculpture in Florence, Paris, Rome, and Berlin, and he exhibited at the Paris Salons and at the Royal Academies of London and Berlin. Upon his return to America he established studios in Milton, Massachusetts, and then in New York City. A number of his monumental public works are found in New York, including a Pietá in St. Patrick's Cathedral and commemorative statues of Samuel Tilden, General Grant, and Alexander Hamilton. He made his exhibition debut at the Columbian Exposition of 1893 in Chicago, where he showed busts of Shakespeare, Edward Everett Hale, James Russell Lowell, and Alexander Hamilton. Other well-known works by Partridge are the Kauffmann Memorial in Washington, the Pulitzer Memorial in Woodlawn, New York, and portraits at Bowdoin College, Columbia University, and the Boston Public Library. Most of his sculptures in both bronze and marble are naturalistic, but by the turn of the century he developed a more impressionistic style, with looser modeling in which he sought the essence of the subject. He lectured on art at Columbia University, the Concord School of Philosophy, and the Brooklyn Institute; he was a professor at George Washington University. He had tried acting in his youth and was also the author of several books of poetry and articles on sculpture.

Marble; 24 3/4 x 10 1/2 x 14 1/4; base, integral with sculpture, 2 in. high; rests on second multiple level base, 12 1/4 in. high; mounted on a marble pedestal 51 1/2 in. high; signed, "Ordway Partridge, " on lower right side. The Bradley file gives date as 1910. Presented by Mrs. Silas Weir Mitchell in 1910. *ST 527*

Dr. Mitchell is shown bust length, with body frontal and head tilted downward and very slightly to the right. His hair has a center part and bangs. Under knitted brows his deepset eyes gaze straight down. His nose has a prominent bump at the bridge. His full moustache curves down to meet a long triangular beard. His slender face is marked by deep lines in the forehead, puffy lower eyelids, and hollow cheeks. The subject wears a shirt, a bow tie, and an academic gown with a V-shaped mantle. The likeness is remarkably similar to that in the oil portraits (see above), even with the same brooding expression and downward tilt of the head. The surface of the sculpture is smooth, with no visible tool marks. The head has been modeled extremely well in subtle gradations of planes and with accurate knowledge of the underlying anatomical structure. Although the effect is imposing and stern, the sculptor has animated the composition in several areas, e.g. in the flowing hair in moustache and beard, and especially in the costume, with its scalloped borders which overlap the base, its deep folds, and projecting bits of cloth. The whole sculpture is organized as a series of triangles, including the beard, the shape of the head, and the mantle.

Artist: J. Otto Schweizer (1863–1955)

Born in Zürich, Schweizer studied art at the Art School there, under Schilling at the Royal Academy of Art in Dresden, under Tuiller in Paris, and also in Rome and Florence. He came to the United States in 1894 and established a studio in Philadelphia. He exhibited sculpture at the Pennsylvania Academy of the Fine Arts, the National Academy of Design, and the National Sculpture Society. His public works include numerous commemorative and allegorical statues of presidents, generals, and civic leaders and are found in Pittsburgh, Gettysburg, Valley Forge, Carlisle, and Milwaukee. The following bronze sculptures are in Philadelphia: General Peter Muhlenberg, 1910, installed at City Hall (now in storage); James Bartram Nicholson Tomb, 1913, Mt. Peace Cemetery; Henry Melchior Muhlenberg Memorial, 1917, Lutheran Theological Seminary; and the All Wars Memorial to Colored Soldiers and Sailors, 1934, Fairmount Park. Schweizer also executed numerous ideal groups, portrait medallions, busts, medals, and plaquettes.

Bronze relief, set in wood frame; 19 3/8 x 24 1/2 x 2; signed in recess of tondo, to left of subject's head, "J. Otto Schweizer/ Phila"; identification of foundry on lower right corner of plaque, "Bureau Bros/Phila." Inscription on scroll beneath, "S. Weir Mitchell." Presented by Dr. Lewis C. Scheffey in 1956. *M 1048*

Dr. Mitchell is shown head-and-neck length, in high relief, in a classically derived tondo which is bordered with traditional egg-and-dart molding and with laurel leaves below. His head is in profile, turned to the right. He has thick, wavy hair brushed onto his forehead, a full moustache, side-whiskers, and a pointed beard. His nose has a pronounced bump at the bridge. The subject gazes in the direction of the head turn. There are heavy lines in the corner and below the deepset eye that is visible; its pupil and iris are carved. The mouth is hidden by the moustache. The subject wears a shirt and a coat. The tondo is set in a rectangular frame with classical-style allegorical figures in the corners. According to the files of the College of Physicians, they represent two muses with scroll and lyre in the upper left, Moral Beauty and Health under the Rainbow of Life in the lower left, Aesculapius attending a fainting girl in the lower right, and a tree and a lamp in the upper right. Mitchell's head is smoothly carved. There are tool marks in the tondo and surrounding areas. The relief is well-carved, with a variety of depths from the delicate, wind-blown drapery of the muse, to the high relief of the subject's head. Although the composition is a little crowded and Mitchell's head seems flattened on top, the plaque sparkles with the play of light and shade, which gives it animation.

John Armentaire Monges (1759-1827)

Born in Thorembasse, Provence, France, Monges began his study of medicine with a physician in Marseilles. After a period as house surgeon in the Royal Marine Hospital at Rochefort, he became a surgeon on a French warship bound for the American colonies. He remained in America until 1785 and then went to Santo Domingo, where he established a medical practice. An insurrection there drove him and his compatriots away, and he returned to America, deciding to settle in Philadelphia. He arrived destitute in the year of a terrible yellow fever epidemic. He was unsparing of his energy in caring for the victims of this disease and soon won the support of the local populace, who liked his kind nature, sound medical judgment, and quiet manner. In the winter of 1798 he had pneumonia, and he suffered from chronic and debilitating complications of this disease for the rest of his life, often having to interrupt his medical practice to take to bed.

Artist: Charles Balthazar Julien Févret de Saint-Mémin (1770–1852)

Born in Dijon to a family of the lesser nobility, Saint-Mémin attended military school in Paris, but his plans for a career in the army were disrupted by the French Revolution and his family fled to Switzerland. When the family property was confiscated, they fled to America, after their hopes for establishing themselves in Santo Domingo were dashed by the insurrection there in 1793. Although Saint-Mémin had art lessons in Dijon and had painted landscapes in Switzerland and New York, he considered himself an amateur artist. He turned away from landscapes and maps and devoted himself to the more lucrative field of portraiture only as a means of supporting his family. He became proficient in the use of the physiognotrace, a device which traced onto colored paper the exact profile of a sitter, details being filled in with black and white crayon or chalk. Usually he reduced the drawing by means of another device, the pantograph, to a small disc of copper, upon which he made engravings. He moved from New

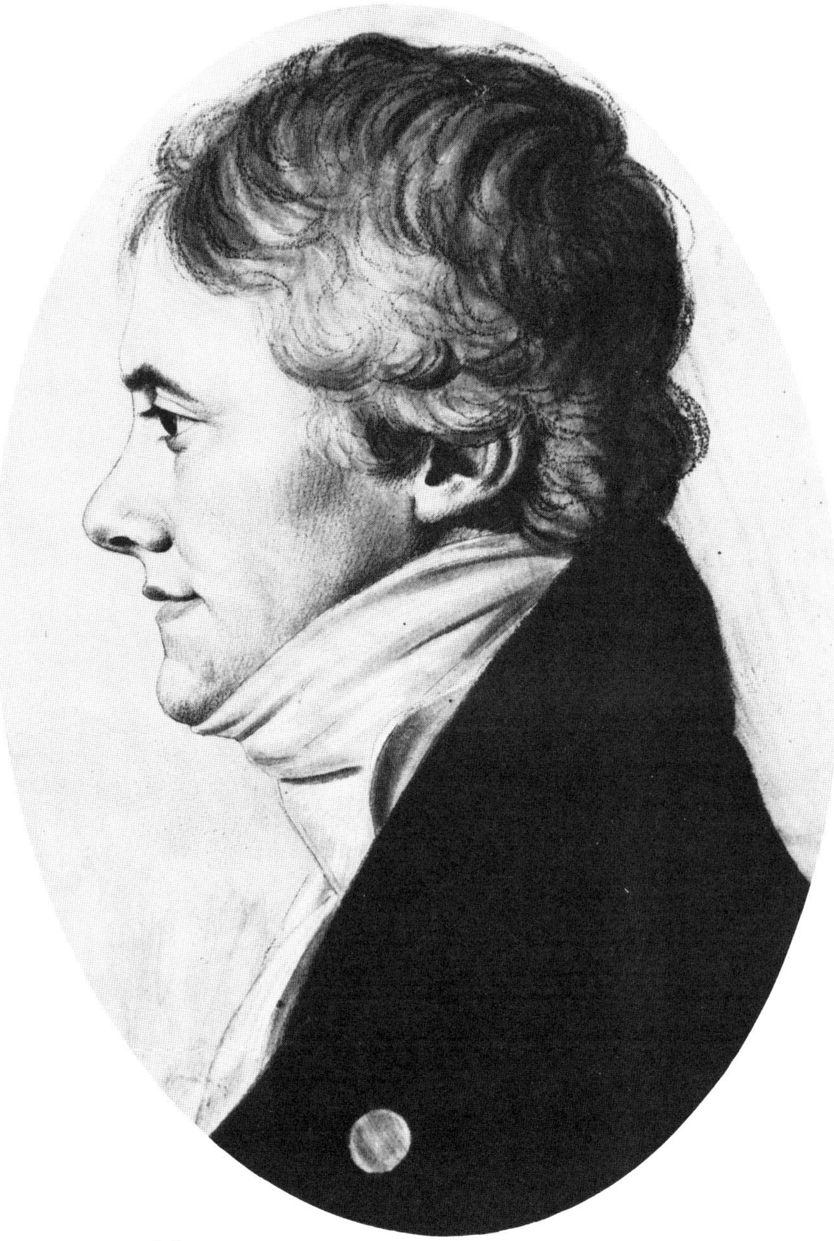

John Armentaire Monges *PH 373*

York to Burlington, New Jersey, in 1798, and then to Philadelphia, where he made likenesses of many notable citizens. He also worked in Baltimore, Annapolis, Washington, Richmond, Norfolk, and Charleston. He made more than 800 portraits of this type. He visited France from 1810 to 1812 and then returned to New York to paint landscapes and portraits. After the restoration of the Bourbons in 1814, he joyfully returned to France, was appointed a lieutenant-colonel by Louis XVIII, and gave up painting to become curator-director of the Museum in Dijon.

Pencil outline, with white and black chalk or crayon and wash on pink prepared paper; oval, 18 3/4 x 14; not signed or dated, but done ca. 1798–1803, when Saint-Mémin probably worked in Burlington and Philadelphia. Presented by bequest of Miss Cora Monges in 1919. *PH 373*

Dr. Monges is shown head-and-neck length, profile to the left. He has a full head of curly hair. His eye looks straight ahead, his nose is tipped up slightly, his mouth is slightly parted, and his chin is firm. He wears a white stock, a white shirt with stand-up collar, a black waistcoat, and a black coat with high collar. The contour of the features is firm but sensitively drawn. The modeling is created by dark crayon or chalk and wash in the hair, coat, and shadows. White is used in the neckwear and on the highlights, and the pink paper becomes the medium tone. The subject is presented as a fashionably dressed, handsome man. There can be no attempt at character depiction by this mechanical technique, although the esthetic effect is very pleasing.

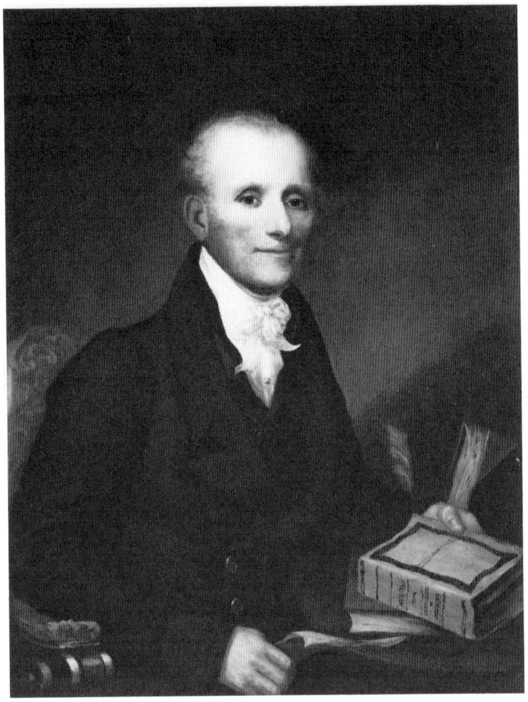

John Armentaire Monges *PA 46*

Artist: Unknown

Oil on canvas; 35 1/2 x 27 1/2; not signed or dated. If painted from life, the portrait would predate 1812, because the book the subject is holding, identified by Miss Christine Ruggere, librarian of the historical collections at the College of Physicians, as Dictionnaire des Sciences Médicales *tome deuxième, was published by C.L.F. Pancoucke of Paris in 1812. The artist's printing on the cover is a combination of English and French words, hence he was most likely an American. Bass Otis has been tentatively suggested by Dr. Ellen Miles, Associate Curator, National Portrait Gallery, and this suggestion will be pursued. Presented by Gordon Monges, date unrecorded, but before 1915, when it was included in the College of Physicians Inventory of 1898–1915.* *PA 46*

Monges is shown half-length, with body and head turned to the right. He is seated in a red upholstered armchair, with both arms resting on the chair arms, his right hand holding a white paper, and his left hand holding a book. On the round table is a quill pen and three books with covers in green, tan, and orange and black. The background is dark brownish-gray above and lighter tannish-brown below. Monges's gray hair is sparse. His triangular face has luminous brown eyes which gaze straight ahead in the direction of the head turn. He has a small nose and a wide mouth with very thin lips. He wears a white shirt, a white neckcloth tied in a bow, a jeweled pin, a black waistcoat, and a black double-breasted coat with an M-notched lapel and a high collar. The paint style of this portrait is difficult to assess because of the ruinous state. The face has suffered great paint loss, and the background has been repainted completely. If the deep folds and tailoring detail on the costume are indications of the original style, most likely the face and hands were modeled carefully and solidly, in a smooth facture. The original facial expression cannot even be guessed.

John Morgan (1735–1789)

The son of a Welsh immigrant, Morgan was born in Philadelphia. He received the A.B. degree from the College of Philadelphia in 1757, at the first commencement of that institution. He also received an A.M. degree in 1760. During these years he began the study of medicine under Dr. John Redman (q.v.) and was a resident apothecary at the Pennsylvania Hospital. He spent the next four years as surgeon to the Pennsylvania troops in the war between Great Britain and France. He sailed for Europe in 1760 and remained for five years of study and travel. In London he attended the lectures and dissections by William Cullen (q.v.) and William and John Hunter (q.v.). In Edinburgh, where he received the M.D. degree in 1763, he studied with Monroe, Cullen , Rutherford, Whyte, and Hope. In Paris he studied anatomy with M. Sue and in 1764 was elected a member of the Royal Academy of Surgery. In the summer of 1764 he made the grand tour of Europe with Samuel Powel; they were probably the first Americans to cross the Alpine pass at Mount Cesnis. Upon his return to London in the fall of 1764, he was made a fellow of the Royal Society of London, a licentiate of the Royal Colleges of Physicians of London and Edinburgh, and a member of the Arcadian Belles-Lettres Society of Rome. While in Europe he visited medical schools in many countries and consulted with many eminent physicians about the founding of a medical school in his native city. When he returned to Philadelphia

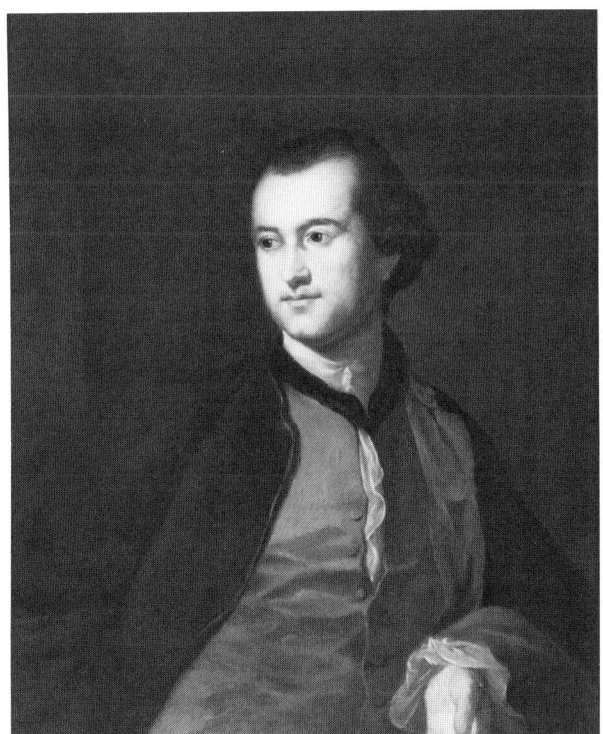

John Morgan *PA 14*

in 1765 he presented a letter from Thomas Penn, the proprietary, to the College of Philadelphia with a plan to establish a medical school. The project was accepted and Morgan was made professor of the theory and practice of medicine. On May 30, 1765, he delivered his famous "Discourse on the Institution of Medical Schools in America." Three years later five students received degrees in medicine, the first given in America. Morgan was on the staff of the Pennsylvania Hospital from 1773 to 1783. He was a member of the American Philosophical Society and a founder of the College of Physicians in 1787, where he was one of its first censors. In his own practice he instituted innovative customs, such as writing prescriptions instead of compounding them himself, practicing medicine to the exclusion of surgery, and charging a fee immediately upon service. In 1775 he was appointed director-general and physician-in-chief of the General Hospital of the Continental army. Two years later he was removed from office without an opportunity to defend himself against the chaotic jealousies, dissensions, and calumnies that existed among his subordinates, including Dr. William Shippen, Jr., who from that time became his bitter rival. Subsequently, Morgan received honorable aquittal from a special committee of Congress, but his dismissal was a crushing blow and he never recovered fully from the public humiliation.

Artist: Isaac Eugene Craig (1830–after 1878)

Born near Pittsburgh, Craig was a painter of portraits and religious and historical paintings. He is said to have studied art in Philadelphia and in Paris. He resided in Philadelphia from 1855 to 1856 and also lived in Pittsburgh and small towns in Maryland and Pennsylvania. He exhibited in annual exhibitions at the Pennsylvania Academy of the Fine Arts frequently between 1855 and 1868, was nominated twice to be an associate, and was instructor in drawing from the antique in 1855. He also exhibited work at the National Academy of Design (1856, 1858–59, and 1868). He left again for Europe in 1868 and was known to have been in Munich and then Florence, his last known whereabouts, in 1878.

Oil on canvas; 31 1/2 x 25 1/2; not signed or dated, but probably painted in 1855–56 when Craig was in Philadelphia; copy after an original portrait by Angelica Kauffmann (1741–1807), painted when Morgan was in Rome in 1764. It is said that a "friendship" developed between the artist and the doctor, and that in return for his treating her when she was ill, Kauffmann gave him a self-portrait. Kauffmann's portrait of Morgan was formerly at the Washington County Historical Society and since 1978 has been at the National Portrait Gallery. Craig's copy was shown in the College of Physicians' Centennial Celebration Loan Collection of Portraits, *1887, when it was owned by Mrs. Amelia C. Shields, who presented it to the College of Physicians at some time before 1915, because when it appeared in the inventory of 1898–1915, it was owned by the College. It was copied by Vincent Desiderio in 1981 for presentation by the College of Physicians to the Royal College of Physicians of Edinburgh.* *PA 14*

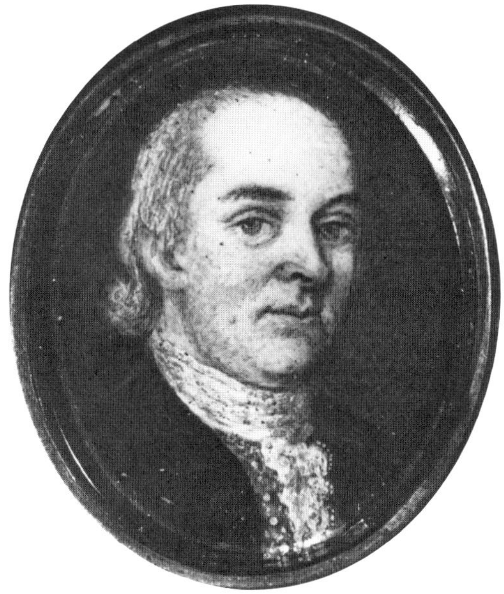

John Morgan *MISC 911*

Dr. Morgan is shown half-length, his body turned slightly from right to left, his head to the left and tilted down. He is standing with his left arm leaning on an unseen piece of furniture. His left hand is bent at the wrist, with the palm facing up. The background is a medium-toned brown, with a lighter vertical strip on the left. Morgan has brown hair with two rows of curls at the ears; it is tied into a black solitaire whose ends are tucked into his shirt front. His large blue eyes look in the direction of the head turn. His square face is wide across his pink cheeks. He has a straight nose, a well-formed mouth, and a cleft chin. He wears a white stock, a white shirt with ruffled cuffs, a white jabot tucked into his yellow-green waistcoat, and a dark green coat lined in a dark pink color and with pink cuffs. The surface of the portrait has been painted smoothly throughout. The head is well constructed with solid and three-dimensional planes. There is some feeling for the bodily forms under the costume. The subject radiates youthful confidence; he has a pleasant, dreamy, romantic expression and an open and inviting gesture. Interestingly, the copyist has reduced the original painting to a closeup study; the original shows the subject three-quarter length in the pose of an aristocratic dandy (weight on one foot, one arm akimbo), in a room whose window affords an outdoor view. Here the subject leans on a high table or desk piled with books and papers, which he studiously ignores.

Artist: Unknown

Miniature water color on ivory; oval, 1 1/8 x 1; not signed or dated. Presented by Miss Julia Morgan Harding, great-granddaughter of John Morgan, in 1913. *MISC 911*

Dr. Morgan is shown head-and-shoulder length, with body and head turned to the right. He has a high forehead, gray hair curled up in the back, blue eyes which look out of their corners directly toward the viewer, a straight nose, full lips, a rounded jaw, and a double chin. His complexion is quite pink, his lips red. He wears a white stock, a white jabot, a gold-patterned waistcoat, and a black coat. The paint style is smooth and the head is solidly constructed. Delicate lines give texture and exquisite detail to the face, hair, and costume. The facial expression is pleasant and direct.

Elliott H. Morse (b. 1916)

Born in New Haven, Connecticut, Morse was graduated from Haverford College in 1938 and obtained the B.S. degree in library science from Drexel University in 1939. He began his library career in 1939 as reference assistant at the University of Pennsylvania. In 1941 he moved to Temple University, where he was named acting reference librarian. During this period he earned the M.A. degree in German at the University of Pennsylvania, where he returned in 1944 as reference librarian. Starting in 1949, he devoted himself to medical librarianship at the College of Physicians, when he was named administrative assistant librarian under W.B. McDaniel II. In 1952 he was appointed administrative associate librarian and in 1953, librarian, a post he held until his retirement in 1981. During his tenure Morse established the Medical Documentation Service to provide detailed reference work on a fee-for-service basis. He formed a local chapter of the Medical Library Association. He oversaw the College's additions to its stacks and he was a driving force which led the College to become the second regional medical library of the National Library of Medicine. Morse has been an active member of the Medical Library Association, serving as chairman of several committees, on the board of directors, as the genéral chairman of the convention held in Philadelphia (1965), and as president (1969–70).

Artist: Ila Junod Capolino (Mrs. J. Joseph Capolino) (b. 1925)

Born in Pittsburg, Kansas, Ila Capolino was awarded the George Innes and Luella Stewart scholarships at the University of Kansas, where she received a B.F.A. degree in 1949. For the following public works, some of which were done in conjunction with her husband, Lieutenant-Colonel J. Joseph Capolino, an artist from Philadelphia, she was awarded letters of commendation from the ranking officers of the U.S. Marine Corps: portraits and murals at the Philadelphia Naval Base; the Navy Building in Washington; the Naval War College in Newport, Rhode Island; the U.S. Marine Corps

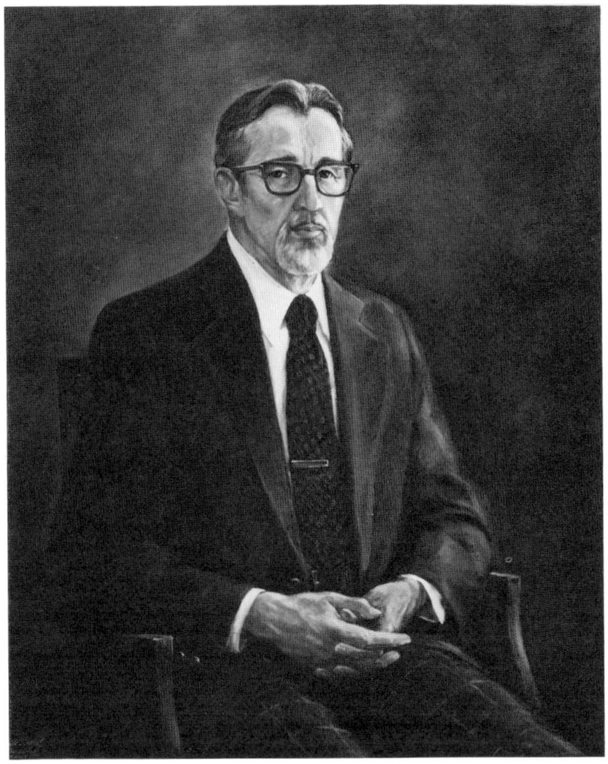

Elliott H. Morse *PA 145*

building in Quantico, Virginia; the War Memorial Building in Camp Lejeune, North Carolina; and the commandant's house in Washington, D.C. In addition to many portraits in private collections, she has recently executed portraits of Alfred Putnam for the Philadelphia Club, of Alfred D'Angelo for the McGee Memorial Hospital, and for the AAA-Keystone Corporate board room.

Oil on canvas; 35 x 29; signed and dated lower left, "Ila Junod Capolino, 1981." Commissioned and presented by friends of Elliott Morse in 1981. *PA 145*

Morse is shown two-thirds length, with body and head turned slightly to the right. He is seated in an armchair set at an angle of 45 degrees to the picture plane. His hands are clasped in his lap. The background is composed of warm gray, brown, red, and yellow areas of color, lighter around the head. The subject has gray hair, parted in the center. Under straight, slanting eyebrows, his brown eyes look directly at the viewer through horn-rimmed glasses. His nose has a bump at the bridge. His small mouth has well-shaped lips. His light gray moustache forms a circular shape in connection with the short beard. He wears a white shirt, a foulard necktie with a dark red background and a red-green pattern, a single-breasted blazer-style sport coat, and plaid trousers with a brown and green background and red and white stripes. The surface of the portrait is fluidly brushed. The head and hands are moderately well constructed in solid, three-dimensional forms, and there is a suggestion of body mass under the costume. Morse's posture is erect but relaxed. His expression is serious and alert. He gazes directly at the viewer and seems to be on the verge of engaging in conversation.

Samuel George Morton (1799-1851)

Son of an immigrant from Clonmell, Ireland, Morton was born in Philadelphia. After an unhappy apprenticeship in a mercantile house, he decided to study medicine. His first experience was as an office pupil of Dr. Joseph Parrish (q.v.) and then at the University of Pennsylvania, where he received the M.D. degree in 1820. That same year he was elected a member of the Academy of Natural Sciences, to which he devoted great effort during the remainder of his life. He went abroad in 1820 or 1821 and continued his studies at the University of Edinburgh, where he received the honors of the University in 1823. When he returned to Philadelphia, he opened a medical practice but pursued his consuming interest in natural science. At the Academy of Natural Sciences he was made auditor, recording secretary, corresponding secretary, vice president, and then president (1849); in 1825-26 he delivered papers there on mineralogy and geology, and he wrote articles for its *Journal* in 1827. He contributed forty articles to the *Transactions of the Academy*, and others to the *Transactions* of the American Philosophical Society and to the *American Journal of Science and Art* on mineralogy, geology, zoology, anatomy, ethnology, and archeology. In 1829 he became physician to the Almshouse Hospital and in 1834 published a book on his pathological research there, called *Illustrations of Pulmonary Consumption.* He was lecturer in anatomy at both the Philadelphia Association for Medical Instruction and at the School of Medicine from 1830 to 1836; he was professor of anatomy at the Pennsylvania Medical College from 1839 to 1843. His great work, *Crania Americana*, published in 1839, is based on his large collection of human skulls, especially of the "aboriginal races" of this continent. This work was followed by *Crania Aegyptica*, published in 1844. His last work was *Human Anatomy, Special, General, and Microscopic*, published in 1849. He was a valued member of the College of Physicians and of medical and scientific societies in Georgia, St. Louis, New York, Copenhagen, Moscow, Edinburgh, and Frankfurt.

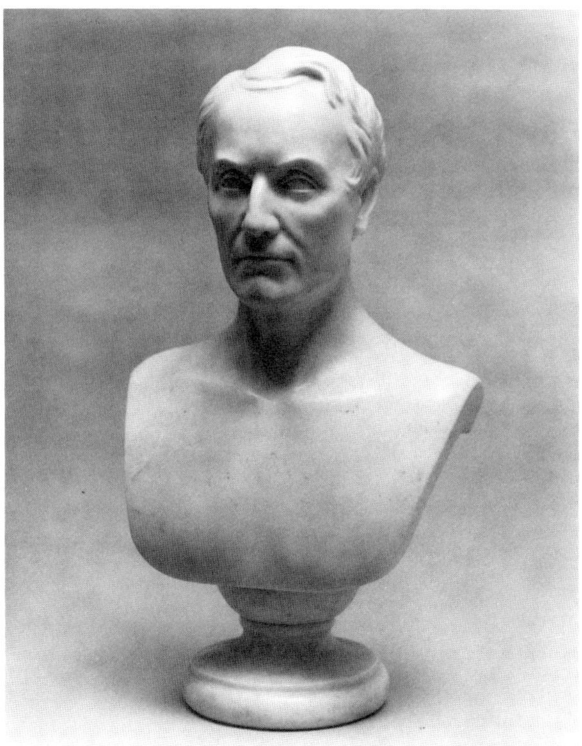

Samuel George Morton *ST 503*

Artist: Unknown

Marble; 26 1/2 x 15 1/4 x 10 5/8; base integral with sculpture, 5 1/2 in. high; not signed or dated. Donor and date of donation unrecorded, but included in College of Physicians Inventory of 1898-1915. *ST 503*

Dr. Morton is shown bust length, head and body frontal. He has wavy hair, a high forehead, arched eyebrows, deepset and blank eyes, a prominent nose with a bump at the bridge, a wide mouth with thin lips, and age lines next to his nose and mouth. Below the clavicle, the body is not rendered anatomically. The marble surface is extremely smooth, with no visible tool marks. The features are deeply cut, and the head is rendered with sensitivity and with understanding of anatomy. The facial expression is severe and somewhat idealized. The only sense of animation in this neoclassical image comes from the differentiated, curving strands of hair.

Thomas George Morton (1835-1903)

Son of the distinguished physician and naturalist, Samuel George Morton (q.v.), Thomas Morton was born in Philadelphia. He received the M.D. degree from the University of Pennsylvania in 1856. Almost immediately thereafter he began a 46-year career at Pennsylvania Hospital, starting as resident physician in 1857, serving as pathologist and curator to its museum from 1860 to 1864, and contining as surgeon from 1864 until his death. He was a founder of the Orthopaedic Hospital and Infirmary for Nervous Diseases and was a trustee and professor of orthopaedic surgery to the Philadelphia Polyclinic and College for Graduates in Medicine. He was also surgeon or consulting surgeon to the Wills Eye Hospital, Pennsylvania Institute for the Instruction of the Blind, the Pennsylvania Institute for the Deaf and Dumb, the Howard Hospital, the Women's and Jewish Hospitals, and others. He was a fellow of the College of Physicians and president of the American Academy of Surgery. During the Civil War he was acting assistant surgeon. With his son, he introduced the new antiseptic technique to the Pennsylvania Hospital, and he performed almost all the major operations of his day. He is best

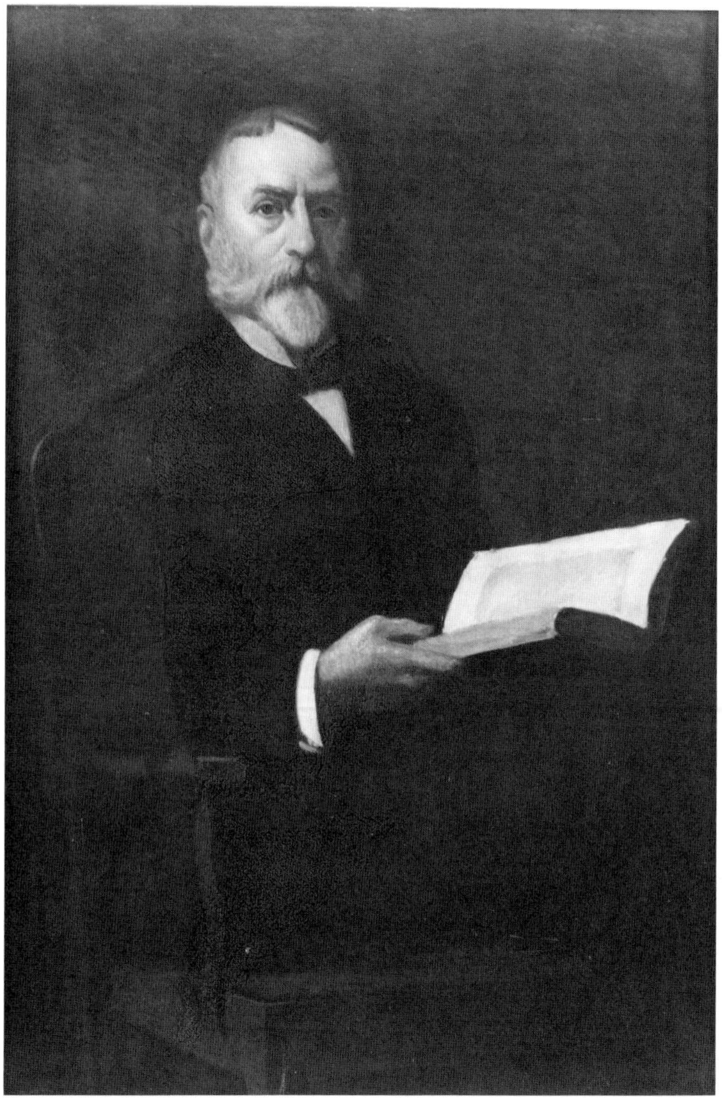

Thomas George Morton PA 71

known for being the first to do a successful laparotomy and appendectomy for appendicitis and the first to describe and cure by surgery an affliction of the foot known as metatarsalgia, later called "Morton's toe" or "Morton's neuralgia." He wrote *Surgery in the Pennsylvania Hospital* (1880) with Dr. William Hunt (q.v.) and *The History of the Pennsylvania Hospital (1895)* with the assistance of Dr. Frank Woodbury. In addition to articles on surgery, Morton wrote on transfusion of blood, antiseptic treatment of wounds, and the care of the insane.

Artist: Hugh Henry Breckenridge (1870–1937)

For biography, see page 38.

Oil on canvas; 49 1/4 x 33 1/4; signed lower left, "H—H Breckenridge." Presented by Arthur V. Morton, son of Dr. Morton, in 1914. Similar to a painting of Morton by Breckenridge at Pennsylvania Hospital. PA 71

Dr. Morton is shown three-quarters length, with head and body turned to the right. He is seated in a Queen Anne-style armchair that is turned at an angle of 45 degrees to the picture plane. His legs are crossed at the knees and his arms rest on the chair arms, while his hands hold an open book. The background is dark gray. The subject has gray hair, a high forehead, light gray muttonchop side-whiskers, a full moustache, and a pointed beard. Under knitted brows his gray eyes look straight ahead in the direction of the head turn. There are deep shadows under his eyes. He has a straight nose; his mouth is hidden. He wears a white shirt and stand-up collar, a black bow tie, and a black vest, coat, and trousers. Because of repeated restorations, it is difficult to judge the surface of this portrait. Even in its present state it can be seen that the head was rendered in solid and three-dimensional forms. At present the costume looks totally flat, with no indication of the body mass underneath. In its original condition the pose must have appeared lively. Although the subject's head and upper body are erect, his hips swivel in the chair so that his thighs are almost parallel to the picture plane. In addition, the figure was painted on a large scale and almost fills the canvas. This closeup bulk, coupled with the imperious facial expression, command the attention of viewer.

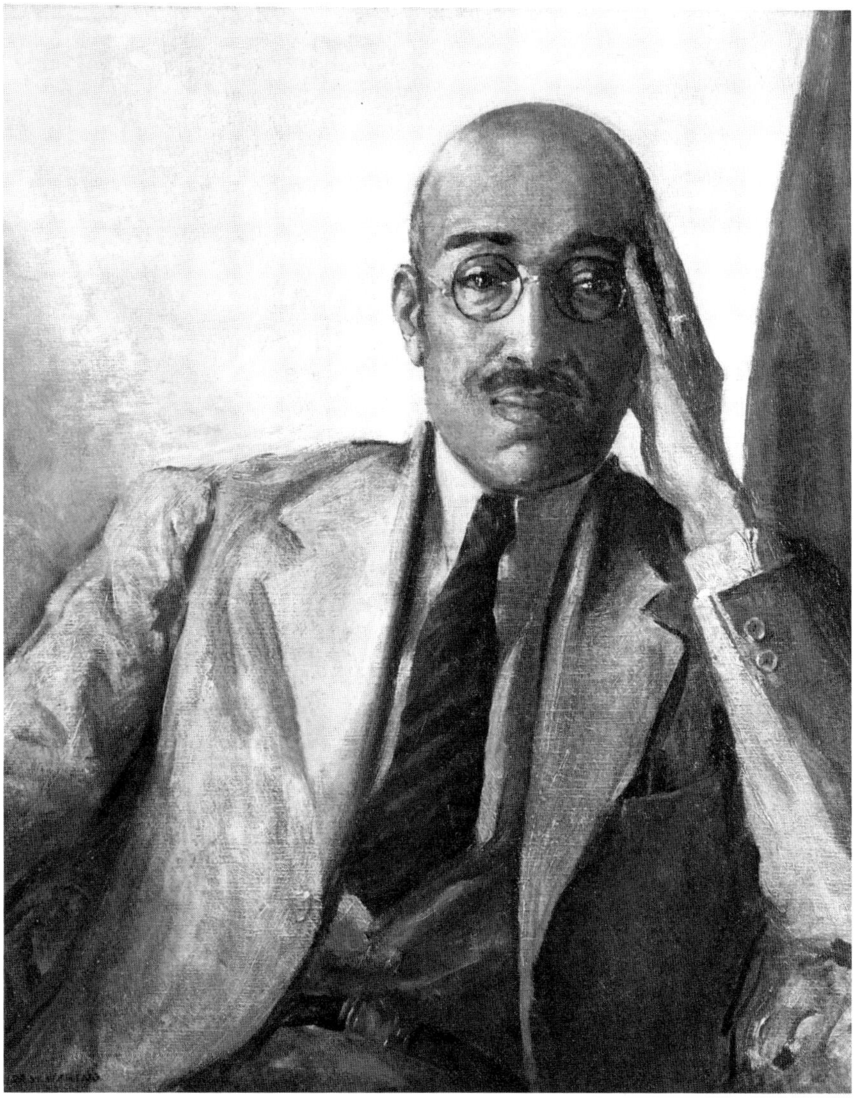

Nathan Francis Mossell *PA 132*

Nathan Francis Mossell (1856-1946)

Born in Hamilton, Ontario, Mossell was the son of free-born natives of Baltimore who had gone to Canada to rear their children in an atmosphere of freedom. He graduated from Lincoln University in 1879 and from the University of Pennsylvania Medical School in 1882, when Dr. James Tyson (q.v.) was dean. He was the first black graduate and finished in the top quarter of his class. After graduation he was admitted reluctantly to the outpatient clinic of the University Hospital, where he spent two years. He took a postgraduate course at the Philadelphia Polyclinic and in 1888 was admitted, again reluctantly and through the sponsorship of Dr. Tyson, to the Philadelphia Medical Society. He continued his education in London, where he studied at Guy's and St. Thomas's Hospitals. Upon his return to Philadelphia in 1895, he confronted the need for a Negro hospital in Philadelphia by becoming the driving force behind the founding of the Frederick Douglass Memorial Hospital and Training School for Nurses, where qualified Negro physicians could practice their profession, where Negro patients could be treated in a sympathetic environment, and where Negro nurses could be trained. Dr. Mossell was the medical director, superintendent, and attending surgeon. Since the hospital was founded to protest racial segregation, its official policy was to admit any patient regardless of race or creed, and it was chosen as one of the hospitals for military patients of the Spanish-American War. Although Dr. Mossell experienced stormy opposition to his dictatorial policies, the hospital flourished under his leadership and he supervised the removal to larger quarters. He was named medical director emeritus in 1933 and given a lifetime annuity. He was a co-founder of the Philadelphia Academy of Medicine and Allied Sciences and the National Medical Association, which he served as president in 1907-08. He received the Golden Harvest award of the Pyramid Club in 1942.

Laura Wheeler Waring (Mrs. Walter E. Waring) (1887–1948)

Born in Hartford, Connecticut, Waring was the daughter of a minister and of a musician-teacher. She studied at the Pennsylvania Academy of the Fine Arts and won a Cresson traveling fellowship to Paris, where she continued her training at the Académie de la Grande Chaumière. She was a consistent exhibitor of her work, mainly portraits and figure studies, at the Pennsylvania Academy, the Corcoran Gallery, the Smithsonian Institution, the Museum of Fine Arts in Dallas, and the Chicago Art Institute. She had one-man shows at the International House, New York, in 1928 and at the Philadelphia Fellowship Commission in 1946. She won first prize at the Exhibition of Colored Artists in 1919 and won the gold medal at the second annual competition of the Harmon Foundation of New York in 1927 for the most distinguished achievement among Negroes in the fine arts. Among the well-known subjects of her portraits are Marion Anderson, Dr. John P. Turner, Paul Robeson, Sadie T. M. Alexander, Raymond Pace Alexander, William D. Dubois, Frederick Douglass, and William H. Hastie. She was head of the art department at Cheyney State Normal School and was a member of the National Advisory Board of Art Movement and the Eastern Arts Association. She was the director of the Negro art exhibit at the Philadelphia Sesquicentennial Exposition in 1926 and the Texas Centennial Exposition in 1935.

Oil on canvas; 29 1/2 x 24 1/2; signed lower left, "Laura W Waring," and dated 1934 on the back of the canvas. Portrait commissioned by Mrs. Sadie T. M. (Mossell) Alexander, who gave it first to Mercy-Douglass Hospital and then presented it to the College of Physicians in 1974. Shown at the exhibitions, A Century of Black Presence at the University of Pennsylvania, 1879–1980, *Van Pelt Library, University of Pennsylvania, 1980–81, and* Three Hundred Years of Black History in the Commonwealth of Pennsylvania, *at the Afro-American Historical and Cultural Museum, 1981–82.* *PA 132*

Dr. Mossell is shown half-length, his body slightly to the left, his face frontal. He is seated in an armchair of multicolored upholstery, with his left elbow leaning on the chair arm and his left hand raised to the side of his head. The background is pale greenish-blue behind his head and medium bluish-violet on the left. There is a medium-toned blue curtain on the right. His oval head is almost bald except for a fringe of gray hair at the sides. His brown eyes look straight ahead through metal-rimmed spectacles. He has a straight nose, full lips, and a neat brown moustache. His complexion is of medium tone. He wears a blue shirt, a striped necktie in two-tone blue, a gray suit with fountain pens in the pocket, cuff links, and a gold ring. The surface of the portrait is painterly, with fluid, visible brush strokes. The head and hand have been constructed solidly in three-dimensional forms. The tailoring of the costume is detailed and there is a suggestion of the underlying bulk of the body. The subject's trunk is in a relaxed position, but his supporting arm and head are rigidly straight. He gazes directly at the viewer with a sober and intense facial expression. By means of the posture and expression, the artist has created a penetrating depiction of the subject's character.

John Herr Musser (1856–1912)

Descended from a family of Swiss Mennonite physicians who first settled in Lancaster, Pennsylvania, in 1710, Musser followed the family tradition and received the M.D. degree from the University of Pennsylvania in 1877. At the University he was appointed medical registrar, chief of the medical dispensary, instructor in clinical medicine, and associate professor, and in 1889 he became professor of clinical medicine, a post he held until his death. He founded and directed the social service department of the University of Pennsylvania Hospital and was named director of the Musser Department of Research Medicine in 1910. He was pathologist to the Presbyterian Hospital and physician to the Philadelphia and Presbyterian Hospitals. His clinical practice was very large, and his reputation as a diagnostician so widespread that he was often called as a consultant by doctors from other cities. In addition to being a fellow of the College of Physicians, he served as president of the American School Hygiene Association, the Philadelphia Pathological Society, the Philadelphia County Medical Society, the American Medical Association, and the National Medical Library Association. He belonged to several foreign medical societies and received an honorary LL.D. from Franklin and Marshall College in 1910. He was the author of at least 200 articles and wrote his monograph, *Medical Diagnosis,* in 1894. He contributed chapters to Hare's *System of Practical Therapeutics* and Osler's *Modern Medicine.* He edited the volume, "Diseases of the Lungs," in Nothnagle's *Encyclopedia* and was co-editor with A.O.J. Kelly of *A System of Therapeutics.*

Artist: John Singer Sargent (1856–1925)

Born in Florence of American parents, Sargent's father was a physician and his mother a watercolorist. An artistic prodigy, John Singer Sargent was enrolled at the Accademia delle Belle Arti in Florence at the age of 14. He went to Paris in 1874, enrolled at the École des Beaux Arts, and entered the atelier of Emile Auguste Carolus-Duran, a popular portrait painter and teacher. Here he quickly mastered the technique of painting directly with the brush. His work soon showed influences from the Impressionists, Whistler, and the 17th century artists, Velasquez and Hals, whose works he saw on trips to Spain and Holland in 1879 to 1880. He started to exhibit at the French Salons in 1877 and won an honorable mention in 1878. He remained in Paris

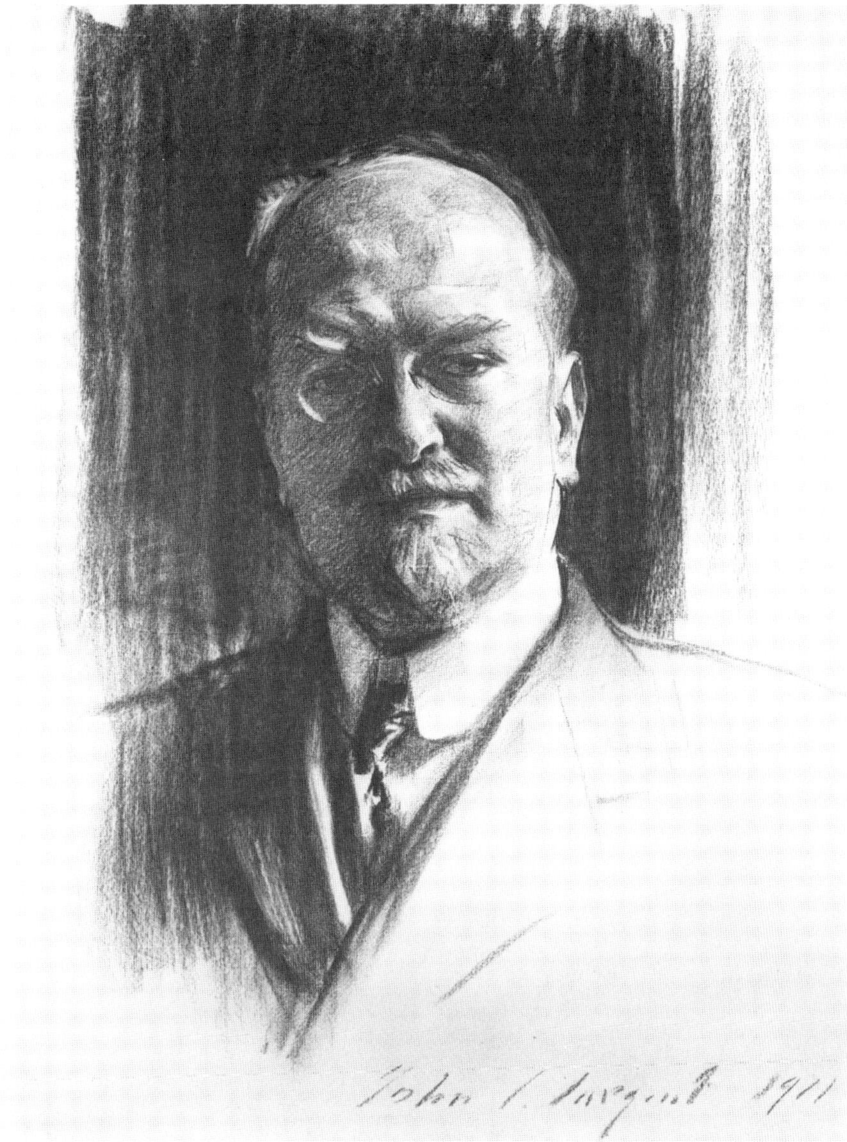

John Herr Musser *PH 212*

until his audacious portrait of *Madame X* (now at the Metropolitan Museum of Art) in the Salon of 1884 caused such a scandal that he moved to London. Although he made London his home from then on, he was a constant traveler, and became best known as a painter of facile, flattering, and elegant portraits of society figures on both sides of the Atlantic. He also did landscapes, still lifes, and genre scenes in both oils and watercolors, many of which show the influence of Japanese art. One of Sargent's best known works is a series of murals for the Boston Public Library tracing the history of Western religion. He also did murals for the Boston Museum of Fine Arts and for the Widener Library at Harvard. His awards were international in scope, and he was elected a member of the National Academy of Design, the Royal Academy of London, and the French Legion of Honor. His paintings are represented in many of the great museums of America and Europe, and during his lifetime he was one of the most acclaimed American artists.

Charcoal drawing on white paper; 23 1/4 x 17 3/4; signed and dated lower right, "John S. Sargent 1911." Bequeathed by Dr. John Herr Musser in 1912. *PH 212*

Dr. Musser is shown bust length, with body and head turned slightly to the left and head tilted slightly to the right. The background is composed of broad vertical strokes, but the left and right borders are blank. The subject has a receding hairline with sparse hair at the top and sides. His eyes look straight out through a pince-nez in the direction of the head turn. He has a small nose, flaring nostrils, a wide mouth, a brush moustache, and a scanty beard. He wears a shirt, a necktie, and a coat. The surface of the drawing is lively; a variety of strokes and tonalities have been used to achieve a masterly likeness and at the same time, a bravura statement by the artist. The modeling of the three-dimensional and solid-looking head is tight and detailed, while the shading of the costume is loose and suggestive. The subject's expression is serious and his gaze is averted, as though he were deep in thought.

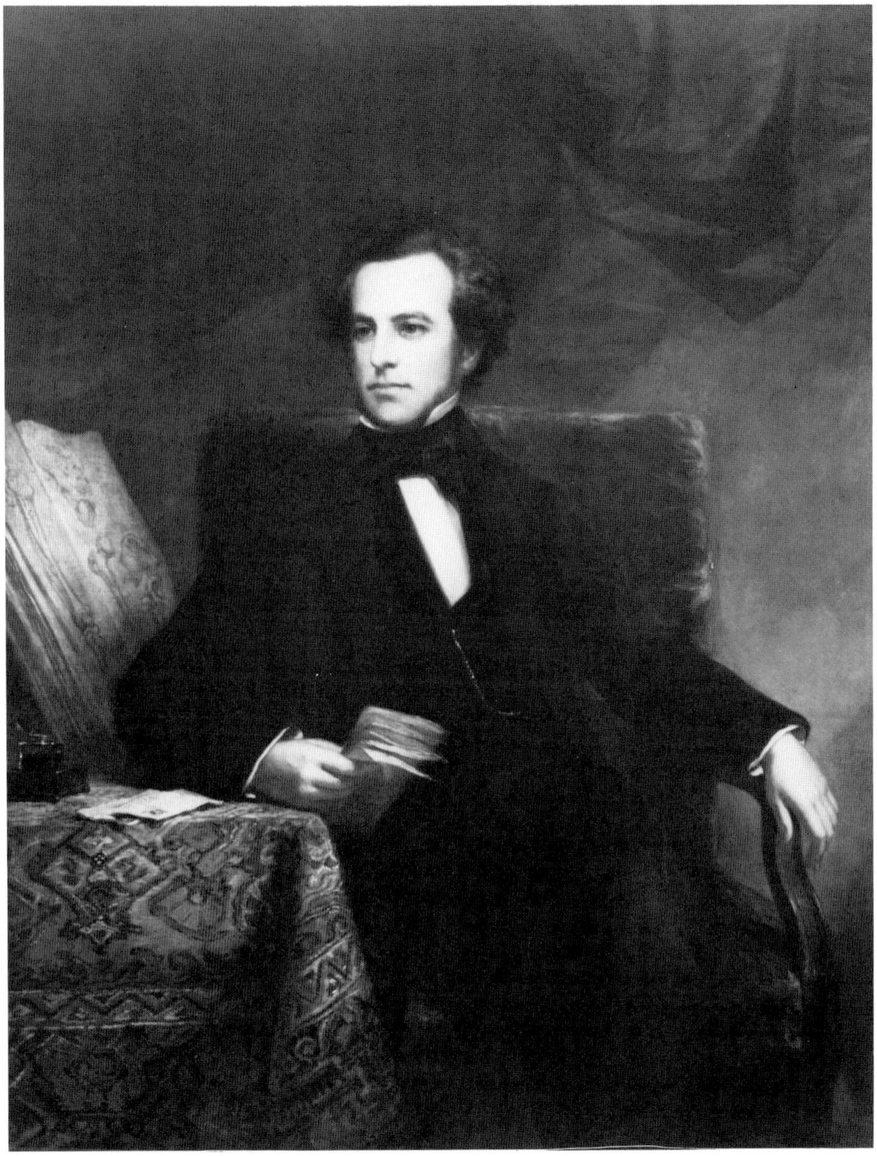

Thomas Dent Mütter *PA 89*

Thomas Dent Mütter (1811-1859)

Descended from Scottish and German forbears who came to America in pre-Revolutionary days, Mütter was born in Richmond, Virginia. He attended Hampden Sydney College and then began the study of medicine under Dr. Simms of Alexandria. He received the M.D. degree from the University of Pennsylvania in 1831 and then studied in Paris and London. Upon his return to Philadelphia he established a medical practice that soon included the most notable families. He held a teaching post at the Philadelphia Institute and in 1841 was named professor of the principles and practice of surgery at Jefferson Medical College, a post he held until his death. He was celebrated for his operations for congenital deformities such as clubfoot and cleft palate and for the repair of traumatic deformities resulting from burns or injuries. Although not a prolific writer, he reported many cases to the *American Journal of Medical Sciences* between 1841 and 1856 and edited an American edition of Lister's *Surgery*. He was a fellow of the College of Physicians and a member of the American Philosophical Society and the Academy of Natural Sciences. In 1856, the time that ill health forced his retirement, he had accumulated an important collection of anatomical and pathological specimens, including bones, wet and dry preparations, casts, wax and papier maché models, and paintings. He left his collection to the College of Physicians with the statement, "I have determined to found a pathological museum which shall be open to all physicians and to all students of medicine without fee or charge of any sort. I hereby offer the guardianship of this museum to the Philadelphia College of Physicians as the body best qualified by the character of its members and the nature of its pursuits for undertaking the trust." Mütter also left a gift of $30,000 for the maintenance of the museum, purchase of additional specimens, and establishment of a lectureship. Today the Mütter Museum is known throughout the world.

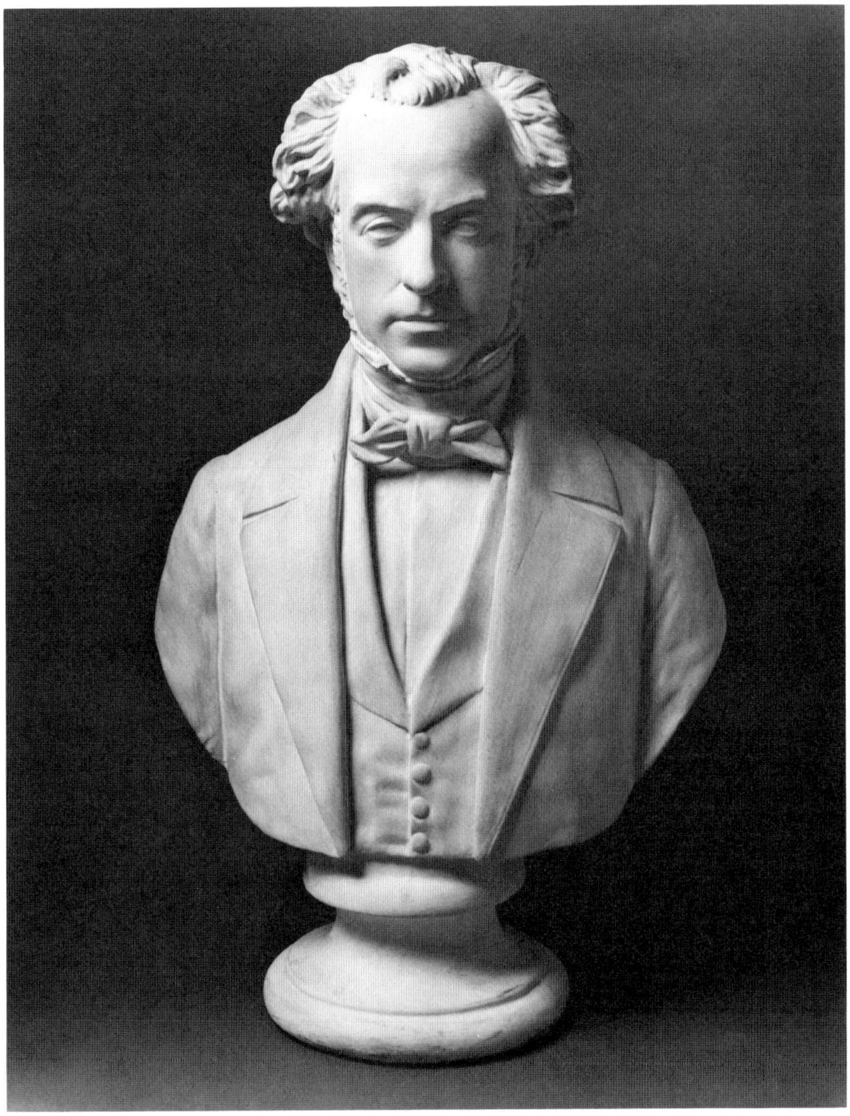

Thomas Dent Mütter *ST 514*

Artist: Daniel Huntington (1816–1906)

For biography, see page 90.

Oil on canvas, mounted on wood; 55 1/2 x 43 1/2; signed lower right, "D Huntington." Donor and date of donation unrecorded. In 1887 the portrait appeared in the College of Physicians' Centennial Celebration Loan Collection of Portraits *(owner, College of Physicians) and in the* Pennsylvania Academy of the Fine Arts Loan Collection of Historical Portraits *(owner, College of Physicians), 1887–88.* *PA 89*

Mütter is shown three-quarter length, with body turned to the right and head to the left and tilted down. He is seated in a brown upholstered armchair with a fringed apron, his upper body leaning diagonally to the left, his legs crossed at the knees and almost frontal. His left arm rests on the chair arm; the left hand is pendent. The right forearm leans on the table and the right hand holds a sheaf of papers. The background contains swags of green drapery stretched from the upper right corner to the middle left behind the figure and has umber atmospheric space to the right. The table is covered with an elaborately worked oriental carpet whose pattern is colored in red, green, umber, and white. The objects on the table are an inkstand, two letters (one of which is addressed to "Mütter"), and a large opened anatomical atlas. The subject's hair is dark brown and curly, with short side-whiskers that meet a short beard under his chin. His oval face has large dark blue eyes which gaze in the direction of the head turn. He has a straight nose, a wide mouth, and full lips. He wears a white shirt with stand-up collar, a black neckcloth tied in a wide bow, a black waistcoat, a gold watch chain, and a black coat and trousers. The surface of the painting is very smooth. The head and hands have great depth and solidity. The costume is less detailed, but there is a feeling for the underlying body mass. The shadows, highlights, and folds are rendered with great care and skill throughout. The subject affects an animated and energetic pose, as he twists his hips in the chair and turns his head in the opposite direction. He looks youthful, with his easy posture, unlined face, and graceful hands, yet he maintains a dignified facial expression and obviously has chosen to be surrounded by the accoutrements of scholarly pursuits and some of the conventional elements of traditional, aristocratic portraiture.

Artist: Peter Charles Reniers (1825-1894)

Reniers was born in Antwerp, Belgium, and studied art in his native city, Brussels, and Paris. He came to America in 1848, first locating in Cincinnati and then three years later in Pittsburgh, where he was connected with the marble-cutting firm of W. W. Wallace and John Lawton. It is said that shortly after his marriage he removed to his wife's city, Philadelphia, on account of his health, and worked with the firm[s?] John Baird and J. F. Jacobi. He returned to Pittsburgh in the early 1860s when he set up in business for himself. He was a sculptor of some note and executed marble portrait busts of Elisha Kent Kane, President Pierce, Charles Spang, Alexander King, and others. A marble bust of Colonel Thomas A. Scott was exhibited at the Centennial Exposition in Philadelphia. Public works in Pittsburgh include an altar at Trinity Church, figures on St. Paul's Cathedral and St. Peter's Church, the General Alexander Hays and Kearney monuments, and his most acclaimed work, the Soldier's Monument, a colossal multi-figured work dedicated in 1871 to the memory of Civil War casualties. He was awarded silver and bronze medals from the Franklin Institute for "meritorious work." For the above biographical information the author is indebted to Mary Mitchell of Lancaster, Pennsylvania, who cited Marilyn Evert's *Discovering Pittsburgh's Sculpture* (University of Pittsburgh, 1983).

Plaster painted white; 27 7/8 x 17 1/2 x 12; base 4 7/8 in. high, integral with sculpture; signed on beveled edge below shoulder on rear, "P Reniers Phdphia." Probably executed in the 1850s, when he resided in Philadelphia. Donor and date of donation are unrecorded but prior to the College of Physicians Inventory of 1898-1915, in which it is included.
ST 514

Dr. Mütter is shown bust length. His body is frontal, his head very slightly to the right and tilted slightly downward. He has a high forehead, thick wavy hair that projects 2 1/2 inches from the sides of his head, and flat side-whiskers that meet a short beard below his chin. His thin, rectangular face has narrow eyes that are blank. The nose is straight; its tip points down slightly. He has a wide mouth with full lips, a prominent jaw, and a square chin. He wears a shirt with stand-up collar, a wide neckcloth tied in a bow, a waistcoat with shawl collar, and a coat with notched lapels and a high collar. The plaster surface of the portrait is smooth. Neither the face nor the body is deeply modeled. The subject looks stiff and lacks vitality, yet the image does bear a resemblance to the Huntington portrait.

Henry Neill (1783-1845)

Born in Snow Hill, Maryland, Neill was descended from Irish forbears who came to North America in 1739. He began his study of medicine with Dr. John Church in Philadelphia and received the M.D. degree from the University of Pennsylvania in 1807. He established a large practice and specialized in obstetrics. He is known to have given a course of lectures in this subject at the Jefferson Medical College. He was physician to the Almshouse, the Walnut Street Prison, and the City Dispensary. At the College of Physicians he was elected a censor in 1818 and a vice-president in 1844. He published several articles in the *North American Medical and Surgical Journal.*

Artist: William E. Winner (ca. 1815-1883)

Winner was born in Philadelphia and resided there during most of his career. At the Pennsylvania Academy of the Fine Arts he was elected associate in 1847 and academician in 1860. He exhibited portraits, religious and genre scenes, and landscapes there between 1836 and 1869 and between 1878 and 1881. He also exhibited work with the Artists' Fund Society from 1836 to 1845 and was a member of its board of control, starting in 1843. He was a member of the Philadelphia Society of Artists and an exhibitor at the Centennial Exposition in Philadelphia. He showed paintings intermittently at the National Academy of Design from 1844 to 1875; he was elected an honorary member, professional, in 1851. He also participated in shows at the Apollo Association, the American Art Union, and the Boston Athenaeum.

Oil on canvas, mounted on wood; 30 x 25, actual size; signed and dated on back of chair, left center, "Winner/ 1867." Presented by Dr. John Neill in 1867. Since the work is posthumous, a probable source for the copy could be a lithograph at the College of Physicians by Albert Newsam, which itself is labeled as being after a daguerrotype by W. & L. Langenheim. *PA 5*

Dr. Neill is shown bust length, with body turned slightly to the right, head slightly to the right and tilted down a little. He is seated in a bright orange upholstered chair. The atmospheric background, dark red along the borders, blends to dark green and then to pale green around the head. The subject has gray hair brushed toward his face in an exaggerated widow's peak. Under knitted brows, his small blue eyes with their heavy upper lids look straight ahead. There are dark shadows around the eyes and deep lines next to the long, thin nose. The mouth is wide with thin lips, a pronounced jaw line, and a cleft chin. The subject wears a white shirt with one collar tip turned up, one down; a black bow tie; a black waistcoat; and a dark gray double-breasted coat with very large lapels. The surface of the portrait is smoothly brushed. The head is constructed in solid and three-dimensional forms. The torso is expansive, almost filling the lower half of the canvas, and therefore suggests the body mass underneath. The facial expression is serious, with a direct and penetrating gaze.

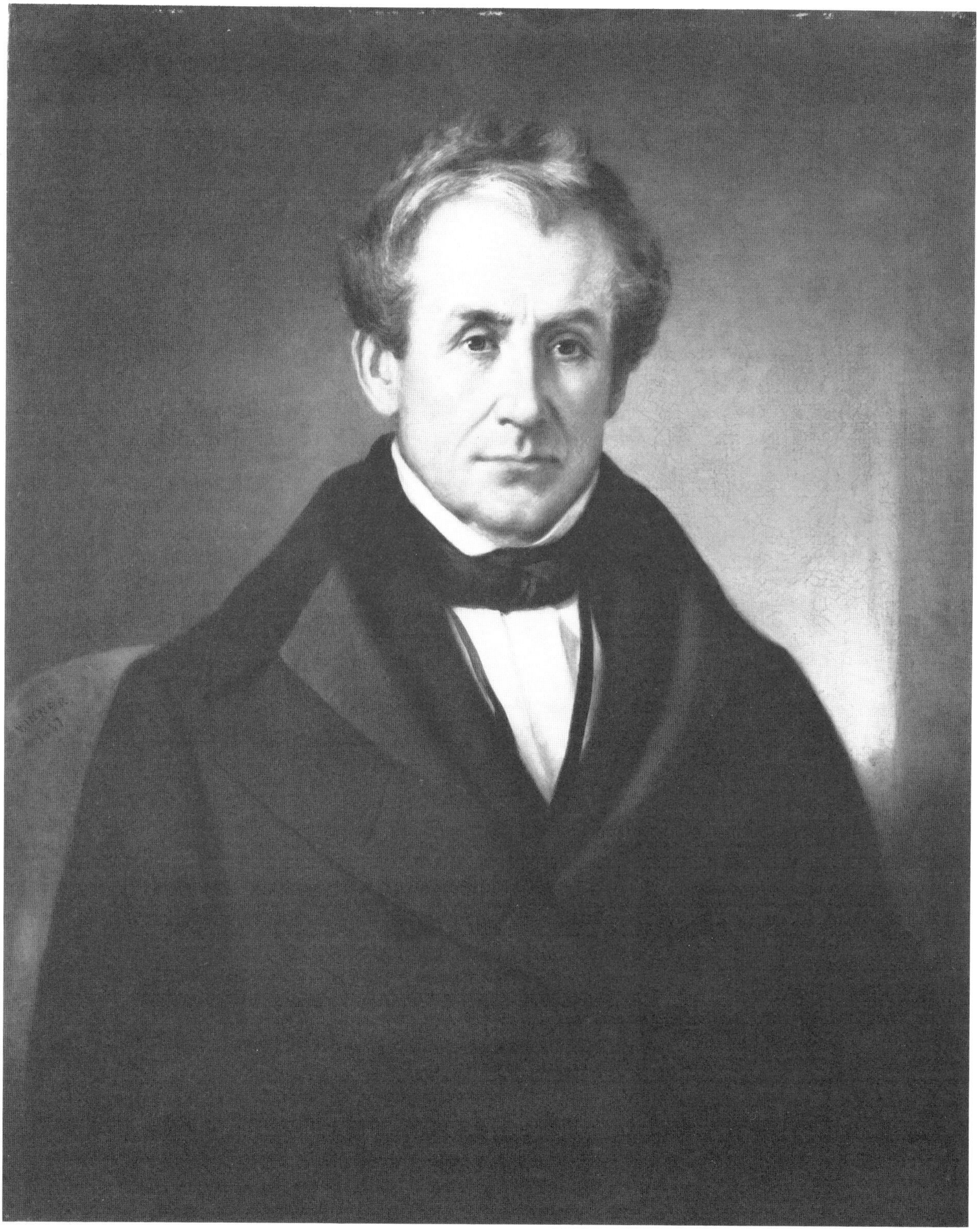

Henry Neill *PA 5*

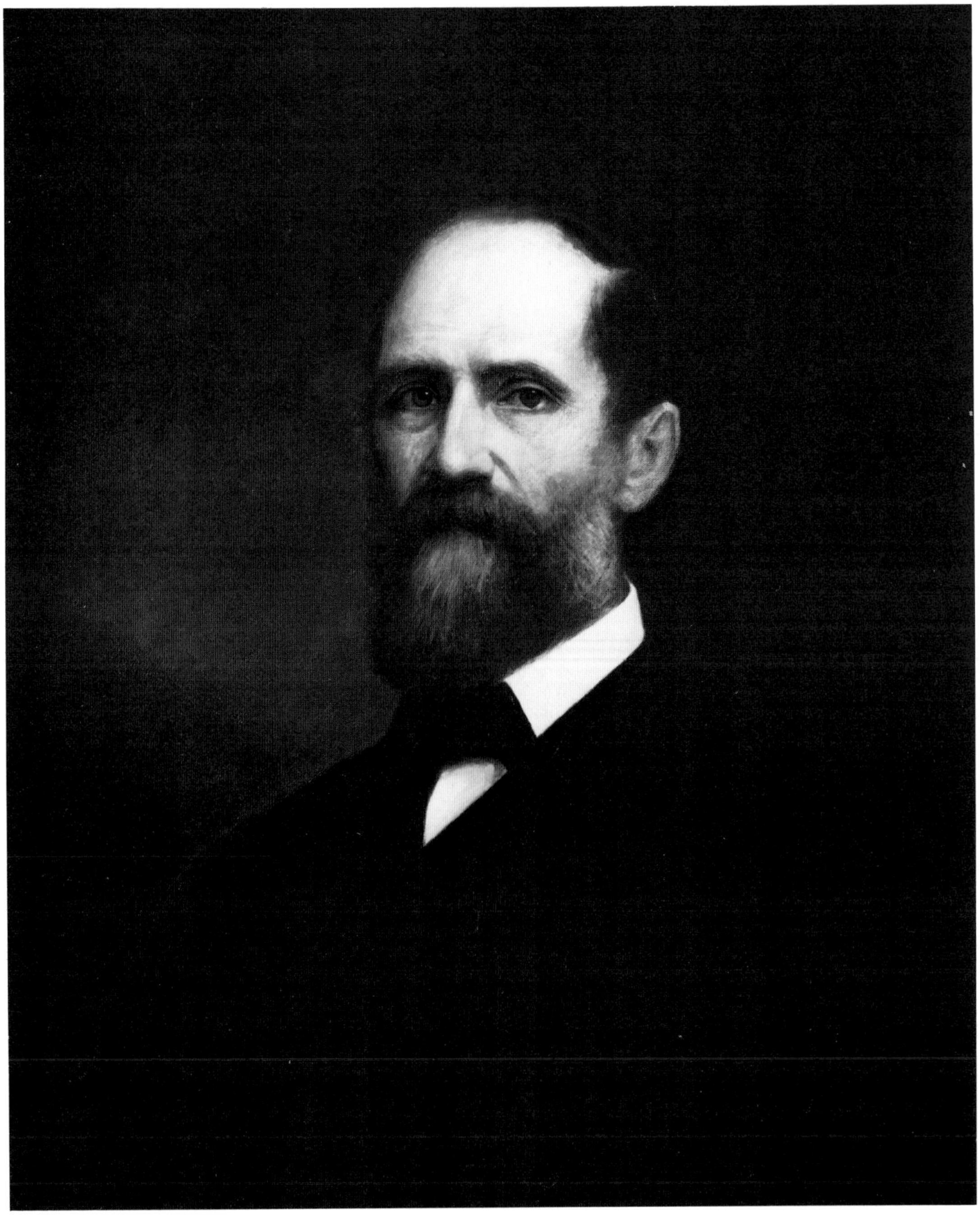

George Washington Norris *PA 44*

George Washington Norris (1808-1875)

Norris, born in Philadelphia, was descended from English Quakers who arrived in America in the 1690s. He earned the A.B. degree from the University of Pennsylvania in 1827 and studied medicine under Dr. Joseph Parrish (q.v.). In 1830 he received the M.D. degree from the University. After becoming a resident physician at the Pennsylvania Hospital, he continued his education in Paris, where he was elected a member of the Société Médicale d'Observation. Upon his return to Philadelphia he established a practice. He became surgeon to the Pennsylvania Hospital in 1836 and served until 1863. He was chosen professor of clinical surgery at the University of Pennsylvania in 1848 and trustee in 1856. He was consulting surgeon to the Orthopaedic Hospital and Children's Hospital, where he presided over the board of managers. He was also vice president of the College of Physicians, the Historical Society of Pennsylvania, and the Philadelphia Medical Society. He was a director of the Mutual Fire Insurance Company and of the Philadelphia Savings Fund Society, a president of the Library Company, and a member of the American Philosophical Society. Dr. Norris was interested in the early history of Philadelphia. The materials he gathered were published posthumously under the title, *The Early History of Medicine in Philadelphia* (1886). Among his other writings are *Contributions to Practical Surgery* (1873) and many articles on surgical procedures and cases, especially fractures, for the *American Journal of Medical Science.*

Artist: Attributed to Mihran H. Kevorkian (1873-1946)

Kevorkian, a native of Istanbul, studied in Paris and then came to America and settled in Philadelphia. He trained at the Pennsylvania Academy of the Fine Arts and at the Spring Garden Institute. He was primarily a portrait painter of local celebrity. He was a Mason and a member of the Union League. Several of his portraits can be found at the League, at the Masonic Temple in Philadelphia, and at the Philadelphia City Hall.

Oil on canvas; 29 x 24; not signed or dated. Donor not recorded but presented in 1909. Included in the College of Physicians inventory of 1898-1915, with the name of the artist omitted. According to the Bradley File and subsequent lists, this portrait is by Kevorkian after a portrait of Norris by Matthew Wilson (1814-1892), possibly the one at the Historical Society of Pennsylvania or at the University of Pennsylvania. The collection at the College of Physicians contains an etching by Hermann Faber and an engraving by T.B. Welch after McClees and Germon that also resemble this portrait; there are similar versions at the Library Company of Philadelphia (unknown artist) and one at the Pennsylvania Hospital, painted by Suzanne Gutherz Warriner, 1933. *PA 44*

Dr. Norris is shown bust length, with body and head turned to the left. The atmospheric background is dark brown on the right, lighter brown on the left, with a dark curving shadow on the lower left. The subject has a high forehead, dark brown hair, and large blue eyes which look directly at the viewer. His nose has a bump at the bridge. His luxuriant gray-brown moustache, side-whiskers, and narrow beard partially obscure his mouth. There are shadows around his eyes and age lines next to the nose. He wears a white shirt and a black bow tie, vest, and coat. Although there is paint loss in the face, the portrait was probably made in a moderately painterly style and rendered in solid and three-dimensional forms. The costume, smoothly brushed and utterly flat, lacks a sense of underlying bulk of the figure. Dr. Norris regards the viewer directly, with a sober and thoughtful expression.

George William Norris (1875-1965)

Grandson of George Washington Norris (q.v.) and son of William Fisher Norris (q.v.), George William Norris was born in Philadelphia, a descendant of English Quakers who came to Philadelphia in the late 1690s. He received the A.B. degree in 1895 and the M.D. degree in 1899 from the University of Pennsylvania. His early professional associations were with the dispensaries of the Episcopal, Orthopaedic, Polyclinic, Pennsylvania, Philadelphia General, and University Hospitals and the Phipps Institute. Later he was made instructor and associate at the University of Pennsylvania Medical School and attending physician to the Pennsylvania Hospital. He was cited by General John J. Pershing for distinguished military service. He was captain and chief of the medical service of Pennsylvania Base Hospital Unit No. 10, which took over the British Hospital No. 16 at Le Tréport, France. He was promoted to major and then lieutenant-colonel and made senior medical consultant in the Toul Sector, to the Fourth Army Corps, and to Base Section No. 3 in England. As full colonel he was commander of troops on the S.S. *Saxonia,* the first hospital ship to return to America after the war. After this service, Norris was elected professor of clinical medicine at the University of Pennsylvania and chief of the medical service at the Pennsylvania Hospital. In addition to numerous articles on cardiac and pulmonary diseases and on the use of the sphygmomanometer, he published three books: *Studies in Cardiac Pathology* (1911), *Blood Pressure, Its Clinical Applications* (1914), and with H.R. Landis, *Diseases of the Chest and the Principles of Clinical Diagnosis* (1917). The last of these was used widely and is still valuable. He was founder of the National Tuberculosis Association, a founder and president of the Heart Association of Southeastern Pennsylvania, a fellow of the College of Physicians, a trustee of the Mutual Assurance Company, and a member of the American Philosophical Society and other medical, social, and scientific organizations.

Artist: John Lambert, Jr. (1861-1907)

For biography, see page 6.

Oil on canvas; 23 3/4 x 17 3/4; signed at upper right, "John Lambert, Jr." Presented by Dr. Francis C. Wood in 1967. *PA 127*

Dr. Norris is shown bust length, his body turned three-quarters to the left, with head to the left and tilted down. The background consists of broad greenish-gray strokes over an umber undercoat. The face is oval. The hair is auburn. Large blue eyes gaze out toward the viewer. The slender nose flares slightly at the nostrils and the chin is narrow. Full red lips hint at a smile. The subject wears a white shirt, a brown necktie with tie-pin, a white vest, and a brown coat with a large white carnation in the lapel. Although restored, the surface of the portrait is still extremely painterly with a bravura style of quick, broad, visible brush strokes and sharp contrasts of light and shade. The head appears solid and three-dimensional, and there is feeling for body mass under the costume. The youthful swagger of posture and the dashingly fashionable appearance accord with biographers' descriptions—they attribute to his Viennese mother his good looks, linguistic fluency, and interest in wildlife and nature, as well as his fondness for dancing, art, music, photography, and composing verse.

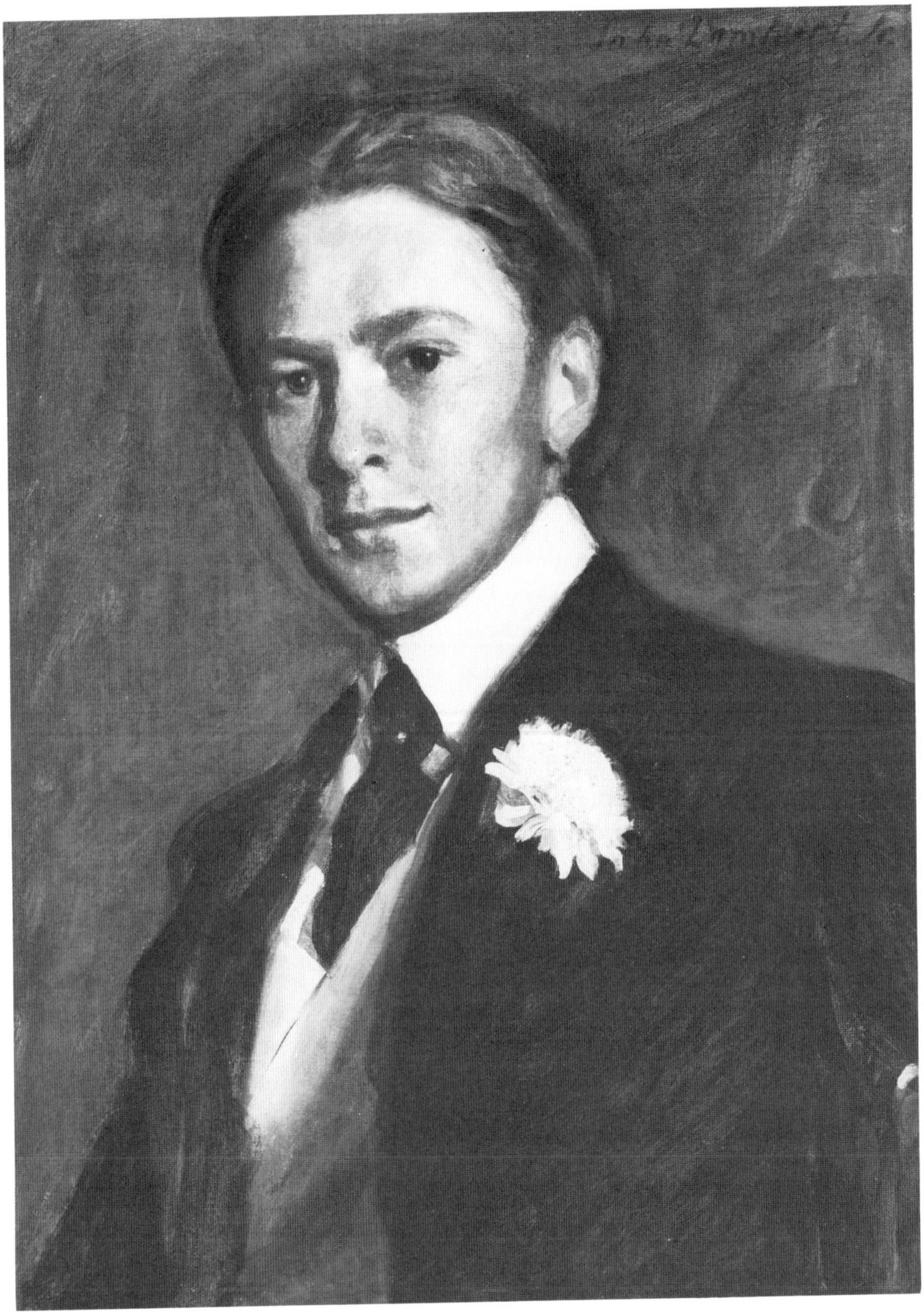

George William Norris

PA 127

Artist: *Lazar Raditz (1887–1958)*

For biography, see page 73.

Pastel drawing on buff paper, backed with board; 20 3/4 x 16 3/4; signed and dated at the lower right, "Lazar Raditz, 1938." Presented by Mrs. William Fisher Norris in 1939. Drawn in the same year as, and probably a study for, the portrait of Norris by Raditz at the Green Tree Collection, Mutual Assurance Company, Philadelphia. *PA 549*

The subject is shown bust length, his body very slightly to the left, the head frontal and tilted diagonally down. The background consists of thick diagonal black lines behind the head and extending to the shoulders of the subject's suit, with most of the borders left blank. All colors in the face and costume are lightly suggested with a few dashes, not filled in solidly. The face is oval; the hair is brown. The subject has large blue eyes that look out at the viewer, a straight nose, a wide mouth with the hint of a smile, and skin tones whose highlights are indicated by traces of warm yellow, red, and orange and by shadows which are sienna brown. Dr. Norris wears a white shirt, a blue tie, a vest, and a coat with a striped lapel pin. The subtle calligraphic style of the drawing uses a variety of strokes, from delicate hatching, to light and firm contours, to heavy lines. The paper acts as a middle tone throughout. The head is rendered in a solid and three-dimensional, detailed style. The costume is barely indicated, with no suggestion of the underlying body. Compared with the youthful portrait of Norris by Lambert, the subject has assuredly matured, but he radiates the same attractive, confident, and energetic personality as before.

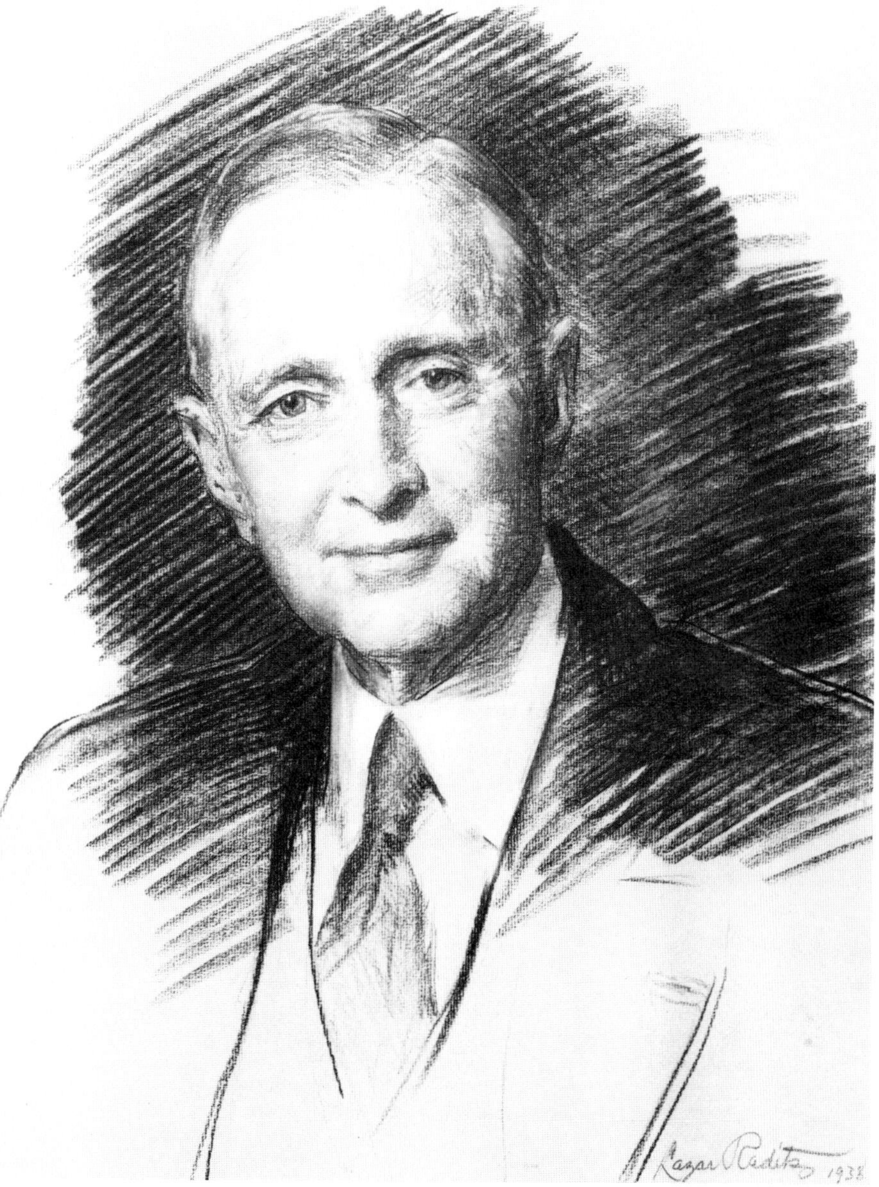

George William Norris PA 549

William Fisher Norris (1839–1901)

Born in Philadelphia, Norris was the son of George Washington Norris (q.v.) and a descendant of English Quakers who came to Philadelphia in the 1690s. He received the A.B. degree in 1857 and the M.D. degree in 1861 from the University of Pennsylvania. During the Civil War he was assistant surgeon in charge of Douglas Hospital in Washington. In addition to carrying out his official duties, he joined Dr. William Thomson (q.v.) in experiments on microscopic photography and on the use of photography to record the appearance of wounds and diseases. After the war he went abroad to study ophthalmology in Vienna with Arlt, Jaeger, Mauthner, and Stricker. Upon his return to Philadelphia he became a lecturer in ophthalmology at the University of Pennsylvania (1870) and a member of the staff at Wills Eye Hospital. In 1873 he was appointed clinical professor of diseases of the eye and in 1876 became full professor. He was president of the American Ophthalmological Association, vice-president of the Philadelphia Pathological Society, a fellow of the College of Physicians (and a founder of its Section on Ophthalmology), a director of the Mutual Assurance Society, a member of the American Philosophical Society, and a founder and president of the Board of Managers of the Hospital of the University of Pennsylvania. His best known medical works are a chapter on "Medical Ophthalmology" in Pepper's *System of Practical Medicine* and two books written with Dr. Charles A. Oliver, *Textbook of Ophthalmology* and *A System of Diseases of the Eye, by Foreign and American Authors.* Dr. Norris was a skillful and devoted surgeon, teacher, and consultant. The list of his assistants and students reads like a "Who's Who" of ophthalmology in Philadelphia.

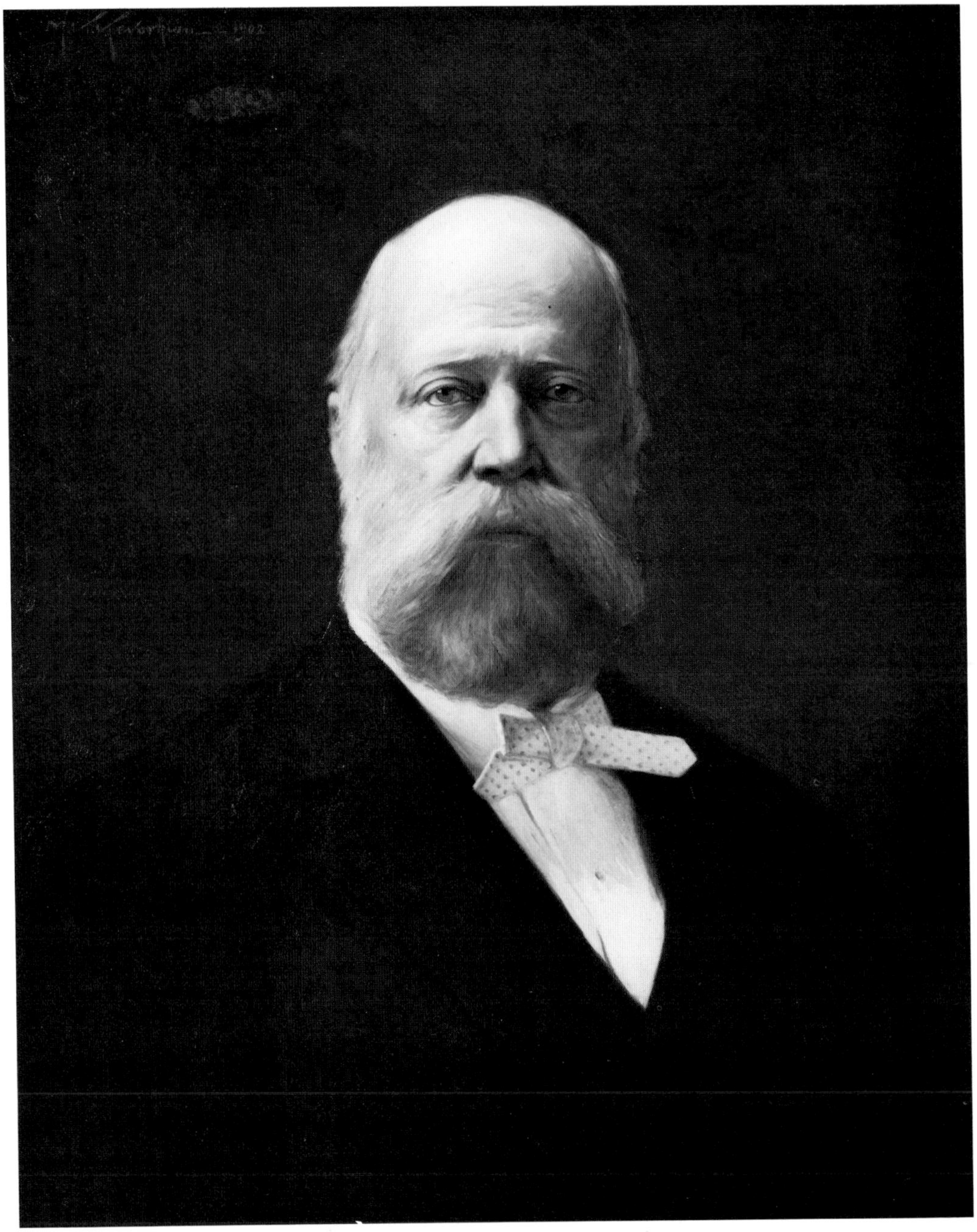

William Fisher Norris

PA 45

Artist: Mihran H. Kevorkian (1873-1946)

For biography, see page 147.

Oil on canvas; 29 x 24; signed and dated at upper left, "M.H. Kevorkian—1902." Donor not recorded, but presented in 1909. According to the Bradley File, it was painted by Kevorkian after an original portrait by Matthew Wilson (1814-1892). It resembles another portrait of Dr. Norris by Kevorkian at the University of Pennsylvania, painted in 1916. PA 45

Dr. Norris is shown bust length, his body turned slightly to the right and his head frontal and slightly tilted. The mottled background consists of gray strokes over a warm brownish-orange undercoat, darker at the top, and with a dark shadow in the right corner. The subject has a high, bald crown with a fringe at the sides of his head of grayish-white hair that joins grayish-blond side-whiskers, a full mustache, and a rounded beard. His light blue eyes, small and narrow-set, gaze directly ahead toward the viewer; his nose has a bump at the bridge and his mouth is partially obscured by the flowing moustache. There are age lines in his forehead, his puffy lower eyelids, and next to his nose. The subject wears a white shirt, a white bow tie with tan polka dots, and a black vest and coat. The surface of the portrait is painterly, especially the visible strokes of the face and hair. The head is rendered in solid and three-dimensional volumes. The costume is smoothly brushed and flatter, but by its unbuttoned coat suggests the ample girth of the subject whose torso almost fills the width of the canvas. The subject looks like the massive, vigorous, fair-haired, and handsome figure described by his biographers, and he gazes toward the observer with a direct and thoughtful expression.

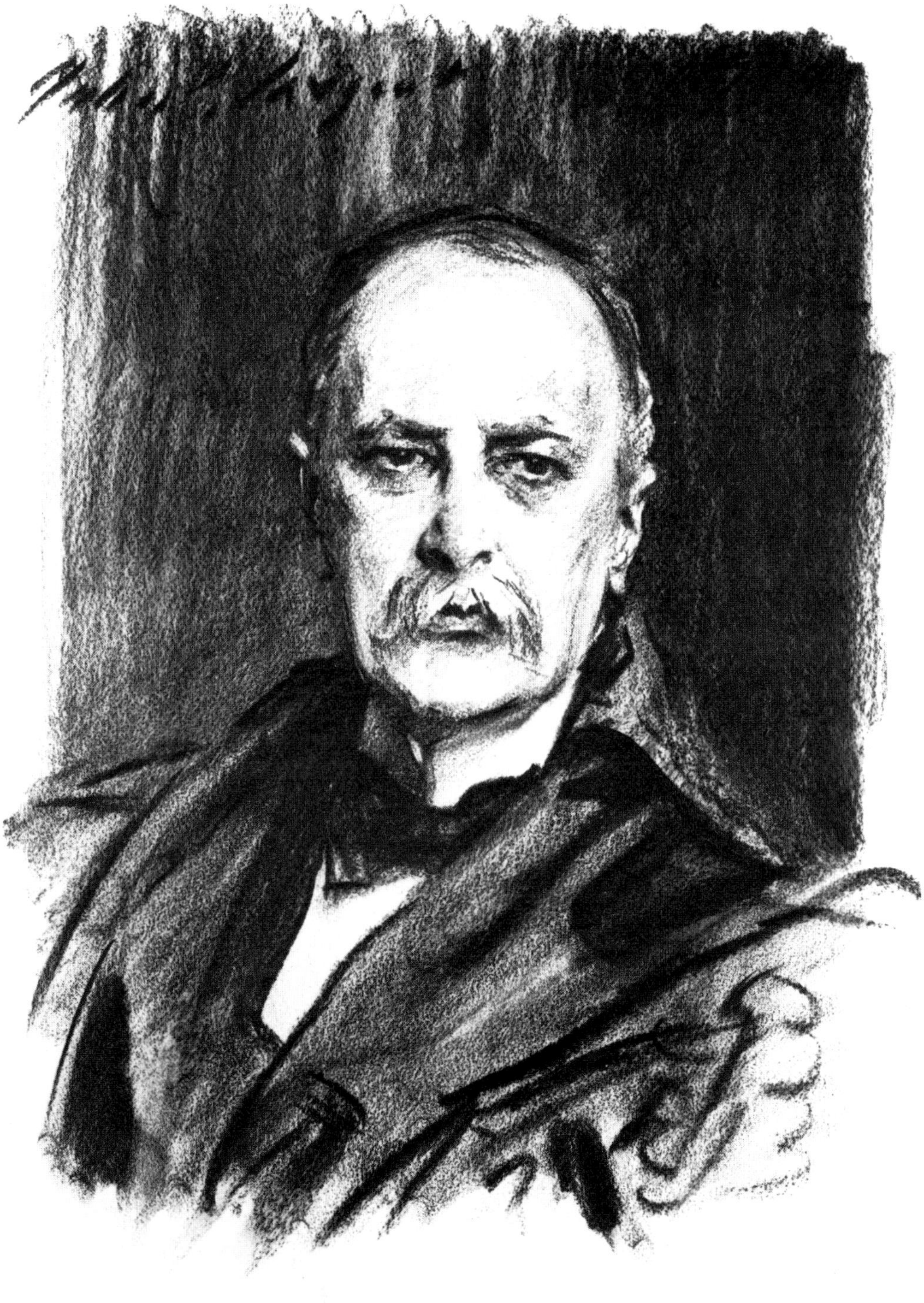

William Osler *PA 213*

William Osler (1849–1919)

Born in Bond Head, Ontario, Canada, Osler was the son of English missionary parents. Although urged to follow the clerical tradition of his family, he was graduated in arts from Trinity College, Ontario, in 1868 and received the M.D. degree from McGill University in 1872. He continued his education in London, Berlin, and Vienna. After returning to Canada, he was appointed lecturer in the institutes of medicine at McGill, where he taught pathology and physiology and engaged in research in pathology. He was appointed professor of medicine in 1875 and then pathologist and physician to the Montreal General Hospital. In 1884 he accepted an appointment as professor of clinical medicine at the University of Pennsylvania. During his four years in Philadelphia he conducted pathological research, but he is best remembered for what was then considered an unorthodox approach to teaching. Instead of delivering declamatory lectures, he taught at the bedside, in the wards of Blockley (Philadelphia General Hospital), at the Orthopaedic Hospital and Infirmary for Nervous Diseases, and in the lecture rooms, to which patients were brought for students to observe and record. The material for later publications, *The Cerebral Palsies of Children* (1889) and *On Chorea and Choreiform Affections* (1894), was gathered in Philadelphia. While in Philadelphia, Osler was elected a fellow of the College of Physicians and served on its library committee, where he was instrumental in urging expansion of its acquisitions in medical history. He also was a generous donor of medical incunabula. He urged the formation of the Samuel D. Gross library to honor donations made to the library of the College by the Gross family. In 1888 Osler became physician-in-chief of the recently organized Johns Hopkins Hospital and professor of the principles and practice of medicine. At Hopkins he initiated a revised curriculum and established new standards of training for medical students, interns, and residents. He wrote a famous textbook, *The Principles and Practice of Medicine* (1892), based on the latest advances in medicine and on classifying diseases according to pathogenesis or anatomical location. In that same year he married Grace Revere Gross, the widow of Samuel W. Gross (q.v.). He founded the Laennec Society for the study of tuberculosis, was president of the American Association of Physicians in 1895, and was a founder of the National Medical Library Association. In 1905 he accepted the Regius professorship of medicine at Oxford. He was elected a fellow of the Royal College of Physicians and of the Royal Society and was a founder of the Association of Physicians of Great Britain and Ireland and of the *Quarterly Journal of Medicine*. In 1911 he was created a baronet by King Edward VII. He was elected president of the Classical Association of Oxford in 1919 and was a curator of the Bodleian Library and a founder of the *Bodleian Quarterly Record*. An internationally known bibliophile, he was president of the Bibliographical Society of London. His elaborate monograph, *Incunabula Medica*, was published posthumously in 1923. A bibliography of his own magnificent library of 7600 medical volumes, most of which were left to McGill University, was published under the supervision of Lady Osler by Oxford University Press and was entitled *Bibliotheca Osleriana*. His own writing consists of 770 items; many of them are articles on his scientific investigations and collections of his addresses, including *Aequanimitas* (1904), *An Alabama Student* (1908), and the Silliman lectures at Yale, *The Evolution of Modern Medicine* (1921). His research and descriptions of typhoid fever, malaria, pneumonia, amebiasis, tuberculosis, and cardiovascular and other diseases are noteworthy, and he was without peer as a teacher and clinician, author, and bibliophile. He is called by many "The Father of Modern American Medicine."

Artist: John Singer Sargent (1856–1925)

For biography, see page 140.

Charcoal drawing on buff paper; 231/2 x 181/2; signed at upper left, "John S. Sargent"; dated in upper right, "1914." Presented by Lady Osler in 1914. Shown at The Art of Philadelphia Medicine *exhibition, Philadelphia Museum of Art, in 1965.* *PA 213*

Dr. Osler is shown bust length, his body turned slightly to the left, his head frontal. The background consists of dark, wide, vertical strokes, heavier on the right, the irregular borders being left blank. His rectangular face has a high forehead, with sparse hair at the top and sides. His dark narrow eyes, which look straight out toward the spectator, have shadows underneath. He has a straight nose, a light moustache with ends turned down, full lips, and a square jaw line. He wears a shirt with stand-up collar, a bow tie, and a dark academic robe. The bravura draftsmanship of this portrait consists of lines which vary from delicate to heavy, straight to curving, and thin to thick. The head has been rendered skillfully by means of precisely and delicately modeled features and appears as a solid three-dimensional form. The costume, more fluidly drawn, has fewer details. The facial expression is one of serious, almost mournful dignity, in contrast to the dramatic and somewhat decorative style of drawing.

Herman W. Ostrum (1892–1970)

Ostrum was reared in Philadelphia and graduated from the Philadelphia College of Pharmacy in 1913 and from the Medical School of the University of Pennsylvania in 1917. From 1918 to 1920, in the interval between an internship and a residency in radiology at Philadelphia General Hospital, he served as lieutenant in the Marine Corps. His professional titles included radiologist at Philadelphia General Hospital from 1922 to 1962, professor of radiology at the University of Pennsylvania and the Graduate School of Medicine, consultant in radiology at Woman's Hospital and at Bound Brook Hospital (New Jersey), and honorary consultant at Philadelphia General Hospital. He was a president of the Philadelphia Roentgen Ray Society and vice-president of the Philadelphia County Medical Society. He wrote many case reports and described a variety of conditions and treatments for *Radiology*, the *American Journal of Roentgenology and Radium Therapy*, and the *American Journal of Roentgenology, Radium Therapy and Nuclear Medicine.*

Artist: Ben Solowey (1900–1978)

Born in Warsaw, Solowey came to the United States in 1914. He studied art at the Spring Garden Institute, the Graphic Sketch Club, the Pennsylvania

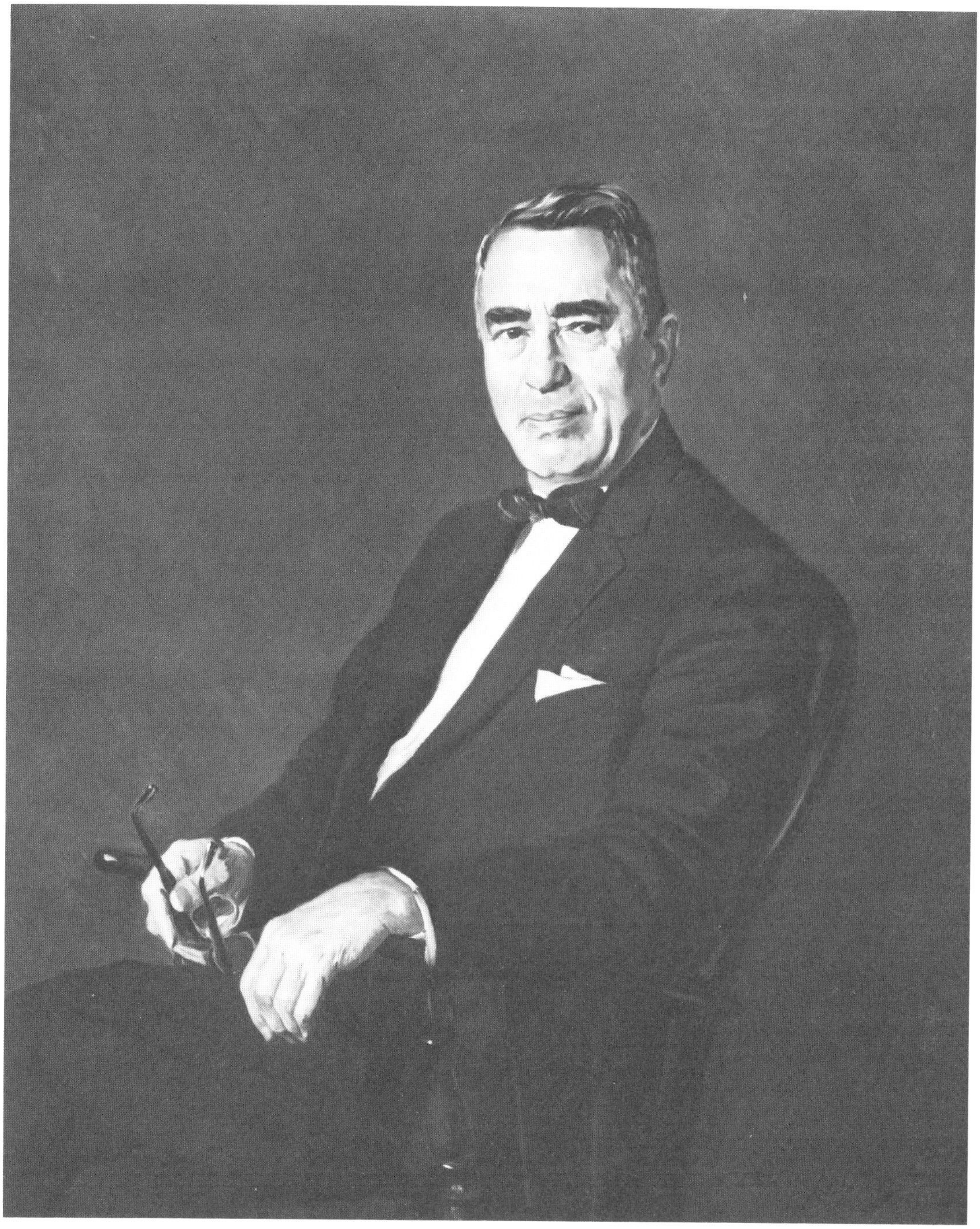

Herman W. Ostrum *PA 140*

Academy of the Fine Arts, and later in France. Upon his return to America he opened a studio in New York and then removed to a farm in Bedminster, Bucks County, where he converted a barn into a studio. As his career as an artist and teacher developed, this farm became a gathering place for artists, students, and patrons. Solowey taught painting at the Philadelphia Museum College of Art and at the Fleisher Memorial Foundation. Although he also painted still lifes and landscapes, he is best known for representational portraits and figure studies. His collection "Theater Greats of the 30's" was shown at Lincoln Center in New York and was widely reproduced in newspapers. He participated in many major exhibitions at the Pennsylvania Academy, the National Academy of Design, the Chicago International, and the Allentown Art Museum. He had one-man shows at the Allentown Art Museum and Lehigh University and a memorial exhibition at Woodmere Art Gallery in 1979. His prizes include the Dawson medal of the Philadelphia Water Color Club, the gold medal of the fellowship of the Pennsylvania Academy, and awards from the Philadelphia Sketch Club, the Wilmington Fine Arts Society, and the Ligonier Art Association. In addition to being in private collections, some of his works are on public view at the Treasury Building, Harrisburg; Thomas Jefferson University; Delaware Art Museum; New Britain (Connecticut) Museum of Art; and the Reading Museum and Art Gallery.

Oil on canvas; 35 x 29; signed and dated at lower right, "Ben Solowey 1961." Commissioned by the Blockley Radiological Society; presented to the radiology department of Philadelphia General Hospital and then to the city of Philadelphia which, in turn, presented it to permanent loan to the College of Physicians in 1977. *PA 140*

Ostrum is shown two-thirds length, his body turned three-quarters to the left, head slightly to the left and tilted down. He is seated in a Windsor-style armchair which is turned three-quarters to the left. His legs are crossed at the knees. His arms rest on the chair arms, his left hand is pendent, and his right hand holds his horn-rimmed eyeglasses. The atmospheric background is green, lighter on the left. The subject's face is rectangular. The hair is steel-gray, and the black eyebrows are thick and straight. The gray eyes look out of their corners to the right. He has a bulbous nose, a wide mouth with full lips, and a chiseled, cleft chin. He has puffy lower eyelids and lines next to his nose. He wears a white shirt, a gray bow tie with diagonal tan stripes, a brown suit, and a white pocket handkerchief. The surface of this portrait is painted fluidly within precisely defined contours. The head and hands are well constructed in solid, three-dimensional volumes. The costume shows details of tailoring and folds and gives a sense of the underlying body. The unusual composition has a blank border on the right and a horizontal thrust of the body toward the left, where the subject's legs are cut off by the left edge. His posture is erect, but relaxed. The pose is active, and he appears to have removed his eyeglasses momentarily and turned his head as though to address an unseen visitor. His thick, dark, knitted eyebrows and tightly pursed lips contribute to the solemn, alert expression.

Francis Randolph Packard (1870-1950)

Born in Philadelphia and descended from distinguished Puritan forbears, Dr. Packard was the son of the surgeon, John Hooker Packard (q.v.), and brother of Frederick A. Packard (q.v.). He was graduated from the biological department of the University of Pennsylvania in 1889 and from its medical department in 1892. He did postgraduate work at Johns Hopkins under William Osler (q.v.). He served as resident physician at the Children's and Pennsylvania Hospitals and became quizmaster in therapeutics at the medical school. In 1895 he began to practice privately and after three years he specialized in diseases of the ear, nose, and throat. He was professor of laryngology and otology at the Philadelphia Polyclinic and College for Graduates in Medicine and was laryngologist and otologist to the Pennsylvania, Children's, Bryn Mawr, and Chestnut Hill Hospitals, the Pennsylvania Institution for the Deaf and Dumb, the Eastern State Penitentiary, and the State Asylum for the Insane at Norristown. He saw military service in two wars, first in the Spanish-American War in 1898 as lieutenant and assistant surgeon to the Second Regiment, Pennsylvania Volunteer Infantry, and secondly in World War I as captain with Pennsylvania Base Hospital No. 10 in Le Tréport, France, and as officer in charge of British General Hospital No. 16. He also served in Belgium and was discharged with the rank of major in 1919. He served as president of the American Otological Society and the American Laryngological Society and as a founder of the Laryngological, Rhinological and Otological Society. At the College of Physicians he was secretary, honorary librarian, vice-president, president (1931-33), and censor. He bequeathed his extensive collection of medicohistorical books to the College. He was a scholarly man, and he is remembered as the author of 97 articles, numerous addresses, and his books on medical history: *A History of Medicine in the United States* (1901), *The History of the Pennsylvania Hospital Unit (Base Hospital No. 10, U.S.A.)* (1921), and *Some Account of the Pennsylvania Hospital from the First Rise to the Beginning of the Year 1938* (1938). He served long and ably as editor of the *American Journal of Medical Sciences* and *The Annals of Medical History.* His literary proficiency being recognized by cultural institutions in the city, he served on the library boards of the Library Company, the Philadelphia Free Library, the Athenaeum, the Pennsylvania Hospital, and the American Philosophical Society. He wrote a medical text, *Textbook of Diseases of the Nose, Throat and Ear* (1908), and received the Newcomb Award of the American Laryngological Association. He was awarded an honorary LL.D. from the University of Pennsylvania.

Artist: Justin Anthony Pardi (1898-1951)

Born in Castelli, Italy, Pardi came to the United States in 1905. He studied at the Boston Museum School of Fine Arts and won two Tiffany scholarships. Most of his career was spent in Philadelphia, where he was widely known as a portraitist and as a restorer of oil paintings. He was an instructor of drawing and painting at the Pennsylvania Museum and School of Industrial Art, a lecturer on artistic anatomy at the Pennsylvania Academy of the Fine Arts, and an instructor at the Woodmere Art Gallery. He exhibited his work at the Pennsylvania Academy, the Warwick Art Gallery, Woodmere, the Philadelphia Art Alliance, and the Philadelphia Sketch Club. He won the Da Vinci gold medal in 1940.

Oil on canvas mounted on wood; 49 1/2 x 39; signed and dated at upper right, "Pardi/1938." Presented in 1942 by Dr. Francis R. Packard, who stated in a letter retained in the files of the College of Physicians that Dr. Romeo A. Luongo [Sr.] "had the portrait painted and gave it to me several years ago." It was shown at the Pennsylvania Academy of the Fine Arts annual exhibition in 1939. *PA 109*

Dr. Packard is shown two-thirds length, with his body turned to the right and his head almost frontal and tilted down slightly. He is seated with his left arm resting on a

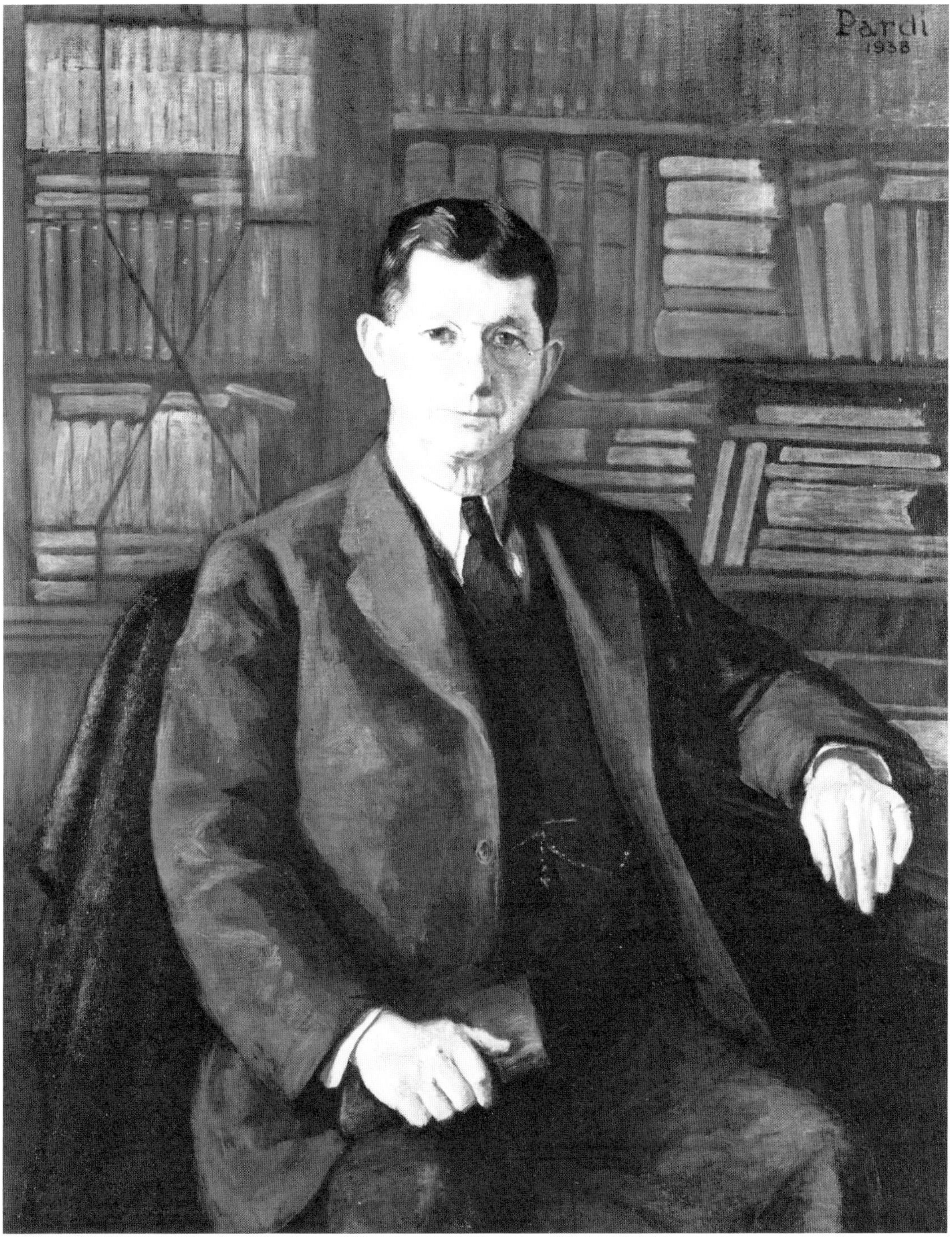

Francis Randolph Packard *PA 109*

table top and his right hand holding a green book which is placed on his thigh. The complex architectural interior contains a breakfront with glass door on the left separated by a vertical post from bookshelves on the right. Both sides have shelves lined with books of various widths, lengths, and colors, placed side by side or stacked vertically. At the lower right there is a table with two books lying on it. Folded over the back of the chair there is green drapery, perhaps an academic gown. The subject has black hair tinged with gray, light brown eyes that look straight ahead through wire-rimmed spectacles with magnifying lenses, a nose with a bump at the bridge, a wide mouth with a thin upper lip, full cheeks, and a pointed chin. There are age lines on his forehead, next to his nose, and on his neck. He wears a white shirt, a dark blue necktie, a dark gray three-piece, single-breasted suit, a gold watch chain, and a gold ring. The surface of the portrait is painterly throughout; the head and hands, done in small strokes, appear solid and three-dimensional. The costume, more broadly painted, suggests the underlying bulk of the body. The light skin tones of the face and hands make them stand out boldly against the animated background. This device, combined with the fact that the subject is seated in the foreground in a close-up view, portrays Dr. Packard as a forceful, energetic figure who has turned away from the table and put down his book; he seems eager to converse with the viewer.

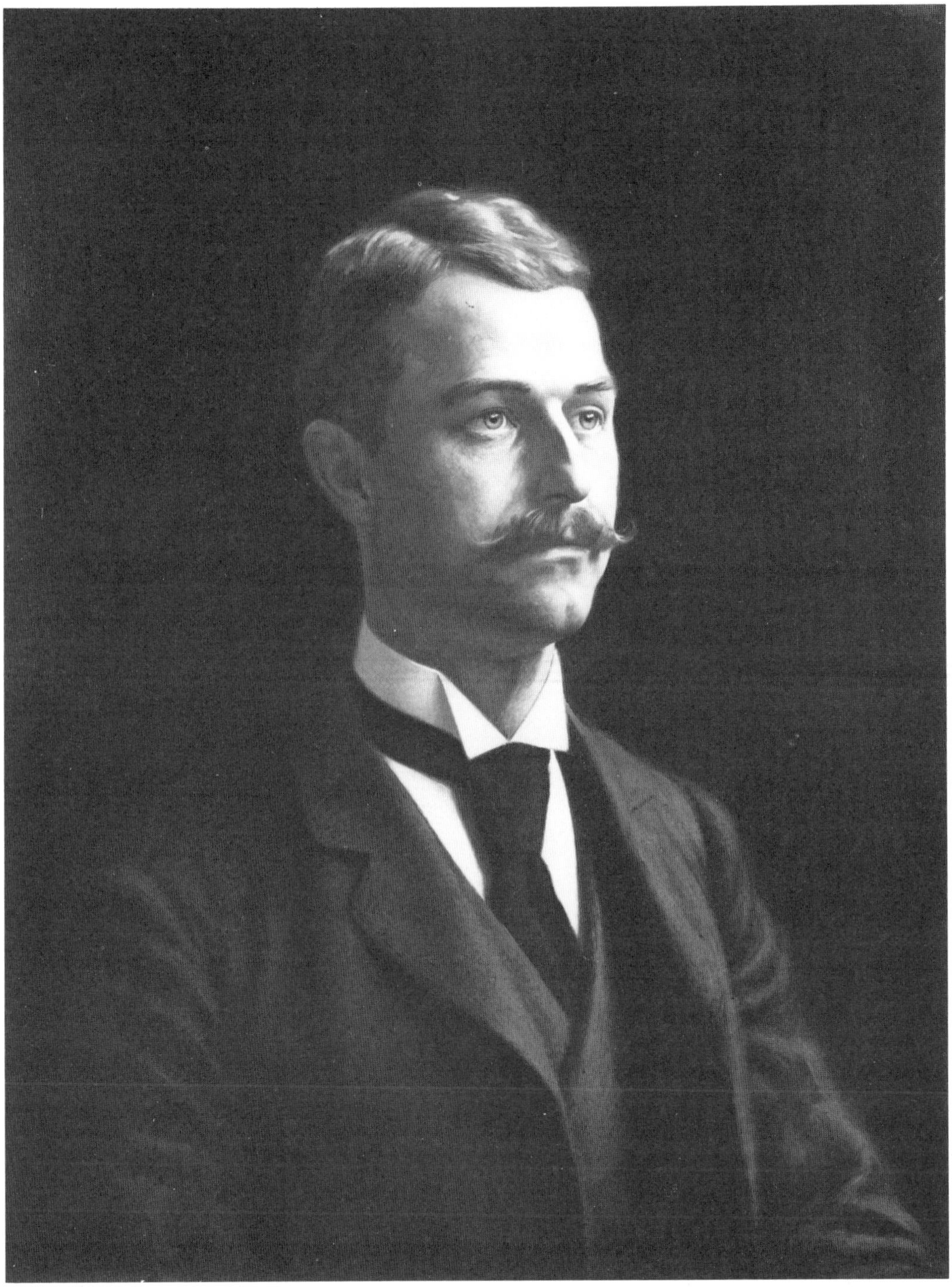

Frederick Adolphus Packard *PA 90*

Frederick Adolphus Packard (1862-1902)

Dr. Packard was born in Philadelphia, a descendant of distinguished Puritan forbears, son of the surgeon John Hooker Packard (q.v.) and brother of Francis R. Packard (q.v.). He received the baccalaureate degree in 1882 and the M.D. degree in 1885 from the University of Pennsylvania. He was an outstanding medical student. After serving as resident physician to the University and Pennsylvania Hospitals, he entered private practice and for three years was an assistant to Dr. William Pepper. He was appointed physician to the Pennsylvania and Children's Hospitals and visiting physician to the Episcopal, Methodist Episcopal, and Philadelphia Hospitals. He was an instructor in clinical medicine at the University of Pennsylvania, president of the Pathological Society of Philadelphia, a founder and president of the Philadelphia Pediatric Society, and chairman of the section on general medicine at the College of Physicians. His writings include papers devoted to tonsilitis, rheumatism, thermic fever, acromegaly, poliomyelitis, osteitis deformans, lead poisoning, and sarcoma of the lungs. Shortly before his death from typhoid fever, he was elected a trustee of the University of Pennsylvania.

Artist: James Longacre Wood (1867-1938)

For biography, see page 96.

Oil on canvas; 29 1/2 x 22 1/2; signed and dated lower left, "J.L. Wood/1903." Presented by fellows of the College of Physicians in 1903. This posthumous work resembles a portrait of Packard by James B. Sword, 1903, at the University of Pennsylvania. *PA 90*

Dr. Packard is shown bust length, with head and body turned to the right. The atmospheric background is dark blue. His face is oval. He has blond hair, light blue eyes that look straight out in the direction of the head turn, a slightly hooked nose, a wide mouth, a reddish-blond moustache, and a cleft chin. He wears a white shirt with wing collar, a black necktie, and a gray vest and coat. The surface of the portrait has been painted smoothly except for the hair and moustache, in which individual strands are differentiated by visible brush strokes. The planes of the head are well modulated with careful gradations from light to dark; they render solid and three-dimensional, almost sculptural forms. The costume shows attention to folds and gives a sense of the underlying body. The contours of the shoulders and arms blend into the background, not unlike some contemporary photographs which might have been a source for this posthumous portrait. The subject's unlined face expresses the gentle, quiet, and optimistic disposition for which he was praised by his biographers.

John Hooker Packard (1832-1907)

Dr. Packard was born in Philadelphia, a descendant of distinguished Puritans, including Thomas Hooker, the founder of Springfield, Massachusetts, and Samuel Packard, founder of Bridgewater, Massachusetts. He received the A.B. degree in 1850 and the M.D. in 1853 from the University of Pennsylvania and continued his education in Paris. Upon his return to Philadelphia he completed a residency at the Pennsylvania Hospital, established a private practice, and was a teacher and demonstrator of anatomy at the University of Pennsylvania. During the Civil War he was acting assistant surgeon in the United States Army, serving in Philadelphia, New Jersey, and Gettysburg. In 1863 he was elected surgeon to the Episcopal Hospital, where he served until 1884, when he was appointed surgeon to the Pennsylvania Hospital. He was also surgeon to St. Joseph's Hospital and to Woman's Hospital. He was a founder of the Philadelphia Academy of Surgery and a founder and president of both the Philadelphia Pathological Society and the Philadelphia Obstetrical Society. He was an original fellow and treasurer of the American Surgical Association. At the College of Physicians he served as secretary, vice-president, and first Mütter lecturer. His contributions to the surgical literature include a translation of Malgaigne's *Treatise on Fractures* (1859), an American edition of Holme's *System of Surgery* (1881), chapters on poisoned wounds and on fractures for Ashhursts's *International Encyclopedia of Surgery*, and chapters on fractures and dislocations for Keating's *Cyclopedia of Diseases of Children.* He wrote *Lectures on Inflammation* (1865), *Handbook of Minor Surgery* (1863), and *Handbook of Operative Surgery* (1870), as well as three editions of the *Philadelphia Medical Directory* (1868, 1871, and 1873). He contributed several articles on ether anesthesia, oblique incision of the skin to lessen scarring, radical cure for hernia, amputation of the hip-joint, and ligation of the internal iliac artery. He was greatly interested in art and was an accomplished draftsman. He was a member of the board of directors of the Pennsylvania Academy of the Fine Arts, where he served also as chairman of the committee on instruction. In 1896 he was infected during an operation and consequently was obligated to give up active medical practice.

Artist: Hugh Henry Breckenridge (1870-1937)

For biography, see page 38.

Oil on canvas; 40 1/2 x 32 1/2; signed at lower left, "Hugh H. Breckenridge." Presented by his son, Dr. Francis R. Packard, in 1917. *PA 21*

Packard is shown two-thirds length, his body to the right, his head frontal and tilted down slightly. He is seated in an armchair with his legs crossed at the knees and twisted around so that his thighs are parallel to the picture plane. His hands are folded and rest on his thigh. The background has a drapery on the left side with a blue, green, and violet pattern over tan. The wall is scumbled tones of gray, violet, and green, lighter on the right; a chair-rail molding divides this portion from the darker area below. The subject has medium-gray hair flecked with light-gray highlights. His face is rectangular. His blue eyes look straight ahead through rimless spectacles. The tip of his nose points down to his red lips, gray moustache, and pointed beard. He wears a white shirt, a dark blue necktie with gold tie pin, a dark gray vest and coat with wide lapels, and medium-gray trousers. The surface of this portrait has loosely brushed, fluid strokes. In the skin tones there are green shadows that relate to the background colors. The head is well constructed in solid and three-dimensional forms. The costume is flatter, with some feeling for the underlying body volumes. The subject sits erectly but his posture is active—the hips are twisted, the upper body is turned, the lips are pursed, and the hands are tightly clasped. This produces an energetic but tense expression, which is reinforced by the barrier of the elongated thigh between subject and viewer. The combination of intimidating posture and sober facial expression makes the viewer feel as though he might expect a reprimand.

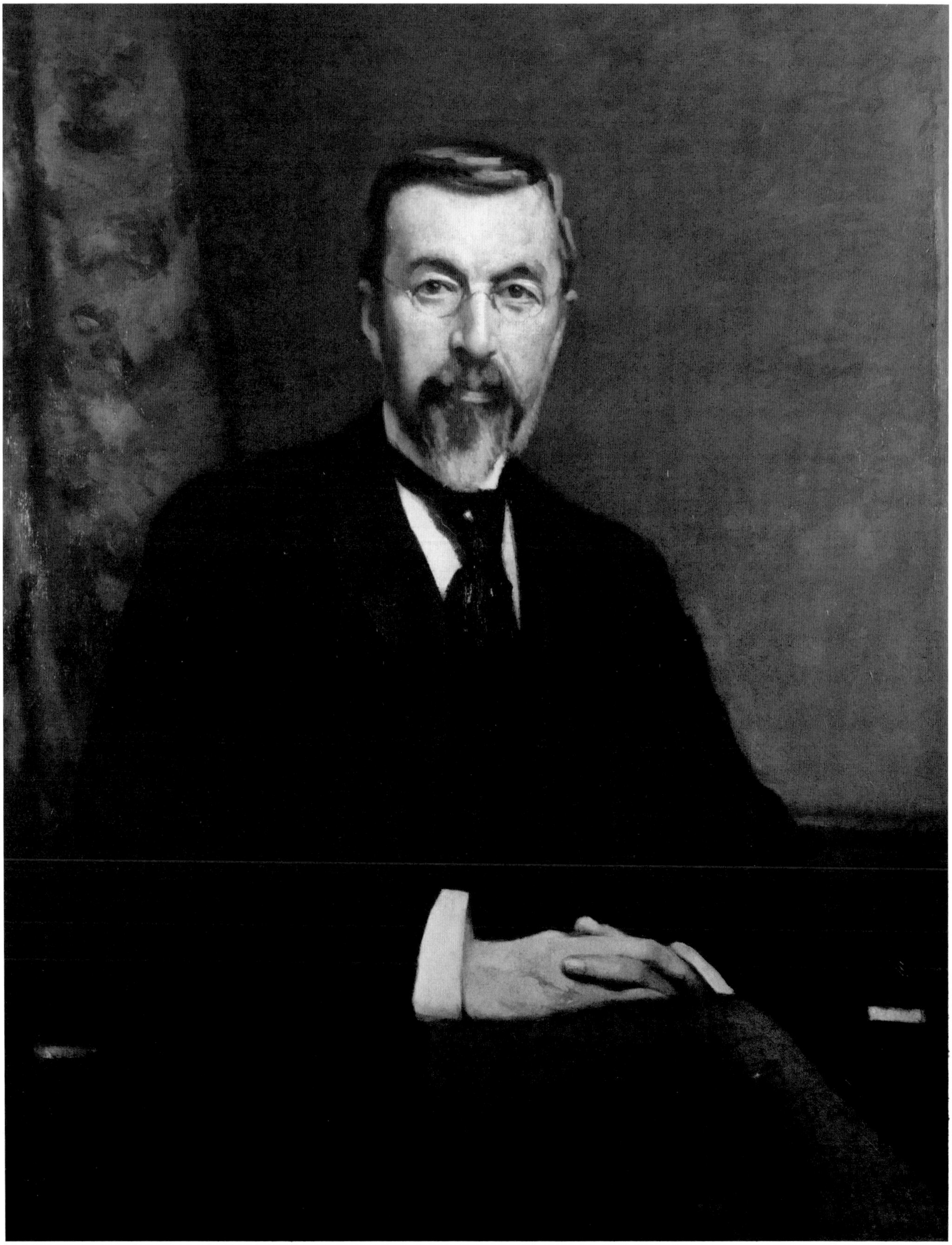

John Hooker Packard *PA 21*

Joseph Pancoast (1805-1882)

Born near Burlington, New Jersey, Pancoast was a descendant of English forbears who came to America with William Penn. He received the M.D. degree from the University of Pennsylvania in 1828 and began a surgical practice immediately thereafter. He was an instructor at the Philadelphia School of Anatomy and was elected physician to the Philadelphia Hospital in 1835, being transferred at his request to the surgical staff in 1837 and remaining there until 1845. In 1838 he became professor of surgery at Jefferson Medical and in 1847 was transferred to the chair of anatomy, which he held until 1874. He was on the staff of the Pennsylvania Hospital from 1854 to 1864. He was a fellow of the College of Physicians and a member of many other societies, including the American Philosophical Society. Dr. Pancoast, an innovative surgeon, devised new techniques for operating on soft mixed cataracts, exstrophy of the bladder, tic douloureux, empyema, strabismus, and occlusion of the naso-lacrimal duct. He performed a lumbar operation for large abscesses and invented an abdominal tourniquet to shut off arterial blood from the lower limbs during amputations. He was the author of several translations and editions of older works, including *System of Anatomy* by Caspar Wistar and William Horner. He contributed many articles to the *American Journal of Medical Sciences*, the *American Medical Intelligencer*, and the *Medical Examiner*. His chief work was his *Treatise on Operative Surgery* (1844).

Artist: Unknown

Marble; 24 1/4 x 13 5/8 x 10 1/8; base integral with sculpture, 4 3/4 in. high in front; not signed or dated. Presented by Dr. William H. Pancoast, his son, in 1887. *ST 541*

Dr. Pancoast is shown bust length, with body and head frontal and sides and lower edges of the torso squared off. His thick hair is curled forward around the ears to offset a receding hairline. His rectangular face has knitted brows and deepset, narrow eyes, in which the carved irises and pupils are directed upward. Under a slightly hooked nose, the mouth is partly obscured by the long, flowing moustache, which connects with side-whiskers at the square chin. There are deep lines on the forehead, near the puffy lower lids, and next to the nose. Below the neck the body is not described anatomically. The surface of the marble is smooth, without visible tool marks. The head has been carved skillfully, with knowledge of the underlying anatomy. Although the sculpture resembles contemporary photographs of Pancoast, especially in the hairstyle, it is rendered in a neoclassical manner with upraised eyes and neutral expression. The sculpture has idealized the subject's bulbous nose, receding chin, and portly round face.

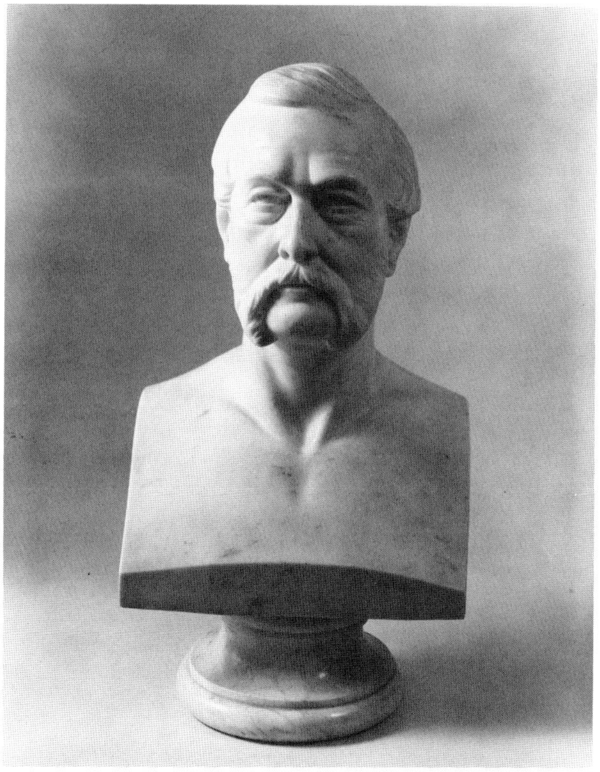

Joseph Pancoast *ST 541*

William Henry Pancoast (1835-1897)

Descended from English forbears who came to America with William Penn, Pancoast was born in Philadelphia, the son of surgeon Joseph Pancoast (q.v.). He was graduated from Haverford College in 1853 and from Jefferson Medical College in 1856. He continued his education in London, Paris, Vienna, and Berlin. Upon returning to Philadelphia he established a general practice, specializing in surgery. In 1859 he was appointed visiting surgeon to the Charity Hospital, where he organized a large surgical clinic. He resigned in 1869 and was then elected consulting surgeon and made a member of the board of trustees. During the Civil War he was surgeon-in-chief and second officer in charge of a military hospital in Philadelphia. At Jefferson Hospital he was demonstrator of anatomy from 1862 until 1874, when he succeeded his father as professor of anatomy; he held the post until 1886. He was also visiting surgeon to the Philadelphia Hospital and lecturer on surgical anatomy in the summer school at Jefferson. From 1886 until his death he was professor of general, descriptive, and surgical anatomy at the Medico-Chirurgical College of Philadelphia, an institution he had helped to found. He was president of the Philadelphia County Medical Society, vice-president of the Pennsylvania State Medical Society, vice-president of the American Medical Association, a fellow of the College of Physicians, and a member of the American Philo-

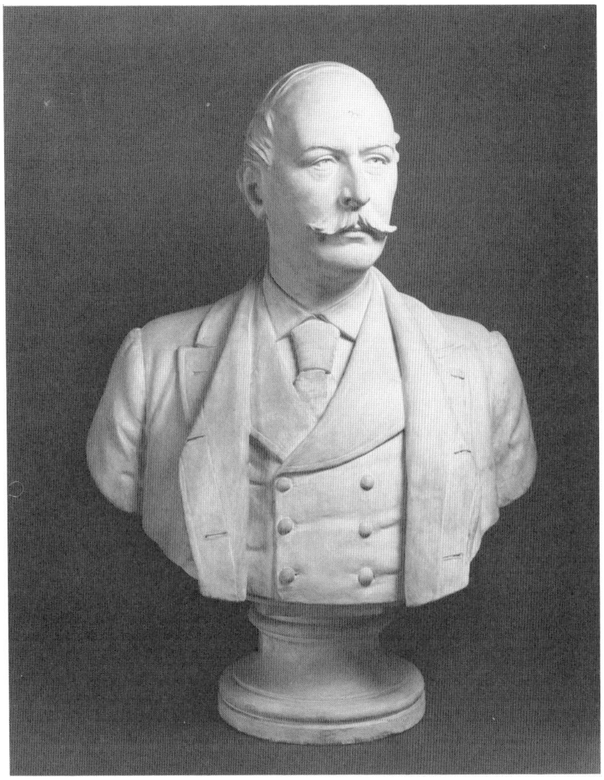

William Henry Pancoast *ST 515*

sophical Society. He presided over the section on anatomy of the Ninth International Medical Congress. In 1874, after the death of the famous Siamese twins, Chang and Eng Bunker, he took an active part in bringing their bodies to the College of Physicians for an autopsy, which he performed with Harrison Allen (q.v.); he also wrote the report that was presented at a special meeting of the College in 1874.

Artist: Castor Berbera (?) or Barberd (?)

Plaster, painted white; 31 3/8 x 11 3/8 x 13 3/4; base integral with sculpture, 6 in. high; signed and dated on the right side of the bottom of the base, "Castor Berbera/Sculptor 12/M/ 1889 [the spelling is partly illegible]." Presented by Mrs. William H. Pancoast in 1897. *ST 515*

Dr. Pancoast is shown bust length, with body frontal and head turned to the right. He has a high forehead with sparse hair combed over the top of his head and curled forward. His face is oval. The eyes have carved irises and pupils that look out in the direction of the head turn. He has a curved nose, round cheeks, and a full moustache that curves upward over a wide mouth and rounded chin. He wears a shirt, a necktie, a double-breasted vest, and an open coat with notched lapels and two lapel pins. The clothes are arranged artfully in layers that project forward in different degrees of depth and show an unusual amount of tailoring details. The sculpture has the uneven surface characteristic of plaster, but no tool marks are visible. The head is carved with understanding of the underlying anatomical structure. The costume covers an expansively proportioned body. The figure is rendered naturalistically and is dramatic in scale and dignity. Although the facial expression is impassive, the total conception conveys a message of confidence, energy, and vitality.

Thomas Parke (1749-1835)

Born in East Caln Township, Chester County, Pennsylvania, Parke was the son of Irish Quaker farmers who came to America in 1724. In Philadelphia he studied medicine under Dr. Cadwalader Evans, and in 1770 he received the Bachelor of Medicine degree from the College of Philadelphia. There he studied under Drs. William Shippen, Jr. (q.v.), Adam Kuhn (q.v.), John Morgan, (q.v.), Benjamin Rush (q.v.), and Thomas Bond (q.v.). He continued his education in London, where he registered as a physician-pupil under Dr. Richard Huck at St. Thomas's Hospital and took a course in obstetrics from Dr. Colin McKenzie, and in Edinburgh, where he studied with William Cullen (q.v.) and others. Returning to Philadelphia, he joined his former preceptor, Dr. Cadwalader Evans, in practice. Dr. Evans died shortly thereafter, and Parke inherited a large and lucrative practice. In 1777 he was made physician to the Pennsylvania Hospital, a post that he held until his retirement in 1823. He is celebrated for devoting long and industrious service to other institutions as well, including the Library Company, of which he was an active director from 1778 until 1834; the American Philosophical Society from 1778 until he resigned in 1817; and the College of Physicians, where he was senior founding fellow, member of the library committee, censor, president (1818-34), and a delegate from the middle states region to the national meeting convened for preparation of a national pharmacopoeia. His biographers agree that Parke performed his duties faithfully and well but without brilliance or innovation.

Artist: Unknown

Oil on canvas; 35 1/4 x 28 1/2; not signed or dated. Presented by Dr. George Bacon Wood in 1866. Copy after original portrait by Thomas Sully, 1822, Library Company of Philadelphia. Both the original at the Library Company and the copy owned by the College of Physicians were shown in 1887 at the College's Centennial Celebration Loan Collection of Portraits. *Consultants have tentatively suggested James Reid Lambdin or John Neagle as the copyist, and further research must be done in order to assign an attribution conclusively.* *PA 15*

Parke is shown half-length, his body turned slightly to the right, his head to the left. He is seated in a green upholstered chair, with his left forearm resting on a table and his left hand holding a sheaf of papers. The atmospheric background is mottled green, lighter on the right, with a curving shadow on the lower right. The subject has a high forehead with wispy gray hair on the sides and back, thick curving eyebrows, large blue eyes that look up and out in the direction of the head turn, an aquiline nose, pink cheeks, a wide mouth with lips slightly parted, and a round chin. He wears a white shirt, a wide white neckcloth tied in a bow, a white waistcoat with a standing collar, and a brown, single-breasted coat with an M-notched collar and horizontal folds stretched over his abdomen. The surface of the portrait is brushed smoothly, especially in the well-constructed, solid, three-dimensional head. The costume, which reveals the underlying body forms, is more fluidly brushed. The posture is relaxed. Dr. Parke appears to have turned his head away from his papers to address an unseen visitor, and he has a curious and lively facial expression. The copyist has made Parke's body more upright than it is in Sully's painting and has reduced the proportions of the torso. The contours of his coat have been made more regular, the highlights on the hands and the paper are more muted, the facial expression is softened, and the total effect is calmer and less dramatic.

Joseph Parrish (1779-1840)

Dr. Parrish was born in Philadelphia and was a descendant of the surveyor-general of the Province of Maryland who served under Lord Baltimore. In his early years he was forced to serve an apprenticeship under his father, a hatter, but eventually was allowed to follow his own inclinations and begin studying medicine with Caspar Wistar (q.v.) in 1802. In 1805 he received the M.D. degree from the University of Pennsylvania and that same year was appointed resident physician to an emergency yellow fever hospital set up by the Board of Health. He was physician and later manager of the Philadelphia Dispensary and served it as consulting physician from 1835 to 1840. He was on the staff of the Philadelphia Almshouse hospital, first as physician (1807-11) and then as surgeon (1811-21); he was also surgeon to the Pennsylvania Hospital (1816-

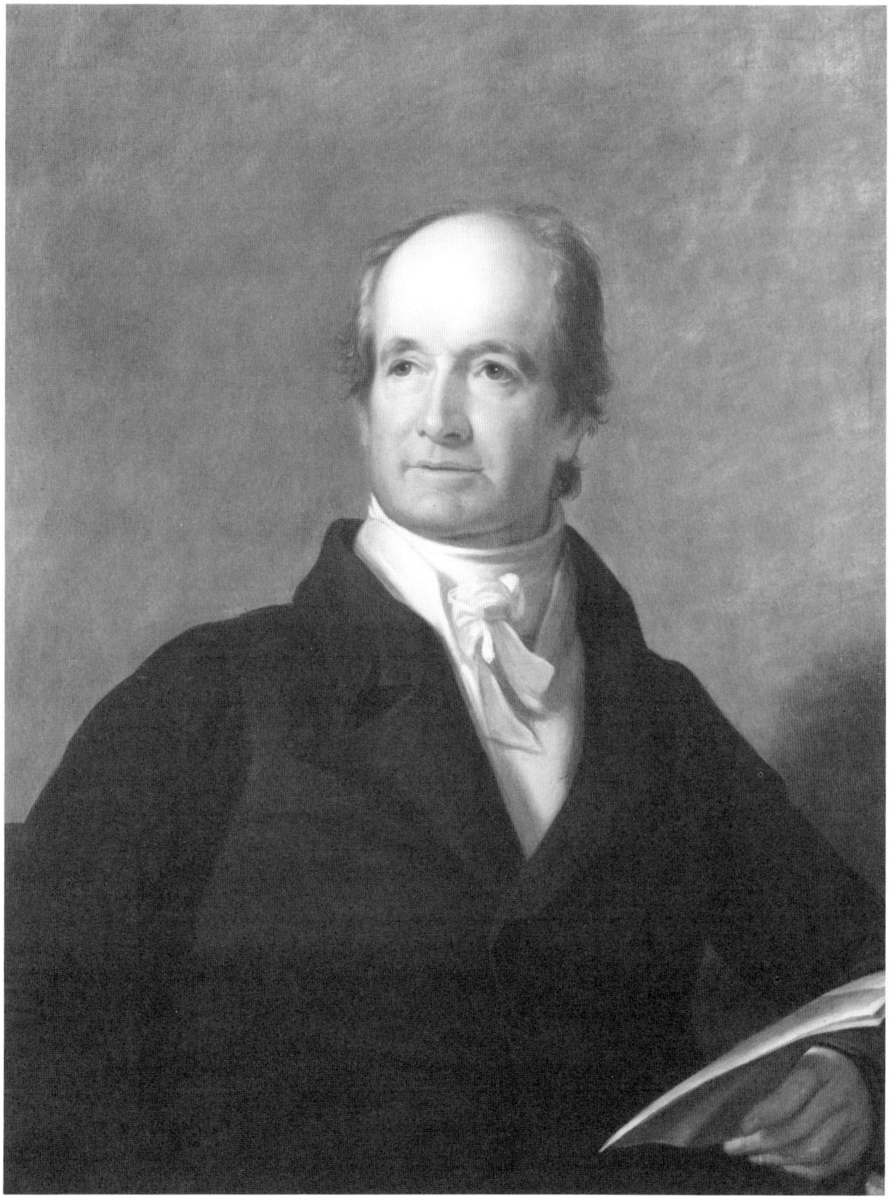

Thomas Parke *PA 15*

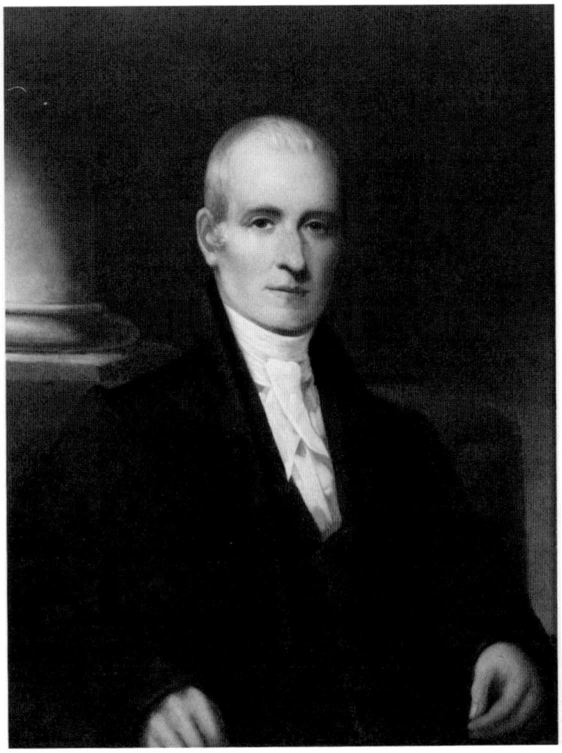

Joseph Parrish *PA 27*

29). He was associated with the establishment of the Wills Eye Hospital and was the first president of its board of managers. He was also vice-president of the College of Physicians and of the Philadelphia Medical Society and a member of the American Philosophical Society. It is said that he declined the chair of anatomy at the University of Pennsylvania in 1818 on the grounds that it would interfere with his manifold religious duties in the Society of Friends. He was a staunch advocate of the abolition of both capital punishment and slavery, and he was president of the Pennsylvania Abolition Society. In recognition of services performed during the cholera outbreak of 1832, he was given a silver pitcher by the civil authorities. Early in his career he delivered a popular course of lectures on chemistry which led several years later to systematic courses of lectures in chemistry, anatomy, and materia medica. In addition to his extensive private practice and civic, religious, and institutional duties, he was a private medical teacher and usually had ten to thirty students at one time. He made numerous contributions to the *North American Medical and Surgical Journal* and to the *Eclectic Repertory and Analytical Review*, of which he was editor. His most noteworthy work was *Practical Observations on Strangulated Hernia, and Some of the Diseases of the Urinary Organs* (1836).

Artist: Attributed to Rebekah T. Furness

Rebekah Furness was a student at the Pennsylvania Academy of the Fine Arts from 1876 to 1877 and from 1879 to 1882. She exhibited work at the Academy in 1881, 1884, and from 1887 to 1890.

Oil on canvas; 35 1/4 x 27 1/4; not signed or dated. Presented by Susanna Dillwyn Wharton (Mrs. Rodman Wharton) in 1910. Although the Bradley File and subsequent inventories list this portrait as a copy by R.I. Furness, it is most probably the work of an artist named Rebekah T. Furness. Bradley adds that it is a copy of an original portrait by Robert Street (1796–1865), owned by the Parrish family. This is presumably the portrait that was shown at the College of Physicians' Centennial Celebration Loan Collection of Portraits, *1887, in which the artist is listed as "Street" and the owner as Miss Sarah Parrish. In the book by Susanna Parrish Wharton,* The Parrish Family, *(Philadelphia, 1925), this portrait is reproduced but the artist is said to be unknown. An identification of Street as the artist is found in an etching in the College of Physicians' collection by Albert Rosenthal, labeled "Street Pinxit/Albert Rosenthal Fecit/from the original painting in the possession of the Family." The copy was probably commissioned by the Parrish family, which owns at least one other copy. The original portrait by Street may be the one in the collection of Maxfield Parrish, Jr., the artist and lineal descendant of Joseph Parrish, according to a letter from the files of the College of Physicians.* *PA 27*

Dr. Parrish is shown half-length, his body turned slightly to the right, head to the right and tilted sideways. He is seated in a red upholstered armchair, his arms resting on the arms of the chair and his fingers loosely curved. The atmospheric background is dark greenish-gray, lighter at the bottom. At the left are the base and plinth of a light brown column, used symbolically, but not explained architecturally. The subject has smooth silver-white hair brushed toward his forehead. Under rounded eyebrows his hazel eyes look out toward the viewer. His long, thin nose has a bump at the bridge and a tip that points down to a wide mouth and full lips. The face is relatively unlined. He wears a wide, white neckcloth with loosely tied ends. His single-breasted, russet-brown waistcoat has very long lapels. The single-breasted coat, of the same color, has a high collar. The portrait is smoothly

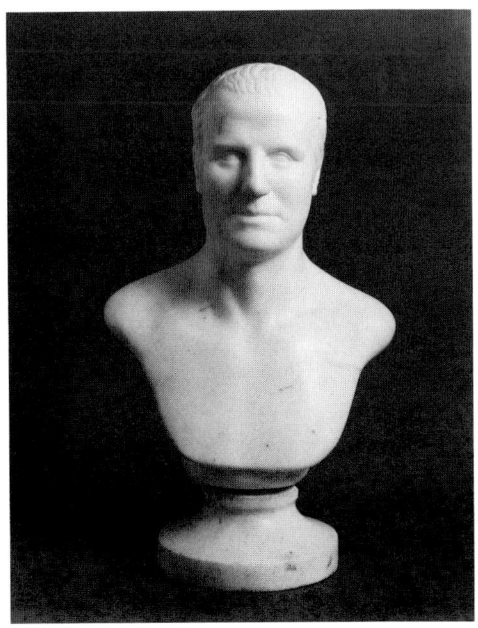

Joseph Parrish *ST 543*

painted throughout. The head and hands appear only moderately solid and three-dimensional. The costume is fairly well described but does not suggest the underlying body. The subject's facial expression is neutral and bland. Comparing this portrait with the original portrait by Street, one can see that the copyist has changed the attitude of the head and hands, softened the edges of contours, and reduced a forceful and energetic expression into a limp and lifeless one.

Artist: Unknown

Marble; 16 1/2 x 10 1/4 x 6 1/2; rests on base 2 1/2 in. high; not signed or dated. Presented by his son, Dr. Joseph Parrish, in 1887. *ST 543*

The subject is shown bust length, with body and head frontal. He has a high forehead with horizontal wrinkles and flat hair with stylized strands combed forward. Under soft brows his deepset eyes, with irises and pupils incised, look straight ahead. The nose has a bump at the bridge and a long tip which points down toward the wide mouth. The jaw is broad, the chin rounded. Below the neck the torso is described only rudimentarily. The surface of the marble is very smooth. The head is moderately well rendered in terms of the underlying anatomy. The facial expression is neutral and bland. The concept of the bust is neoclassical. Although the features have been somewhat regularized and idealized, there is a fleeting resemblance to the subject's likeness, as noted in the painting and etching mentioned above, especially in the hair and nose.

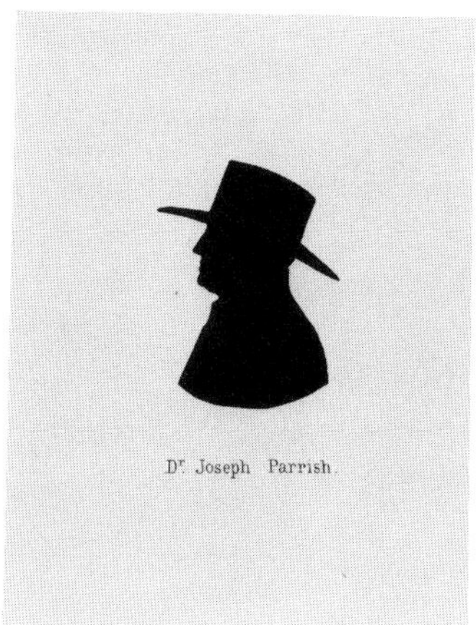

Joseph Parrish *PH 100*

Artist: Unknown

Silhouette, black ink on buff paper; 11 x 8 1/2; not signed or dated. Neither donor nor date of donation is recorded; but it is included in the College of Physicians Inventory of 1898–1915. Closely resembles a full-length silhouette of Joseph Parrish with hat, illustrated in The Parrish Family, *by Susanna Parrish Wharton (Philadelphia, 1925), the artist being unidentified. This silhouette could be a detail, copied from the original; the identification below the figure is not an autograph by Joseph Parrish.* *PH 100*

Parrish is shown bust length, with profile to the left. His features are more regular than those shown in other likenesses. The broad-brimmed "Friends" hat is the most distinguishing characteristic of this work.

Oliver Hazard Perry Pepper (1884–1962)

Born in Philadelphia, Dr. Pepper was a descendant of a family well known for its distinguished intellectuals, including many physicians. His grandfather, Dr. William Pepper, Sr., was professor of medicine at the University of Pennsylvania. His father, Dr. William Pepper, Jr., was professor of medicine and provost at the University. His brother, William Pepper III, was professor of medicine and dean at the University. Dr. O.H. Perry Pepper received the B.S. degree in 1905 and the M.D. degree in 1908 from the University. After completing his residency at University Hospital, he worked in the laboratory and wrote many articles describing his research in hematology. During World War I he was a lieutenant-colonel and chief of medical services of Base Hospitals 34 and 69 in Nantes and Savenay, France. After his return to Philadelphia he established a medical practice and turned to teaching. He instituted a series of "correlation clinics" in which first-year medical students could observe patients and correlate practical diagnosis and treatment with knowledge of the preclinical sciences. He became an associate professor of clinical medicine in 1928 and full professor in 1934. He succeeded his brother-in-law, Dr. Alfred Stengel (q.v.), as departmental chairman in 1937, a post which he held until his resignation in 1945. He was also chief of the medical clinics at the University Hospital. Pepper had a distinguished military record in the Second World War. He was drafted by the National Research Council in Washington and made chairman of its committee on medicine, which advised the surgeons general of the army and navy. He was chosen chairman of an advisory council of the National Academy of Sciences that was created to advise the war department about biological warfare. He was also chairman of the army's epidemiological board, which advised the surgeon general of the army about epidemic diseases. After the war he was chosen by the Veterans Administration to be chairman of the committee on veterans' medical problems. He served as president of the College of Physicians (1943–46), the Philadelphia Pathological Association, and the American College of Physicians. He also served on the boards or councils of the Association of American Physicians, the American Climatological and Clinical Association, the National Board of Medical Examiners, and the American Board of Internal Medicine. He wrote numerous articles and sections in textbooks and with David L. Farley was co-author of *Practical Hematologic Diagnosis.*

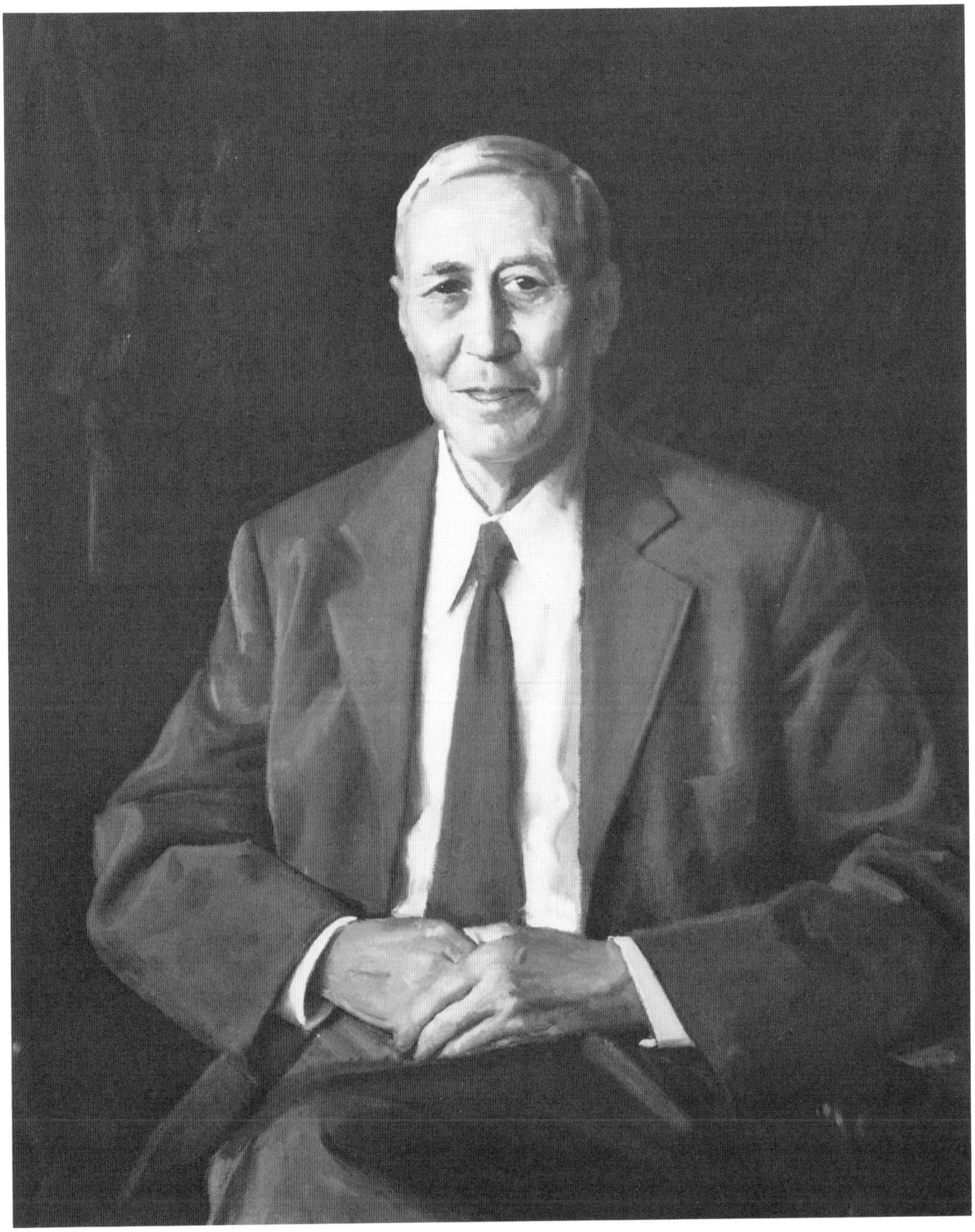

Oliver Hazard Perry Pepper *PA 124*

Artist: Sean O'Sullivan

O'Sullivan, an Irish portrait painter, worked in Philadelphia in the fall and winter of 1955, when an exhibition of his portraits was held at the Philadelphia Art Alliance. According to a contemporary article on the social page of the *Evening Bulletin*, he is best known for portraits of eminent persons such as Eamon De Valera, American-born former president of Ireland; Monsignor P. Browne, President of Galway University; James Joyce; and William Howard Taft III, ambassador to Dublin. He is a member of the Royal Hibernian Academy.

Oil on canvas; 35 1/4 x 29; signed and dated at lower right, "Sean O'Sullivan Philadelphia/1955." Presented by Dr. O.H. Perry Pepper in 1955. *PA 124*

Dr. Pepper is shown two-thirds length, his body and head being almost totally frontal. He is seated in an upholstered armchair which is turned at an angle of 45 degrees to the picture plane. His legs are crossed at the knees, his forearms rest on the chair arms, and his clasped hands rest on his lap. The black background has drapery folds at the upper right and a green tassel and stripes of an academic robe and hat in the upper left. The subject has smooth gray hair, narrow and hooded brown eyes which look straight ahead at the viewer, a wide-based nose, high cheek bones, dimples, and a wide mouth with the lips parted in a full smile. He wears a white shirt, a reddish-brown necktie, and a tan-brown, single-breasted suit. The surface of the portrait is loosely brushed with visible strokes. Although the strokes are very free and fluid, the head is described in solid three-dimensional volumes, and there is a suggestion of the big-framed body under the costume. The pose and background are conventional, but the subject's smiling and benign facial expression and his unbuttoned coat contribute informality. This is emphasized by the close-up view. The direct and energetic force of his presence radiates a kind of welcome to the viewer; this accords with biographers' descriptions of his ready wit and charm.

George Edward Pfahler (1874–1957)

Dr. Pfahler was born in Numidia, Pennsylvania. His family traced its lineage to German royalty. He was educated at an ungraded country school and worked as a school teacher in 1892. He was graduated from the Bloomsburg State Normal School in 1894 and from the Medico-Chirurgical College, Philadelphia, in 1898. After a fifteen-month internship at Philadelphia General Hospital, he served as chief resident physician (1899–1902) and also became the first director of the department of radiology (1899–1903). At the Medico-Chirurgical Hospital he was made director of the department of radiology from 1902 until 1918. He became clinical professor of radiology in 1909 and was the first full professor of radiology from 1911 until 1916, when the institution merged with the University of Pennsylvania. At the University he was appointed professor of radiology and vice-dean of the department of radiology in the Graduate School of Medicine, a post he held for thirty years. He was also director of the radiological departments of the Graduate Hospital (1916–32) and the Misericordia Hospital (1916–43), and he was consulting radiologist to the Philadelphia General Hospital, Hahnemann Hospital, and Woman's Medical College. He was an inspiring teacher and administrator and the author of more than 330 contributions to the medical literature. He was president of the American Roentgen Ray Society, the American Electro-Therapeutic Association, the American Radium Society, the American College of Radiology, the Medical Club of Philadelphia, and the Dermatological Society of Philadelphia. He was president of the Aid Association and chairman of the committee on cancer control of the Philadelphia County Medical Society. He was chairman of the executive committee and a member of board of the directors of the Philadelphia chapter of the American Cancer Society. He served as member of the executive committee or as vice-president of six international congresses of radiology between 1925 and 1956. He was a member of the College of Physicians. His stature was international, as shown by his honorary memberships in radiological societies in France, Germany, England, Russia, Scandinavia, Austria, Cuba, Mexico, Panama, and Peru. He won many medals and other honors, including the Strittmatter gold medal of the Philadelphia County Medical Society, the gold medal of the American Radium Society, the gold medal of the Radiological Society of North America, the gold medal of the American Roentgen Ray Society, the first medal of the Centre Antoine Béclère of Paris, and awards of merit from the American Cancer Society, the Medico-Chirurgical College Alumni Association, the American Medical Association Foundation, and the American Society of X-ray Technicians. Two important early textbooks in radiology, *Lehrbuch der Röntgen Diagnostik* and *Radiodiagnostico En La Infancia*, were dedicated to world leaders in radiology, including Pfahler. A building at Ursinus College was named the Pfahler Hall of Science. It is said that he had singleness of purpose and devotion to his specialty. He died of leukemia, probably caused by many years of exposure to radiation. He bequeathed almost his entire estate to endow scholarships for deserving medical students, the funds to be administered through the Philadelphia County Medical Society.

Artist: Robert Susan (1888–1957)

Robert Susan studied art at the Pennsylvania Museum School of Art, the Graphic Sketch Club, and the Pennsylvania Academy of the Fine Arts, where he won two Cresson traveling scholarships. He studied in France and Spain from 1911 to 1913. He was a frequent exhibitor at Pennsylvania Academy annual exhibitions. He won the fellowship prize in 1923 and the popular award in 1932. He was the first president of the Graphic Sketch Club when it incorporated, and he belonged to the Philadelphia Art Alliance, the Pen and Pencil Club, and the California Art Club. He was a fashionable portrait painter who included among his patrons Cardinal Dougherty, Governor Gifford Pinchot, William Draper Lewis, Dean of the University of Pennsylvania Law School, and many judges, corporate leaders, and members of society. His work hangs at the Philadelphia City Hall, the Capitol at Harrisburg, and in the United States Supreme Court in Washington. He was the father of the novelist, Jacqueline Susann.

Oil on canvas; 41 1/4 x 34 1/4; signed and dated in upper right, "Robert Susan/1942 [the last two digits are unclear]." The portrait hung in Dr. Pfahler's home. His will stipulated that Mrs. Pfahler should present it to the Philadelphia Roentgen Ray Society and that it should be hung in their meeting hall, located at the College of Physicians. It was presented to the College in 1978 on the occasion of the sixth annual Pfahler Oration, co-sponsored by the Philadelphia Roentgen Ray Society and the Philadelphia County Medical Society. *PA 142*

Dr. Pfahler is shown two-thirds length, his body turned slightly to the left, his head very slightly to the left. He is seated in a red upholstered armchair, with his left forearm resting on the volute end of the chair arm and his right arm resting on a table. Both hands hang loosely from the wrists, and a little material of his academic gown is held between his fingers. The interior setting has a

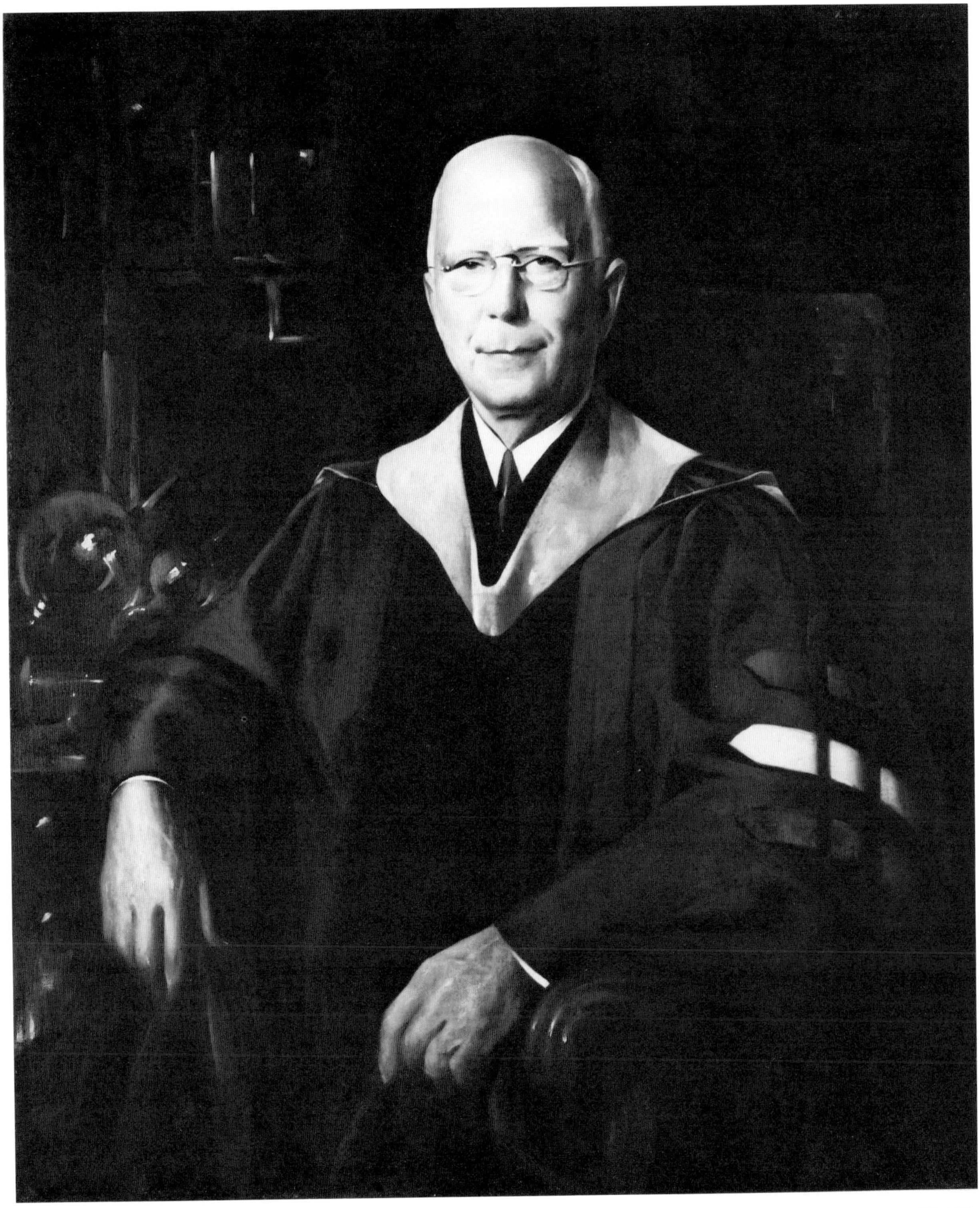

George Edward Pfahler *PA 142*

dark, brownish-black background; cylindrical X-ray tubes are seen in the upper left corner and there is a radiological apparatus on the table. The subject has a high forehead; smooth, silver-white hair and eyebrows; and narrow, dark blue eyes which look straight ahead through rimless glasses. The broad span between his slender aquiline nose and wide mouth is accentuated by the lines in his cheeks. His complexion is high-keyed, with the cheeks, lips, and square chin colored emphatically pink. He wears a dazzling white shirt, a brilliant blue necktie, a black suit, a black academic robe with vivid purple, yellow, and green stripes on the sleeves, and a yellow hood with red lining. The surface of the portrait is very smoothly painted; the head and hands are solid and three-dimensional, though the robe is too voluminous to indicate the underlying body. The subject's facial expression is fixed in a pleasant smile. The meticulously smooth paint style, especially in the head, hands, and laboratory apparatus, lends the portrait an almost surreal quality. This style, in addition to the close-up view, the use of brilliant color, and the presence in the background of spectral objects that appear to float, creates a dramatic presentation.

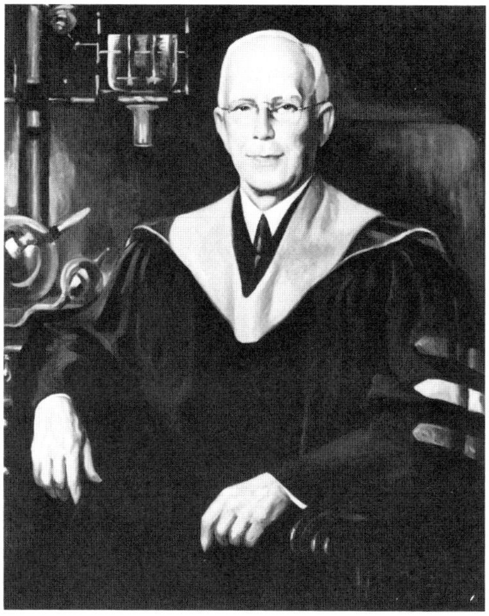

George Edward Pfahler PA 138

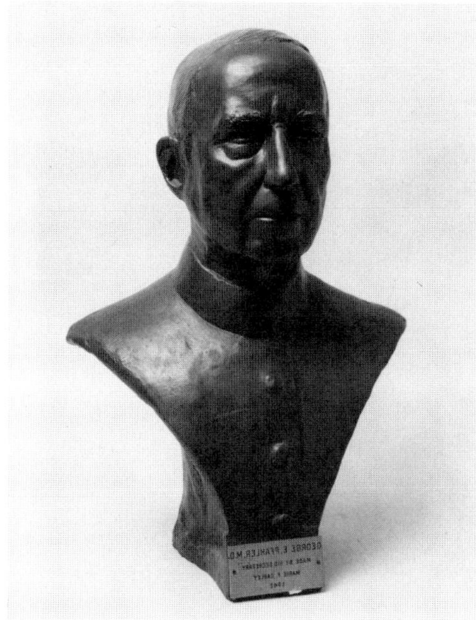

George Edward Pfahler ST 561

Artist: Martha Fleck Brown

Oil on canvas; 35 1/2 x 29 1/2; signed at lower right, "Martha Fleck Brown/after/Robert Susan." Donor, Mrs. George E. Pfahler, in 1977. This portrait hung in the Pfahler Sanctum at Philadelphia General Hospital and was presented to the College of Physicians with the rest of the contents of the room when the hospital was closed. PA 138

In this reduced portrait the copyist has included all the details of the original by Robert Susan (see above). However, an all-over painterly style, together with a less advanced command of anatomy, the garish color, and differing emphasis of various objects, creates a portrait whose total effect is quite different from that of the original. This artist, forsaking the atmospheric spatial depth, has moved all the elements of the painting to the same plane. As a result the figure, chair, X-ray apparatus, and table all compete for the viewer's attention. This copy lacks the subtlety of the original.

Artist: Marie F. Carley

Plaster, painted brown; 20 1/2 x 14 1/4 x 9 1/8; base, 2 1/2 in. high; not signed or dated, but a brass plaque attached to front of base states, "George E. Pfahler, M.D./made by his secretary/Marie F. Carley/ 1942." Presented by the estate of Dr. George E. Pfahler in 1957. The original bronze sculpture was bequeathed to the Philadelphia County Medical Society. ST 561

Dr. Pfahler is shown bust length, with body and head frontal. He has smooth hair. The narrow eyes, with deeply carved irises and pupils, look straight ahead. The lower lids are puffy and there are deep lines next to the nose. The mouth is wide with thin lips. The subject wears a military coat with standup collar and three large buttons. The anatomy of the head has been portrayed superficially and the stern expression is stiff, even wooden. Nevertheless, the image bears a striking resemblance to the painted portraits described above and to contemporary photographs.

Philip Syng Physick (1768-1837)

Born in Philadelphia, Dr. Physick was the grandson of the famous silversmith, Philip Syng, and the son of the receiver-general of the Province of Pennsylvania, who after the Revolution was agent for the Penn estates. He received the A.B. degree in 1785 and the A.M. degree in 1788 from the University of Pennsylvania. After studying medicine under Adam Kuhn (q.v.), he went abroad in 1788 with his father, who wished to give him every opportunity to continue his medical education. In London he lived with John Hunter (q.v.), who arranged for him the post of house-surgeon at St. George's Hospital. He was awarded membership in the Royal College of Surgeons and was so outstanding that Hunter offered him a partnership. For unknown reasons he refused this honor in favor of going to Edinburgh, where he received the M.D. degree in 1792. After his return to Philadelphia he slowly established a practice. Special opportunities arose during the yellow fever epidemic of 1793, when he made careful notes and performed autopsies in order to investigate the causes and treatment of the disease. This work brought him to the notice of Benjamin Rush (q.v.), who began to refer his surgical patients to Physick. Through his post-mortem examinations Physick became convinced that yellow fever was not contagious and that its causes were local. This work, in addition to the service he rendered at the Bush Hill yellow fever hospital, and his appointment in 1794 as surgeon to the Pennsylvania Hospital and to the Almshouse Infirmary in 1801, brought him into prominence. He is considered to be the originator of pathological anatomy in this country. In 1800, students at the University asked him to deliver a course of lectures on surgery at the Pennsylvania Hospital. His reputation as teacher, surgeon, and pathologist was so great that by 1805,

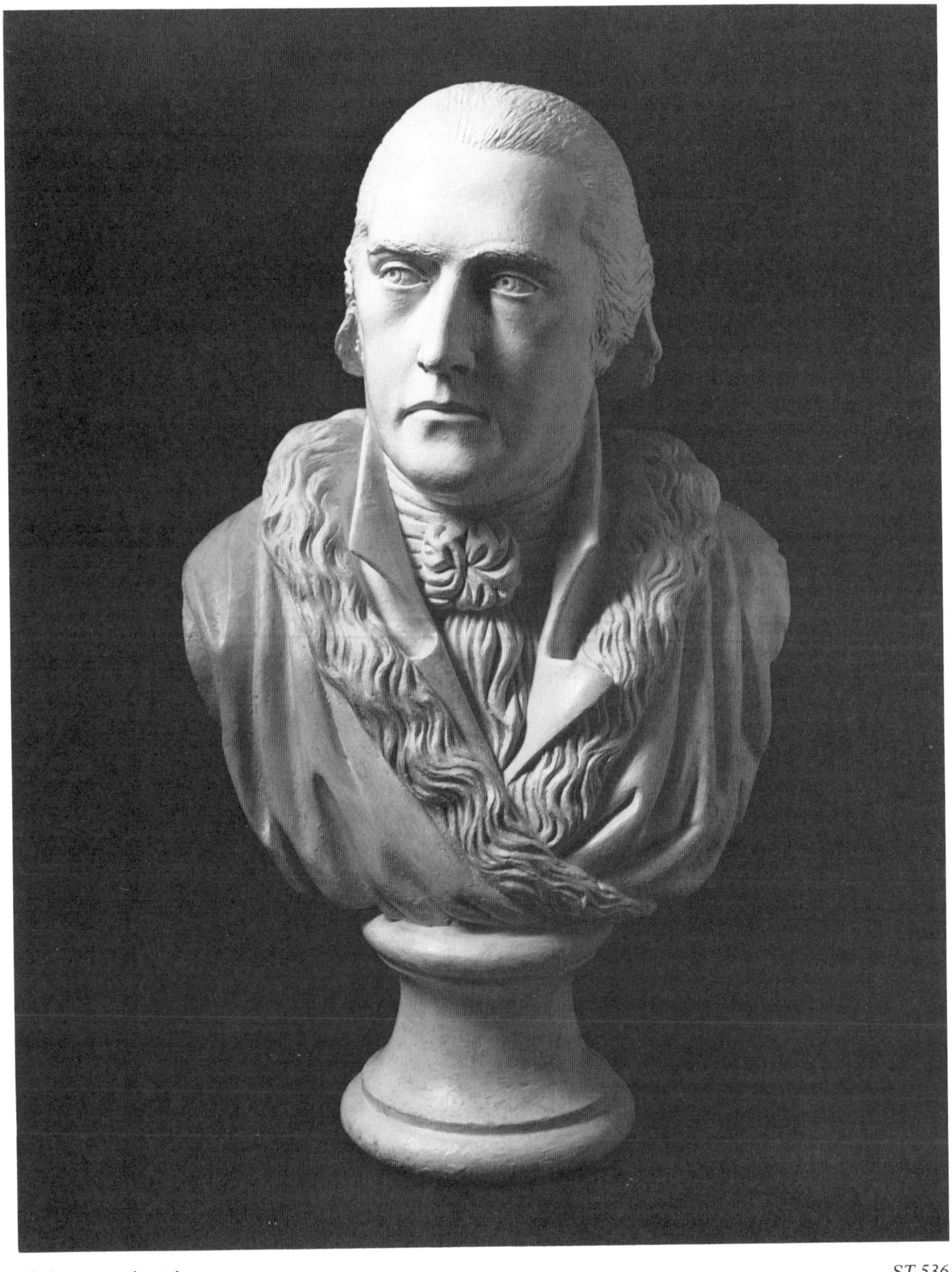

Philip Syng Physick *ST 536*

when the University created its first chair of surgery—previously this subject had been an adjunct of anatomy—Physick was appointed. The next three decades saw him at the peak of his fame. His practice was immense and he was in constant demand as consultant and correspondent. This is all the more remarkable since he himself was allegedly a victim of yellow fever twice, and in addition had had typhus and suffered chronically from dyspepsia, renal calculi, and catarrh. His many contributions to surgical technique include new methods for extracting poisonous substances by means of a stomach pump; new methods for treating ulcers; the use of setons for cases of ununited fracture; the use of splints, rest, and low diets in treatment of diseased hip joints; an operation for artificial anus; and a procedure for enucleation of the cataractous lens. Among his contributions to instrumentation are the double cannula for removal of tonsils and hemorrhoidal swellings, a curved needle for deep-seated arteries, the improvement of Desault's splint for fractures of the thigh, a dental forceps, an appliance for outward displacement of the foot, improved lithotomy instruments, and a catheter and bougie combined in one instrument to improve the procedure of bladder drainage. Physick was one of the first surgeons to use catgut sutures. In 1819 he was transferred to the chair of anatomy at the University, which he filled until 1831, when he was made emeritus professor of anatomy and surgery. He was president of the Philadelphia Medical Society, the Philadelphia Academy of Medicine, and the Philadelphia Phrenological Society. He was a member of the American Philosophical Society and the French Royal Academy of Medicine and honorary fellow of the Royal Medical and Chirurgical Society of London. He never composed any major literary works, but his surgical lectures were published in 1813 by his nephew, John Syng Dorsey, as one of the first American textbooks of surgery. During his lifetime he was called the "Father of American Surgery."

Artist: William Rush (1756–1833)

William Rush, born in Philadelphia, was the son of a ship's carpenter. It is said that as a youth he carved ships out of wood and drew figures in chalk or paint. In his early years he was apprenticed to Edward Cutbush, an English carver who worked in Philadelphia. He also studied modeling with Joseph Wright, the sculptor and painter. Rush served as an ensign in the Philadelphia militia starting in 1777. For more than a decade he worked on merchant vessels and small warships, for which he carved figureheads as well as stern ornaments that represented national heroes, Indians, and allegorical figures; only one of these early figures has survived. By 1794 he had enough stature as an artist to be one of forty artists, including members of the Peale family, who founded the Columbianum, one of America's earliest academies of art; however, it disbanded after one exhibition. Rush was introduced into Philadelphia's scientific and medical community in the early years of the 19th century, when he helped Charles Willson Peale carve missing bones of the famous mastodon that Peale had exhumed in 1801. Under the supervision of Caspar Wistar (q.v.), professor of anatomy, he collaborated with Peale in the construction of large-scale wooden anatomical models. This project started in 1808 and continued until 1820. Rush was elected to both the common and the select councils of Philadelphia. He served on the committee that oversaw the Philadelphia waterworks and he designed a wooden fountain, entitled *Allegory of the Schuylkill River* or *Water Nymph and Bittern,* in 1809 for the front of the Pump House at the original site at Centre Square. His *Allegory of the Schuylkill River in Its Improved State* and *Allegory of the Waterworks* in 1825 were used for the entrances of the second location of the Pump House at Fairmount. He served on the committee that supervised the festivities for Lafayette's triumphal visit to Philadelphia in 1824. He was a founder of the Pennsylvania Academy of the Fine Arts in 1805, and he served on its building committee and its committee on instruction; he was one of only two artist-members on the board of directors. He was made an academician in 1812. He was also a founder, first president, and professor of sculpture at the Society of Artists, organized in 1810 independently of the Academy. He resigned in 1812 from the Society because of differences between the two organizations. He was also a founder of the Franklin Institute (1824). At the end of the first decade of the 19th century, the shipbuilding industry declined and Rush turned to architectural statues and portraiture. His first architectural statues were *Comedy* and *Tragedy,* carved in 1808 for the façade of the Chestnut Street Theater. Other works were allegorical figures carved in 1820–21 for the Masonic Hall in Philadelphia. Most of these statues were painted white to imitate marble. Rush showed his awareness of ancient sculpture in his antique-style draperies, his depiction of hair, and his use of columns. He exhibited portrait busts at the Pennsylvania Academy frequently between 1811 and 1833. In this period of chauvinistic patriotism, it was fashionable for middle-class homes to display busts of contemporary heroes. It was Rush's usual practice to model from life a terra-cotta original, which he then exhibited in the hope of obtaining subscriptions for replicas made in plaster. In a letter of May 22, 1815 (New-York Historical Society), he told Benjamin West to expect the plaster cast of a clay model of Benjamin Rush, and that in a few days after the execution of the original terra-cotta "fifteen hundred dollars was subscribed principally for him, some for Dr. Physick at $10 per cast. . . ." The existence of this letter and much of the preceding biographical material has been derived from an essay by Linda Bantel in the *William Rush, American Sculptor* exhibition catalogue, Pennsylvania Academy of the Fine Arts, 1982. Among his most famous portrait busts in wood, plaster, and terra-cotta (in addition to those of Rush and Philip Syng Physick) are those of Dr. Caspar Wistar (q.v.), Samuel Morris, Benjamin Franklin, Carolus Linnaeus, George Washington, the Marquis de Lafayette, a self-portrait, and now-missing busts of Andrew Jackson, Thomas Jefferson, James Madison, Commodore Perry, and General Winfield Scott. His most ambitious portrait was a full-length wooden statue of George Washington (1815, Independence National Historical Park), which failed to bring him the expected subscriptions for plaster casts. Although Rush was awarded honorary membership in New York's American Academy of Fine Arts (1825), his reputation as America's first worthy sculptor has had mercurial ups and downs from his own day to the present. The exhibition of 1982 at the Pennsylvania Academy was the first retrospective since the exhibition of 1937 at the Pennsylvania Museum of Art.

Plaster, painted white; 19 1/4 x 15 x 11 7/8; round base integral with sculpture 5 1/2 in. high; not signed or dated, but probably made shortly after the original terra-cotta from which it was cast (1812–13; Pennsylvania Academy of the Fine Arts). Neither donor or date of donation is recorded; no documentation could be found in the files of the College of Physicians, and the portrait bust is first mentioned in an article on College treasures in the 1937 Transactions and Studies of the College of Physicians of Philadelphia. *Other plaster replicas are at the American Philosophical Society, the Library Company of Philadelphia, and the collection of Dr. Robert Erwin Jones. Shown at the* William Rush American Sculptor *exhibition, Pennsylvania Academy of the Fine Arts, 1982. As with the College of Physicians' plaster casts of Benjamin Rush and Caspar Wistar, this plaster cast of Philip Syng Physick was taken by means of piece molds from a terra-cotta original freely modeled from life. The original version was hollowed out and rested on clay supports at the back. The busts of all*

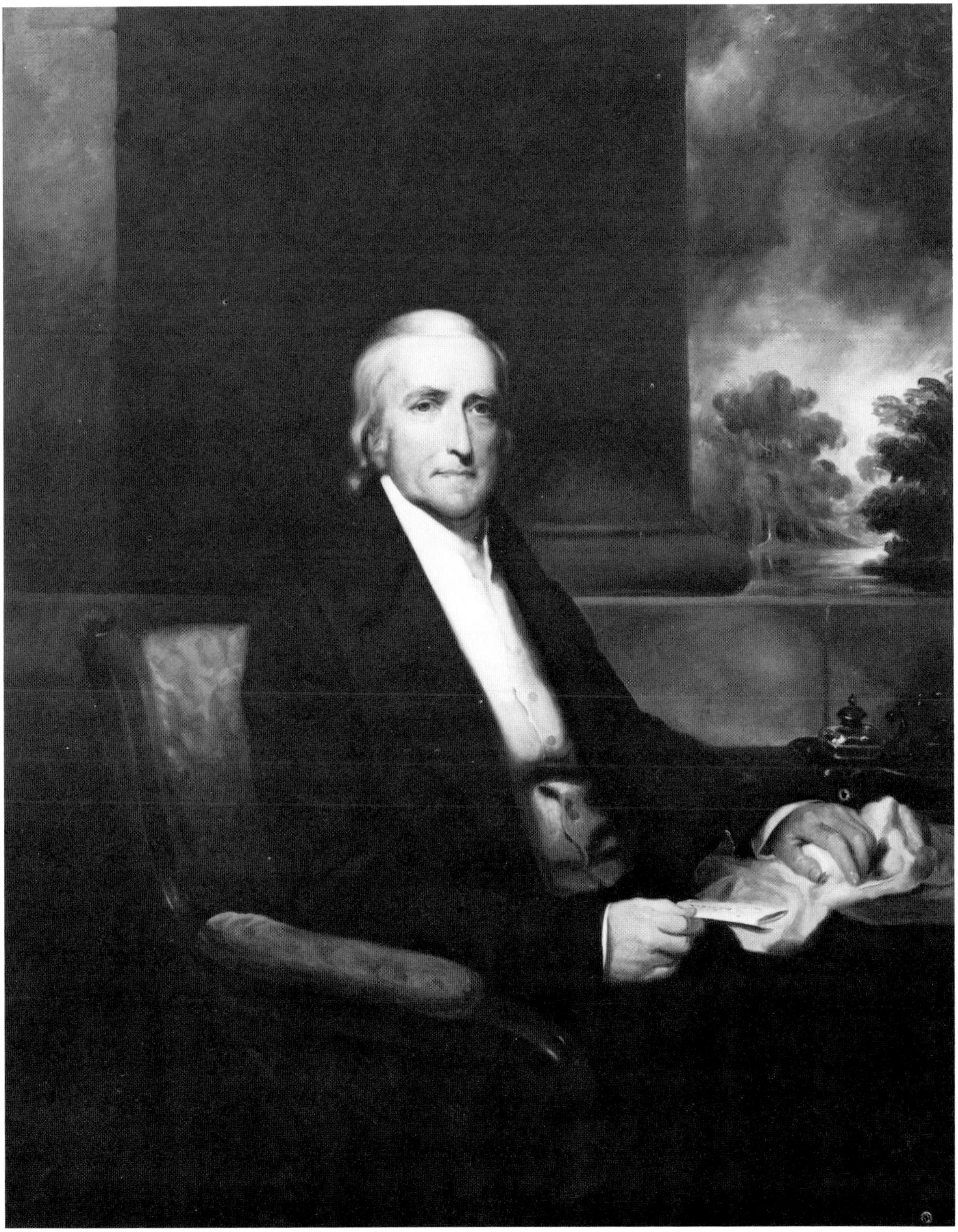

Philip Syng Physick *PA 113*

three physicians were fired without their protruding collar points, for ease in making the casts in piece molds. After casting, the replicas received individual attention in defining details and in attaching collar points or jabots. Since the casts were hollow, each had to be attached to a base so that it could stand. All the casts were painted at some period with multiple layers of white or black paint, "but whether the intention of using paint to imitate a bronze or marble bust originated in Rush's studio we cannot yet say." This quotation and the above technical description of casting come from the essay by Virginia Naudé, "Toolmarks and Fingerprints: A technical discussion," in the catalogue of the exhibition, William Rush American Sculptor, *Pennsylvania Academy of the Fine Arts, 1982. According to a conservation report by Virginia Naudé (1982), at some time this plaster bust of Physick had been covered with gesso and then layers of bronze, cream, and white paints that obscured the sculptural detail. Because of disfiguring discoloration on the plaster and the remaining bits of gesso, the bust was later painted with white reversible paint after the aforementioned layers were removed in a conservation procedure before the 1982 Academy show.* *ST 536*

Dr. Physick is shown bust length, with body frontal and head turned slightly to the left. His smooth, finely striated hair is brushed away from his face, formed into a queue in the back, and tied in a round bow. His rectangular face has wavy eyebrows that overhang deepset eyes with sharply defined lids. The eyes, which look to the left and upward, are carved in Rush's characteristic style, with incised irises and depressed pupils. The aquiline nose has a sharp tip. The lips of the wide mouth turn down. The jaw is wide and the chin is pointed. The somewhat fanciful costume consists of a wide stock or neckcloth fastened by a round-topped jabot with curving ends. The next layer is a waistcoat or coat with sharply angled and turned collar and lapel points. The uppermost layer of coat or overcoat has a fur-trimmed shawl collar with deep curving folds. The surface of the sculpture has the uneven texture characteristic of plaster. The naturalistic head is moderately well-rendered in its anatomical planes; the costume does not reveal the underlying body volumes. The subject's facial expression is dignified and austere, in contrast to the animated and decorative effect of the costume. As in most translations from terra-cotta original to plaster cast, some of the verve of facial expression and the crisp details of the carving are lost.

Artist: Robert F. Reynolds (b. ca. 1818)

Little is known about Reynolds except that he was a portrait painter and lithographer; he was active in Philadelphia in the 1840s and 1850s.

Oil on canvas; 49 3/4 x 39 3/4; signed and dated at lower right, "R.F. Reynolds 1840[?; the last two digits are not clear]. Presented in 1946 by Mrs. Frances R. Brooks, who inherited the painting from Dr. Emlen Physick, Jr. It is a copy of the portrait of Physick by Henry Inman (1801-1846), who painted it for the graduating class of 1836 at the University of Pennsylvania. Reynolds's copy was shown at the Artists' Fund Society's sixth annual exhibition, held at the Pennsylvania Academy of the Fine Arts in 1841, the owner being listed as Emlen Physick (son of Dr. Physick). It resembles a copy after Inman at the Pennsylvania Hospital. *PA 113*

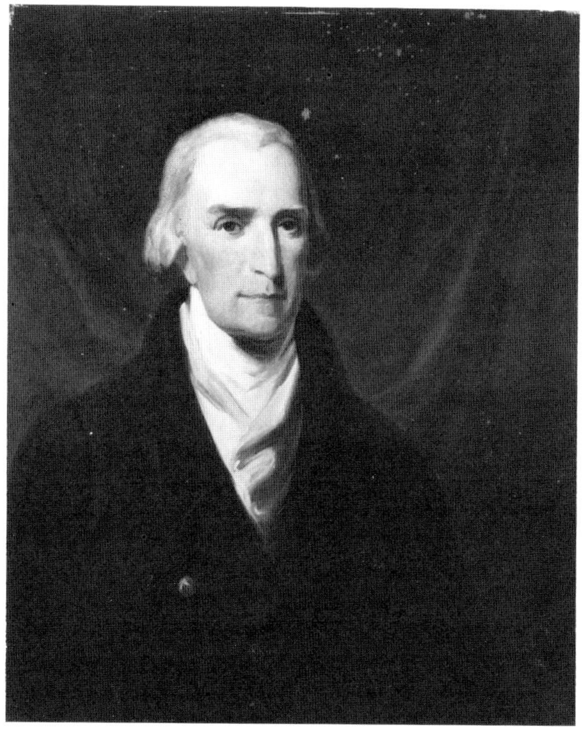

Philip Syng Physick *PA 94*

Physick is shown three-quarters length, with body turned three quarters to the right and head slightly to the right. He is seated in a square-backed, red upholstered armchair with volute hand holds and caned sides. His legs are crossed at the knees. His left hand crumples a piece of white material on top of a writing table. His right hand, which rests on his thigh, holds a pamphlet. The subject has smooth, long, silver hair brushed back from his forehead. His brown eyes look out toward the viewer. His long, aquiline nose has a tip which points down toward a wide mouth with thin lips. He has a prominent jaw, a pointed chin, and age lines beneath his eyes and on his cheeks. He wears a white stock and waistcoat with a high collar, and a black coat with high collar, M-notched wide lapels, and tight sleeves. He is wearing black breeches. Except for the loosely brushed landscape, the portrait is very smoothly painted. The head and hands are rendered in solid and three-dimensional forms, while the folds and wrinkles of the costume help to suggest the underlying forms of body. The elaborate setting suggests an outdoor terrace or porch. Behind the figure is a buff-colored stone parapet which divides the composition horizontally. This supports a buff column which rises to the upper border of the painting. At the left of the column there is an unexplained dark, rectangular, vertical shape; the section to its left suggests foliage. To the right is a view into the distance, with heavy clouds and green trees reflected in the water below. The rectangular writing table is covered with green cloth; on it are a silver inkstand and writing implements. Although the setting is illogical in terms of spatial depth, its various elements—elegant furniture, column, silver inkstand, pamphlet, and landscape background—suggest Dr. Physick's social status, erudition, and wisdom. He looks up from his writing and turns his head to regard the viewer with a dignified and sober facial expression. His posture is erect and energetic. The copyist has been faithful to the original.

Artist: Albert Rosenthal (1863–1939)

For biography, see page 54.

Oil on canvas; 29 1/4 x 24 1/4; not signed or dated on front of canvas. Inscription on back, "Dr. Philip Syng Physick/ copied by Albert Rosenthal 1916/for Dr. J. Cheston Morris." Presented by Dr. J. Cheston Morris, in 1925. The painting is a copy after the original by Thomas Sully, listed in his own Register of Portraits *as having been painted for Dr. William P. Deweese [sic] in 1809; it was formerly at the U.S. Medical War Museum, Washington, and now owned by the Ehrich Galleries, New York City.* *PA 94*

The subject is shown bust length, with head and body turned slightly to the right. A dark red drapery falls in diagonally curved folds behind the figure and fills the entire background, except for a brown vertical strip at the right. The subject's long gray hair has a pronounced widow's peak and is full over the ears. His brown eyes have heavy upper lids and look out toward the viewer. His rectangular face has a long, aquiline nose whose tip points down toward a wide mouth. He has a pronounced jaw line and pointed chin. His complexion is high-keyed; the cheeks are pink, the lips red. He wears a white stock or neckcloth, a white waistcoat, and a black single-breasted coat with brass buttons. The surface of the portrait is smoothly brushed. The head is moderately well rendered in solid and three-dimensional volumes. The flat costume gives no suggestion of the underlying body volumes. Although this portrait is a recognizable likeness of its subject, the serious facial expression is bland and neutral, without animation and vitality.

Artist: Unknown

Oil on canvas; actual size 26 x 20 1/4; not signed or dated. Inscription on back of canvas in later hand, "Dr. Philip Syng Physick/Born 1768 Died 1837." Presented by Dr. S. Weir Mitchell in 1885. This portrait has been the subject of much debate. It was shown at the College of Physicians' Centennial Celebration Loan Collection of Portraits, *1887, where the subject was listed as Physick, the owner as College of Physicians, and the artist as unknown. It was shown also at the Pennsylvania Academy of the Fine Arts* Loan Collection of Historical Portraits, *1887–88, in which the subject was listed as anonymous, the owner as the College of Physicians, and the artist as "R.E. Pine?" These two exhibitions prompted two letters from Philip Syng Physick Conner, a grandson of Dr. Physick. One was dated Jan. 9, 1888, and addressed to* The Evening Bulletin. *The other, a long letter dated Feb. 1, 1888, and addressed to the Historical Society of Pennsylvania, protests that the subject of this portrait does not resemble Philip Syng Physick or any of his portraits and that Robert Edge Pine died when the subject was only twenty years old. The writer continues: "This is the portrait that was bought at Brentano's in New York by Dr. S. Weir Mitchell on the chance of it being a likeness of Dr. Philip Syng Physick . . . no one knows whose likeness it really is nor anything about it save that it reached New York from Maryland." Subsequent records at the College are not helpful. The inventory of 1898–1915 lists this portrait as a work by Pine and quotes from Philip Syng Physick Conner, "This is not Philip Syng Physick, but probably his nephew Dr. Theodore Physick of Cecil County, Maryland." This identity and precise location go beyond the information offered in Conner's letters. The catalogue of the College Collections of 1940 continues to call this a work by Pine, but says that the subject "has been proved not to be that of Doctor Physick." In the exhibition catalogue,* Robert Edge Pine, British Portrait Painter in America 1784–1788, *National Portrait Gallery, 1979, Robert G. Stewart lists this painting as definitely not by Pine, a judgment based on its stylistic qualities as well as the age conflicts. Among the experts consulted, one suggested Matthew Pratt (1734–1805) as the artist. Another felt that the portrait was not by Pratt, but possibly was the work of another English or English-trained artist. Further research is needed to establish the identities of both artist and subject.* *PA 84*

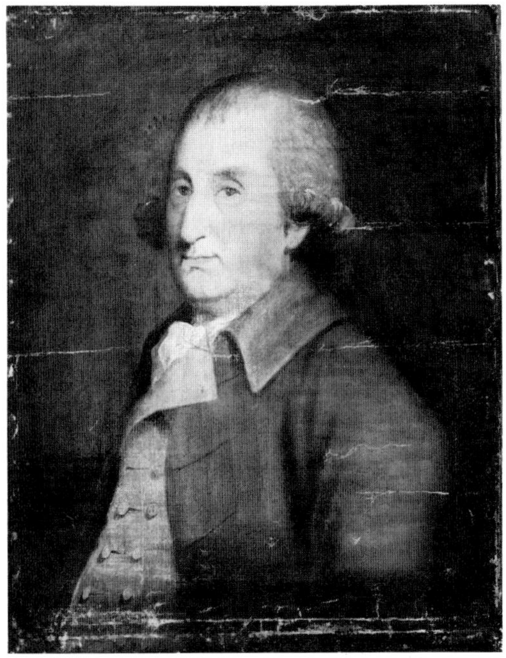

Formerly identified as Philip Syng Physick PA 84

The subject is shown bust length, with body and head turned to the left. The dark brown background is lighter on the left. The subject has gray hair, brushed forward onto his high, sloping forehead and rolled into a single formal curl at the ears. Under straight eyebrows, his narrow, gray eyes with heavy upper lids look out of their corners toward the viewer. His very long, hooked nose has a tip which points down to a small pursed mouth with a thin upper lip and protruding lower lip. His face is wide across the cheeks and narrow at the rounded, double chin. The subject wears a white neckcloth and a yellowish-tan, double-breasted waistcoat in which the lapel and collar fold over the open, bluish-gray coat. Because the painting was painted thinly and has been severely over-cleaned, the damage makes it difficult to judge the surface. Probably it was painted smoothly. The remaining paint indicates that the head was probably rendered in three-dimensional solidity. The costume, too, shows depth and emphasizes the girth of the abdomen. The face is very individualistic; its expression is somewhat aggressive and almost sly. Experts feel that the portrait was probably contemporary with the subject (i.e., 18th century) and probably was painted from life.

Joseph Price (1853-1911)

Born on a plantation in Rockingham County, Virginia, Dr. Price studied at Union College, read medicine with his brother Mordecai, and was graduated from the Medical Department of the University of Pennsylvania in 1877. He worked at the Philadelphia Dispensary, where he became head of the obstetrical division and organized a gynecological department that established what was considered to be the largest and best clinic in the United States for women. In 1887 he was appointed director and resident physician of the Preston Retreat, a philanthropic maternity hospital in Philadelphia. The following year he and Dr. C.B. Penrose founded the Gynecean Hospital. He resigned three years later to found his own hospital in association with Dr. J.W. Kennedy. Later called the Joseph Price Memorial Hospital, it was the largest private institution for abdominal surgery in the United States. Although he frequently contributed short articles to journals, he never wrote a major treatise and never held a professorial position. Yet he had great influence in his field and taught by example; doctors came to his hospital from great distances to observe his methods. He advocated asepsis and careful cleansing of the operative field. He made safe the radical operation for the treatment of pelvic suppurations and hysterectomy for fibroid tumors. He advised immediate operations for ectopic pregnancy and for appendicitis. His only elected office was president of the American Association for Obstetricians and Gynecologists in 1895. He was a fellow of the College of Physicians. A month before his death he received an honorary LL.D. from Union College, New York. His reputation as a brilliant pioneer in gynecological surgery still stands today.

Artist: Charles Grafly (1862-1929)

Grafly was born in Philadelphia, the son of poor Dutch-German parents. In his youth he was an apprentice carver in a stoneyard and helped carve some of the ornamental detail for the new City Hall. He attended evening classes at the Spring Garden Institute in 1882. He enrolled at the Pennsylvania Academy of the Fine Arts in 1884, where he was a pupil of Thomas Eakins in the anatomy and life drawing classes, and he later studied with Thomas Anshutz. He continued his education in Paris from 1888 to 1891 and in 1895, studying with Henri-Michel Chapu at the Académie Julien and later with Jean Dampt. In 1890 he won a student prize and had two sculptures exhibited at the Paris salon. It is not known whether or not he ever succeeded in passing the rigorous entrance examination for the École des Beaux Arts, but his life-size allegorical female nude won an honorable mention in the salon of 1891. In that year he returned to Philadelphia and accepted a teaching post at Drexel Institute, which he held until 1895. In 1892 he joined the faculty of The Pennsylvania Academy and served as instructor in sculpture until his death in 1929. At the Academy he was on the fellowship board of directors for three terms, was a member of the committee on casts, and won the gold medal in 1899, the Widener memorial medal in 1913, and Lea Prize in 1916. He also taught modeling at the Boston Museum School of Fine Arts. Grafly was a frequent exhibitor at national and international expositions and was a consistent winner of prizes, including a medal at the Columbian exposition of 1893 in Chicago, a gold medal for an allegorical work, *Vulture of War,* at the Paris Exhibition of 1900, gold medal at the Charleston Exposition of 1902, grand prize at the Buenos Aires Exposition of 1910, Watrous gold medal of the National Academy of Design in 1918, and the Potter Palmer gold medal of the Chicago Art Institute in 1921. Grafly was commissioned to create monumental, allegorical sculptural groups for the Pan-American Exposition in 1901 in Buffalo (where he won a gold medal), the Louisiana Purchase Exposition of 1904 in St. Louis, and the Panama-Pacific Exposition in San Francisco in 1915. His important public works include three colossal bronze busts of Civil War heroes for the Smith Memorial in Philadelphia, the marble memorial to General George Gordon Meade in Washington, D.C. (dedicated in 1925), and the statue of James Buchanan for Lancaster, Pennsylvania (1927). He also did portrait busts of Admiral Farragut, John Paul Jones, and Jonathan Edwards for the Hall of Fame in New York (1925-28). In addition to creating these public works, Grafly was sought after for more intimate busts of family members, friends, and patrons, including businessmen and professional persons. These works were rendered in a more naturalistic style, with penetrating characterizations. Grafly was elected to the National Academy of Design in 1905 and to the National Institute of Arts and Letters. He was a member of the Municipal Art Jury of Philadelphia and was a charter member of the National Sculpture Society in 1893. In addition to private collections and locales already mentioned, his work can be found at the Pennsylvania Academy and at major museums in Boston, Detroit, St. Louis, Pittsburgh, Cincinnati, and Baltimore. In 1930 a memorial exhibition was held at the Pennsylvania Academy. In 1971 the sculptor's daughter, the noted art critic Dorothy Grafly, donated a collection of 213 plaster casts of her father's work to the Ulrich Museum of Art at Wichita State University in Kansas. In 1981 this museum acquired the Charles Grafly papers.

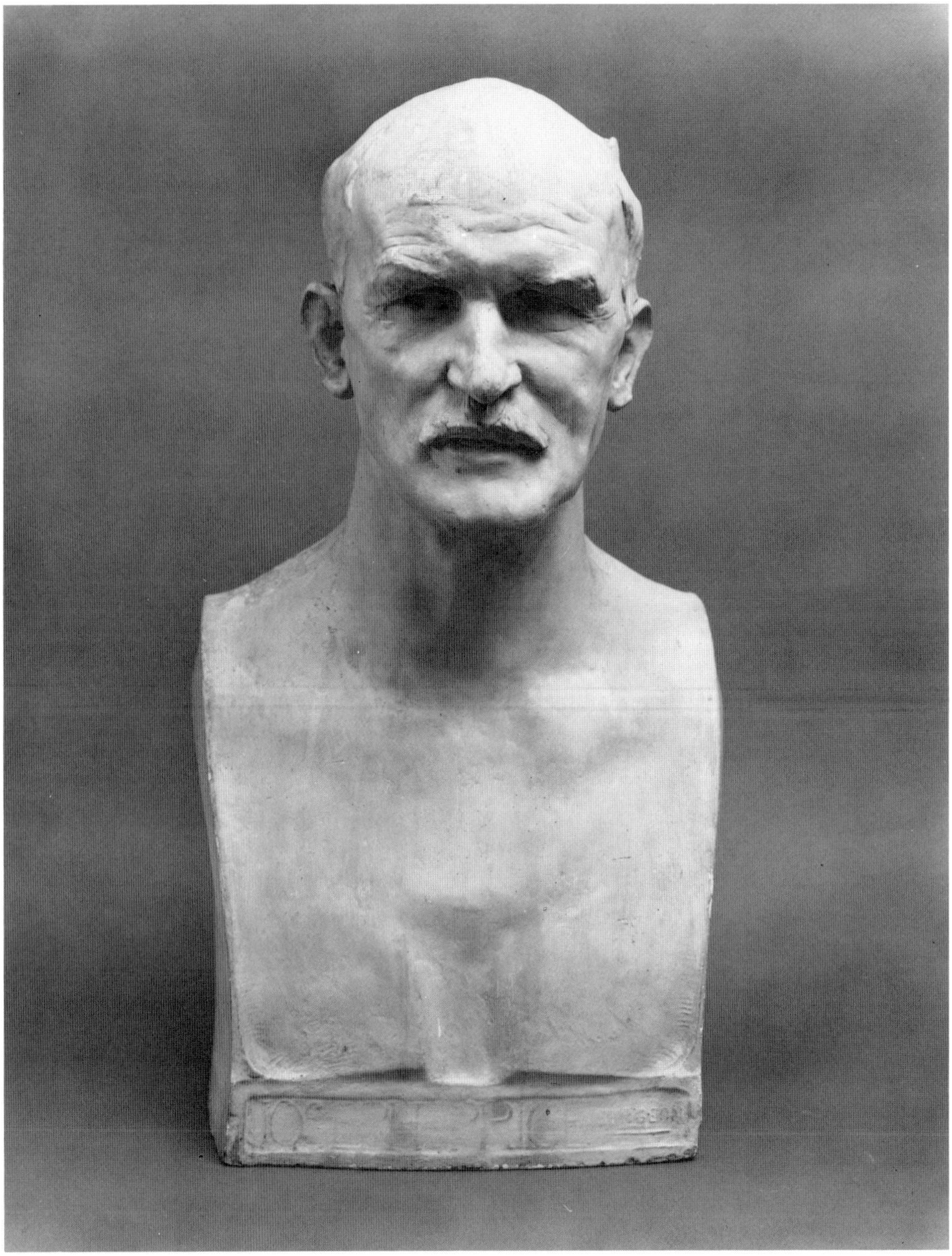

Joseph Price — *ST 578*

Plaster, painted buff; 24 5/8 x 13 1/4 x 11; rectangular base integral and flush with bust, 2 in. high; signed and dated on back below shoulder, "Charles Grafly/Jan. 1906." Inscription on front of base: "Joseph Price Surgeon." Purchased in 1981 by the College of Physicians through Samuel T. Freeman & Co. Auctioneers, 1981, from the consignor, Roy Pederson of Berrus Galleries, Lambertville, New Jersey, which had acquired it from the estate of Frederick Newlin Price. Dr. Price was Mrs. Grafly's physician and this created the contact between artist and subject. The original bronze was presented to the Pennsylvania Academy of the Fine Arts in 1914 by Mrs. Price. Another plaster cast is at the Ulrich Museum of Art, Wichita State University, Kansas.
ST 578

Price is shown with body and head frontal. The area below the sternum is not described anatomically but acts as a base, in the style of antique busts. The subject's head is almost totally bald, except for a flat fringe of hair above his ears. His forehead is wide and lined with deep furrows. Under thick, shaggy eyebrows, his deepset eyes, with irises and pupils carved, look out of their corners to the left. There are wrinkles in the corners. His long, aquiline nose has a tip that points down to a thick brush moustache which partially hides his wide upper lips. He has high cheekbones and a square jaw. The tendons in his thick neck protrude. The plaster bust has the characteristic uneven surface of that medium. The naturalistic portrayal is rendered with skillful understanding of the anatomy. Dr. Price looks strong and energetic. His lips are parted as if to speak, and he looks to the side as if he has just noticed someone. The sculptor has successfully suggested the aggressive personality and strength of the subject, who is said to have been dogmatic and undiplomatic in professional relations and physically powerful enough to engage in boxing.

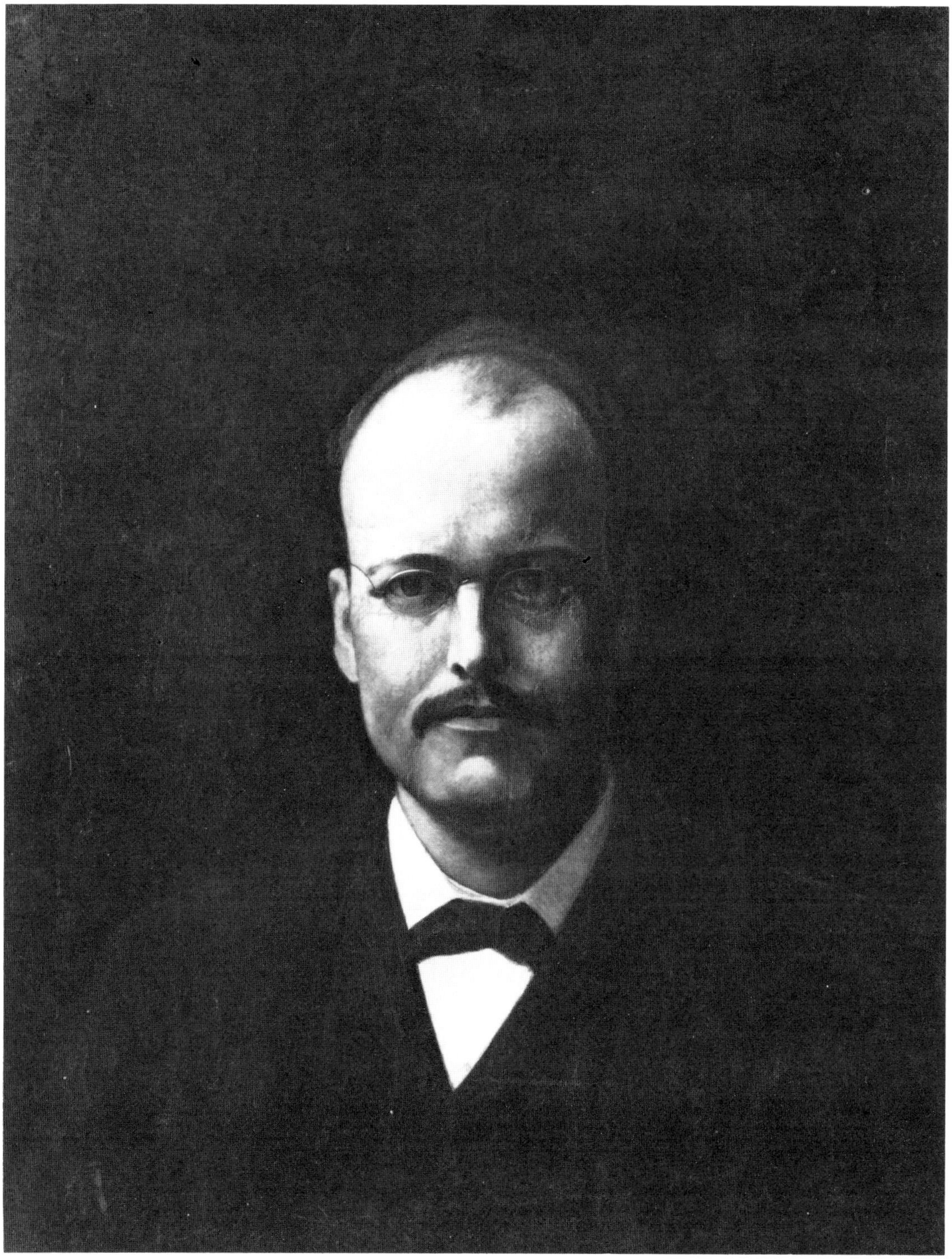

Nathaniel Archer Randolph *PA 69*

Nathaniel Archer Randolph (1858–1888)

Dr. Randolph was born in Philadelphia and studied at Swarthmore College and Cornell University before receiving the M.D. degree from the University of Pennsylvania in 1882. At the University he held the following appointments: assistant demonstrator of physiology in the medical department (1882); instructor in physiology in the Towne Scientific School (1883); instructor in biology in the department of biology (1884); and professor of hygiene in the auxiliary department of medicine (1886). He was a fellow of the College of Physicians and a member of the American Philosophical Society, The Academy of Natural Sciences, and many other societies. From 1885 to 1887 he was assistant editor of *Medical News.* In 1887 he became chief editor of *Medical and Surgical Reporter.* During his short but promising career he published fifteen articles on his research in the physiology and hygiene of digestion. His death was due to drowning in the ocean at Longport, New Jersey.

Artist: Attributed to James Longacre Wood (1867–1938)

For biography, see page 96.

Oil on canvas; 26 1/2 x 21 1/2; not signed or dated. Presented by Dr. Horatio C Wood in 1889. The portrait is included in the College of Physicians inventory of 1898–1915, which lists the artist as "Wood." Subsequent inventories list the artist as James L. Wood, but no convincing documentation has been discovered as yet. James L. Wood usually signed his paintings, but this portrait is in bad condition with varnish bloom and much paint loss. It differs in brush style and conception of pose from the portraits of Drs. Keen (q.v.), Leidy (q.v.), and F.A. Packard (q.v.), yet it has fundamental similarities with the portrait of the artist's father, Dr. Horatio C Wood (q.v.), with its close-up view of the head, dramatic contrast of light and dark, flat costume, and sensitive facial expression. *PA 69*

Randolph is shown bust length, with head and body frontal. The dark, mottled background is black over deep purple. The oval face has a high forehead, with sparse brown hair on the top and sides of the head. The brown eyes look straight ahead through wire-rimmed spectacles. The nose is straight; there is a dark brown curved moustache over the full lips. The jaw line is pronounced. The subject wears a white shirt, a black bow tie, and a black vest and coat. Probably the surface of the portrait was brushed smoothly. The planes of the head, subtly modeled, form a solid three-dimensional structure. The head is illuminated from the left, and there is a dramatic contrast of light and shadow on the face. The costume is totally flat and reveals nothing of the body. The close-up frontal view, the penetrating gaze, and the unusual placement of the figure at the lower portion of the canvas create a striking portrait. Most important is the sensitive and meditative facial expression confronting the viewer, who is tempted to return that relentless scrutiny. The face is unlined, but the subject's age appears greater than the age he is known to have attained.

John Redman (1722-1808)

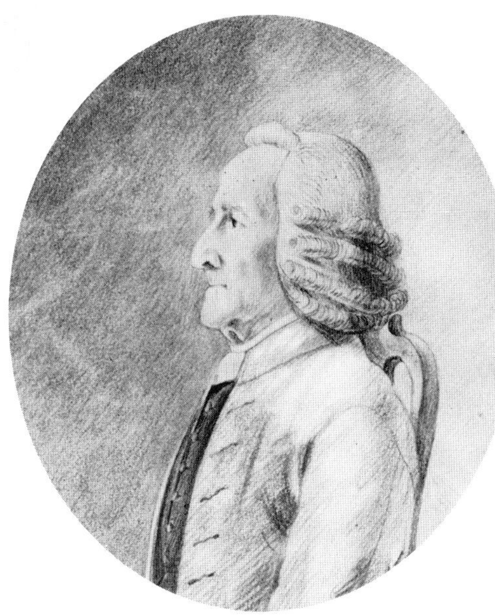

John Redman *PH 273*

Born in Philadelphia, Dr. Redman studied medicine under Dr. John Kearsley. For several years he practiced medicine in Bermuda, and from there he went to Great Britain and Europe. He attended lectures of Alexander Monro, Charles Alston, and John Rutherford at Edinburgh University in 1746–47 and received an M.D. degree in 1748 from the University of Leyden after studying with Bernhard Siegfried Albinus and Hieronymous David Gaubius, the successor to the great Boerhaave. For practical experience he visited hospitals in Paris and walked the wards at Guy's Hospital in London (1748–49). He returned to Philadelphia in 1849 as one of the best-educated of American physicians, and he established a deservedly large and lucrative practice. He was a consulting physician to Pennsylvania Hospital from 1751 to 1780, where he first practiced surgery and midwifery. Because of his rather delicate health, he turned to the practice of physic. He was a senior founding fellow of the College of Physicians and served as its first president (1787–1805). His few published papers include *De Abortu* (1748), *Defence of Inoculation* (1759), and *An account of the yellow fever as it prevailed in Philadelphia in the autumn of 1762.* He was preceptor to a number of pupils, whom he called his "professional children" and who became equally celebrated. They included Benjamin Rush (q.v.), William Shippen, Jr. (q.v.), John Morgan (q.v.), Caspar Wistar (q.v.), and John Redman Coxe. He was elected a member of the city council in 1751. He was a trustee of Princeton University and of the College of Philadelphia (the latter from 1762 to 1791), a member of the American Philosophical Society, and an elder of the Second Presbyterian Church. Redman is alleged to have survived two attacks of yellow fever. He also had rheumatism and liver disease, and in 1784 these ailments compelled him to retire.

Artist: Unknown

Crayon, pencil and chalk miniature drawing, on buff paper; tondo, actual size 5 7/8 in diameter; not signed or dated. Presented by estate of John Redman Coxe in 1864. Experts at the National Portrait Gallery feel that the work is contemporary with the subject and is typical of drawings done by French emigrés in the 1790s. Further research is needed. *PH 273*

Dr. Redman is shown bust length with body and head in profile to the left. He is seated in a yoke-back, Queen Anne-style armchair. The shaded background is darker on the left. Dr. Redman wears a gray wig with a tight, formal curl at the forehead and a row of four curls at the sides. His profile is distinctive. The forehead is high and the gaze of the brown eye is directed straight ahead. The nose is long and hooked. The mouth is tight, and the thin lips are scarcely visible. The chin is sharp and juts forward. The neck shows loose folds of skin. The subject wears a white shirt with a rounded, hemmed collar, a white cravat, a black collarless waistcoat, and a blue jacket with high collar and no lapels. The contours of the head, costume, and chair are outlined. Shading is accomplished by delicate parallel strokes; touches of local color in the drawing include gray in the hair, reddish-brown in the face, and bluish-gray with white highlights in the coat. The old-fashioned style of hair and costume should not lead the modern historian into misjudging the date of this drawing. The subject was described by his contemporaries as looking like "an antiquated old gentleman." The sensitive face shows poignant signs of age, the burdens of heavy duties, and, perhaps, illness.

Artist: Unknown

Oil on canvas; 35 1/2 x 28 1/2; not signed or dated. Presented by Dr. George Bacon Wood in 1865. Shown in 1887 at the College of Physicians' Centennial Celebration Loan Collection of Portraits *with artist listed as unknown. Shown also at* The Art of Philadelphia Medicine, *Philadelphia Museum of Art, 1965. This oil portrait is probably a mid-19th century copy of the drawing described above.*
PA 13

The painter shows the sitter from the same view and with almost identical details of face, costume, and chair. He has lengthened the figure and added to the left arm a forearm and hand; the latter holds a book, which rests on the thigh. The subject is now placed in an interior setting, which includes paneled walls, a lowboy or bureau at the lower left, and a secretary-bookcase or bookshelves with two rows of books at the right. The portrait is painted smoothly. The head is moderately well-constructed in three-dimensional volumes. The costume gives a slight suggestion of the underlying body forms. The copyist has taken a distinctive and chiseled profile of an old man and translated it into a face that borders on the grotesque. The figure has been cut off awkwardly at the elbow and legs, and the long tapered fingers seem boneless. The interior appears flat, yet it is crowded with objects which do not have enough space to exist in depth. The additions of book, elegant furniture, and paneled walls convey a message of social status and learning. Instead of describing age and sensitiveness, the new facial expression is one of wooden tenseness, unrevealing of character.

Artist: Joseph Sansom (1767–1826)

For biography, see page 23.

Silhouette, black ink on buff paper; 4 3/4 x 3 3/4; inscription in black ink beneath the figure, "John Redman, of Philad^{a} M.D./President of the Colledge [sic] of Physicians;/aged 69"; written in pencil by another hand and not shown in the photograph, "By Jos. Sansom 1789." The date is incorrect because this silhouette is one in a group done between 1790 and 1792 by Sansom, and Redman would have been 69 years old in 1791. However, the identity of the artist and subject are correct, because although this silhouette is missing from Sansom's manuscript book at the Historical Society of Pennsylvania, it is listed in the

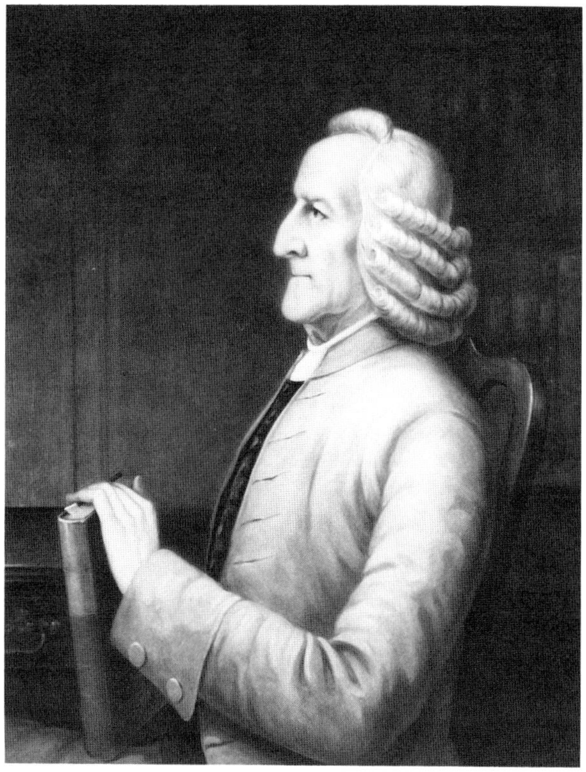

John Redman *PA 13*

table of contents, with the statement "John Redman. Short. Philadelphia. 1722—." There are copies in the Gilpin Collection and by Auguste Edouart. Presented by Hampton L. Carson in 1909.
PH 293

Dr. Redman is shown bust length, with profile to the left. His famous cocked hat has a wide brim that covers his eye. He has a very long, hooked nose, a retracted mouth, and a pointed chin. His fluffy hair has round curls in the back, texture being indicated by delicate, wavy lines. The profile is distinctively Redman's, as shown by the drawing and oil painting described above. The silhouette is solidly opaque except for the hair. The outlines are crisp and clear, and the bust has the conventional concave shape and sharp points.

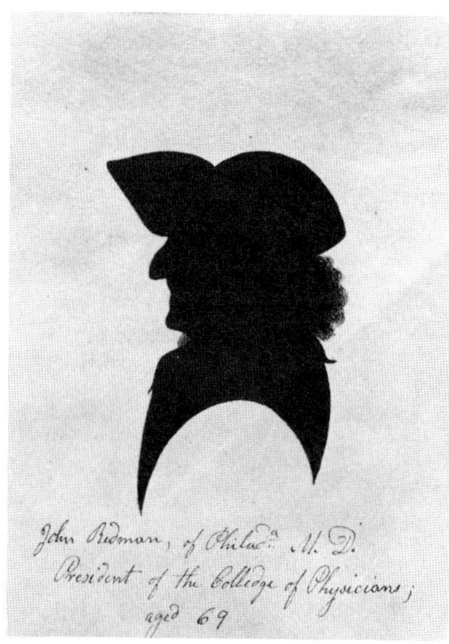

John Redman *PH 293*

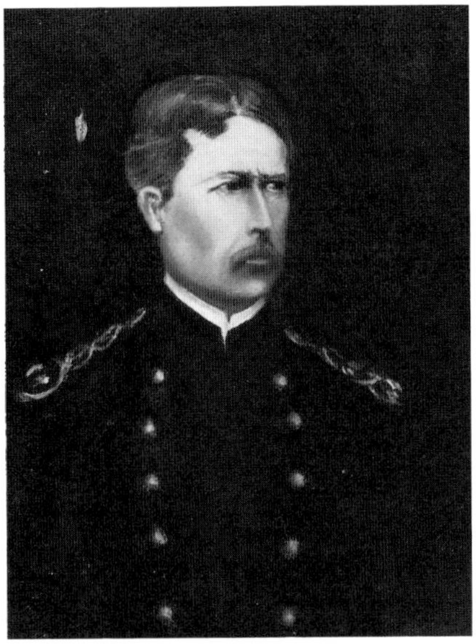

Walter Reed *PA 129*

Walter Reed (1851–1902)

Born in Gloucester County, Virginia, Walter Reed was the son of an itinerant Methodist minister. He entered the University of Virginia and in 1869 received the M.D. degree there at the age of 17; he was the youngest medical graduate in the history of the university. He continued his medical training at Bellevue Hospital Medical College in New York, where he received a second medical degree in 1870. In 1874, after serving as an intern at King's County Hospital and as an inspector for the Brooklyn Board of Health, he enlisted in the United States Army Medical Corps. After serving in New York and filling a long assignment in the frontier of Arizona, he maneuvered a change to Baltimore. There he was permitted to conduct research at Johns Hopkins in the laboratory of Dr. William Welch, professor of bacteriology and pathology, who had assembled a brilliant group of investigators. This was the impetus that inspired Reed to a decade of teaching, intense scientific study, and the publication of a steady stream of papers. In 1893 he was ordered to the surgeon general's office, where he became curator of the Army Medical Museum and professor of bacteriology and clinical microscopy in Surgeon General Sternberg's Army Medical School. After the outbreak of the Spanish-American War, Reed was made chairman of a committee to study the causes and modes of propagation of typhoid fever. Severe epidemics at military camps were found to be caused by the common fly, which carried contagion to susceptible persons from infected patients and from contaminated bedding and waste. The commission also found that the water-borne factor was not as important as had been believed. The final report was not published until 1904. Reed's most important assignment was as head of a commission to investigate the transmission of yellow fever. Along with Drs. James Carroll, Jessie W. Lazear, and Aristides Agramonte, he arrived in Cuba in the summer of 1900. After a series of human experiments with immune and non-immune volunteers, it was found that mosquito, *Stegomyia fasciata,* (now known as *Aedes aegypti*) was the intermediate host for yellow fever. This proved what had been conjectured by Dr. Carlos Finlay in 1882. It was shown also that yellow fever was transmitted to non-immune persons by the bite of a mosquito that had previously fed on the blood of a patient with the disease. The commission instituted mosquito-control methods that were adopted all over the world, wherever yellow fever was endemic. In 1901, Reed presented the conclusions of the commission in an address before the Pan-American Congress. He returned to teach at both the Army Medical School and the Columbia Medical School (now George Washington University). Before his death, caused by periappendiceal abscess, he received an honorary A.M. degree from Harvard and an honorary LL.D. degree from the University of Michigan. He was unquestionably one of the great military physicians. His memory is perpetuated by the Walter Reed Army Medical Center in Washington.

Artist: Unknown

Oil on canvas; 81/2 x 61/2; signed lower right, but name is undecipherable. Presented by Dr. Claude P. Brown, 1971, through Dr. Fred B. Rogers, who gave the following information: the portrait was found in a New York bookstore by Dr. Arthur Parker Hitchens, an Army medical officer who was professor of public health at the University of Pennsylvania and a colleague of Dr. Brown. *PA 129*

Major Walter Reed is shown bust length, his body frontal, his head turned to the right. The background is dark reddish-brown. The subject has light brown hair, brown eyes which look out in the direction of the head turn, a straight and slender nose, and a brown brush moustache that hides his upper lip. He is dressed in a military uniform of a white shirt with standup collar and a blue double-breasted coat with gold epaulets and brass buttons. The portrait is smoothly painted. The head is minimally described in three dimensions. The coat is flat and does not suggest the underlying body forms. The subject's posture is ramrod straight. His knitted brows and tight mouth give him an expression of preoccupied severity.

Joseph Gibbons Richardson (1836–1886)

Richardson was born in Philadelphia, a descendant of English forbears (including the renowned silversmith, Joseph Richardson) who came to America in 1681. He received the M.D. degree from the medical department of the University of Pennsylvania in 1862. His first medical practice was established in Union Springs, New York, where he remained for

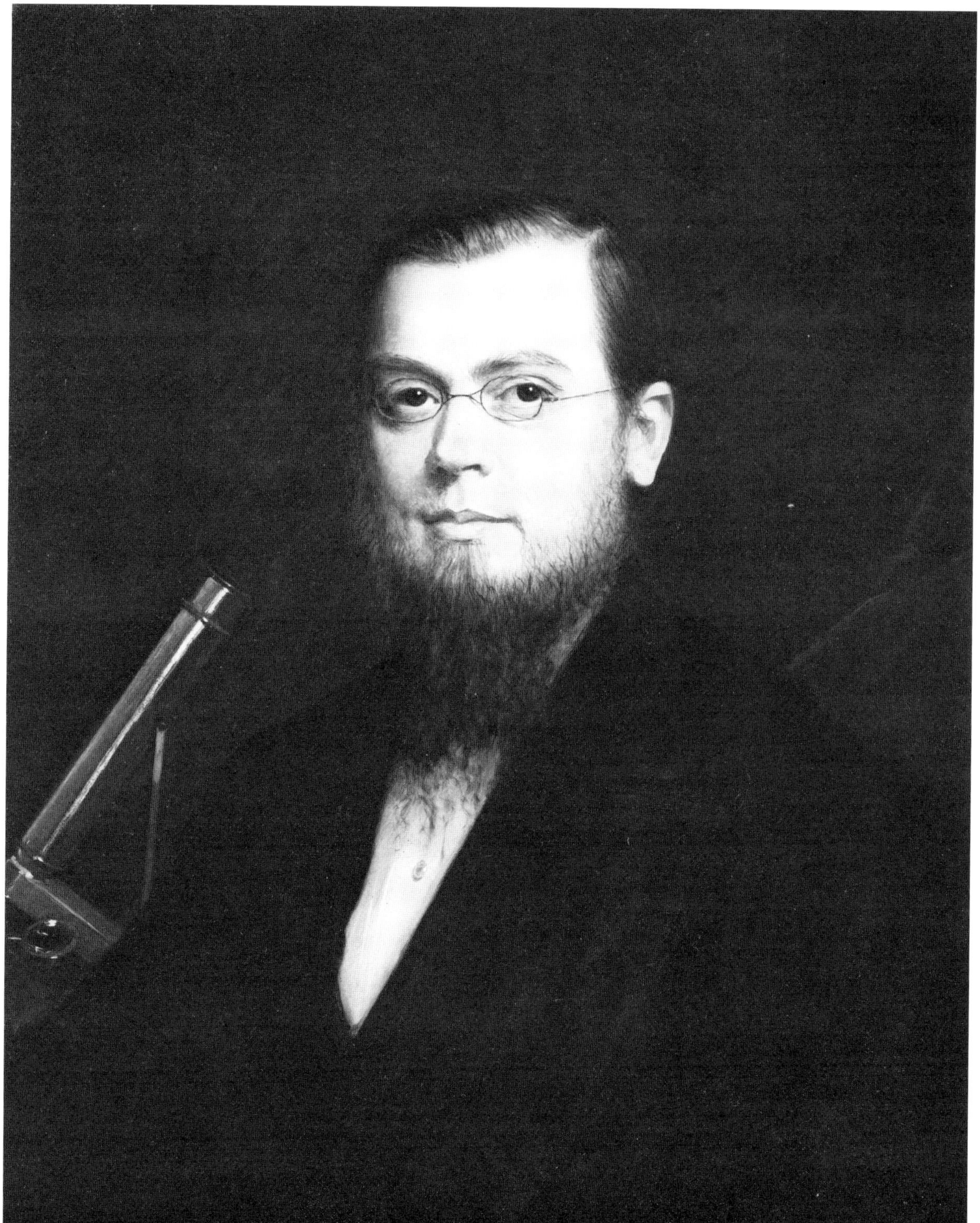

Joseph Gibbons Richardson

PA 115

five years and served as vice-president of the Cayuga County Medical Association. Returning to Philadelphia, he specialized in microscopy and was made microscopist to the Pennsylvania Hospital and visiting physician to the Presbyterian Hospital. In 1877 he became professor of hygiene in the medical department of the University of Pennsylvania. In addition to being a fellow of the College of Physicians, he was secretary of the biological and microscopical sections of the Academy of Natural Sciences. He wrote many articles, including "Cellular Structure of the Red Blood Corpuscle," "Identity of Red Blood Corpuscles in Various Races of Mankind," "The True Nature and Origin of the Salivary Globules," and "The Detection of Elastic Tissue in the Sputum of Phthisis." His most important treatise was his *Handbook of Medical Microscopy* (1871).

Artist: Attributed to [?] Wilson

Oil on canvas; 26 1/4 x 21 1/2; not signed or dated. Bequeathed in 1947 by Miss Josephine Richardson Howell, granddaughter of Dr. Richardson. According to a letter kept in the files of the College of Physicians and written by Mrs. Sara Binder Moore, a friend of the donor, this portrait was listed in the notebook of Mrs. Elizabeth Randolph Richardson Howell, daughter of Dr. Richardson and mother of Miss Josephine Howell, in the following way: "Portrait of my father Joseph Gibbons Richardson, M.D., painted by ——— Wilson in Philadelphia." For unexplained reasons, Mrs. Moore suggested the date of 1869. Since the bequest, inventories at the College of Physicians have listed this portrait either as a work by an unknown artist or by Matthew Wilson (1814–1892), a portrait painter and miniaturist who was born in London and came to Philadelphia in 1832 to study with Henry Inman (1801–1846). After additional study in Paris under Claude-Marie Dubufe in 1835, he returned to America and worked in several East Coast cities and in Ohio; then he settled in Brooklyn. In 1843 he was made an associate of the National Academy of Design and exhibited there frequently in the years 1841–46 and 1861–85. Later he was called to Washington to paint portraits of several Civil War leaders, including one of President Lincoln made two weeks before the assassination. Portraits by Wilson in Philadelphia institutions can be found at the Historical Society of Philadelphia, the University of Pennsylvania, and the Union League. At least four lesser-known artists named Wilson lived in Philadelphia during this general period and their portraits are also represented in Philadelphia collections: Jeremy Wilson (1824–1899), Stephen D. Wilson (b. 1825), Mrs. Jessie Sartell Wilson, and an artist who signed his work, "J. Wilson." More research will have to be done on this work and on these artists before secure attribution can be made. PA 115

Dr. Richardson is shown bust length, with body and head turned slightly to the left. The greenish-brown background has a small triangle of dark red drapery on the center right border. The left edge has a dark brown vertical strip, under which is a table with a brass microscope. The subject has medium brown hair. His dark brown eyes gaze straight out toward the viewer through metal-rimmed spectacles. He has a straight nose and full lips. His round cheeks have a pink complexion. His most prominent characteristics are reddish-brown side-whiskers and an uncut, scraggly beard, depicted in particularized detail. He wears a white shirt with a gold stud, a black bow tie, a black vest, and a black coat. The surface of the portrait has smooth brush strokes except for the linear treatment of the hair. The naturalistic portrayal of the face is rendered in solid and convincing three-dimensional volumes. The flat costume does not suggest underlying body forms. Although the microscope has been placed in the background, it is important iconographically, since it identifies the subject's profession. The strong highlights on the brass attract the viewer's attention. The subject has a pleasant, open, and approachable facial expression, and he does not seem perturbed by the interruption of his work. The artist has created a convincing sense of a vital and energetic figure.

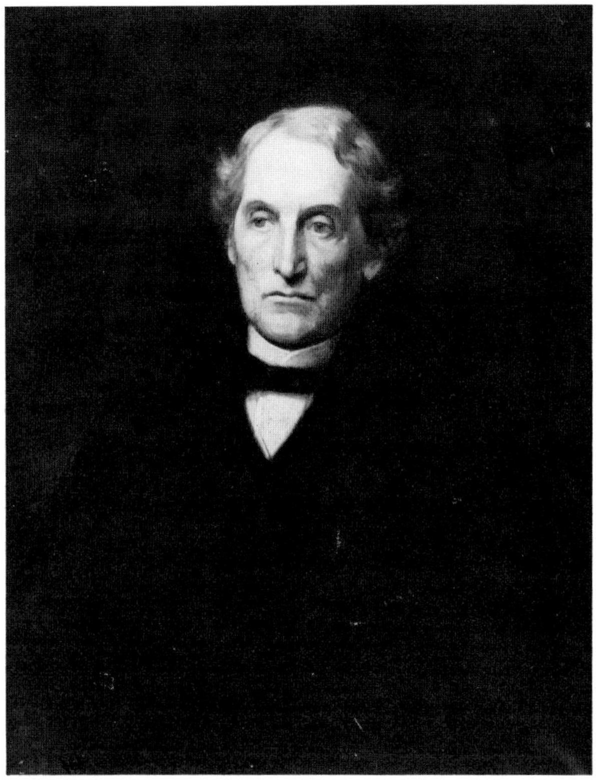

Lewis Rodman *PA 53*

Lewis Rodman (1806–1890)

Born on a large country estate in Eddington, Bucks County, Pennsylvania, Dr. Rodman was a descendant of Irish Quaker forbears who left their homeland to settle in Barbados and then came in 1675 to Newport, Rhode Island. He studied medicine under Dr. Joseph Parrish (q.v.) and was graduated from the medical department of the University of Pennsylvania in 1827. After finding country practice in Moorestown, New Jersey, excessively "laborious," he removed to Philadelphia and joined the obstetrical and general practice of Dr. John Ruan, an uncle by marriage. He was a consulting physician to the Preston Retreat and a manager of the Philadelphia Dispensary. He was a fellow of the College of Physicians, which he served as a censor for almost thirty years. A memorial biography read at the College by Dr. William G. Porter in 1892 wistfully enlogizes: "With him has passed away one of the strong links which bind us to a past generation of physicians, when medicine was practiced more as a profession, and less as a trade. . . . He was essentially one of the old-time family physicians, now fast disappearing from the public gaze, who were almost members of the families in which they practiced."

Artist: Unknown

Oil on canvas; 31 1/4 x 24 1/4; not signed or dated. Presented by Mrs. Lewis Rodman in 1892. PA 53

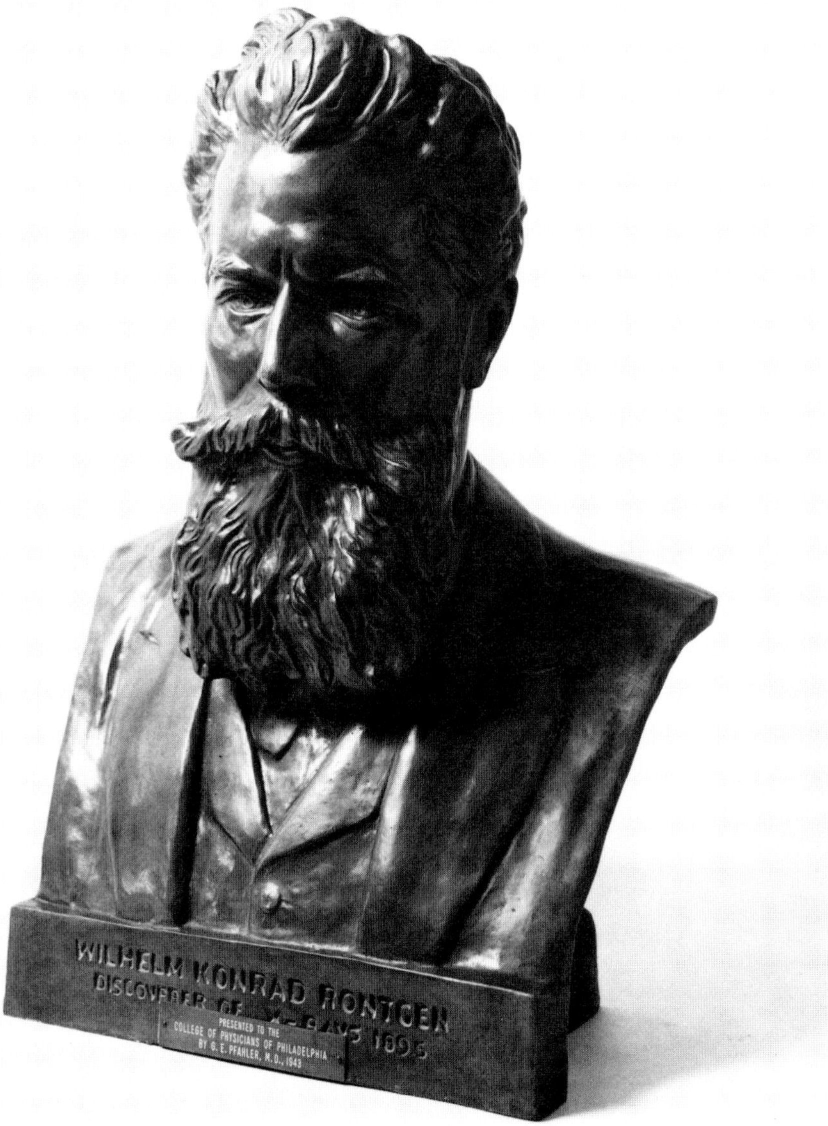
WILHELM KONRAD RONTGEN
PRESENTED TO THE
COLLEGE OF PHYSICIANS OF PHILADELPHIA
BY G. E. PFAHLER, M.D., 1943

Wilhelm Conrad Röntgen *ST 555*

Dr. Rodman is shown bust length, with head and body turned very slightly to the left. The background is dark brownish-maroon. He has gray wavy hair, heavy-lidded blue eyes that look to the left, high cheekbones, a long, aquiline nose whose tip points down to a wide mouth with thin lips, and a firm chin. He wears a white shirt with stand-up collar, a black bow tie, a black vest, and a black coat with wide lapels. Although the portrait has suffered paint loss as well as other damage, it is evident that the surface was painted smoothly and that the head was formed in solid and three-dimensional volumes. The costume is flat and does not suggest the underlying body forms. One feels that the representation is a naturalistic likeness of the subject, who "filled a quiet, modest, unassuming place," but was "actuated by high desires, noble impulses and a profound sense of duty."

Wilhelm Conrad Röntgen (1845–1923)

Röntgen, the son of a textile merchant, was born in Lennep, Germany. He received a diploma as a mechanical engineer at the Polytechnical School in Zürich in 1868 and a Ph.D. from the University of Zürich in 1869. He filled a succession of academic posts at the Universities of Würzberg and Strasbourg and at the Hessian University in Giessen. In 1888 he returned to Würzburg's brilliant scientific circle to succeed Kohlrausch, the great experimental physicist, as professor of physics and director of the physical institute. In 1894 he was elected rector of the University. His early experiments concerned the compressibility of liquids, the conductivity of electrolytes, and the thermal coefficients of expansion. In 1888 he published a paper on what was subsequently called the "Röntgen current," a major discovery of the magnetic effects produced in a dielectric when it is moved between two electrically charged condenser plates. He also published papers on the physical properties of crystals, their electrical conductivity, and the influence of radiation on them. His fame with the general public rests on his discovery of X-rays, as he called them, or as they are called in Germany, Röntgenstrahlen. Although he was preceded by the work of Hittorf, Crookes, Hertz, and Lenard, it was Röntgen who found that X-rays are emitted by the part of the glass wall of the tube that is opposite the cathode and receives the beam of cathode rays; he also found that X-rays travel in straight lines, cannot be refracted or reflected, are not deviated by magnets, can travel approximately two meters in the air, and have penetrating properties that can produce images. During his experiments Röntgen was astonished to notice the outlines of the bones of his own fingers, as well as objects in the laboratory. He repeated the experiment by imposing the hand of Frau Röntgen between the Hittorf-Crookes tube and the photographic plate. He reported his findings first to the editors of the Physical and Medical Society of Würzburg on December 28, 1895. In January the sensational news was released to a world which responded quickly to its earliest applications in medicine and metallurgy. For this discovery Röntgen received scores of prizes, medals, decorations, and honorary degrees, including the Prussian Order of the Crown, second class, an honorary M.D. degree from the University of Würzburg, and the first Nobel prize in physics. A statue of him was placed on the Potsdam Bridge in Berlin. He was extremely reticent socially and never sought a patent or entered into any contracts for the commercial manufacture of his apparatus. In 1899, succumbing to royal pressure, he removed to the University of Munich to become professor of physics and director of a new physical institute. He wrote 58 papers, most of which were published in *Annalen der Physik und Chemie.*

Artist: Christabel Cummings

Cummings is a sculptor and painter who worked and taught art in Washington, D.C.

Bronze; 24 x 16 1/2 x 11 5/8; base integral with sculpture 2 3/4 in. high; signed and dated on back of base, "Christabel Cummings 1940/©"; inscription on front of base, "Wilhelm Konrad Röntgen/ Discoverer of X-rays 1895." Presented by Dr. George E. Pfahler in 1954. In 1943 Dr. Pfahler had presented to the College a plaster cast of a sculpture by Cummings. According to letters on file at the College of Physicians, he removed it in 1954 and had it cast in bronze at the Roman Bronze Co, Inc., of Corona, New York. This work is the bronze cast. The plaque attached to its base was made for the plaster cast presented in 1943. ST 555

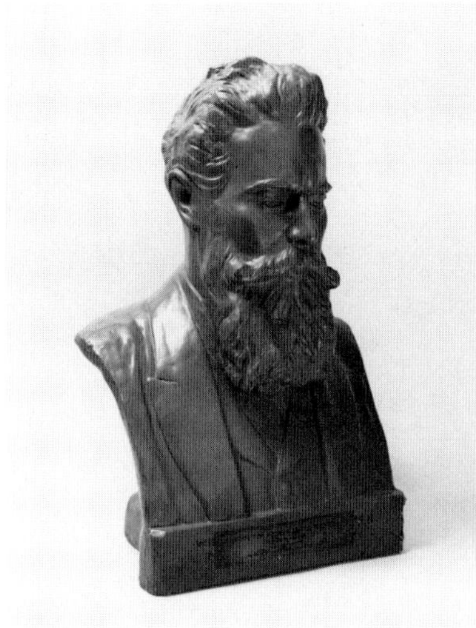

Wilhelm Conrad Röntgen ST 577

Professor Röntgen is shown bust length, with body frontal and head turned slightly to the right and tilted down when seen frontally. The accompanying photograph was taken from an angle. The larger than life-size head has very thick, wavy hair brushed away from the protuberant forehead. The sharply incised eyebrows surmount eyes with carved irises and pupils which look straight out in the direction of the head turn and tilt. The subject has hollow cheeks, a straight nose, a very long, bushy moustache which joins side-whiskers, and a luxuriant, long, square beard. He wears a shirt, vest, and coat. The bronze sculpture is carved smoothly except for the texture of the hair. The depressions and projections produce a rippled effect of light and shade. The head is modeled with knowledge of anatomy. The naturalistic likeness is an image of strength because of its large scale and its expressive features, especially the scowling eyebrows, riveting gaze, and pursed lips. The linear description of thick hair and the play of light and shade give additional animation to a lively and energetic portrayal.

Artist: Christabel Cummings

Plaster, painted brown; 24 7/8 x 16 3/4 x 11 1/2; base integral with sculpture, 2 7/8 in. high; signed and dated on back of base, "Christabel Cummings 1940/©"; inscription on base, "Wilhelm Konrad Röntgen/ Discoverer of X-rays 1895." Presented by the Blockley Radiological Society in 1977. A bust of Röntgen was presented to the United States government by the American College of Radiology on July 20, 1956, to commemorate the sixtieth anniversary of the discovery of X-rays. That bust was provided for the presentation by Dr. George E. Pfahler, who had it in his Philadelphia office. The association of that bust with Pfahler and the label on the bust now in the College suggest that the bust given by Pfahler to the College in 1943, the bust presented to the government by the ACR in 1956, and the one received by the College after the closing of Philadelphia General Hospital in 1977 might be one and the same. No supporting documentation has yet been found. ST 577

The plaster cast is naturalistic and expressive but lacks the sharp linear definition of forms and the contrast of light and shadow seen on the gleaming surface of the bronze sculpture above.

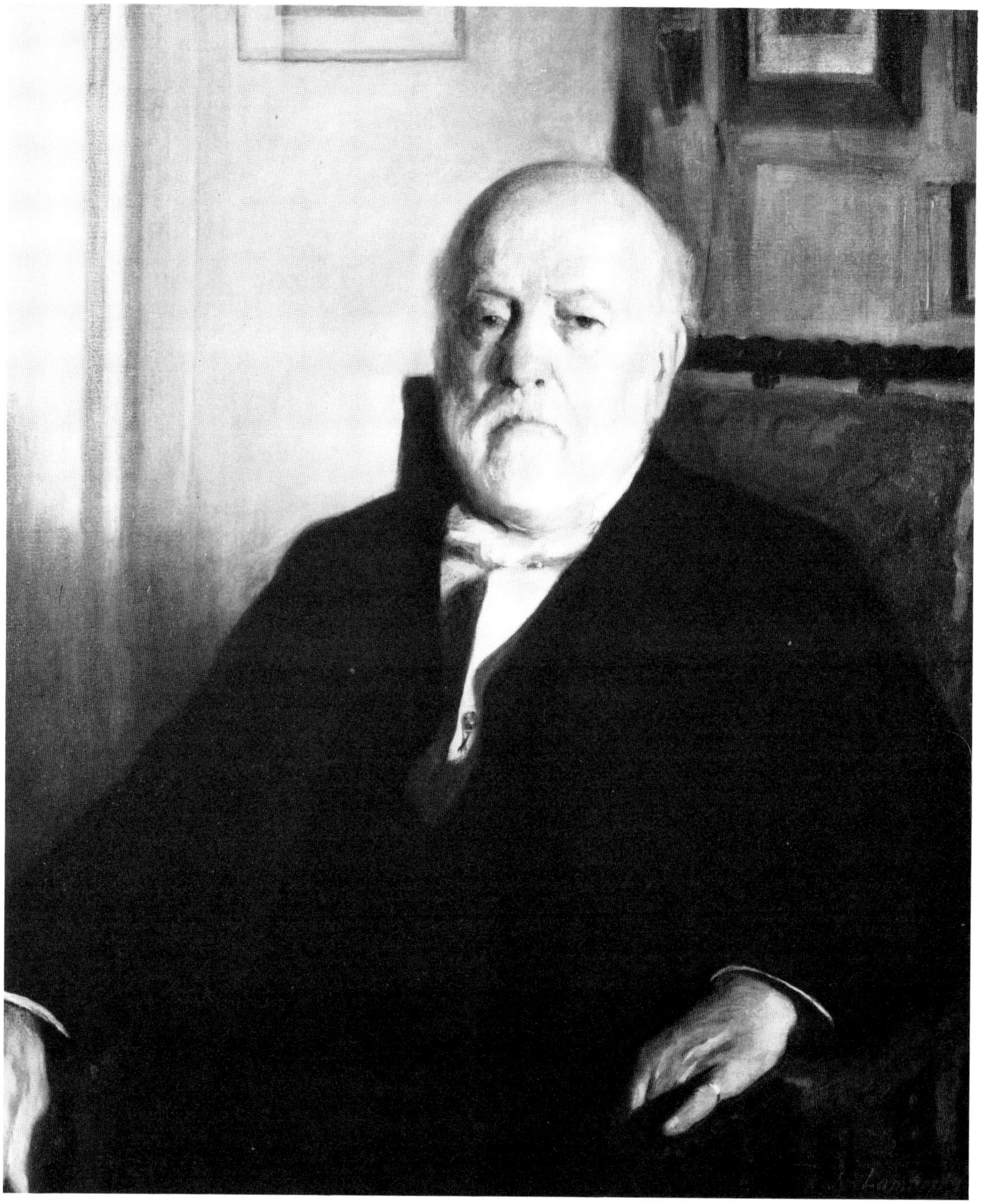

William Samuel Waithman Ruschenberger *PA 18*

William Samuel Waithman Ruschenberger (1807-1895)

Dr. Ruschenberger was born on a farm in Bridgeton, New Jersey. At the age of nineteen he enlisted in the United States Navy, but he soon returned to academic life and entered the Medical Department of the University of Pennsylvania, graduating in 1830. In 1831 he rejoined the Navy and was commissioned as surgeon. This was the start of 64 years of continuous service in the medical corps, with a total of 43 years of active duty, which ended with his commission as medical director with the rank of commodore, bestowed after his retirement in 1869. During his naval career he organized the United States Naval Laboratory and published several widely read chronicles of his long voyages in the Pacific, South America, and the East. He served as president of the Academy of Natural Sciences for twelve years and as vice-president of the American Philosophical Society for ten years. He was president of the College of Physicians from 1879 to 1883 and wrote *An Account of the Institution and Progress of the College of Physicians of Philadelphia during a Hundred Years, from January 1787*; this was published in the Centennial Volume of the College *Transactions* in 1887. He also wrote a popular series of small books on the natural sciences, *First Books of Natural History.*

Artist: John Lambert, Jr. (1861-1907)

For biography, see page 6.

Oil on canvas; 30 1/4 x 25 1/4; signed at lower right, "John Lambert Jr." According to his biography by John Ashhurst, Jr., in the Transactions and Studies of the College of Physicians of Philadelphia, *vol. 18, 1896, a number of fellows of the College "asked the privilege" of having a portrait of him painted, and that he, though "feeble in body," acceded, "only stipulating that... he should be given sittings at his home." The portrait was completed in five weeks, exactly ten days before Ruschenberger died. It was presented by the fellows in 1895. It was exhibited twice at the Pennsylvania Academy of the Fine Arts—at the annual exhibition of 1895-96 and at the Lambert Memorial Exhibition in 1930.* *PA 18*

Dr. Ruschenberger is shown half-length, with body and head turned to the left. He is seated in an armchair with spiral turned moldings above the back which is upholstered in a leafy green patterned fabric. He sits well back in the chair, with both arms resting on the chair arms. His hands are partly hidden—his pendent right hand by the edge of the painting, the left hand by the handhold of the chair. The background of the interior setting has a pale green wall and an asymmetrical arrangement of small pictures. The subject's head is bald except for wispy, white hair at the sides. His small, heavy-lidded blue eyes look straight ahead into the far distance in the direction of the head turn. The tip of his nose points down to a small mouth with thin lips turned down. He has sparse white side-whiskers, moustache, and beard. He has puffy lower lids and deep lines next to his nose. He wears a white shirt with stand-up collar, a white bow tie, a black vest, and a black coat. His jewelry includes shirt studs, cuff links, and a gold ring. The surface of the portrait is painterly, with all-over visible strokes, soft contours, and pervasive green shadows. The head is well-constructed in three-dimensional, solid volumes. The costume, though flat and more fluidly painted, manages to suggest the underlying bulk of the body. The artist was singularly sympathetic to his subject, who was near death. Although the feeble body sinks back into the chair, it is attired fashionably. The face shows unmistakable signs of age and decline, but the head is erect and the meditative expression gives a sense of dignity and elevation of spirit.

Benjamin Rush (1745-1813)

The famous Dr. Benjamin Rush, a descendant of English Quakers who arrived in Pennsylvania in 1683, was born on a farm near Philadelphia. He was taken two years later to the city, where his father carried on his trade as a gunsmith. He graduated from the College of New Jersey (later Princeton University) in 1760 and then studied medicine for six years with Dr. John Redman (q.v.). He also attended the first course of lectures on anatomy given by Dr. William Shippen, Jr. (q.v.). He continued his education at the University of Edinburgh under Dr. William Cullen (q.v.) and received an M.D. degree there in 1768. In 1769, after spending several months attending hospitals and lectures in London and France, he returned to Philadelphia. He began to practice medicine and became professor of chemistry at the College of Philadelphia. He soon became involved in social and political issues of the colonies. He was a member of the Pennsylvania delegation to the second Continental Congress in the momentous years 1776 and 1777, and he signed the Declaration of Independence. In 1777 he was appointed physician general of the military hospitals in the medical department of the American army, resigning the following year because of conflicts with the director general, William Shippen, Jr. His last public office was as treasurer of the United States Mint (1797-1813). In 1783 Rush was elected physician to the Pennsylvania Hospital, a post he held until his death. He was placed in charge of the insane and mentally ill, and in the next several decades he campaigned against the atrocious care of patients and wrote a systematic description of mental illness and its treatment under the title *Medical Inquiries and Observations Upon the Diseases of the Mind* (published in 1812). For this he later was called "The Father of American Psychiatry." Unlike most physicians of his day, Rush believed that mental illness had a physical basis. He felt "the cause of madness to be seated in the blood vessels of the brain," with the brain and nerves being the secondary seat of madness. He recognized that environmental causes such as isolation, fear, guilt, and grief might result in mental illness; he also believed that madness could be hereditary. He divided madness into three groups: "hypochondriasis" (brought on by the patient himself), "melancholia" (brought on by outer events or circumstances), and a miscellaneous category of "general intellectual derangement." His therapeutics included bloodletting, purges, emetics, occupational and physical treatment, travel, and exercise. Upon the death of John Morgan in 1789, Rush succeeded him as professor of the theory and practice at the College of Philadelphia. When that institution merged with the University of the State of Pennsylvania to become the University of Pennsylvania in 1791, Rush was appointed professor of the institutes of medicine and clinical practice. In addition to these duties he always had a large number of private students, estimated at 2250 in the course of 44 years. He belonged to the American Philosophical Society, of which he was curator, secretary, councillor, and vice-president; he also was a founder and attending physician of the Philadelphia Dispensary, a senior founding fellow and a censor of the College of Physicians and president of both the Society for the Abolition of Slavery and the Bible Society. He was a founder of Franklin and Marshall College and of Dickinson College, and he received an honorary LL.D. degree from Yale in 1812. Rush had a dogmatic personality and was often at the

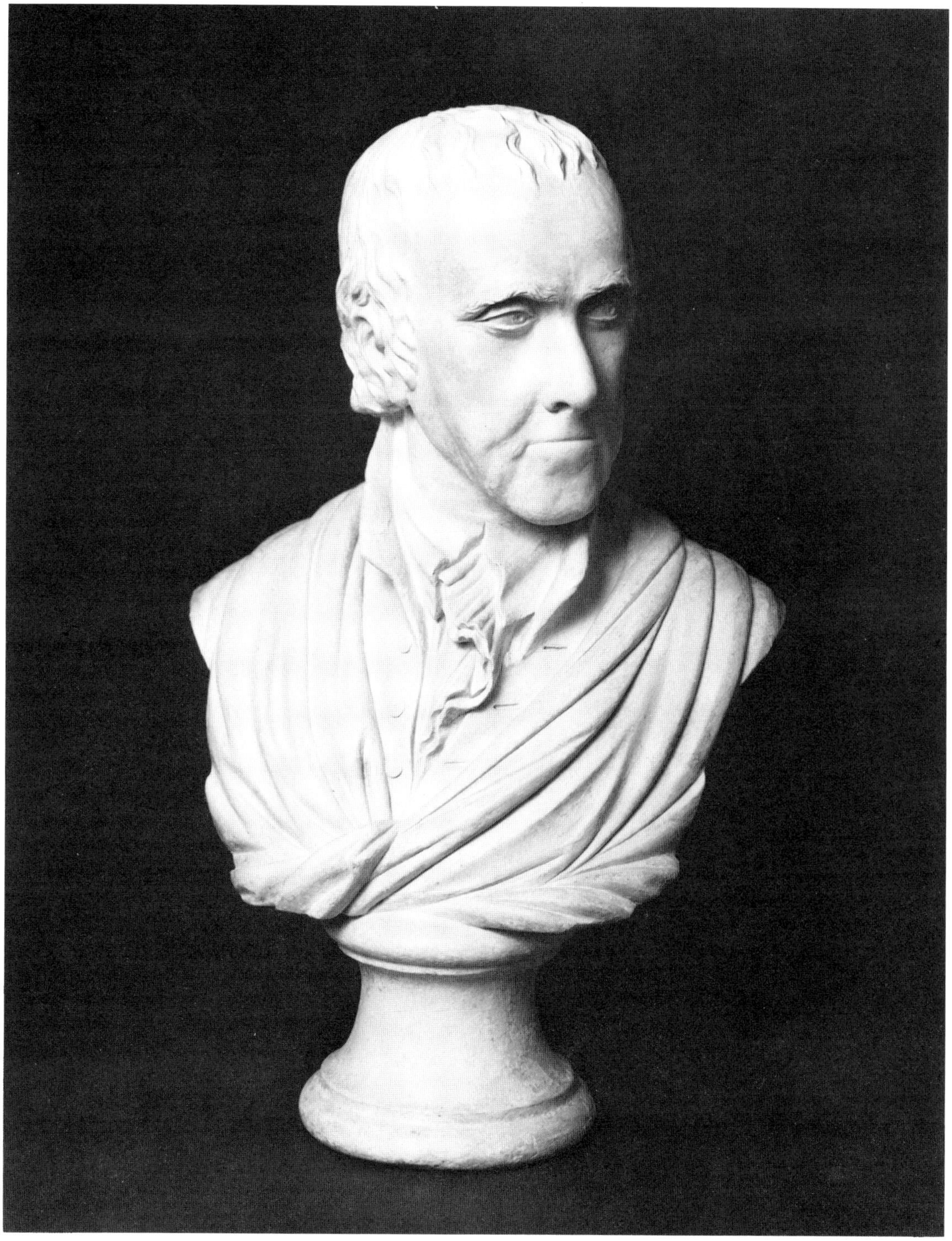

Benjamin Rush *ST 542*

center of controversy. He campaigned for some unpopular causes, including freedom and education for slaves, broader education for women, temperance in alcohol and tobacco, a system of public education, prison reform, and abolition of capital punishment. For his advocacy of bleeding and purgation in the treatment of yellow fever during the epidemics of 1739 and 1797 and his belief that the disease resulted from filth in the streets and was not imported, he was attacked in the press by his professional colleagues and others. These disputes with other fellows of the College of Physicians led to his resignation from that body and the loss of public favor. Rush's contributions to the medical literature include the popular work entitled *Medical Inquiries and Observations.* In 1948 his memoirs were edited by George W. Corner and published as *The Autobiography of Benjamin Rush: His "Travels through Life" together with his Commonplace Book for 1789–1813.* In 1951 Lyman H. Butterfield edited the *Letters of Benjamin Rush.* One epithet of Rush is "the American Sydenham," but unlike the latter, his medical reputation has experienced periods of both decline and ascent from his own day to ours.

Artist: William Rush (1756–1833)

For biography, see page 169.

Plaster, painted white; 187/8 x 15 x 11; round base integral with sculpture, 56/8 in. high; not signed or dated. Neither donor nor date of donation has been recorded. Included in College of Physicians Inventory of 1898–1915. A plaster cast made after the original terra-cotta in 1812 is at the Pennsylvania Academy of the Fine Arts. Other plaster casts are at the Library Company of Philadelphia, the Pennsylvania Hospital, and the private collection of Andrew Oliver of Boston. (For description of piece-mold casting technique, see entry on Rush's bust of Physick.) An inscription in pencil was found on back of the base, "Do^r^ John C. Otto," a pupil of Benjamin Rush, and probably refers to the person for whom the plaster cast was made. That Rush thought highly of this sculpture and of his other portrait busts is evident in a letter to Benjamin West, dated March 12, 1815 (New-York Historical Society), which reads: "I expect you will receive for the Royal Academy, a plaster cast taken from a clay model of Do^r^ Rush, which I executed 8 or 9 months before his death. The likeness you may judge must be tolerable, when in a few days fifteen hundred dollars was subscribed principally for him, some for Do^r^ Physick at $10 per cast—The size of the cranium appears large, but that, with the whole of the head, and profile is correct from actual measurement . . . I have . . . considerable part of my time in modeling several busts of Do^r^ Physick, Do^r^ Wistar . . ." (reference to this letter and much of the above information is courtesy of Linda Bantel, chief organizer of the William Rush American Sculptor *exhibition at the Pennsylvania Academy of the Fine Arts, 1982, and to her essay in the exhibition catalogue). The conservator at the Pennsylvania Academy, Virginia Norton Naudé, who discovered the name of Dr. Otto on the raw plaster surface, reasoned that successive layers of gesso and three colors of paint had been added after the cast had left Rush's studio. These layers were therefore removed for historical and artistic reasons, expecially since they obscured sculptural detail. Since many stains could not be removed in the time allowed and since the surface was irregular, the surface was consolidated for exhibition by the application of two thin coats of reversible white paint. The bust owned by the College of Physicians was included in the exhibition* William Rush, American Sculptor *at the Pennsylvania Academy of the Fine Arts, 1982. ST 542*

Dr. Rush is shown bust length, with body frontal and head turned sharply to the right. His thin hair, which is brushed in wavy individual strands on to his forehead, is full around the ears and then descends into a long queue tied with a bow. The narrow face is surmounted by long, undulating eyebrows. The eyes, carved with the irises and pupils characteristic of William Rush's technique, look sharply away from the viewer in the direction of the head turn. The cheeks are hollow, the nose is aquiline. The lips are closed so tightly that the upper lip is virtually hidden and the lower lip protrudes. The chin is squared off. There are age lines in the forehead, the corners of the eyes, and next to the nose and mouth. The subject wears a shirt, a jabot that falls in undulating curves, a waistcoat with stand-up collar, and an outer garment with deep, curving parallel folds tied together at the bottom. The surface of the plaster cast has the characteristically uneven texture of that medium. The head has been rendered in moderately solid, three-dimensional volumes. The costume does not reveal underlying body forms. The sculpture is a naturalistic rendering of the subject, who was a second cousin of the artist. As in several other portrait busts by William Rush, the severity of the facial expression contrasts with the animation suggested by the arrangement of the hair and the somewhat fanciful costume, with its active movement in the jabot and in the folds of the outer garment. The bust is an impressive portrait of a controversial figure in Philadelphia medical and social circles, shown in the twilight of his life.

Artist: Adele von Helmbold

For biography, see page 11.

Oil on canvas; 411/2 x 331/2; not signed or dated. Inscription on back of relined canvas reads, "Portrait of Benjamin Rush, M.D./from an Original Picture by Sully/copy by Adele von Helmbold." Presented by Catharine Rush and Mary Rush in 1888. Thomas Sully made five oil portraits of Benjamin Rush, all with the same posture, but in different lengths and with different backgrounds. The source for this copy is the Sully portrait of 1812, once owned by Rush's son, Richard, and now in the collection of the Benjamin Rush Estate. Sully also made a small watercolor resembling this version. In addition to the oil copy by von Helmbold, the Sully portrait was engraved by James B. Longacre, R.W. Dodson, Christian Gobrecht, and David Edwin, and it was drawn by Albert Newsam. PA 17

Dr. Rush is shown two-thirds length, with head and body turned to the right and head tilted diagonally down. He is seated in an upholstered chair with volute hand holds and a wooden cresting rail. His right arm is bent loosely; his right hand and wrist rest on a writing table, the fingers holding the pages of an open book. His left arm is bent sharply with the elbow leaning on the table and the thumb and index finger of his hand supporting his tilted head; the other three fingers are curved. The interior setting is complex. Behind his head there is a maroon drapery drawn back in a triangular shape. The wall on the right is grayish-green. In the lower left corner leaning against the chair there is a portion of a black portfolio with red corners, tied loosely with cloth straps to show a sheaf of white papers. The writing table is covered with a brown cloth. On the table there are standing and stacked books, a quill pen, and an open book. Rush's wire-rimmed spectacles rest on his high forehead. His sparse gray hair is tied in the back in a queue. Under thick, dark eyebrows his large blue eyes gaze into the distance in the direction of the head tilt and turn. His aquiline nose points down toward a tightly closed mouth and a pointed chin. What can be seen of his costume is a white neckcloth tied in a bow, a grayish-green, double-breasted coat with high collar and M-notched lapel, and breeches with buttons. The surface of the portrait has been brushed smoothly. The face and hands are rendered in solid and three-dimensional volumes, and the costume gives an impression of the underlying bodily bulk. The copyist has been faithful to the composition and content of

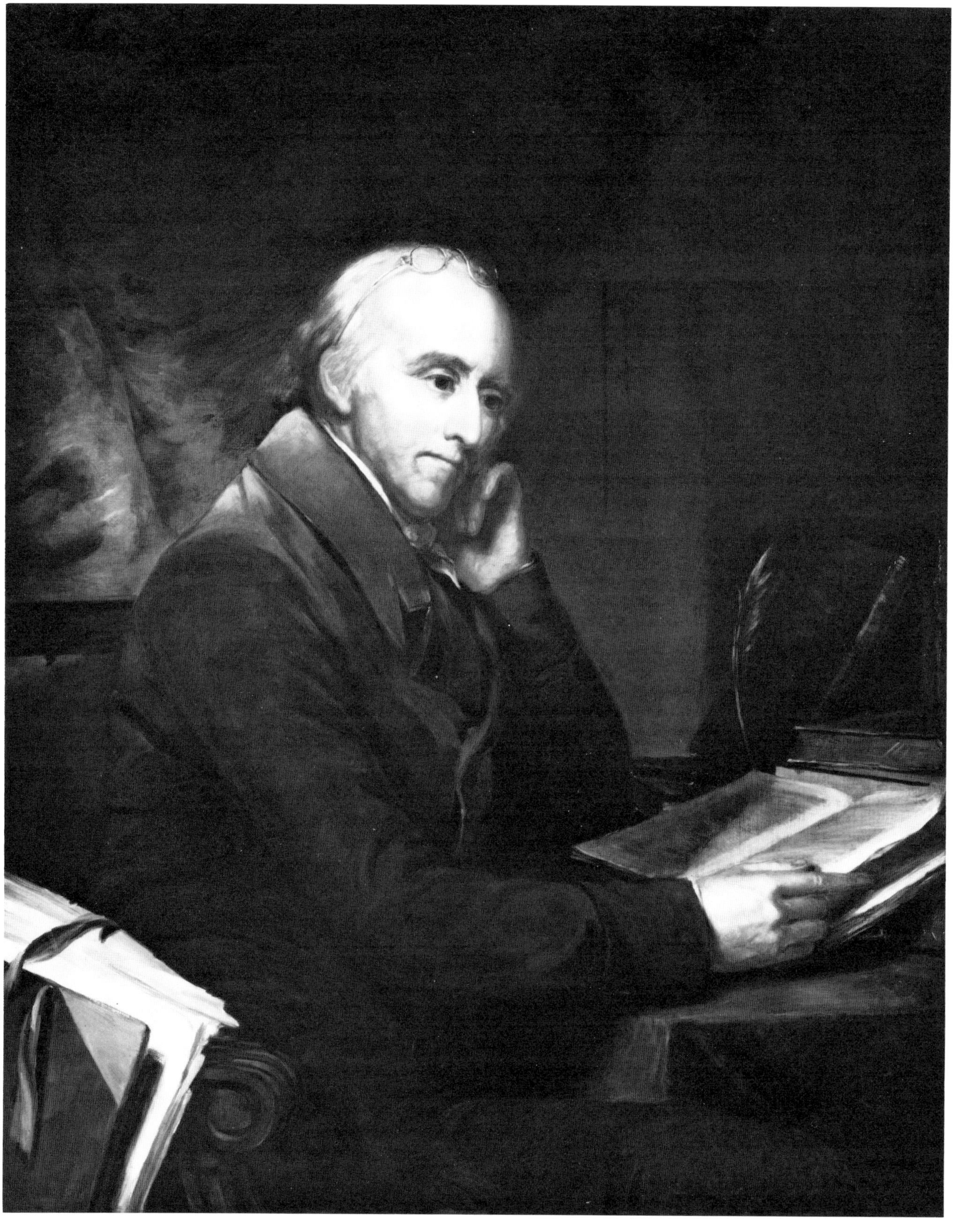

Benjamin Rush *PA 17*

Sully's painting, if not to its emotion and power. Crowded with iconographical objects that refer to the subject's erudition and elevated social status—portfolio, books, pen, furniture, drapery, and costume—it is a striking portrayal of a scholar in repose, the subject having just looked away from his book in order to gaze into the distance and pause before turning the page. The viewer is not included in the subject's thoughts but is merely an observer outside the action.

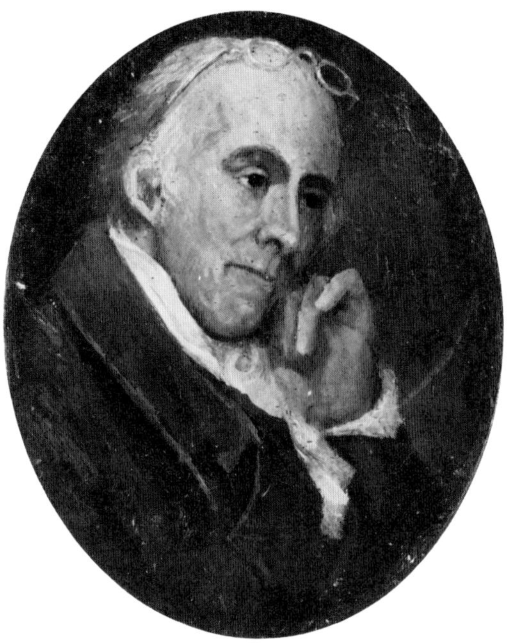

Benjamin Rush *PA 105*

Artist: Unknown

Miniature; oil on wood; oval, 3 x 21/2; not signed or dated. Presented by Dr. George P. Müller in 1939. This work is a copy made after the characteristic Rush pose used in five portraits by Thomas Sully between 1809 and 1815. *PA 105*

Dr. Rush is shown bust length in a pose similar to that in von Helmbold's portrait, described above. In this version the artist has regularized the features by shortening and straightening the nose, widening the mouth, and rounding the chin. He has also changed the color of the eyes from blue to brown. The miniaturist has elaborated the costume by showing more of the shirt collar, cuffs, and jabot. The style of painting is smooth and the head and hand have been constructed reasonably well in solid volumes. The artist has cleverly composed the contours and shape of the subject's head, neck, shoulders, and back to conform to the oval shape of the wooden panel.

Artist: Unknown

Silhouette, either black ink on white paper or black paper glued onto a grayish-white cardboard backing; 3 x 21/2; not signed or dated. Presented by Dr. George P. Müller in 1939. *PH 547*

Dr. Rush is shown bust length, with body and head turned in profile to the right. There is an irregular contour to his long hair which is tied back by a ribbon into a queue. He has a sloping forehead, a prominent eyebrow ridge, a long, aquiline nose whose tip points down to a pinched mouth, and a receding, rounded chin. All that is described of his costume is the jabot, which stands away from his chest with angular contours. The bust has been finished off in a slightly curving line between two sharp points. The outline of the silhouette has been drawn skillfully in irregular contours to make a dramatic, black opaque form against the light background.

Artist: Unknown

Oil on canvas; 36 x 28, top corners rounded; not signed or dated. Presented by Mrs. Louis A. Biddle in 1943. Shown at the College of Physicians' Centennial Celebration Loan Collection of Portraits, *1887, with the subject being identified as Benjamin Rush, the artist as Benjamin West, and the owner as Dr. A. W. Biddle. "Evidence" in the files of the College of Physicians in favor of this attribution is the mention in* History of Philadelphia, 1609–1884, *by John Thomas Scharf and Thompson Westcott (Phila, 1884), vol. 2, p. 1031, of "a portrait of Dr. Benjamin Rush, painted by West while Rush was prosecuting his studies in London, belonging to Dr. W. Kent Gilbert. It is a kit-cat and handsomely executed." Later records of the College of Physicians and its 1940* Catalogue of the College Collections *cast doubt on the identities of subject and artist. Although Rush and West were acquainted when Rush was in London in 1768 and 1769, Rush was then only 23 or 24 years old, and West was busy with royal commissions. Hence it seems improbable that he would have painted a young colonial physician. Experts doubt both attributions on the ground of style and likeness. The painting does not look like the work of West and does not sufficiently resemble other portraits of Rush. Further, it is not mentioned in Rush's memoirs and is not known in West's oeuvre. However, it could be a late 18th or early 19th century portrait. Additional research is needed to establish the identity of both subject and artist.* *PA 110*

The subject is shown half-length, with body turned to the left and head turned to the left and tilted diagonally down. The right hand rests on the crown of a skull. The left forearm lies on what appears to be a table top, while the left hand holds a book upright. Because of bloom on the varnish and extensive loss of paint followed by repair, it is difficult to judge the background, but the color is brownish-gray on the left and a warm brown on the right. On the table there is a green book with a paper marking the place. The subject's hair, strangely puffy, dense, and solid-looking, projects 31/2 inches from his

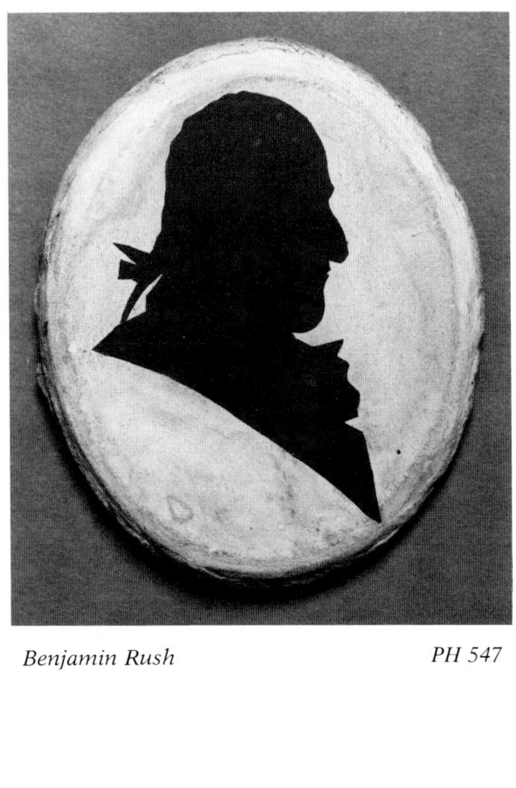

Benjamin Rush *PH 547*

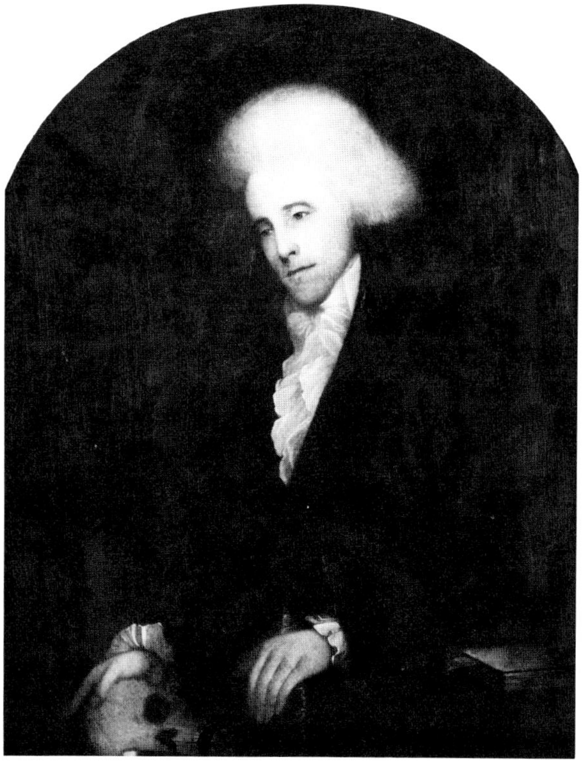

Formerly identified as Benjamin Rush *PA 110*

head. The narrow face has dark eyebrows, heavy-lidded blue eyes which look down in the direction of the head turn, a slender nose, a wide mouth with a very thin upper lip, and a narrow chin. The subject wears a white shirt with stand-up collar and ruffled cuffs, a white neckcloth tied in a bow, a white jabot, a yellow waistcoat, and a black coat. Although in lamentable condition, this portrait in all probability was smoothly painted. The head, hands, and skull are modeled in solid and three-dimensional volumes. The flat costume does not suggest the underlying body forms. The presence of a skull is unusual but is by no means unique as an iconographic symbol used to identify the profession of a physician. The bottom of the painting is crowded; it is unclear how the various objects could exist in the space depicted. The subject's narrow face, tight mouth, averted gaze, and strange hair give him an ascetic, introspective expression.

Charles Eucharist de Medicis Sajous (1852-1929)

Born at sea off the coast of France, Sajous was descended from the French-Flemish branch of the noble de Medici family and was the son of Count Charles Roustan de Medicis-Jodoigne. He added the name of his stepfather, Sajous, when his widowed mother remarried. After receiving his early education in Mexico and California, he was graduated from Jefferson Medical College in 1878. He was successively clinical lecturer in laryngology at Jefferson (1883-91), dean of the faculty and professor of laryngology at the Medico-Chirurgical College (1897-98), professor of applied therapeutics at Temple University (1910-22), and professor of applied endocrinology at the University of Pennsylvania's Graduate School of Medicine, a post he held from 1921 until his death in 1929. Although specializing in laryngology, he wrote books on hay fever and diseases of the nose and throat and invented several surgical instruments. When he became interested in the new field of endocrinology, he studied the subject in Paris from 1891 to 1897. He wrote more than 80 articles, and his treatise, *The Internal Secretions and the Principles of Medicine* (1903), was influential in the introduction and development of endocrinology and was the first comprehensive work on the subject. He was editor of *The New York Medical Journal* from 1911 to 1919. In addition to his teaching posts and his work as a writer and editor, he was a member of 22 societies, including the College of Physicians and the American Philosophical Society. He was president of the American Medical Editors Association, the American Association for the Study of the Internal Secretions, and the American Therapeutic Society. In addition to receiving an honorary LL.D. from St. Joseph's College and an honorary Sc.D. degree from Temple University in Philadelphia, he was awarded many foreign decorations and titles, including officer of the French Academy, knight of the Legion of Honor of France, member of the Gold Medal Humane Society of Belgium, knight of the Order of Leopold of Belgium, commander of St. John of Jerusalem of Spain, and a member of the Order of the Liberator of Venezuela.

Artist: Charles L. Sasportas

Oil on canvas; 29 1/2 x 24 3/4; signed and dated at lower left, "Ch. L. Sasportas. 1919." Presented by the estate of Dr. Sajous in 1942 through the efforts of Miss Louise Weissgerber, secretary at the F.A. Davis Co., where the portrait had hung. *PA 108*

Dr. Sajous is shown bust length, with body turned slightly to the left and head frontal. The atmospheric background is a medium tone of brown, lighter around the head. The subject has a high forehead, blondish-gray hair, medium-gray diagonally placed straight eyebrows, a wide-based nose, thin lips, and a white moustache and short white goatee. His large and luminous brown eyes gaze directly toward the viewer. His high-keyed complexion is rendered in various shades of orange. The center part, the curving hairline, and the pointed goatee give his face a heart shape. The subject wears a white shirt with stand-up collar, a black necktie, a black vest, and a black coat with a bright red circular lapel pin. The surface of the portrait shows a painterly style in the well-constructed head and a smoother style in the background; the flat costume does not suggest the underlying body forms. The subject's penetrating, intense, direct gaze engages the viewer's attention and almost demands a response. The dark sloping eyebrows give him a Mephistophelean look.

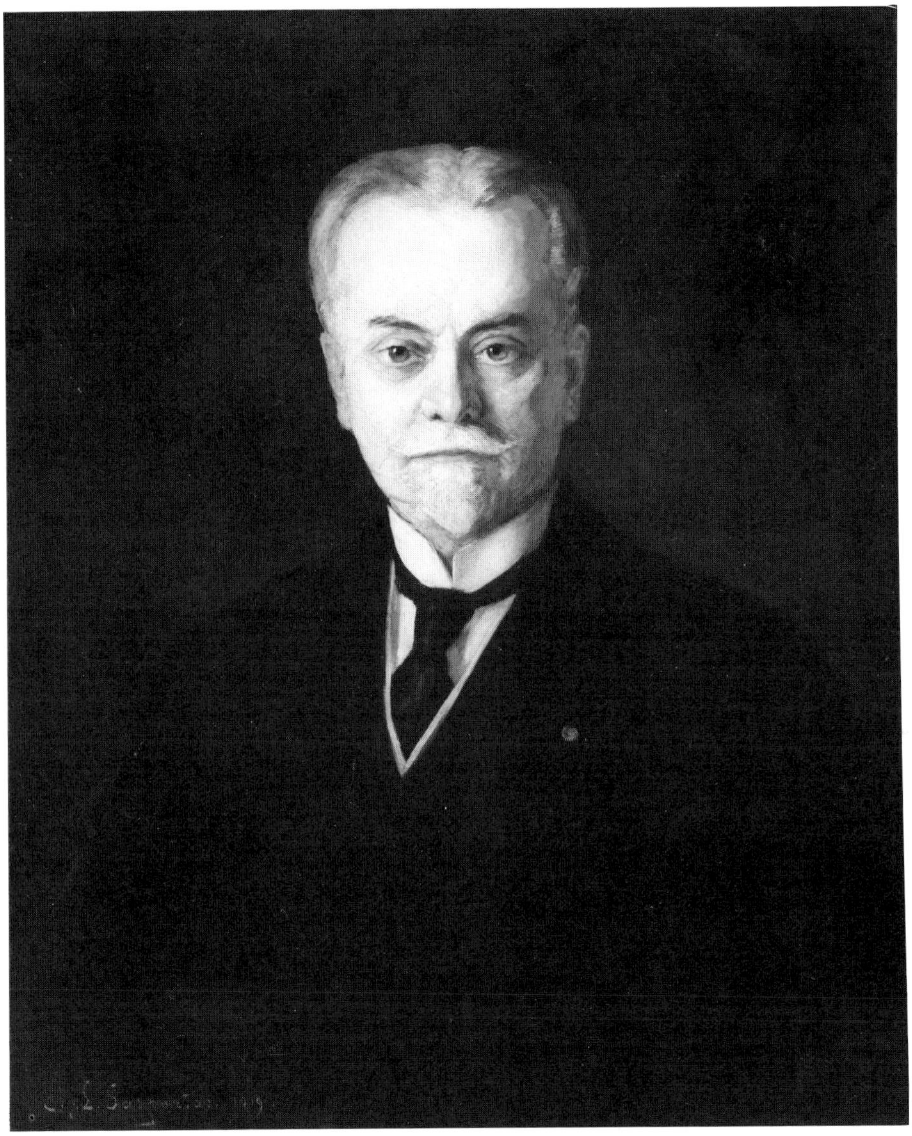

Charles Eucharist de Medicis Sajous *PA 108*

Lewis Cass Scheffey (1893–1969)

Dr. Scheffey was of German ancestry and was born in Hartford, Connecticut. His graduation with honors from the Philadelphia College of Pharmacy in 1915 made it possible for him to earn his tuition at Jefferson Medical College by working as an assistant pharmacist until he received the M.D. degree in 1920. After internship in the Jefferson Medical College Hospital he became an assistant demonstrator of gynecology at Jefferson and private assistant to Dr. Brooke M. Anspach, professor and head of the department of gynecology. He received successive academic appointments, culminating in his succession to Dr. Anspach's position in 1940. Five years later he became the first administrative head of the combined department of obstetrics and gynecology and director of the division of gynecology. He had a lifelong interest in pelvic cancer and became a recognized authority on this subject. In 1928 he established the clinic for pelvic cancer at Jefferson. He was an early advocate of the value of vaginal cytology in the diagnosis of pelvic malignancy. A founder (1951) of the Inter-Society Cytology Council, he served as its president in 1956 before it became the American Society of Cytology. He was president of the Philadelphia division of the American Cancer Society and was awarded the gold medal of that organization in 1962. He was president of the American Gynecological Society, the Obstetrical Society of Philadelphia, and the Philadelphia County Medical Society, which in 1958 gave him its Strittmatter Award for distinguished service to Philadelphia medicine. At the College of Physicians he served as counselor, vice-president, president (1955–58), and censor, and he was a generous donor. He was a trustee of the Philadelphia College of Pharmacy and recipient of its alumni award. He was president of the Jefferson Medical College Alumni Association, which awarded him an honorary L.H.D. degree in 1959, and he received an honorary Sc.D. degree from Ursinus College.

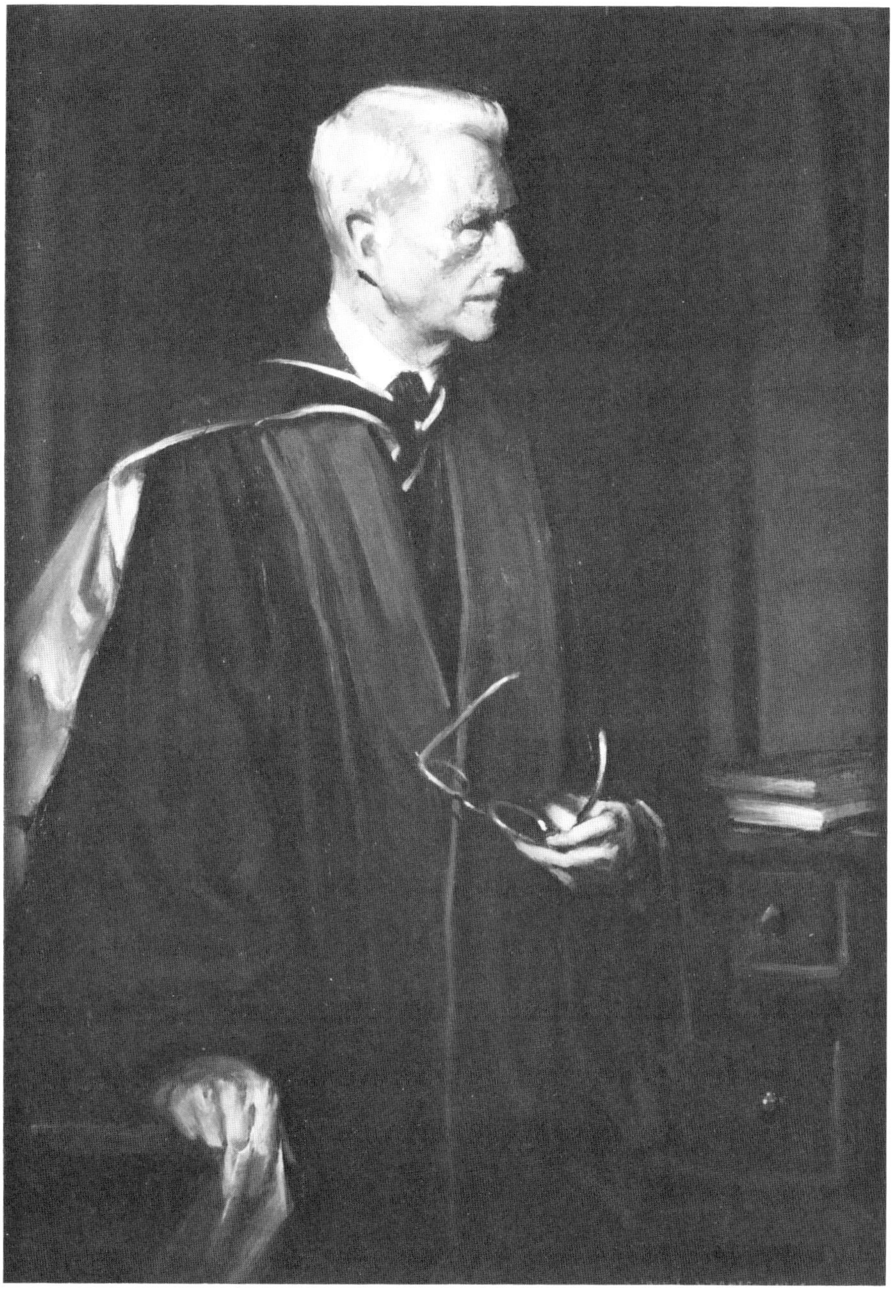

Lewis Cass Scheffey *PA 126*

Artist: John Christen Johansen (1876–1964)

Born in Copenhagen, Johansen was brought to America as a child and studied at the Art Institute of Chicago, in Paris at the Académie Julien with Jean Joseph Benjamin-Constant and Jean-Paul Laurens, and with Frank Duveneck at the Art Students' League in New York. He specialized in portraits. After a period of teaching at the Art Institute in Chicago, he set up a studio in New York. He was made an associate member of the National Academy of Design in 1911 and a full member in 1915. He was a member of the National Society of Portrait Painters, the National Institute of Arts and Letters, and the American Federation of Arts. He frequently won prizes in national expositions, including the Municipal League purchase prize and Young fortnightly prize at the Art Institute of Chicago (1903); silver medal, Chicago Society of Artists (1904); bronze medal at the St. Louis Louisiana Purchase Exposition (1904); gold medal at the Buenos Aires Exposition (1910); Saltus gold medal at the National Academy of Design (1911); Harris silver medal at the Chicago Art Institute (1911); honorable mention at the Carnegie International in Pittsburgh (1912); gold medal at the Panama-Pacific Exposition in San Francisco (1915); silver medal at the Sesquicentennial Exposition in Philadelphia (1926); French memorial gold medal at the Art Institute of Chicago (1928); and the Beck gold medal at the Pennsylvania Academy of the Fine Arts (1927). His portraits hang in many of America's important museums, including the Art Institute of Chicago, the National Gallery of Art, the Metropolitan Museum of Art, the Pennsylvania Academy of the Fine Arts, the National Collection of Fine Arts, the Corcoran Gallery of Art, the Wadsworth Atheneum, and the New-York Historical Society, as well in universities, clubs, and other institutions. He was one of the eminent portrait painters selected by the National Art Committee to execute portraits of leaders of the Allies in World War I.

Oil on canvas; 47 1/2 x 33 1/4; signed and dated at lower right, "John C. Johansen 1963." Presented by Dr. James Monroe Thorington in 1963. *PA 126*

Dr. Scheffey is shown two-thirds length, with body turned to the right and the head almost in profile to the right and tilted down slightly. He stands with his right hand leaning on a table and holding a white paper between his fingers. His left arm is flexed and he holds his spectacles in front of his body, the temple pieces upright. The upper part of the background is dark olive-green and black and vaguely suggests architectural moldings or a curtain. At the lower right there in a country-style chest of drawers painted olive green, with two books lying on top. The subject's face is narrow. He has white hair, puffy lidded dark brown eyes which look straight ahead, a thin nose with a bump at the bridge, hollow cheeks, thin lips, and a sharp chin. He wears a white shirt and a black necktie under a black academic robe with full sleeves, dark green panels down the front, and a black, blue, and white mantle with a pale blue lining. The surface of the portrait is painterly, with visible, short, choppy strokes in the well-modeled head and more fluid strokes in the background and in the academic gown. The latter is too full to reveal the underlying body. The hands are depicted very sketchily. The subject is tall and thin, with an angular face, long bony fingers, and a slightly stooped posture; these features give him a somewhat ascetic appearance. However, the pose is full of action, as if the doctor had just removed his eyeglasses, turned away from the table on which the paper was located, and was about to address an unseen visitor.

Albert Schweitzer (1875-1965)

Born in the Alsatian town of Kaysersberg, Dr. Albert Schweitzer was the son of a Protestant minister. From his early days he showed a multiplicity of interests; he studied theology and philosophy at the University of Strasbourg and music in Paris and Berlin. In addition, he was ordained in the Lutheran ministry, becoming curate of St. Nicholas church in Strasbourg. At the University of Strasbourg he served as private-docent and as principal of St. Thomas College, its theological seminary. During this time he was acclaimed as an organist at the Société Johann Sebastian Bach in Paris and at the Orféo Catalá in Barcelona. When he decided to dedicate himself to the "direct service of humanity" by becoming a physician, he paid for his tuition through organ recitals and royalties from his books on organ-building. After receiving the M.D. degree at the University of Strasbourg in 1913, he joined the Paris Missionary Society and was sent to the mission station in Lambaréné in Gabon, French Equatorial Africa. For the next four years he worked to build a hospital in the middle of the jungle. Since he and his wife were considered German aliens in French territory, they were interned in France during the last year of World War I. Schweitzer used the time to prepare a draft of his great work, *The Philosophy of Civilization*, the first two volumes appearing in 1923, and an account of his early work in Lambaréné called *On the Edge of the Primeval Forest* (1921). After the war he returned with a new staff, and they built a larger hospital in a healthier location, although access was by canoe only, as there were no roads. By 1965 this hospital-village contained 72 buildings on 225 acres, and the hospital had 500 beds. The hospital welcomed patients with almost every known ailment, but it was for the treatment of lepers that it made medical history and attracted patients from as far away as 600 miles. Although he was criticized in some circles for lack of administrative efficiency and poor standards of hygiene, Schweitzer felt that his methods had to adapt to the prevailing jungle and tribal conditions, and his credo is inscribed on a lamp outside the hospital—"Here, at whatever hour you come, you will find light and help and human kindness." In addition to the books already mentioned, his other works attest to his widespread interest in theology, peace, philosophy, and music, and include *The Quest of the Historical Jesus* (1906), *Paul and His Interpreters* (1911), *J.S. Bach* (1908), *J.S. Bach: Complete Organ Works, A Critico-Practical Edition* (1912-14), *Memoirs of Childhood and Youth* (1924), *My Life and Thought* (1931), *From My African Notebook* (1937), and *Peace or Atomic War?* (1958). Schweitzer's innumerable awards included honorary degrees from universities in Zürich, Prague, Tübingen, Edinburgh, Oxford, St. Andrews, Cambridge, Capetown, and Chicago. He won the Goethe Prize of the City of Frankfurt, the first Paracelsus medal of the German Physicians Congress, and the Nobel peace prize, awarded in 1953 for his humanitarian work in the African jungle and for his philosophy of reverence for life. In 1955 he received the British Order of Merit from Queen Elizabeth II. He was an honorary member of medical societies in many countries, including the College of Physicians of Philadelphia.

Artist: Louis Michelotti

Plaster, painted bronze color; 11 3/4 x 7 1/4 x 6; rectangular base integral with sculpture, 1 3/8 in. high in front; signed and dated on rear of base, "By Louis Michelotti.©.59" Inscription on front of base; "Dr. Albert Schweitzer." Presented by Dr. Douglas Macfarlan in 1960. *ST 564*

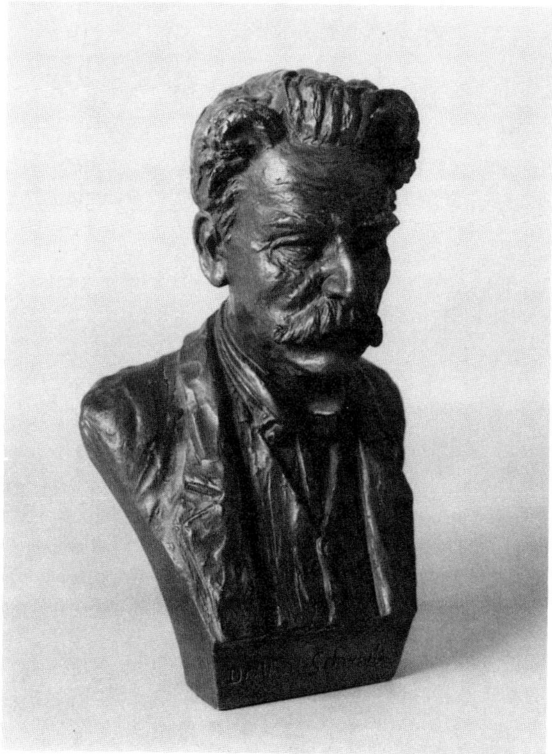

Albert Schweitzer *ST 564*

Dr. Schweitzer is shown bust length, with body and head frontal. He has very thick, wavy hair which curves around his high forehead. His deep-set, narrow eyes are like slits, and their incised pupils and irises are scarcely visible. He has hollow cheeks, a long nose with a bump in the middle and a long tip which points down to his mouth, and a bushy, long moustache. There are deep age lines in his forehead, around his eyes, and next to his nose. The subject wears a shirt with stand-up collar, a bow tie, a vest, and a coat. The surface of this sculpture is usually irregular and active for the medium of plaster. The head is well constructed in its modeling of planes. The costume is flat and does not suggest underlying body forms. The portrayal is naturalistic, and the hair and moustache provide instant recognition of this world-famous physician. Although the wrinkles give a physical indication of old age, the subject's facial expression is neutral and no effort has been made to interpret his character.

William Shippen, Jr. (1736–1808)

Dr. William Shippen, Jr., born in Philadelphia, was the son of an eminent physician. After receiving the A.B. degree from the College of New Jersey (later Princeton) in 1754, he studied medicine with his father until 1758 and then continued his medical education abroad. In London he studied anatomy under John Hunter (q.v.) and midwifery with William Hunter and Colin McKenzie; he was on friendly terms with John Fothergill (q.v.), who was greatly interested in Shippen's plans to establish courses in midwifery and anatomy in Philadelphia. At the University of Edinburgh he studied with Alexander Monro Secundus and William Cullen (q.v.) and obtained the M.D. degree in 1761. When he returned to Philadelphia he carried with him a number of superb anatomical drawings by Jan Van Riemsdyk and anatomical casts, placed in his care by Fothergill for use in teaching at the Pennsylvania Hospital. In 1762 he began a series of lectures in anatomy at the home of his father to students of medicine and other selected gentlemen. In 1765 he began his lectures on midwifery. These were the first systematic courses in those subjects given in this country. In 1765 he was elected professor of surgery and anatomy at the newly founded medical school of the College of Philadelphia. When the College became the University of Pennsylvania in 1791, he held the chair of midwifery in addition to the chairs of anatomy and surgery. He was physician to the Pennsylvania Hospital from 1778–1802, except during absences for military service. In 1776 he had been appointed chief physician and director-general of the hospital of the continental army in New Jersey. Later he was made director-general of all the hospitals on the west side of the Hudson River, after John Morgan's dismissal from this portion of his duties. The result was a breach between the two men. In 1777 Shippen was appointed to succeed Morgan as director-general of the continental army hospital and chief physician of the American army, having submitted to Congress a plan for reorganization of the Army medical department. Shippen, accused of appropriating military funds and medical supplies, was subjected to court martial. After acquittal he had a second session before the tribunal. In 1781 he resigned, returning to medical practice and teaching in Philadelphia. Aside from his doctoral dissertation and lecture notes, Shippen did not contribute to the medical literature. He belonged to the American Philosophical Society and to the College of Physicians, of which he was a senior founder, vice-president, censor, and president (1805–08).

Artist: Unknown

Oil on canvas, mounted on wood; 35 1/2 x 28 1/2; not signed or dated. Presented by Dr. George B. Wood in 1866. Shown in the College of Physicians' Centennial Celebration Loan Collection of Portraits, *1887, the College of Physicians being listed as owner. Copy after a portrait of Shippen by Gilbert Stuart, ca. 1789, owned by Edward Shippen. Consultants have offered two suggestions for the identity of the copyist—James Reid Lambdin (1807–1889) and Rembrandt Peale (1788–1860)—but further research is needed on this point. At least four oil copies of the Stuart portrait by other artists are known to exist, as well as several engravings.* *PA 19*

Dr. Shippen is shown half-length, seated, with body and head turned to the right. His right arm sweeps across his body and his right hand holds a folded white paper or pamphlet. The background includes a reddish-maroon

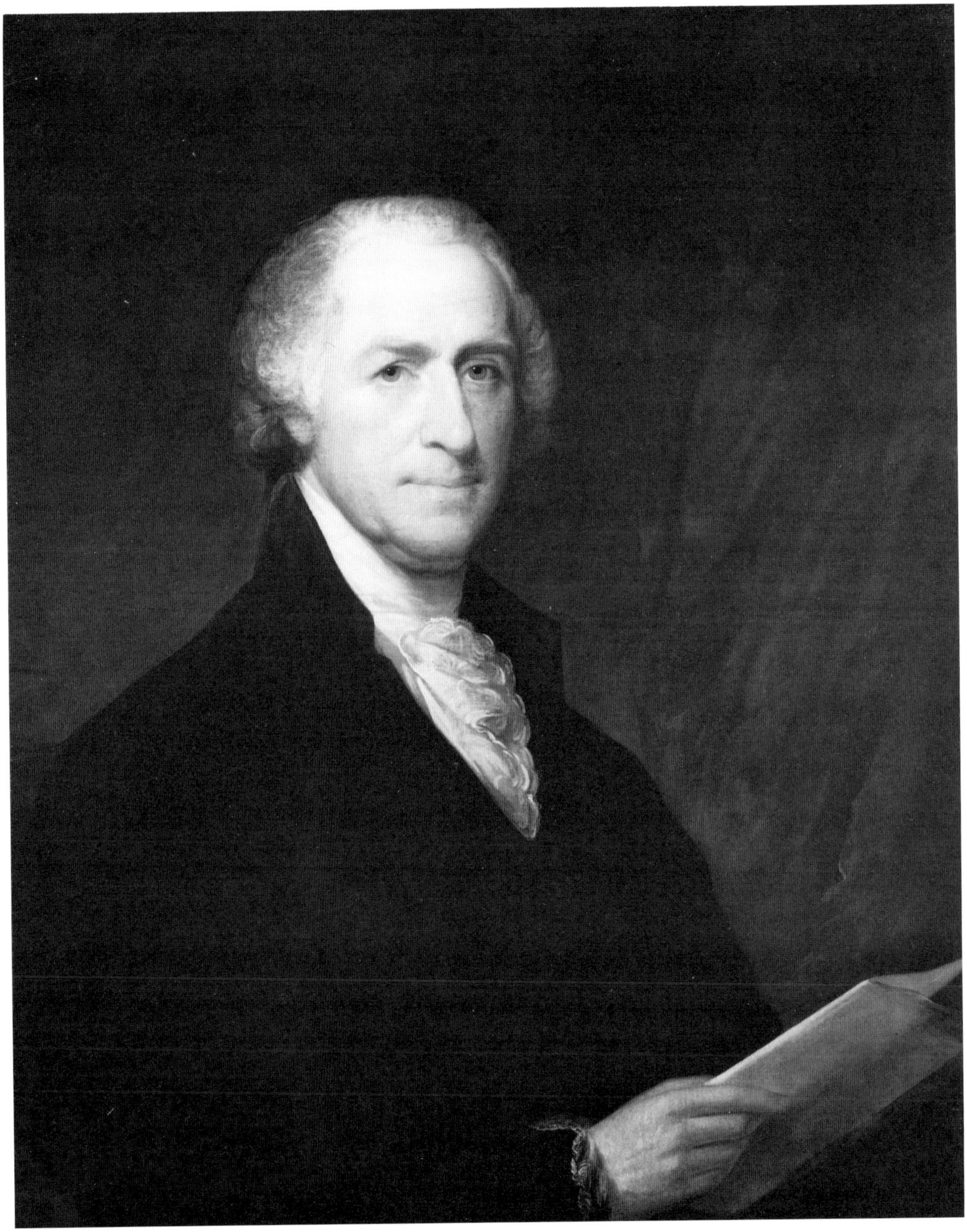

William Shippen, Jr. *PA 19*

drapery and a rounded chair back. The subject's face is rectangular. The gray hair was probably worn long in the back. Light blue-gray eyes look out of their corners toward the spectator. The long straight nose has a tip which points down to a full mouth, a prominent jawline, and a square (and doubled) chin. The complexion is distinctly fair. The subject wears a white stock, a white jabot, a black waistcoat, and a black coat with white ruffles showing at the cuff. The surface of the portrait is very smooth, without visible brush strokes. The head has been rendered in solid and three-dimensional volumes, with skillful and subtle modeling of planes. The costume is flat and does not suggest the underlying body forms. The facial expression is open and direct, engaging the spectator's attention as though in conversation. A disquieting feature is the right arm and hand, which are not present in the Stuart original. The arm was painted disproportionately short in order to fit into the lower right corner, and the hand looks wooden, especially in the schematic, diagonal line of the knuckles. Furthermore, the white paper distracts from the primary focal point of the face.

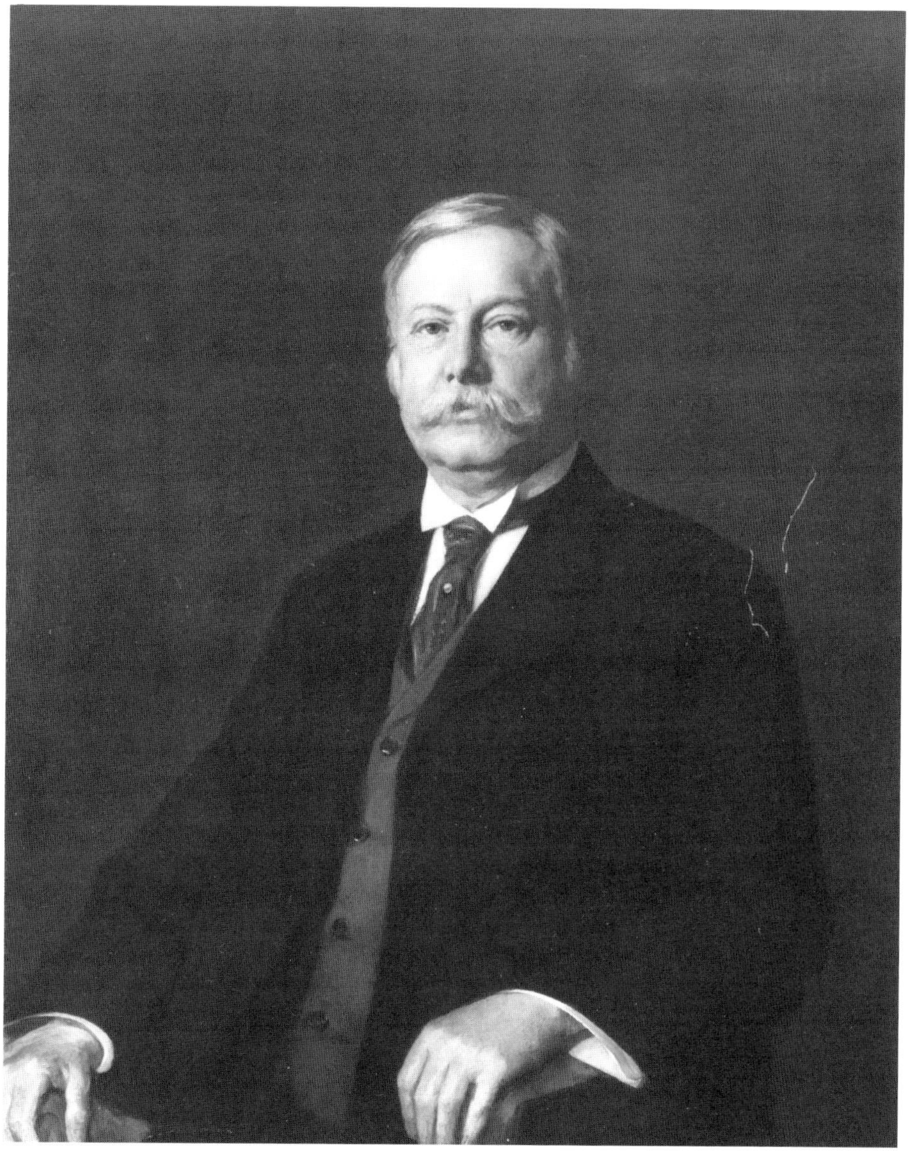

Wharton Sinkler

PA 9

Wharton Sinkler (1845-1910)

Dr. Sinkler was born in Philadelphia but was raised on a South Carolina plantation that had been in his family for several generations. His education at South Carolina College having been interrupted by the Civil War, he served in the Charleston Little Dragoons and the Second South Carolina Cavalry. After the war he came to Philadelphia and was graduated from the medical department of the University of Pennsylvania in 1868. At Episcopal Hospital he served as resident physician, attending physician (1872-79), and manager (1886-10). Although he engaged in the general practice of medicine, he began to devote himself especially to the study of nervous diseases. In 1870 he became an assistant physician to the recently organized Philadelphia Orthopaedic Hospital and Infirmary for Nervous Diseases and in 1872 was made attending physician there. He was devoted to this institution and patients came to him from distant parts of this country and Canada. He was also neurologist or consulting neurologist to the Philadelphia Hospital, the State Hospital for the Chronic Insane at South Mountain, the Widener Home for Crippled Children, and the Bryn Mawr and Germantown Hospitals. He served as chairman of the section on nervous and mental diseases of the American Medical Association, president of the American Neurological Association, and president of the National Association for the Study and Care of Epileptics. His other important positions include vice-president of the College of Physicians, trustee of the University of Pennsylvania, president of its medical department's Alumni Society, president of the Philadelphia Medical Club, trustee of the Eastern Pennsylvania Institute for Feeble-Minded and Epileptic, and president of the board of managers of the Pennsylvania Epileptic Hospital and Colony Farm. He contributed many papers on infantile paralysis and nervous diseases to the medical literature and co-authored several important systems of medicine.

Artist: Alice Mumford Roberts (Mrs. Stewart Culin) (1875–1955)

Born in Philadelphia, Alice Mumford was the granddaughter of Edward William Mumford, an artist of Newport, Rhode Island. She studied at the Pennsylvania Academy of the Fine Arts, the Philadelphia School of Design for Women, and also in Paris (1897–1900), and Spain (1901–02). She exhibited at the Paris salon in 1900 and in London at the Ville de Gant (1901) and at Earl's Court (1902). In the United States she exhibited at the National Academy of Design, the Society of American Artists, the Carnegie Institute, the Chicago Art Institute, the Minneapolis Art League, the Philadelphia Art Club, and the Pennsylvania Academy of the Fine Arts, where she won the Mary Smith prize in 1906 and 1910 and where she served on the board of the fellowship from 1902 until 1905. She won a bronze medal at the Panama-Pacific Exposition in San Francisco in 1915. She was married to her first husband, Jacob Roberts, from 1905 until his death in 1910 and then was married to Stewart Culin from 1917 until his death in 1929.

Oil on canvas, mounted on board; 38 1/4 x 31 1/4; signed and dated at upper right, "Alice Mumford Roberts/1912." Presented by the family of Dr. Sinkler in 1912. Obviously painted posthumously, the original source of this portrait has not yet been traced. *PA 9*

Dr. Sinkler is shown half-length, with body turned three-quarters to the left and head slightly to the left. His armchair is turned at an angle to the picture plane. His forearms rest on the chair arms and his hands rest on the hand holds. The atmospheric background is dark gray on the left, lighter gray-green on the right. His face is square; his hair is silvery-gray. His small blue eyes look straight ahead toward the viewer and have puffy lower lids. The nose is straight and the mouth is full-shaped but partly hidden by the long, curving, blondish-gray moustache. The jaw line is prominent, the cleft chin is square. The full cheeks have a ruddy complexion. The subject wears a white shirt with wing collar, a brown and gray patterned tie with a red tie pin, a brown vest, and a black coat. The surface of the portrait has painterly brush strokes in the beautifully modeled head and hands, which have been rendered in solid and three-dimensional, almost sculptural, forms. The costume and background are more smoothly brushed. The costume is flat but the angle and line of the buttoned vest and open coat lend a sense of the underlying body forms. The figure has great solidity and seems to occupy space in a convincing way. The subject's posture is erect. His direct gaze and confident expression offer a sense of energetic and immediate presence, which inspires a response from the viewer.

Jacob da Silva Solis-Cohen (1838–1927)

Dr. Solis-Cohen was born in New York, the descendant of a distinguished intellectual family whose da Silva Solis forbears were in the first small band of Sephardic Jews that arrived in New York in 1654. He was also a descendant of the Hays family, which reached New York in the early 18th century and moved to Philadelphia at about the time of the Revolutionary War, in which they participated. After attending Jefferson Medical College in 1857–58, Solis-Cohen entered the University of Pennsylvania Medical School, from which he received the M.D. degree in 1860. During the Civil War he served as assistant surgeon in the 26th Regiment, Pennsylvania Volunteers, as acting assistant surgeon with the U.S. Navy, and then as acting fleet surgeon with the U.S. Navy in the South Atlantic squadron. After the war he established a medical practice in Philadelphia and specialized in laryngology. In 1866 he organized a series of lectures on laryngology at the Philadelphia School of Anatomy, the first systematic course for undergraduates on this subject in the United States. He was soon appointed lecturer on electrotherapeutics and later on laryngology and diseases of the throat and chest at the Jefferson Medical College. He was also visiting physician to the German (now Lankenau) Hospital, St. Mary Hospital, the Jewish Hospital, and the Home for Consumptives. At the Franklin Institute of Philadelphia and later at the Stevens Institute of Technology in Hoboken, New Jersey, he gave popular illustrated lectures on acoustics, another of his major interests. He was a founder and co-editor of the first journal of laryngology, the *Archives of Laryngology*. He was the first president of the Philadelphia Laryngological Society and a founder and second president of the American Laryngological Association. He was twice president of the Philadelphia County Medical Society, president of the Northern Medical Association, vice-president of the Philadelphia Pathological Society, and treasurer of the Congress of American Physicians and Surgeons. He was a member of the American Philosophical Society, a fellow of the College of Physicians, and a generous donor to its Mütter Museum. He was awarded a Congressional medal of honor in recognition of his wartime service and received honorary LL.D. degrees from Temple University and Jefferson Medical College. In 1867 he wrote an important book, *Inhalation in the Treatment of Disease—Its Therapeutics and Practice,* based on research commissioned by the American Medical Association. In the same year he did a laryngotomy for a large fibrous tumor of

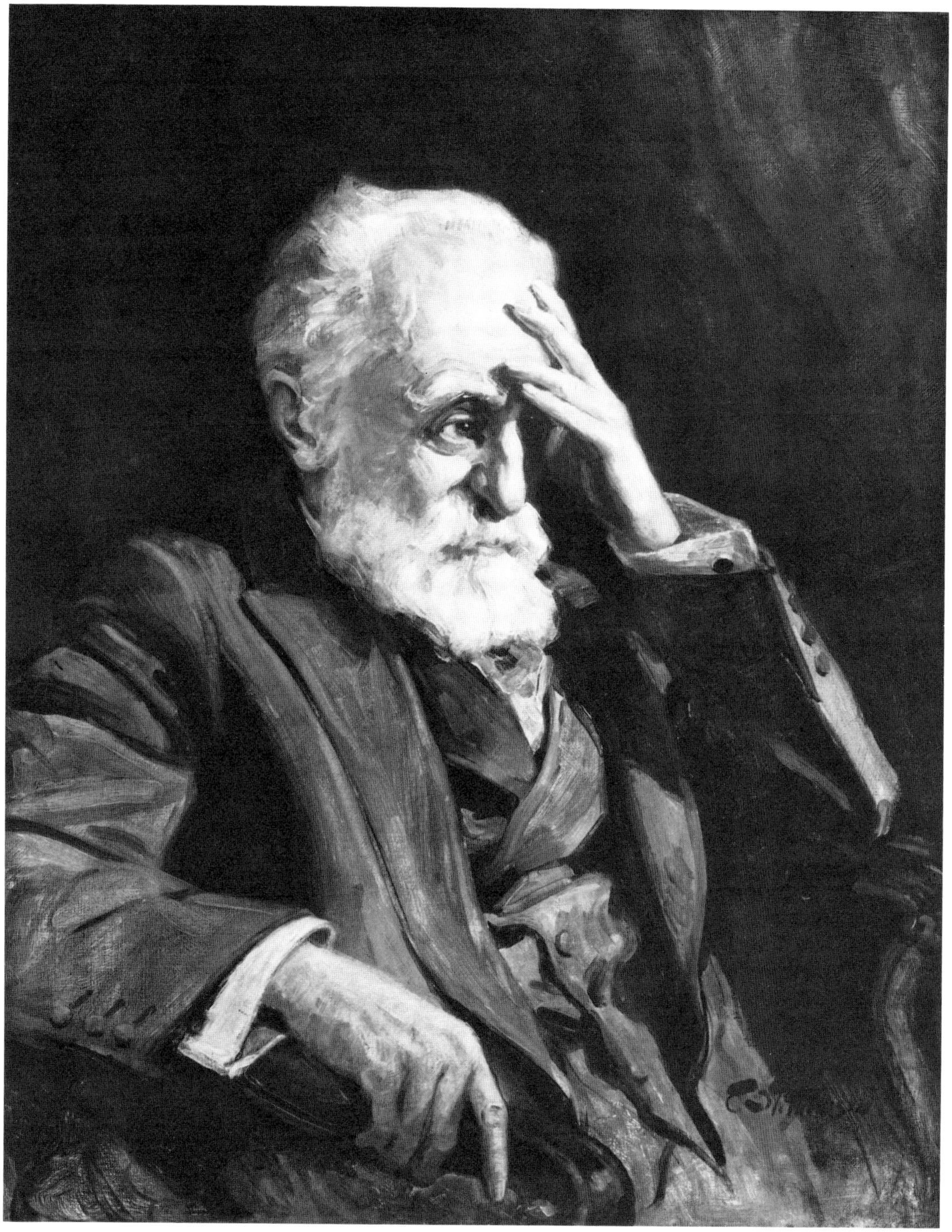

Jacob da Silva Solis-Cohen *PA 104*

the vocal cord and the next year performed the first successful laryngotomy in the world for cancer of a vocal cord. He also performed the first complete laryngectomy in America. His most famous work, *The Diseases of the Throat and Nasal Passages,* published in 1872, became a standard text. His monograph, *Croup in Relation to Tracheotomy* (1874), proposed a treatment which is credited with saving the lives of many children. Another important work is his *Surgical Treatment of Cancer of the Larynx.* He also contributed chapters to several medical encyclopedias and systems.

Artist: William Taylor Thomson (1858–1941)

Born in Philadelphia, Thomson was a well-known painter and illustrator who studied at Drexel Institute and at the Pennsylvania Academy of the Fine Arts. He was a member of the Academy's fellowship, the Art Club of Philadelphia, the Philadelphia Sketch Club, and the Philadelphia Art Alliance. He exhibited at the Academy, the Philadelphia Art Club, the Philadelphia Sketch Club, the American Art Society, the Newspaper and Illustrators' Club, and in Cincinnati and Chicago. He made illustrations for periodicals and books, and he executed numerous decorations.

Oil on canvas; 29 3/4 x 23 3/4; signed at lower right, "W.T. Thomson." Presented by the section on otolaryngology of the College of Physicians in 1939, through the efforts of Dr. George Morrison Coates, who stated the provenance of the portrait in a letter in the College of Physicians files. The portrait was found in the studio of the artist by his physician, Dr. E.J. Beardsley, who was a fellow of the College and who suggested to Dr. Coates, an influential member of the section on otolaryngology, that it be purchased. The artist told Dr. Beardsley that it was painted in the last year of the doctor's life "simply because of the interest of the artist in the subject" and the portrait had remained in the studio in the intervening years. At Jefferson Medical College there is a copy, made by Agnes Allen.

PA 104

Dr. Solis-Cohen is shown half-length, his body turned to the right, the head to the right and tilted down. He is seated in a French-style armchair turned at an angle of 45 degrees to the picture plane. His right arm and hand rest on the chair arm; his left arm rests on the chair arm and the fingers of his left hand support his head. The background is reddish-brown. The subject has a high forehead with parallel, curving wrinkles. He had thick white hair and luminous brown eyes that look out in the direction of the head turn and are surrounded by wrinkles and shadows. His very long nose has a bump at the bridge and a tip that points down to the slash of a mouth almost totally hidden by the bushy white moustache, which joins white side-whiskers and a square beard. His complexion is fair and his cheeks are pink. He wears a white shirt and green cuff links, a pink and green tie, and a gray vest and coat. The surface of the portrait is extremely painterly; the forms have calligraphic contours and the shapes have been brushed loosely, with rapid, visible strokes. The head and hands are skillfully constructed in solid and three-dimensional volumes. The costume is more freely painted but its undulating folds and shadows give a sense of the underlying bodily forms. Adding to the drama of this bold expressionistic portrayal is the contrast of light and shadow, especially the dark area of the face under the left hand, next to the highlighted nose. Although the 89-year-old subject sinks back in his chair in the traditional pose of the philosopher or melancholiac, the modernist style of the painting, with its bold color and animated brush strokes and linear contours, is in accord with the mood. The doctor is not really quiet and reflective but seems to radiate energy and alertness as one hand grips the arm of the chair and the other holds his head, as if these gestures are metaphors for deep thoughts that have been brought to the surface of his consciousness and to the surface of the painting.

Louis Starr (1849–1925)

Descended from English Quakers who arrived in Wilmington, Delaware, in 1710, Dr. Starr was born in Philadelphia. He received the A.B. degree from Haverford College in 1868 and the M.D. degree from the University of Pennsylvania in 1871. After establishing a large medical practice he began to specialize in pediatrics. He was made visiting physician to the Episcopal and Children's Hospitals and was clinical professor of the diseases of children at the University of Pennsylvania from 1884 to 1890. He was a fellow of the College of Physicians, which he served as councillor and censor, and a fellow of the Royal College of Physicians in London. He received an honorary LL.D. degree from Haverford College in 1910. He assisted Dr. William Pepper in the editing of *A System of Practical Medicine by American Authors* (1885–86) and worked with T.S. Westcott in editing *An American Text-book of Diseases of Children by American Teachers* (1894). He wrote *Diseases of the Digestive Organs in Infancy and Childhood* (1886), *Hygiene of the Nursery* (1888), and *The Adolescent Period: Its Features and Management* (1915). In 1911, when he retired from professional duties because of serious heart disease, he removed to England with his family. He spent the period of the first world war in England, mainly in London, and acted as a consultant to English doctors. Following the death of his younger son in the battle of the Somme, he sought comfort in developing his artistic talent, eventually becoming very skilled in etching. After the death of his elder son, his grief was so overwhelming that he moved to the coast of Brittany and there pursued his interest in art.

Artist: Charles Grafly (1862–1929)

For biography, see page 173.

Bronze; 17 x 8 3/4 x 9 3/4; base integral with sculpture, 3/4 in. high, resting on 14 1/2 in. high green marble and bronze pedestal terminating in bun feet ornamented with volute and shell carving; signed and dated on rear, on beveled edge at the left, "Portrait by Charles Grafly/Philadelphia 1900–01," and on beveled edge on right, "Louis Starr M.D." Presented by Mrs. Starr in 1921. Shown at the Louisiana Purchase Exposition in St. Louis, 1904, and at the Memorial Exhibition of Work by Charles Grafly, *Pennsylvania Academy of the Fine Arts, 1930, having been lent by the College of Physicians. Plaster cast at the Ulrich Museum of Art, Wichita State University.* *ST 525*

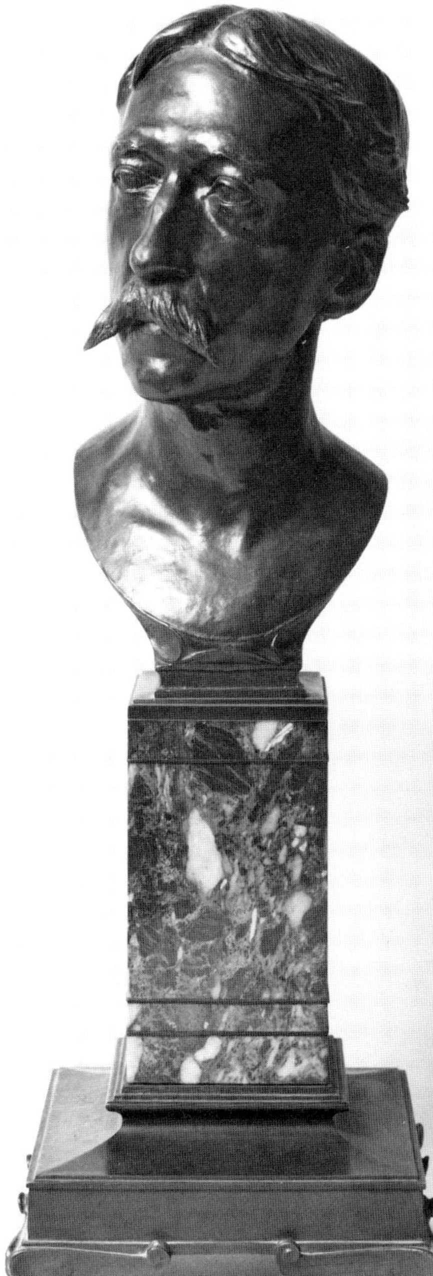

Louis Starr *ST 525*

Dr. Starr is shown head-and-neck length, with the head turned sharply to the left and tilted sideways. His face is thin and elongated. His smooth flat hair is parted at the center and brushed to the sides. His eyebrow ridge protrudes from his sloping forehead; his deepset eyes with puffy lower lids have incised irises and pupils, which look in the direction of the head turn and tilt. His long, thin nose has a bump at the bridge. The long, thick moustache tapers diagonally down to a point extending beyond the irregular jaw line and almost totally obscures the mouth. The chin is pointed. The torso, abbreviated below the neck, seems disproportionately small to balance the weight of the head. The irregular surface of the bronze enhances the play of light and shadow on the skillfully carved forms. The carving of the planes of the head has been rendered with obvious knowledge of the underlying anatomy, and the naturalistic portrayal conveys a sense of energy and vitality, as though the subject has just turned his head for an earnest reply to some unseen visitor.

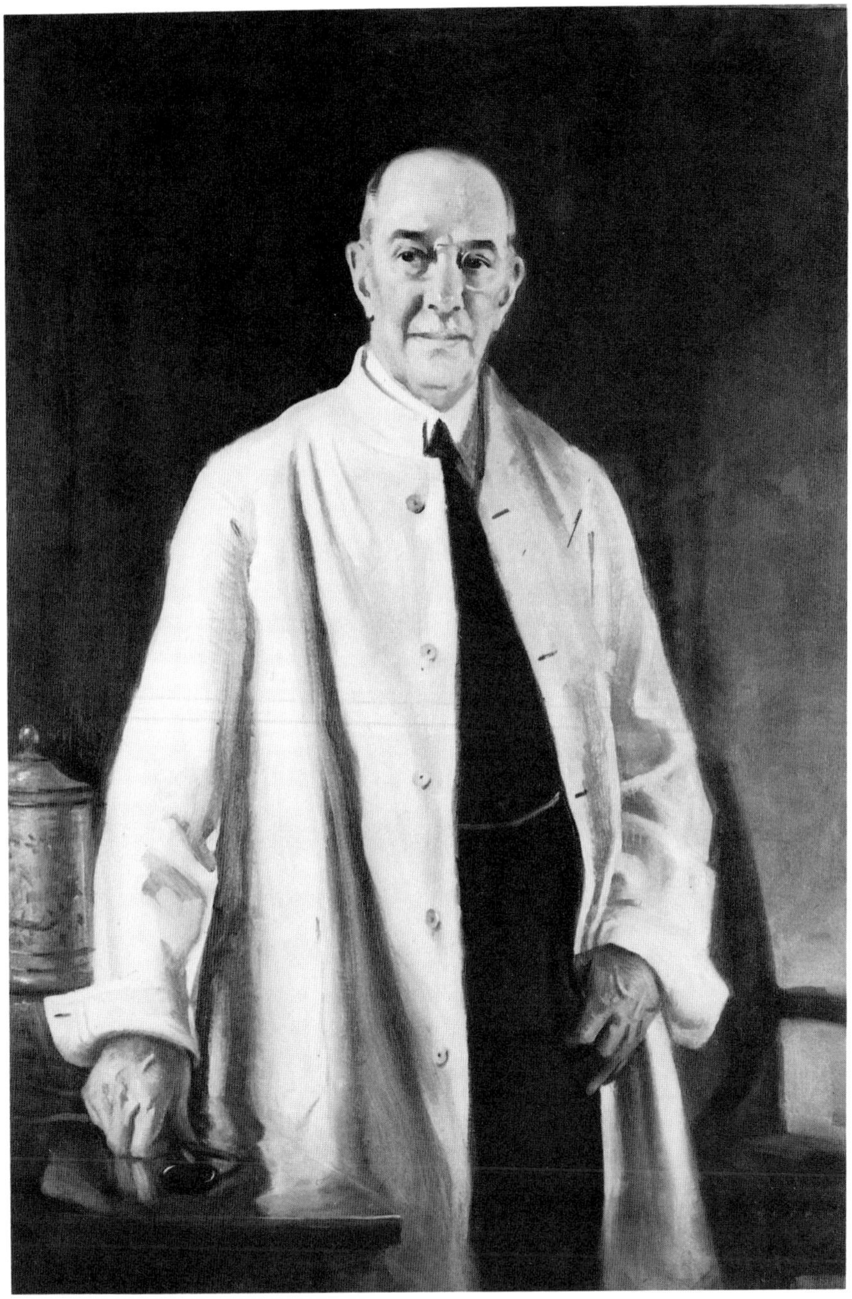

Alfred Stengel *PA 123*

Alfred Stengel (1868–1939)

Dr. Stengel, the son of a German-born civil engineer, was born in Pittsburgh. He received the M.D. degree from the University of Pennsylvania in 1889. After internship at Philadelphia General Hospital he obtained a position in the pathology department at the University. In 1893 he became pathologist to the German (now Lankenau) Hospital. In 1892 he had become the office assistant of Dr. William Pepper, professor of medicine and provost at the University of Pennsylvania, and in 1895 he became assistant director and later director of the newly founded William Pepper Laboratory of Clinical Medicine. At the University, he was successively appointed instructor in clinical medicine (1893), professor of clinical medicine (1897), professor of medicine (1911), and emeritus professor of medicine (1937). He also served the University as trustee, vice-president in charge of medical affairs, manager of its affiliated hospitals, and manager and president of the board of the Wistar Institute; he was also responsible for persuading Martin Maloney to contribute the funds for the Maloney Memorial Building. He was professor of medicine at Woman's Medical College and was physician to the University, Howard, Children's, Pennsylvania, and Philadelphia General Hospitals. He served as president of the American College of Physicians and of the College of Physicians of Philadelphia (1934–37). His contributions to the literature include editorship of the *American Journal of Medical Sciences* and of the American edition of Nothnagel's *Encyclopedia of Practical Medicine* (1902–04). He authored the chapters on diseases of the blood and diseases of the spleen in *Twentieth Century Practice of Medicine,* diseases of the intestines in Osler's *Modern Medicine,* and the chapter on diseases of the liver and gall bladder (with Dr. Richard A. Kern) in *Nelson Loose-Leaf Medicine.* He was sole author of the very successful *Text Book of Pathology* (1898). He received honorary degrees from the University of Pennsylvania, the University of Pittsburgh, and Lafayette College.

Artist: John Christen Johansen (1876–1964)

For biography see page 191.

Oil on canvas; 51 1/2 x 35 1/2; signed at lower left, "John C. Johansen." Presented by friends of Dr. Stengel in 1955. Similar in size and content to a portrait of Stengel at the University of Pennsylvania, signed and dated by Johansen in 1936. *PA 123*

Dr. Stengel is shown two-thirds length, with body turned slightly to the right and head frontal. He stands with his left thumb hooked into his trousers pocket. His right hand, leaning on a table top, grasps a stethoscope with bright red rubber tubing. The background consists of dark green and brown streaks at the top left, fading to a lighter tone at the top right, and tan and yellow streaks at the right center and bottom. A curiously small upholstered armchair is behind the subject at the right. To his left is a glass-topped table with the stethoscope and a white ceramic apothecary jar. The subject has an oval face, a bald crown with fringes of grayish-brown hair, dark brown eyebrows over brown eyes which look to the left through a pair of pince-nez, and a white brush moustache over a wide mouth. His complexion is ruddy. Under a long, white laboratory coat he wears a white shirt, a dark brown necktie, and a dark brown suit with a gold watch chain. The surface of the portrait is painterly, with broadly brushed strokes and few precise details except in the solidly modeled face and hands. Though the costume has deep folds and highlights which reflect the warm yellow tones of the background, it does not reveal the underlying bodily forms. The eminent physician is an impressive figure in his medical coat, which contrasts with the dark background. He stands poised for action, with one arm drawn back and the other thrust forward as if he were about to pick up the stethoscope. His facial expression shows eagerness to begin his work and confidence that he will do it well.

Alfred Stillé (1813–1900)

Dr. Stillé, born in Philadelphia, was descended from Swedish settlers who came to America in 1638. He entered Yale College in 1828, leaving after his sophomore year to attend the University of Pennsylvania. There he received the A.B. degree in 1832 and the M.D. degree in 1836. While house physician at Philadelphia Hospital, he came under the tutelage of Dr. W.W. Gerhard (q.v.). His personal observations of typhus patients during the epidemic of 1836 in Philadelphia and of typhoid patients abroad helped convince European physicians of Gerhard's distinction between typhus and typhoid fever. After completing his medical education in Paris under Louis, he returned to Philadelphia and was named visiting physician to St. Joseph's Hospital. He lectured on pathology and the practice of medicine at the Philadelphia Association for Medical Instruction. In 1854 he was appointed to the chair of the practice of medicine at the Pennsylvania Medical College. In 1864 he succeeded Dr. William Pepper, Sr., as professor of the theory and practice of medicine at the University of Pennsylvania, a post he held until 1884, when he was awarded emeritus professorship. He was an army surgeon in the Satterlee Hospital in Philadelphia during the Civil War. He was a founder and president of the Philadelphia Pathological Society, president of the Philadelphia County Medical Society, president of the College of Physicians (1883–84), and a founder, first secretary, and president of the American Medical Association. His contributions to the medical literature include *The Elements of General Pathology* (1848), *Epidemic Meningitis, or Cerebro-spinal Meningitis* (1867), *Cholera* (1885), *Materia Medica and Therapeutics* (1860), and, with John M. Maisch, the *National Dispensatory.*

Artist: Bernard Uhle (1847–1930)

For biography, see page 3.

Oil on canvas, mounted on board; 45 1/2 x 36 1/2; signed and dated at lower right, "B. Uhle/1892." Presented on behalf of the medical profession in 1892, on the same occasion as the portrait of Oliver Wendell Holmes (see entry on Holmes). *PA 4*

Dr. Stillé is shown three-quarters length, his body turned three-quarters to the left and head slightly to the left. He is seated in a Victorian armchair, turned at an angle of 45 degrees to the picture plane. The chair is upholstered in red velvet and has a carved classical-style head on the arm supports. His arms rest on the chair arms; his left hand holds the hand hold, while his right hand is pendent. The atmospheric space, darker on the right and lighter on the left, reveals the base of an architectural pilaster. At the lower right are bookshelves and three rows of books. At the lower left there is a table with two books, one open and one closed. The subject's face is angular. He has smooth, white hair, short thick eyebrows, and blue eyes which gaze out in the direction of the head turn and have puffy lower lids. His cheeks are hollow. He has an aquiline nose, a full white moustache which joins the side-whiskers, and a long, white, square beard that obscures his mouth. He wears a white shirt, a black cutaway coat, a black vest and trousers, and a gold ring. The surface of the portrait is brushed smoothly. The head and hands have been rendered meticulously in solid and three-dimensional planes that are almost sculptural.

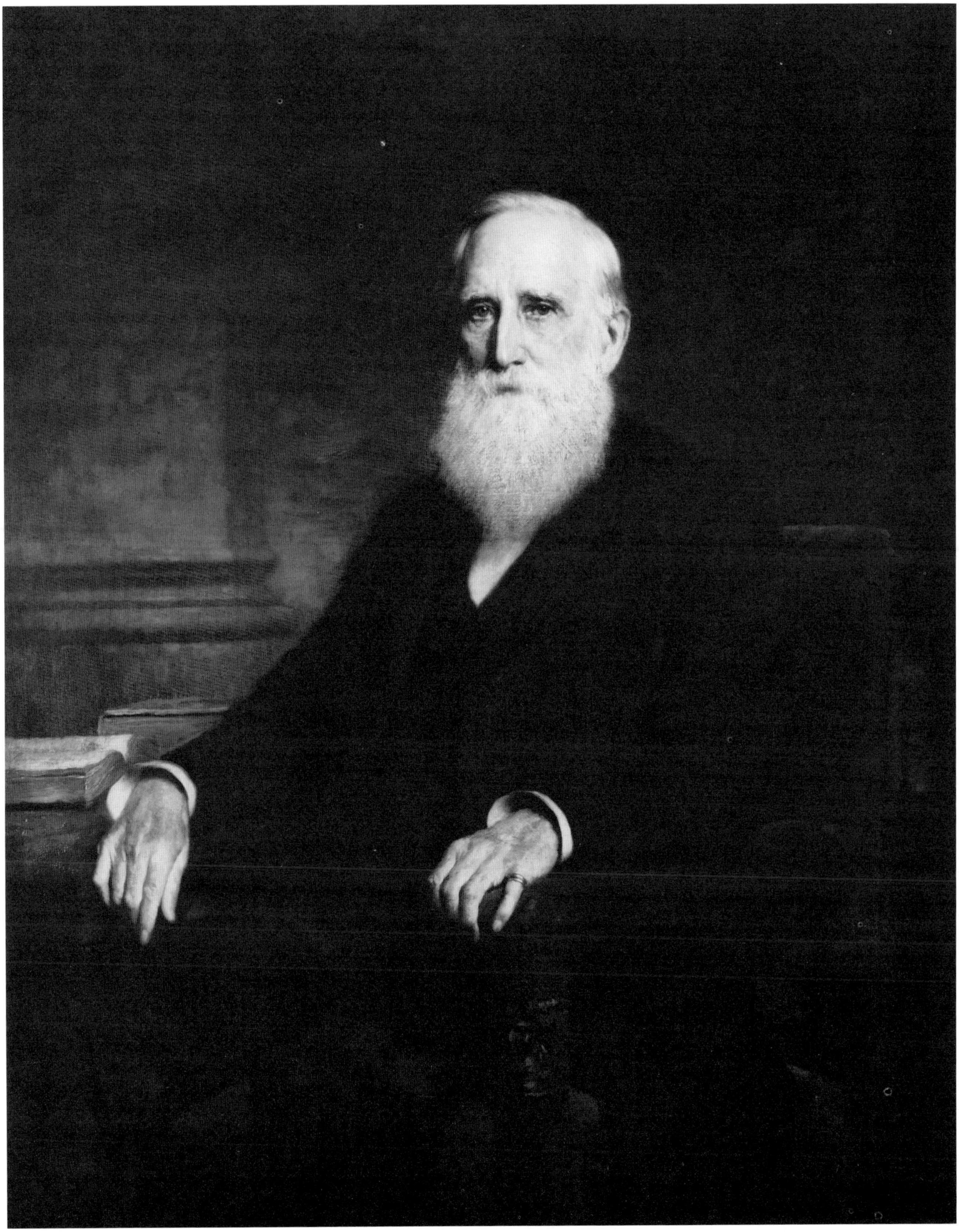

Alfred Stillé PA 4

The costume, more fluidly brushed, suggests the underlying bodily forms. The portrayal of this elderly physician communicates dignity and wisdom accumulated through the years, not only because of the patriarchal beard, but also because of the iconographical content of the pilaster, books, and furniture. Although the facial expression is calm and reflective, energy and vigor are suggested by the erect position of the head and the strength of the hands.

Georg Friedrich Louis Stromeyer (1804–1876)

Born in Hannover, Germany, Dr. Stromeyer was the son of a surgeon who studied in England and introduced Jennerian vaccination into Germany. Like his father, Stromeyer studied not only in Germany but also in England and France. He was professor successively in Erlangen, Munich, Freiburg, and Kiel. He was surgeon-general in the Schleswig-Holstein and Hannoverian armies and was considered the father of modern military surgery in Germany. He wrote extensively on war wounds and field sanitation, his most famous work on that subject being *Maxims of War Surgery*. Although Stromeyer was not the first to perform subcutaneous section of the Achilles tendon, he developed the technique and applied subcutaneous tenotomy in many deformities dependent on muscular defects, such as strabismus, wry-neck, and clubfoot. He is considered one of the founders of modern orthopaedics. He treated more than 350 patients with clubfoot, the most famous being a physician, John William Little, who after his own cure introduced this method into England and established the Royal Orthopaedic Hospital in London.

Artist: Friedrich-Wilhelm Engelhard (1813–1902)

Born in Grönhagen, Germany, Engelhard studied art with Bertel Thorwaldsen and Herman Vilhelm Bissen in Copenhagen and with Ludwig Schwanthaler in Munich. He worked in Paris, London, Munich, Rome, Hamburg, and Hannover. He was a painter and sculptor of portraits, historical and religious subjects, and monumental public works.

Plaster, painted black; 23 1/2 x 18 1/2 x 11; the lower edge of the bust, beveled for about 3 in., is inscribed, "Stromeÿer"; signed and dated on rear of right shoulder, "W. Engelhard/ Hanov. 1876." Presented by contributors to the Stromeyer oration in 1877. *ST 537*

Dr. Stromeyer is shown bust length, with body frontal and head turned very slightly to the right. His square head has thick, deeply carved clumps of hair that project in all directions. His forehead has rows of parallel lines that curve downward to connect with the wrinkles at the outer corner of his eyes. His eyebrows project and overhang his deepset eyes that have carved irises and pupils and that look in the direction of the head turn. The eyes have deeply lined, puffy lower lids. The tip of the aquiline nose almost touches the bushy moustache, which obscures the mouth. The subject has an angular jawline and a square chin. Below the thick neck and the clavicle, the anatomy of the broad torso is merely suggested. The sculpture has the uneven surface characteristic of plaster. The portrayal is one of physical strength and almost fiercely aggressive character, as emphasized by the large scale, massive proportions, leonine hair, piercing gaze, and tightly clenched jaw.

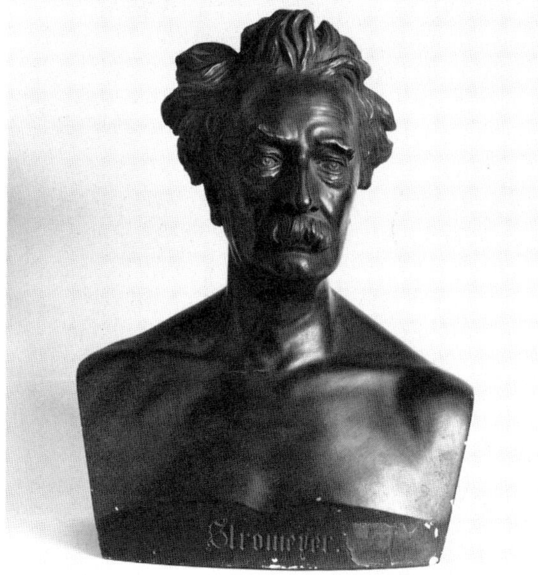

Georg Friedrich Louis Stromeyer *ST 537*

Katharine R. Boucot Sturgis (b.1903)

Dr. Sturgis, born in Philadelphia, studied at the University of Pennsylvania for two years until 1923, when she interrupted her education to marry and raise two children. She completed her premedical studies at Pennsylvania State University in 1935, and in 1942 she received the M.D. degree from Woman's Medical College after recovering from a prolonged attack of tuberculosis. She took an internship at the hospital of the Woman's Medical College and a residency in chest disease at the Herman Kiefer Hospital in Detroit. Returning to Philadelphia, she took charge of chest X-ray surveys for the Philadelphia Tuberculosis and Health Association and then for the City Department of Health. At the Woman's Medical College she became instructor in medicine in 1945 and was promoted through successive appointments to become clinical professor of medicine and chairman of the department of preventive medicine, a post she held from 1952 until 1968. In order to qualify better for the latter position, she took time off to receive a Master of Public Health degree from the Johns Hopkins School of Hygiene and Public Health in 1954 and to become a diplomate of the American Board of Preventive Medicine (1955). In 1969 she was made emeritus professor of preventive medicine. At the Graduate School of Medicine of the University of Pennsylvania, she was special lecturer in radiology and in internal medicine and was associate in medicine from 1951 to 1963. She held other appointments at Philadelphia General Hospital, Jefferson Medical College, Woman's Medical College

Hospital, Veterans Administration Hospital, and Landis State Hospital. From 1945 to 1947 she participated in the Philadelphia Diabetic Survey, a study of tuberculosis in diabetics, and published a number of important papers on her observations. When effective antimicrobial therapy promised to eradicate tuberculosis as a major public health problem, she shifted her attention to cancer of the lung. In 1951 she and David A. Cooper surveyed a population of 6000 older male volunteers for an epidemiologic study of bronchogenic carcinoma and undertook the Philadelphia Pulmonary Neoplasm Research Project, in which each patient was followed for ten years. Careful observation of the findings revealed cigarette smoking to be an important etiologic factor in pulmonary cancer. It was concluded that semi-annual screening was of little help and that prevention was the only way to attack this disease. More than 20 articles were written on this work, which inspired similar studies here and abroad. In more recent years Dr. Sturgis has been in the forefront of the battle against air pollution. Other scientific activities are her work as special consultant to the Solitary Nodule Project of the University of Pittsburgh School of Public Health and the National Cancer Institute and service on the public health and preventive medicine committee of the National Board of Medical Examiners. Although she has always downplayed her role as a pioneering woman physician, she has received the esteem of her male colleagues by becoming the first woman to fill the following important positions: vice-president of the American Thoracic Society, president of the Pennsylvania Thoracic Society, president of the Laennec Society of Philadelphia, vice-president and then president (1972–73) of the College of Physicians, president of the Philadelphia County Medical Society, vice-president of the Association of Teachers of Preventive Medicine, president of the American College of Preventive Medicine, and member of the council of the National Institute of Environmental Health Services. Dr. Sturgis is the author of more than 80 scientific articles. In addition, she wrote sixty-nine editorials for the *Archives of Environmental Health,* of which she was editor from 1960 to 1970. She wrote "Early Detection and Prevention of Lung Cancer" in J.P. Hubbard's *The Early Detection and Prevention of Disease* (1957), "Preclinical Bronchogenic Carcinoma" in E. Naclerio's *Bronchopulmonary Diseases* (1957), and "Diseases of Respiratory System" in the *Encyclopedia Britannica* (1961). Among her awards are the Distinguished Daughter of Pennsylvania, the Philadelphia Gimbel award, the Trudeau Medal of the National Tuberculosis and Respiratory Diseases Association, the Strittmatter award of the Philadelphia County Medical Society, an award from the Philadelphia Division of the American Cancer Society, honor medal of the Daughters of the American Revolution, and an award from the American Academy of Occupational Medicine. She has received honorary degrees from Keuka College, Beaver College, Woman's Medical College, and Thomas Jefferson University. In 1964 she was married to Dr. Samuel Booth Sturgis (q.v.).

Artist: William Arthur Smith (b. 1918)

Smith was born in Toledo, Ohio, and began his study of art at an unusually early age under the tutelage of Theodore J. Keane, former dean of the Chicago Art Institute. He established a studio in New York at the age of 19 and studied at the Art Students' League and later, in Paris, at the École des Beaux Arts and the Académie de la Grande Chaumière. During the next few decades he became an instructor at the Grand Central Art School and Pratt Institute in New York and a lecturer at the Academy of Fine Arts in Athens, the University of Santa Thomas in Manila, the Academy of Fine Arts in Warsaw, and many American universities, including Bucknell and Carnegie-Mellon. An artist of international renown, he works in oil, water color, and graphics, and he is celebrated not only for his portraits but for his landscapes, animal paintings, and figure paintings of both genre and historical subjects. His paintings range from illustrations for magazines and designs for postage stamps, including the well-known Boston Tea Party series, to monumental murals such as the historical series for the Maryland House of Representatives. This includes one panel honoring the contributions of Dr. William Welch to the development of the Johns Hopkins Medical School. Other medical subjects, in addition to many portraits, are Dr. William Morton's first use of anesthesia (John Hancock Collection) and Clara Barton attending the wounded in a wartime hospital (Humble Collection). Smith's paintings and prints have been exhibited in almost every major museum in the United States and are represented in the permanent collections of the Metropolitan Museum of Art, the Los Angeles County Museum, the National Academy of Design, the Library of Congress, and the National Portrait Gallery. One of his most memorable portraits is at the latter museum and depicts his friend, Carl Sandburg, who reciprocated with a poem entitled "Bill Smith." Smith has had more than thirty one-man shows in America, Europe, and Asia. In addition to his studio in Bucks County, Pennsylvania, he maintains one in Paris and has worked for long periods in China, Japan, and Burma. Besides his duties as artist, teacher, and lecturer he is an articulate critic and observer. He has written articles for catalogues and books and two articles on the art scene behind the Iron Curtain and in the Orient for *Harper's Bazaar.* He has served as president of the American Water Color Society and as president of the UNESCO-sponsored International Association of Art. His awards for oil painting, watercolors, and prints are

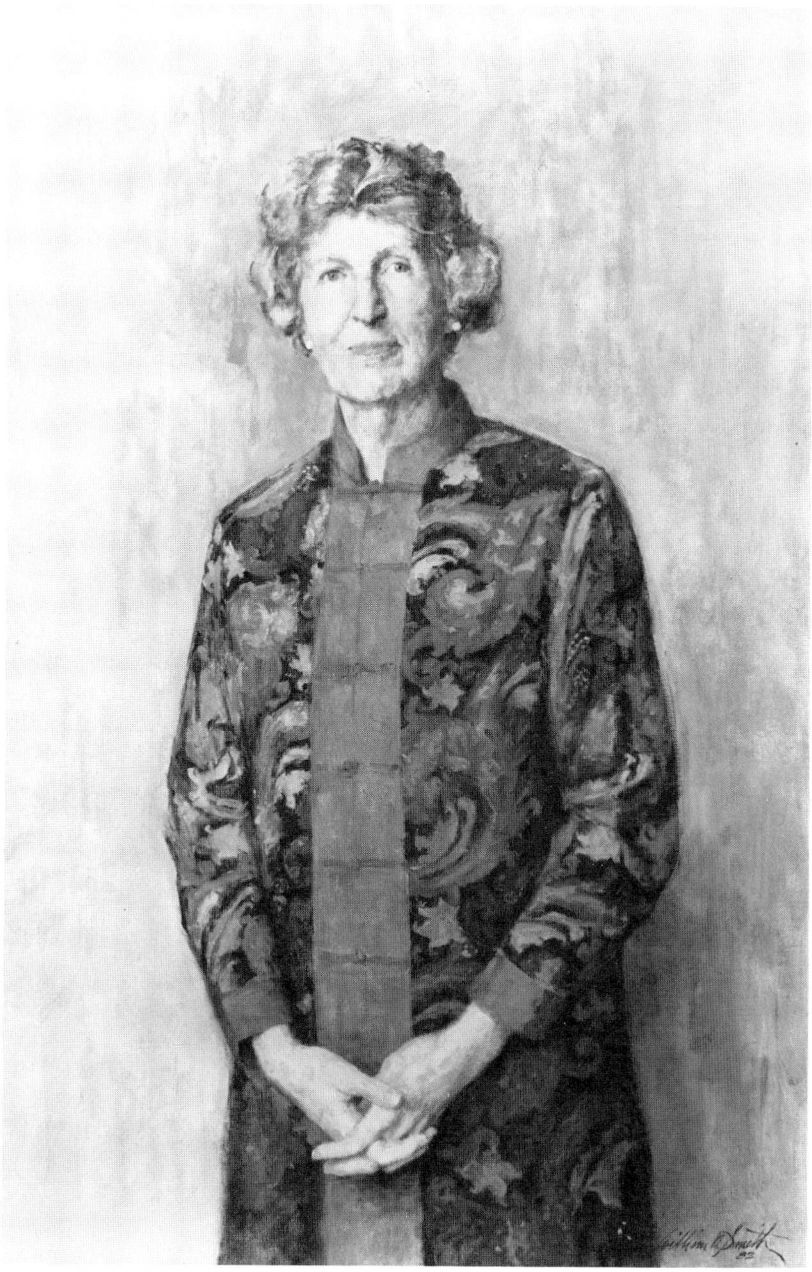

Katharine R. Boucot Sturgis *PA 146*

almost innumerable. He was the first painter ever to win twice both the gold medal and the grand prize of the American Water Color Society. He has also won prizes at the National Academy of Design, where his election to membership in 1952 made him the youngest member at that time.

Oil on canvas; 39 1/4 x 25 3/4; signed and dated lower right, "William A. Smith/82." Presented by Dr. Katharine R. Boucot Sturgis in 1982. *PA 146*

Dr. Sturgis is shown three-quarters length, her body turned slightly to the left and her head slightly to the right and tilted up. She stands with hands loosely clasped in front of her body. The mottled background has rectangular, vertical strokes of light grayish-violet over a layer of light umber-yellow. Her round face has short, curly blond hair with brown-violet shadows. Her bright blue eyes look out in the direction of the head turn and tilt. Her nose is straight with a pointed tip. She has a small full-shaped mouth, wears bright red lipstick, and has a round jawline and chin. She wears an oriental-style dress which has an all-over floral pattern in colors of turquoise, purple, violet, yellow-green, and dark blue. The dress has long sleeves and frog closings. Its mandarin collar, central vertical panel, and cuffs are bright pinkish-red. She wears white pearl button earrings and pink nail polish. The surface of the portrait is painterly, with quickly executed, visible brush strokes. The face and hands are extremely well modeled in solid and three-dimensional planes. Their color is related to that of the background. Although the costume has straight lines and an all-over pattern, it still suggests the underlying body forms. The subject stands erect and calm and has an engaging smile. Her expression radiates eagerness, poise, and confidence, enhanced by the slight turn and tilt of her body and head. This adds a sense of energy and alertness.

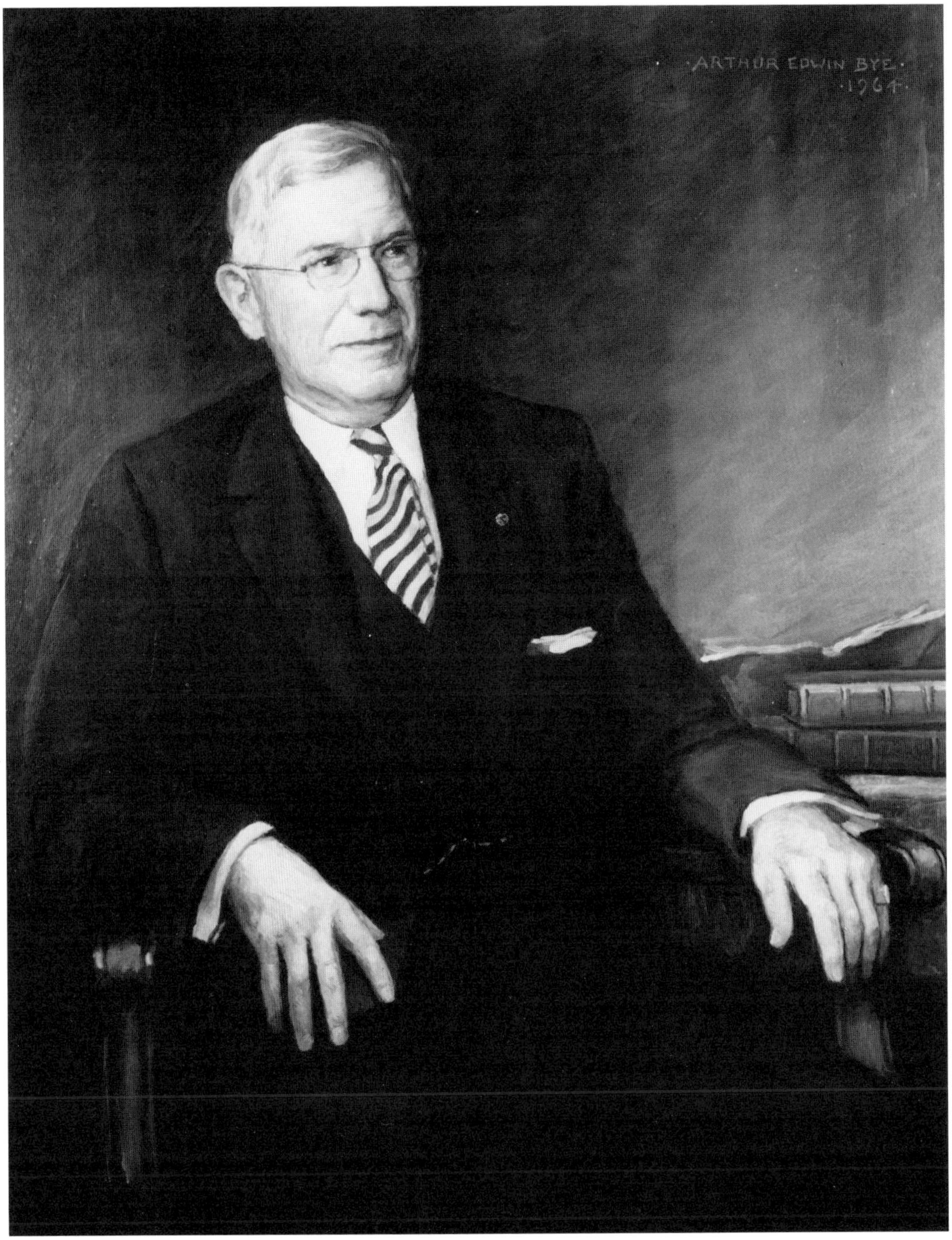

Samuel Booth Sturgis *PA 136*

Samuel Booth Sturgis (1891–1983)

Born near Philadelphia, Dr. Sturgis was descended from a distinguished family which came to America in 1643. While preparing for a career in the ministry at Haverford College, he was stricken with typhoid fever. After his recovery he changed his course of study to medicine. He was graduated from Haverford in 1910 and received the M.D. degree from the University of Pennsylvania in 1914. After interning at Easton Hospital (Pennsylvania), he was named director of Foothills Sanatarium, a small hospital in the Blue Ridge country of Lenoir, North Carolina. In addition to his duties at the hospital, he had an office over the local drug store and made house calls to his mountain-folk patients by horse and buggy or on horseback. In 1916 he married Dr. Margaret Castex Jones, who was descended from a 17th century North Carolina family and who had graduated from Woman's Medical College of Philadelphia. She joined him in practice in North Carolina, until he was commissioned as a first lieutenant in the army medical corps in 1917 and was sent to the University of Pennsylvania for special training in neurosurgery. He was assigned to Base Hospital No. 65 in South Carolina and then sent to Kerhuon, France, to care for the sick and wounded of the American Expeditionary Forces who were waiting to be evacuated. After being mustered out in 1919, he returned to Philadelphia, where he and his wife established a medical practice. In addition, he worked at the surgical dispensary at the University of Pennsylvania, was an instructor in operative surgery under Astley P.C. Ashhurst (q.v.), worked in the office of Dr. M. Howard Fussell (professor of therapeutics at the University of Pennsylvania), became an assistant in the private practice of Dr. George McLeod, was a physician for the Lower Merion Township school system, managed a dispensary for employees of Sears Roebuck, and did liability examinations for the Insurance Company of North America. During the next twenty-five years his Main Line practice grew to enormous proportions, but in addition to including the carriage trade and many physicians among his patients, he took care of many who could not afford to pay, especially during the Depression. Dr. Margaret Sturgis forged her career at Woman's Medical College, where before her death in 1962, she had risen to be chairman of the department of gynecology. She was also chairman of the department of obstetrics and gynecology at Philadelphia General Hospital. Dr. Samuel Sturgis was a noted collector of medical and historical prints and was generous in his gifts to the College of Physicians (where he was named honorary curator at medical art), the Historical Society of Pennsylvania, and the Philadelphia Museum of Art. Another major interest was genealogy; he thoroughly researched his Huguenot, Swedish, and English ancestors and was a member and officer of many genealogical societies. In 1964 he married Dr. Katharine Boucot (q.v. Katharine Boucot Sturgis).

Artist: Arthur Edwin Bye (1885–1969)

Born in Philadelphia, Bye was descended from a noble English family that traced its origins to the 14th century. The family property in Bucks County, Pennsylvania, had been a land grant from William Penn. Bye studied art at the Philadelphia School of Industrial Art, the Pennsylvania Academy of the Fine Arts, the University of Pennsylvania (where he received the A.B. degree in 1911), Oxford University, and, in Paris, the Académie de la Grand Chaumière and the Sorbonne. He received the Ph.D. degree in art history and architecture from Princeton University in 1916. While studying in Europe and on frequent subsequent trips he paid special attention to the work of the 16th and 17th century old masters. Upon his return to Philadelphia he was named curator of paintings at the Philadelphia Museum of Art, a position he held for ten years; during this time he wrote many scholarly articles on the collections. From 1927 until 1939 he was in the business of restoring paintings and also was proprietor of an art gallery in center-city Philadelphia. After relocating in Bucks County he continued the work of restoration for many institutions, including Princeton University. As an artist, Bye was best known for his impressionistic paintings of still lifes and landscapes and for his sensitive portraits of friends and patrons. In addition to his multifaceted career as curator, conservator, and artist, he was an instructor of art and architecture at Lafayette, Vassar, and Bryn Mawr Colleges and the Universities of North Carolina and Pennsylvania. He was a member of several local historical societies and both the Baronial Order of Magna Charta and the Baronial Order of Runnymede. He wrote many articles on art and architecture and he catalogued the art collection of the Union League of Philadelphia. He wrote the following books: *Pots and Pans, or Studies in Still-Life Painting; A History of the Bye Family; A Friendly Heritage along the Delaware; Tales of Bucks County;* and *Magna Charta, King John and the Barons.*

Oil on canvas; 35 1/4 x 28 1/2; signed and dated at upper right, "Arthur Edwin Bye/ 1964" Presented by Dr. Samuel B. Sturgis and Dr. Katharine B. Sturgis in 1978. PA 136

Dr. Sturgis is shown two-thirds length, with body turned to the right and head turned to the right and tilted up. He is seated in a green upholstered armchair, with both forearms resting on the chair arms and both hands pendent. The background consists of streaky tones of brownish-green, darker on the top and around the head, lighter at the right center. At his left there is a table covered with a red cloth, on which there are three books; the closed books are bound in green and yellow, the open book has a gray paper cover. The subject has gray hair, bluish-gray eyes which look in the direction of the head turn through metal-rimmed glasses, a full nose with a bump at the bridge, a wide mouth whose thin lips form a smile, a prominent jawline, and a square chin. His complexion is fair. He wears a white shirt, a blue and white striped necktie, a three-piece dark blue suit, a white pocket handkerchief, a round lapel button, and a gold watch chain and gold ring. The surface of the portrait is painterly, with small, visible strokes. The head and hands have been rendered in moderately three-dimensional and solid forms. There is a suggestion of the body forms under the costume. The subject sits rather stiffly well back in his chair, with his weight leaning on his left arm; his large hands are positioned awkwardly. His smile is reserved and his facial expression is a bit tentative as he looks away from his books and off into the distance.

Thomas Sydenham (1624–1689)

Born in Wynford Eagle, England, the famous Sydenham was the son of a Dorset squire whose family went back to the time of King John. His education at Oxford was interrupted by the civil war, in which he fought as a captain on the side of the parliamentarians. He was made a Bachelor of Medicine at Oxford in 1648. He removed to London in 1656 and became licentiate of the Royal College of Physicians in 1663. He was not made an M.D.

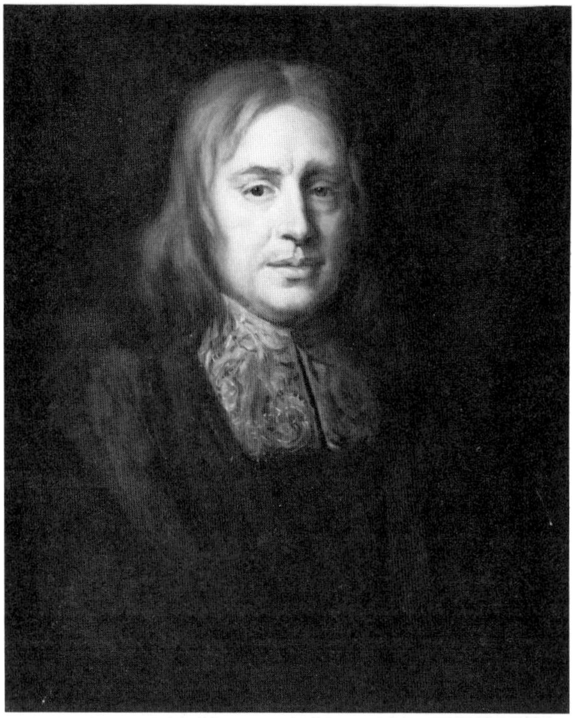

Thomas Sydenham *PA 32*

until 1676 (Pembroke College, Cambridge) and never moved beyond his status as licentiate in the Royal College, yet his reputation was so great in his own day that he was known as the English Hippocrates. His philosophy was that "the art of medicine was to be properly learned only from its practice and exercise." His magnum opus, *Medical Observations Concerning the History and Cure of Acute Diseases* (1676), was based on his observations of the Great Plague of 1665 and on outbreaks of smallpox, continued fevers, and intermittent fevers. In it he set forth his premises for therapeutic reforms—belief in the healing power of nature, nature's orderly production of diseases by species, the need for more refined delineation of the seasonal and annual varieties of diseases, the possibility of deriving treatment from the observable phenomena of a disease, and the desirability of making repeated trials of treatment before declaring them effective. He helped to establish the use of Peruvian bark, or cinchona, as a specific remedy for ague. He also wrote classic descriptions of gout, epidemic diseases, venereal diseases, dropsy, and the minor form of St. Vitus' dance, also called "Sydenham's chorea."

Artist: Anna Lea Merritt (Mrs. Henry Merritt) (1844–1930)

For biography, see page 70.

Oil on canvas; 29 1/2 x 24 1/2; not signed or dated. Information on brass plaque attached to frame is in accord with contemporary records of the College of Physicians: "Thomas Sydenham/ Artist Mary Beale/copied by Anna Lea Merritt/ by permission of/The Royal College of Physicians of London/ presented by John Kearsley Mitchell, M.D. 1899." Included in checklist of paintings in Galina Gorokhoff's Love Locked Out: The Memoirs of Anna Lea Merritt *(Museum of Fine Arts, Boston, 1982). According to* The Royal College of Physicians of London: Portraits *(edited by Gordon Wolstenholme, written by David Piper, London, 1964), the source for Anna Merritt's copy is now considered to be a copy of a missing portrait by Mary Beale (1632–1697), a distinguished English portraitist.* *PA 32*

Dr. Sydenham is shown bust length, his body and head turned slightly to the right. The background is maroonish-brown. His face is rectangular. His straight, grayish-blond hair falls to his shoulders. He has knitted eyebrows, blue eyes which look toward the observer, a slender nose, a small mouth with full lips, and a square jawline and chin. The subject wears a reddish-maroon gown and a white lace falling-band collar. Although the surface of the portrait has undergone several restorations and the gown and background show extensive paint loss, the head has been rendered in painterly style and is well constructed in solid and three-dimensional volumes. Lively painting of the face and collar add to the vitality of the physical presence and to the sober dignity of Sydenham's facial expression.

William Johnson Taylor (1861–1936)

Born in Worcester County, Maryland, Dr. Taylor was descended from early settlers along the eastern shore of Maryland and Virginia. He was graduated from the medical department of the University of Pennsylvania in 1882. After establishing a private surgical practice in Philadelphia, he attracted the attention of Dr. W.W. Keen (q.v.), who engaged him as an assistant in his own practice and in his work at the Orthopaedic Hospital and Infirmary for Nervous Diseases. Later Taylor became attending surgeon to the Orthopaedic Hospital, which he served for fifty years. His other hospital positions were surgeon at St. Mary and St. Agnes Hospitals and consulting surgeon to Woman's and Abington Hospitals. He was also professor of orthopedic surgery at the Philadelphia Polyclinic. During World War I he was commissioned as first lieutenant and sent to Le Tréport, France, with the Pennsylvania Hospital Unit, Base Hosptial No. 10. He rendered exemplary service as surgeon and, for much of the time, as senior surgeon of the unit. He was discharged in 1919 with the rank of lieutenant colonel. Taylor was president of the Philadelphia Academy of Surgery (1908–09). At the College of Physicians he was president from 1919 to 1922 and served as a member of the council, censor, member and chairman of the library committee, chairman of the finance committee, and secretary of the building committee. At the Library Company of Philadelphia he was a director or board member from 1909 to 1935. He wrote many scientific papers, including the article on hernia in Keating's *Cyclopedia of Diseases of Children.*

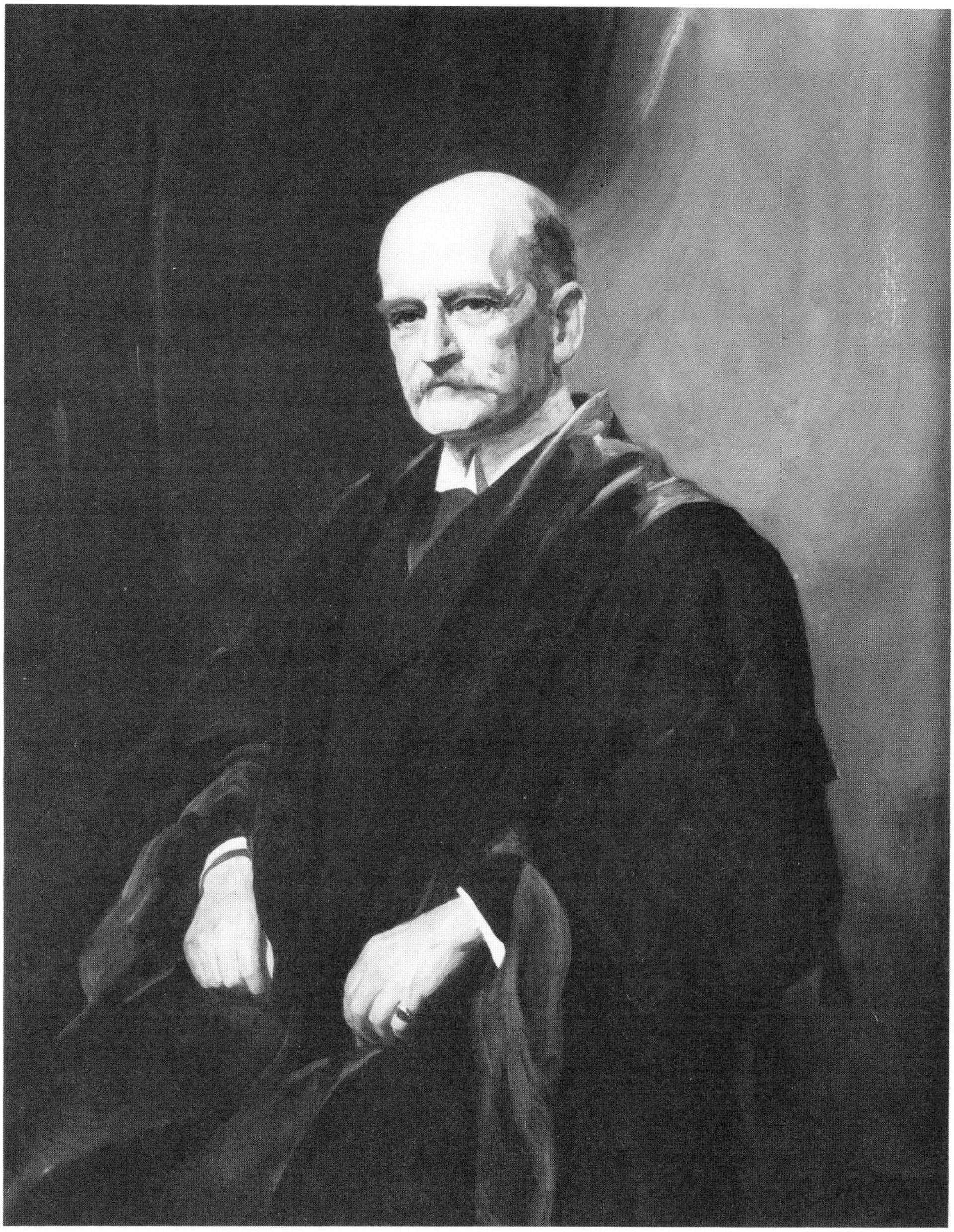

William Johnson Taylor PA 2

Artist: Lazar Raditz (1887–1958)

For biography, see page 73.

Oil on canvas; 43 1/2 x 35 1/4; signed and dated at lower right, "Lazar Raditz/1924." Presented by fellows of the College of Physicians in 1924. Shown at the Pennsylvania Academy of the Fine Arts annual exhibition of 1925, at the Philadelphia Art Alliance (date unknown), and at Raditz's one-man exhibition at McClees Gallery in 1935. PA 2

Dr. Taylor is shown two-thirds length, his body turned three-quarters to the left, his head to the left and tilted downward and sideways. He is seated with both hands resting on his lap, palms down. The background has a brownish-umber curtain that stretches diagonally from the center to the lower left. The wall on the right is in lighter tones of green, yellow, and brown. The subject's face is square. He has a bald head with short brown hair at the sides. His narrow blue eyes gaze in the direction of the head turn and tilt. He has a straight nose, a gray moustache, a small mouth, and a square jawline and chin. He wears a white shirt with wing collar, a gray vest, a black coat, and a gold ring. His black academic robe has green vertical panels down the front and voluminous sleeves with a green lining and green stripes. The surface of the portrait is painterly, with fluid strokes throughout. The head and hands are rendered in very solid and three-dimensional forms. The features seem chiseled, with visible curving and geometric patches of paint which describe the highlights and shadows of the planes. The green of the background and the costume is repeated in the hair, eyebrows, and moustache. One can sense the bulk of the bodily forms underlying the carefully depicted folds of the costume. The bravura style of painting seems more expressive of the artist than of the subject. The pose is conventional and the facial expression is dignified but neutral or even bland.

William Thomson (1833–1907)

Born in Chambersburg, Pennsylvania, Dr. Thomson was descended from Scotch-Irish settlers who came to America early in the 18th century. In 1855, after graduating from Jefferson Medical College, he started a general medical practice in the suburbs of Philadelphia. He had a distinguished military career, first serving as a lieutenant with the army of the Potomac and then as chief of staff to the office of General McClellan's medical director. For his work at the battle of South Mountain, where he was left in sole charge of 2500 wounded men, he was complimented by President Lincoln. His subsequent proposals for change in the supply systems of field hospitals and for formation of division hospitals were adopted throughout all the Union armies. In 1863 he was placed in charge of Douglas Hospital in Washington. Under his reorganization it became a model for other army hospitals. In the following year he was appointed inspector of all hospitals in the Washington area. He was especially active in the recently organized Army Medical Museum, contributing a major portion of the first published catalogue, including valuable descriptions of osteomyelitis and wounds of the joints. In collaboration with William F. Norris (q.v.) he was a prime mover behind the establishment of a photographic bureau at the museum by demonstrating the practical value of photographic surgical records of wounds. This bureau evolved into the Medical Illustration Service of the Armed Forces Institute of Pathology. In addition, Thomson and Norris began experiments in photomicrography, demonstrating that prints of microscopic fields magnified 15 to 250 times could be made. After the war, Thomson's interest in photography led him to the study of optics and he began to limit his practice to ophthalmology. At Jefferson Medical College, he was appointed clinical lecturer on diseases of the eye and ear in 1873 and was subsequently made honorary professor, professor, and emeritus professor of ophthalmology. He was also surgeon and later emeritus surgeon to the Wills Eye Hospital. His contributions to medical literature include the editing of the American edition of Nettleship's *Diseases of the Eye*. He wrote the chapters on diseases of the eye in Samuel D. Gross's *System of Surgery* (fifth edition) and in the *American Textbook of Surgery*, as well as "Detection of Color Blindness" in Norris and Oliver's *System of the Diseases of the Eye*. He also wrote the following articles: "The Use of the Ophthalmoscope in the Diagnosis of Intracranial Lesions" (with S. Weir Mitchell, q.v.), "Astigmatism as a Cause for Persistent Headaches Treated by Correction of Optical Defects" (with S. Weir Mitchell), and "History of the First Brain Tumor Diagnosticated with the Ophthalmoscope in Philadelphia." He was an early worker on refractive problems and the inventor of several instruments, including the ametrometer and a new kind of refractometer used to measure abnormalities of ocular refraction. He called attention to the causal relations between ocular abnormalities and other symptoms. In association with S. Weir Mitchell he published papers on ocular fatigue as a cause of headache and other nervous disorders. Thomson was one of the first to commend the use of the ophthalmoscope, then a relatively new and little-used instrument. He was one of the first to recommend full correction for myopia and to correct conical cornea by spherocylinders. As ophthalmic surgeon to the Pennsylvania Railroad, he simplified tests for color blindness by using colored wool and lanterns to detect the condition in trainmen, whose ability to see colored signals correctly was a critical factor in railroad safety. Thomson was a fellow of the College of Physicians, and his own ophthalmoscopes, correspondence, and fourteen volumes of case books are preserved there.

Artist: Thomas Eakins (1844–1916)

Thomas Eakins, one of this country's most famous painters, was born in Philadelphia to parents of Irish descent. He studied art first with his father, a writing master and professional calligrapher. From 1862 to 1865 he studied at the Pennsylvania Academy of the Fine Arts, taking classes in drawing from casts of antique sculpture, attending lectures in anatomy and perspective, and, in his last year, drawing from life. He also attended anatomy lectures at Jefferson Medical College in 1865–66. He continued his education in Paris at the École des Beaux Arts from 1866 to 1869, where he studied painting with Jean Léon Gérôme and sculpture with Alexandre Dumont. He also studied painting in the private atelier of Léon Bonnat. He traveled in Spain and Italy to study the work of the old masters. Upon his return to Philadelphia, he again attended anatomy classes at Jefferson. In addition to portraits of members of his family, his early paintings were of outdoor scenes of rowing, hunting, and sailing. He exhibited at the American Society of Water Colors in 1874, at the Paris salon of 1875, and at the Centennial Exposition of 1876 in Philadelphia, where five of his works were included in the art section, but his most ambitious painting to date, *The Gross Clinic* (Thomas Jefferson University), was considered too controversial and was hung in the U.S. Army Post Hospital. During the next decade he was optimistic about his career and exhibited regularly at the Pennsylvania Academy of the Fine Arts, the National Academy of Design, and the Society of American Artists. During these years he achieved prominence, but many critics and most of the public found his style too harsh and his subject matter problematic. As early as 1874 he started his teaching career with the evening life class at the Philadelphia Sketch Club and then at the Pennsylvania Academy, where he was soon dismissed from

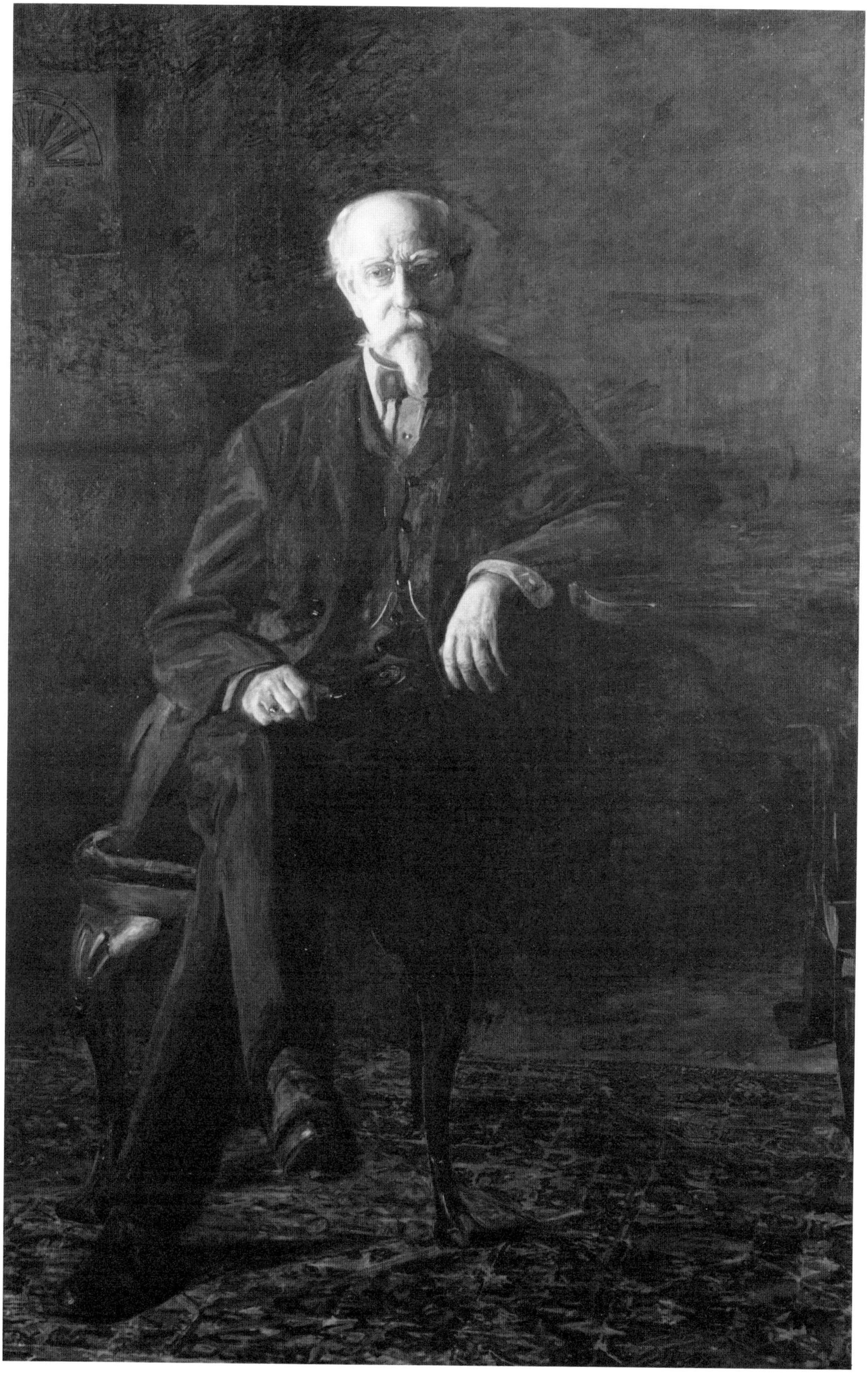

William Thomson *PA 77*

the post of assistant instructor. Nevertheless, he remained as a chief demonstrator of anatomy in a class taught by Dr. W.W. Keen (q.v.). After a year of teaching at the newly formed Art Students' Union, he was reinstated at the Academy and was named professor of drawing in 1879 and director of the Academy school in 1882. In the next four years he reorganized the conservative curriculum to accord with his training at the École des Beaux Arts, emphasing anatomy and dissection to increase understanding of the human form. Because of his insistence that both male and female students study from nude models in the life classes, Eakins was forced to resign from the Academy. Nine years later he was dismissed from the art department of Drexel University for the same reason. He also taught at the Art Students' League of Philadelphia from 1886 to 1892 and held short-term teaching posts in New York, at the Brooklyn Art Guild, the Art Students' League, the National Academy, and Cooper Union. During these years of teaching he continued to paint a variety of subjects, which included scenes of boxing, old-fashioned themes and historical subjects, genre scenes, landscapes, and a *Crucifixion* (Philadelphia Museum of Art). Most of these works were of great seriousness but were not in tune with contemporary taste. They were the product of his desire to paint traditional figural works in native American settings in combination with the results of his scientific researches into perspective, anatomy, and still and motion photography. (Eakins often used photographs as an aid to composition and did pioneering work in serial motion photography in order to study the mechanics of locomotion.) It is a popular misconception to think that Eakins had no positive support to counter his critics, and in addition to his wife, the artist Susan MacDowell Eakins, and his student and constant companion, the sculptor Samuel Murray (q.v.), Eakins had a loyal group of former students and friends who believed in his genius. Nevertheless, because of his failure in teaching and the public neglect or adverse criticism of his subject paintings, Eakins turned to portraiture for the remainder of his career. He favored intellectuals, and many of his subjects were men and women in the sciences, art, music, and the clergy. It is not surprising that among the portraits were those of at least twenty different physicians, counting the group portraits of *The Gross Clinic* and *The Agnew Clinic* (University of Pennsylvania) as one each. Because of his study of anatomy at Jefferson, his creation of at least 17 plaster casts of dissections as an aid for students, and his roles as both demonstrator and arranger for courses in anatomy at the Academy when he was director, Eakins had strong ties to the medical profession, and his portraits of physicians are among his strongest and most penetrating. Throughout this period of his career, he continued to exhibit his work. He even won prizes, including a bronze medal at the Columbian Exposition in Chicago (1893), gold medals at the Pan-American Exposition in Buffalo (1901), the Louisiana Purchase Exposition in St. Louis (1904), and the Temple gold medal at the Academy (1904), where he started to exhibit again in 1894. In 1902 he was finally elected an academician of the National Academy of Design. The first memorial exhibition of his work was held at the Metropolitan Museum of Art in 1916, the year of his death. In the following year his work was shown at the Pennsylvania Academy. Other retrospective exhibitions were at the Philadelphia Museum of Art (three times, in 1944, 1961, and 1982), the Carnegie Institute (1945), the National Gallery of Art and the Art Institute of Chicago (1961–62), and at the Brandywine River Museum (co-sponsored by the University of Delaware, 1980). Most of his works remained in his studio at the time of his death and many were sold to the Metropolitan, Brooklyn, Cleveland, and Chicago Museums, and to the Museum at Phillips Academy in Andover, Massachusetts. The majority of his paintings were presented by Mrs. Eakins to the Philadelphia Museum of Art as a memorial to her husband. The other great repository of Eakins's art and memorabilia is the Hirshhorn Museum and Sculpture Garden in Washington, D.C. Today Eakins is widely regarded as one of America's greatest artists and one of the most important portrait painters of all time.

Oil on canvas, mounted on wood; 73 1/2 x 47 1/2; signed and dated on the right lower center, "Eakins, 1907." Presented by the family of Dr. William Thomson in 1909. This is the second version of an Eakins portrait of Dr. Thomson. The first, ca. 1907, measures 68 x 48 and is unfinished. It is in the collection of Mrs. John Randolph Garrett of Roanoke, Virginia. The portrait at the College of Physicians was also painted in 1907, the year of Thomson's death, but no evidence yet uncovered indicates that it was posthumous. It was shown at two exhibitions at the Philadelphia Museum of Art, the Thomas Eakins Centennial *in 1944, and* The Art of Philadelphia Medicine, *1965. In 1982 it was on temporary loan to the Eakins Gallery at Thomas Jefferson University.* *PA 77*

Thomson is shown full-length with upper body frontal and head tilted down and slightly to the right. He is seated in a Chippendale-style side chair with shell carving on the knees; it is placed perpendicularly to the table on which his left arm rests. His left hand is pendent. His right arm rests on his thigh and holds a Noyes ophthalmoscope. The legs are crossed at the knees. The background wall of the interior setting is in scumbled tones of brown. The chair has been placed on an oriental rug with a complex pattern in muted red, green, blue, and tan. At the right center there is a library table with a pedestal base and with books and a lamp on top. In the upper left corner there is an eye chart for astigmatism, mounted in a wooden frame. The subject has an elongated face and a high forehead, with a fringe of white hair on the top and sides. His forehead is lined and his brows are knitted. His pale blue eyes, which look down in the direction of the head turn and tilt through a pince-nez, are encircled with puffy lids and age lines. There are also deep lines next to his long nose. His mouth is almost obscured by his long, bushy, white moustache and long, narrow Vandyke beard. He wears a white shirt, a maroon bow tie, a rumpled three-piece suit, and brown shoes. His jewelry includes cuff links, a ring, and a watch chain. The surface of this portrait is painterly, with visible brush strokes throughout. The head and hands have been rendered in solid and three-dimensional forms, with exquisite modeling of the planes and sensitive use of contrasts of light and shade. One senses the body masses underlying the costume, which is rendered with careful attention to folds and wrinkles. One reason that the figure shows an unusual degree of vitality and energy is the posture. Although the pose is conventional, the artist has manipulated the subject's figure to show subtle animation. The head tilts downward and sideways and the right shoulder and arm slump downward, while the left shoulder and arm rest on a table made high to force them upward. The hips are placed in the corner of the chair and twist from left to right while remaining frontal. The right foot projects forward, and the right hand grasps the ophthalmoscope firmly. This physical motion is in contrast to the portrayal of the subject as an old man. In addition to the signs of age already noted, the body seems frail and has shrunk, so that the shirt collar gapes at the neck. The face is haggard, its expression being one of weariness and introspection. Even the autumnal tones and colors are a metaphor for the age and character of the subject. The portrait is suffused with brown tones throughout; the spotlighted head and hands and highlights on the furniture are muted, and the bright oriental rug is faded. Eakins was especially sympathetic toward Thomson as a subject because of their common interest in optics and photography. Thomson's biographers also mention his consuming hobby of painting and sketching.

Dr. Tulp's Anatomy Lesson

Artist: Wilhelmus H.P.J. de Zwart (1862–1931)

A Dutch painter and etcher, de Zwart was born in The Hague and studied at the academy there from 1876 to 1880. His best work was produced in that city between 1880 and 1894. He made two short trips to Paris in 1891 and 1908, and he worked in several other cities, including Soest, Hilversum, Laren, Amsterdam, Bloemendaal, Scheveningen, Leiden, and Voorburg. His figures, landscapes, still lifes, and religious scenes are represented in many Dutch museums, in Montreal, and in Belgrade. He won honorable mention in the Exposition Universelle in Paris (1889).

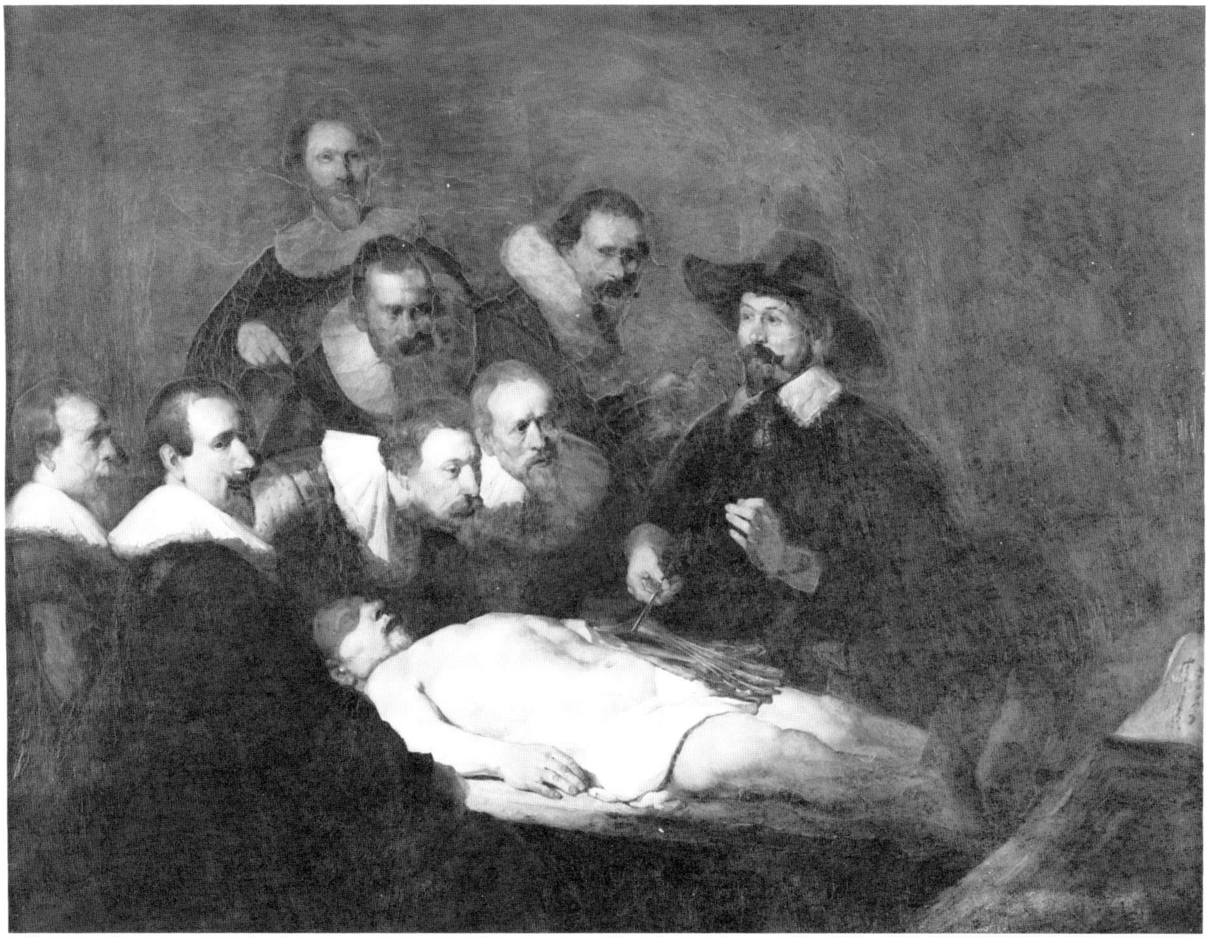

Dr. Tulp's Anatomy Lesson *PA 68*

Oil on canvas; 64 x 84; signed and dated on the back, "W. de Zwart/Haag 1887." Presented by Mary Small and Mary Cadwalader Mitchell in 1887. Copy after Rembrandt's Anatomy Lesson of Dr. Tulp, *1632, The Mauritshuis, The Hague.* *PA 68*

The original painting by Rembrandt has long been the subject of controversy in the art historical literature—whether the setting is imaginary, whether the demonstration was public or private, and whether or not it is a group portrait of the Guild of Surgeon-Anatomists, whose anatomical folio lies at the foot of the cadaver. In addition, the accuracy of Rembrandt's portrayal of the dissected arm has been disputed. The copyist, de Zwart, includes all of the original figures in a generalized portrayal, but it does not capture the intensity of facial expression, details of costume, complex architectural interior details, or the emotional contrast of light and shade that are so characteristic of Rembrandt.

James Tyson (1841-1919)

Dr. Tyson, a native of Philadelphia, was descended from 17th century settlers in Germantown, Pennsylvania. He received the A.B. degree from Haverford College in 1860, the M.D. degree from the University of Pennsylvania in 1863, and the A. M. degree from Haverford in 1864. During the Civil War he was acting assistant surgeon, stationed in army hospitals in Philadelphia and Harrisburg. After a residency at the Pennsylvania Hospital, he began the private practice of medicine. He held a long succession of academic positions at the University of Pennsylvania, starting as quiz-master of a private class of students and then as lecturer in microscopy (1868) and in urinary chemistry (1870). In 1874, when the new University Hospital was organized, he was appointed lecturer on pathological anatomy and histology and, two years later, professor of general pathology and morbid anatomy. In 1889 he was transferred to the chair of clinical medicine and in 1899 to the chair of medicine, from which he was forced to retire because of age in 1910. He served also as secretary and then dean to the faculty of medicine and as manager of the University Hospital. Other staff positions were as those of pathologist, visiting physician, and president of the medical board at Philadelphia Hospital; founder and trustee of the Rush Hospital for Consumption; and consulting physician to the Kensington Hospital for Women and St. Mary Hospital. He was president of several medical societies, including the College of Physicians (1907-10), the Pathological Society of Philadelphia, and the Medical Society of Pennsylvania. He was a founder and president of the Pennsylvania Society for the Prevention of Tuberculosis and a founder of the Obstetrical Society of Philadelphia and the Association of American Physicians. He served as assistant editor of the *Philadelphia Medical Times* and editor of *Transactions of the Pathological Society of Philadelphia.* He wrote *The Cell Doctrine, Its History and Present State* (1870), *An Introduction to the Study of Practical Histology* (1873), *A Guide to the Practical Examination of the Urine* (1875), *A Treatise on Bright's Disease and Diabetes* (1881), *A Manual of Physical Diagnosis* (1891), and *The Practice of Medicine; a Text-book for Practioners and Students* (1896). He received honorary LL.D. degrees from Haverford College and the University of Pennsylvania.

Artist: Joseph Rodefer De Camp (1858-1923)

Born in Cincinnati, De Camp was a student of Frank Duveneck at the Cincinnati Art Academy; he also studied at the Royal Academy in Munich and in Florence. During his career in the United States he was an instructor at the School of the Museum of Fine Arts in Boston and the Pennsylvania Academy of the Fine Arts (1895-96). He was a member of "The Ten American Painters," the National Institute of Arts and Letters, the Philadelphia Art Club, the National Society of Portrait Painters, and the Boston Guild of Artists. His portraits, landscapes, and figure paintings won prizes at the decorative competition of Philadelphia City Hall and at the Pennsylvania Academy of the Fine Arts, where he won the Temple gold medal in 1899, the Beck medal in in 1912, and the Lippincott prize in 1920. At the Paris Exposition of 1900 he won an honorable mention, at the Louisiana Purchase Exposition of 1904 in St. Louis he won a gold medal, at the Corcoran Gallery of Art he was awarded the Clark Prize in 1909, and at the Philadelphia Art Club he won the gold medal in 1915. His works are represented at the Pennsylvania Academy of the Fine Arts and the city museums of Boston, Cincinnati, and Worcester, Massachusetts.

Oil on canvas; 41 1/4 x 33 1/4; signed and dated at upper left, "Joseph De Camp 1910." Presented by friends of Dr. Tyson in 1911. *PA 8*

Dr. Tyson is shown two-thirds length, his body turned to the right and his head slightly to the right and slightly down. He is seated with both arms stretched forward and both hands lying stiffly on his thighs; the right is clenched, the left has fingers spread out rigidly. The background is a warm gray wall with a detail of wooden molding at the lower right. The subject has brown hair, which parts at the center and forms bangs at the forehead. The brows are knitted. The blue eyes look through a pince-nez in the direction of the head turn and tilt and have puffy lower lids. The nose has a bump at the bridge and wide nostrils. His angular face has hollow cheeks, a prominent jawline, and a square chin. He wears a white shirt with stand-up collar and a black necktie, coat, trousers, and academic gown, whose mantle is trimmed in red and blue. The surface of the portrait is smoothly painted, and the head and hands are well constructed in solid and three-dimensional volumes. The body masses are entirely lost under the voluminous robe. The portrayal

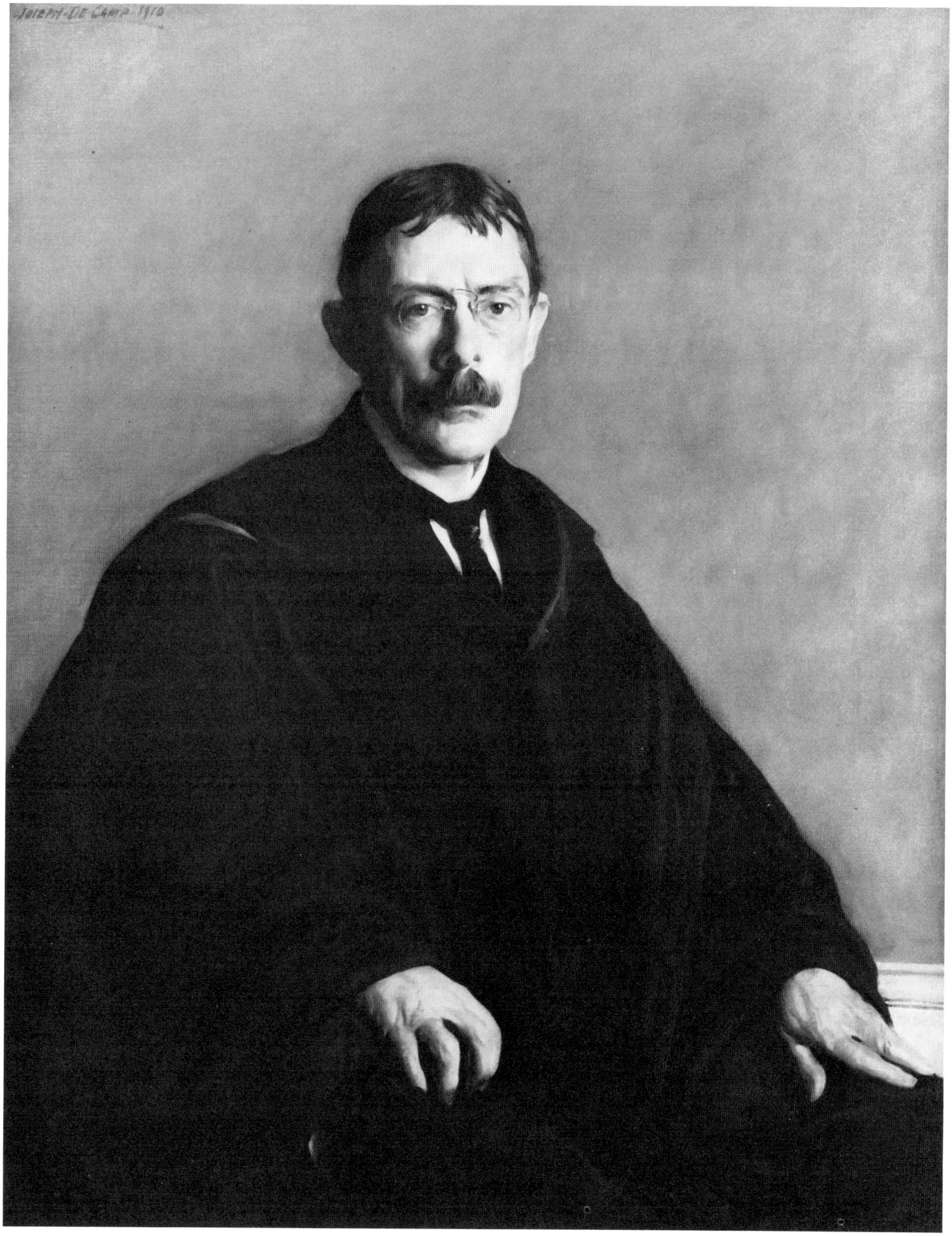

James Tyson PA 8

is rendered with penetrating characterization and power by means of several devices. The composition is pyramidal, with a wide, stable base. The subject's arresting facial expression is mournful and very tense; the jaw is clenched and the mouth is tight. One wonders if the portrait was painted after the subject's forced resignation from the professorship of medicine. The stooped posture and rigidity of hands are probably due to Paget's disease, from which he suffered, in addition to a serious ailment of the heart. De Camp has produced a moving portrayal of a once powerful pillar of the Philadelphia medical establishment in the midst of physical and professional decline.

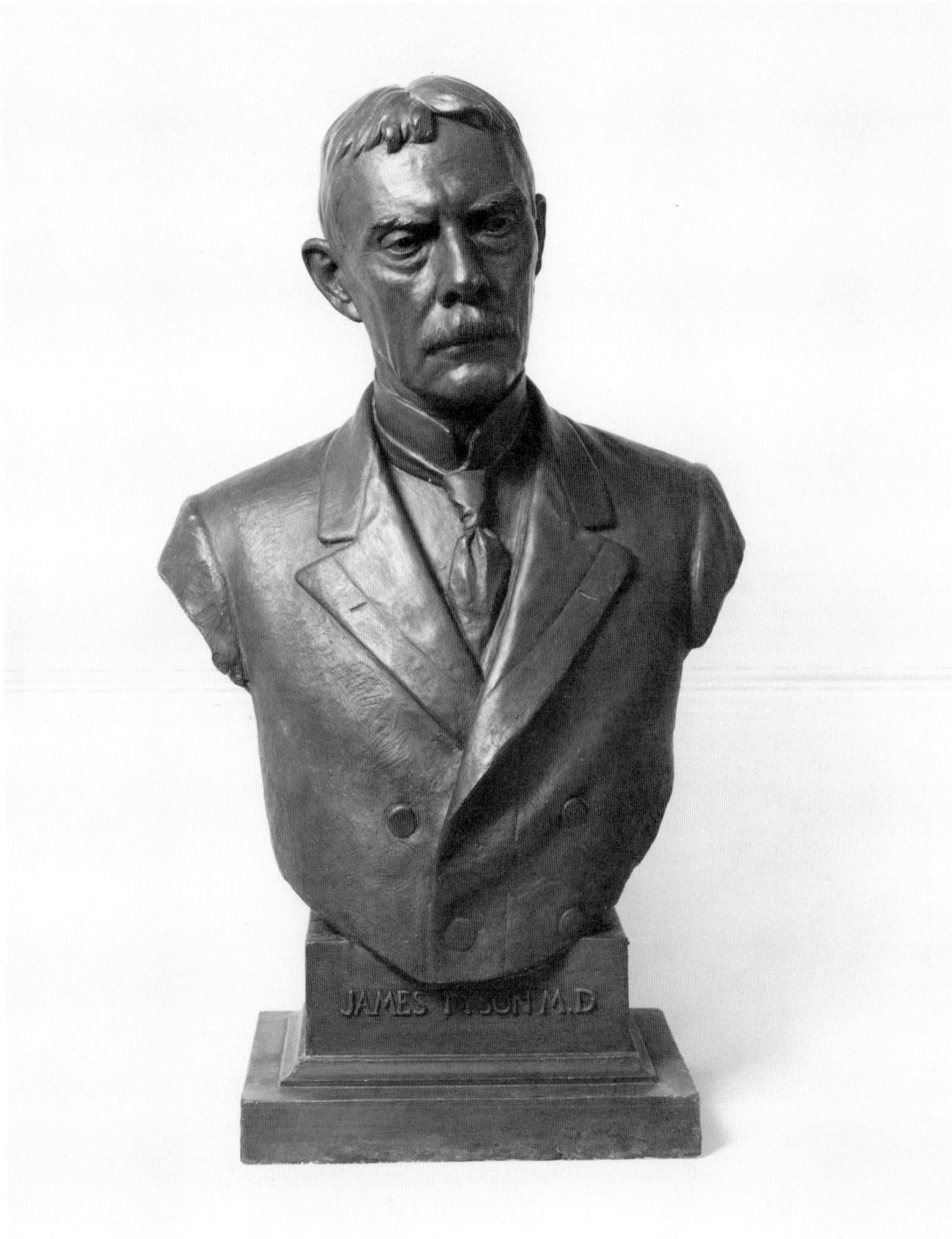

James Tyson *ST 557*

Artist: Samuel Aloysius Murray (1870–1941)

For biography, see page 3.

Plaster, painted brown; 31 1/2 x 19 x 11 1/2; rectangular base integral with sculpture, 6 in. high; signed and dated on rear on beveled edge of shoulder, "Samuel Murray 1914"; inscription on top vertical edge of base, "James Tyson M.D." Presented by Mrs. Samuel Murray, through the efforts of Dr. William Bradley, in 1944. *ST 557*

Tyson is shown bust length. The body is frontal, the head has been turned sharply to the right and tilted diagonally down. The face is rectangular. The hair, parted at the center, forms bangs at the furrowed forehead. The brows are knitted. The eyes, with deeply carved irises and pupils, look in the direction of the head turn and tilt and have deep and puffy lower lids. The thick nose ends in a bulbous tip. The thick brush moustache covers the upper lip of the wide mouth. The cheeks are hollow, the jaw is square. The subject is wearing a shirt with stand-up collar, a necktie, and a double-breasted coat with wide lapels and which overlaps the base. In addition to the characteristically uneven texture on the surface of this plaster bust, the sculptor has made lightly incised parallel lines on the coat. The portrayal has been done with very skillful modeling of the planes of the head and with a feeling for the body masses underlying the costume. As in the painting by De Camp (described above), the subject has a morose and tense facial expression. Here the progression of his Paget's disease is shown in the stiffness of the neck and the diagonal tilt of the shoulders. These naturalistic observations add to the expressiveness and vitality of the figure.

Andreas Vesalius (1514-1564)

Born in Brussels, Vesalius was the grandson of eminent physicians and scholars, and his father was apothecary to Charles V. His medical education at the University of Paris was interrupted by the war between France and the Holy Roman Empire. He continued at the University of Louvain, where he received the degree of Bachelor of Medicine in 1537, and at the University of Padua, where he received the Doctorate of Medicine in the same year. He was immediately named professor of anatomy and surgery at Padua and, contrary to custom, performed the dissections himself. He also introduced, for reference by his students, six large anatomical charts representing the portal, caval, arterial, nervous, and skeletal systems, designated after their publication in 1538 as *Tabulae anatomicae sex.* In the same year he published a dissection manual for his students, *Institutiones anatomicae . . .*, a revised and augmented edition of the Galenically oriented book that had been used by his teacher in Paris, Günther of Andernach. His next book, *Epistola docens venam . . .*, was written in support of the revived classical procedure of venesection, whereby the blood was drawn from a site near, not distant from, the location of the ailment. To support his arguments he proposed that anatomical dissection might be used to test speculation, a major step toward the scientific method of study. His greatest work on anatomy, *De humani corporis fabrica,* was published in 1543 and revised in 1555. In it he demonstrated that much of Galen's human anatomy was fallacious because it was based on the dissection and observation of animals and that human anatomy could be learned only by dissection and investigation of the human body. He hoped also that his verbal descriptions and precisely detailed pictorial representations would persuade physicians to appreciate anatomy as fundamental to all other aspects of medicine. Although his book is replete with errors, Vesalius made many anatomical discoveries, and the fame of the work spread far and wide, earning for the author the epithet, "Father of Modern Anatomy." After the publication of the *Fabrica* and its condensed version, the *Epitome,* Vesalius returned to the practice of medicine and received an appointment as physician to the household of Emperor Charles V. He accompanied the imperial armies to the battlefield and became noted as a surgeon; his most significant contribution was the introduction of surgically induced drainage of empyema. After Charles V abdicated in 1556, Vesalius took service with his son, Philip II of Spain. Returning from a voyage to the Holy Land, his ship was delayed by a storm; it finally reached the island at Zante (Zakinthos), where he went ashore and died on October 15, 1564.

Artist: Adolfo Tagliaferri

Oil on canvas; 40 x 30 1/2; painted in 1963. Presented by Dr. Julian A. Sterling in 1968. Written on the back of the canvas, "Tiziano da Cadore N. 1477 M. 1576/copia del pittore:/Adolfo Tagliaferri/via Quintino Sella 20/Firenze." The files of the College of Physicians contain a letter written to Dr. Sterling by Tagliaferri in which the latter identifies himself as a Florentine and a professional painter who, commissioned by Dr. Sterling in 1963, copied Titian's portrait of Vesalius, which is in the Pitti Gallery. M. H. Speilmann, in The Iconography of Andreas Vesalius *(London, 1925), reviews the controversy over the identities of both subject and painter of the Titian-Vesalius portrait; neither has been settled as yet.* *PA 128*

Vesalius is shown two-thirds length, with head and body turned to the left. He is seated in a Renaissance-style armchair with his right arm resting on the chair arm and right hand holding his pince-nez. His left arm is bent at the elbow to hold a book on the chair arm. The book has a tan leather binding and leather straps, and Vesalius marks the place with his index finger. The background is dark brown. The subject has dark brown hair flecked with gray, brown side-whiskers, a moustache, and a long, square beard which reaches his chest. His forehead shows deep age lines and his brows are knitted. His heavy-lidded brown eyes, which look in the direction of the head turn, have puffy lower lids. There are deep lines next to his long, bulbous nose. Because of severe paint loss, it is hard to distinguish the costume. It is either an open black coat over a brown robe or a black robe with a brown lining. White shirt cuffs show at the sleeves, and there is a ring on the left hand. The surface of the portrait

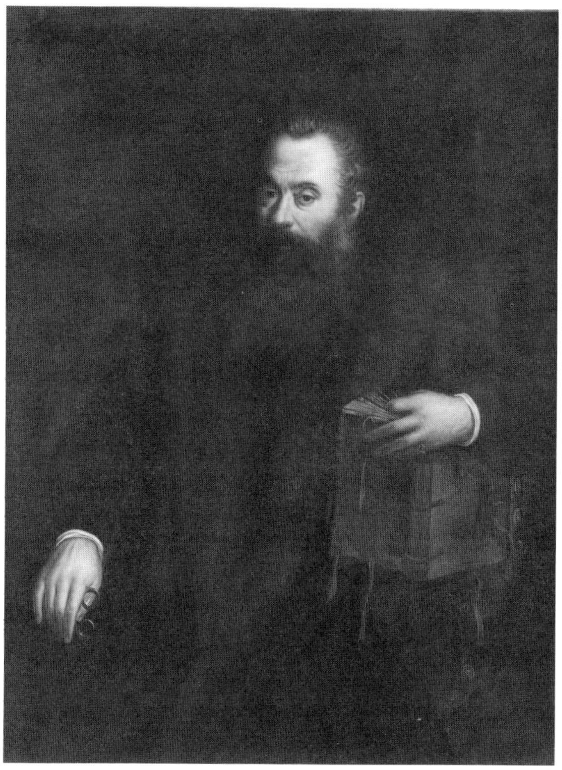

Andreas Vesalius *PA 128*

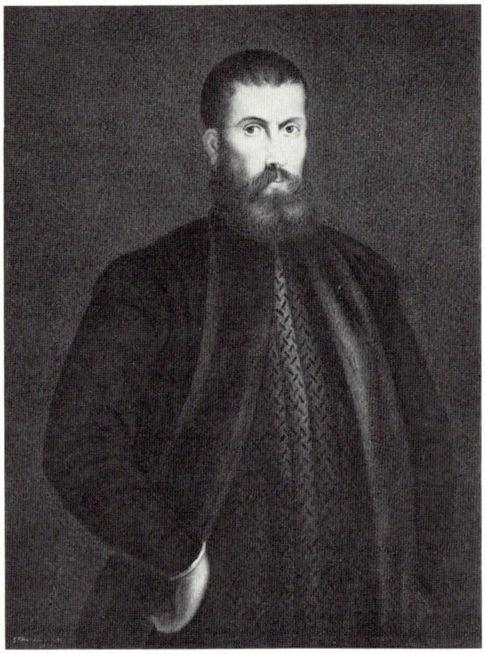

Andreas Vesalius *PH 261*

is smoothly brushed, the head and hands being rendered in solid and three-dimensional volumes. The entire painting is very dark except for the dramatically spotlighted head and hands. It is moving portrait of an elderly academic scholar who has removed his spectacles, looked away from his book, and paused momentarily in weary reflection.

Artist: George Perfect Harding (ca. 1780–1853)

Son of Silvester Harding, the English miniaturist publisher, G. P. Harding was a watercolorist and miniaturist who exhibited at the Royal Academy at intervals between 1802 and 1840. He specialized in watercolor copies of historical portraits located in royal palaces, noble homes, college halls, and professional and civic societies. He made the paintings which were later engraved to illustrate Neale and Bradley's *History of Westminster Abbey*, Moule's *Ancient Oil Paintings and Sepulchral Brasses in the Abbey Church of St. Peter, Westminster*, J. H. Hesse's *Memoirs of the Court of England during the Reign of the Stuarts*, and a book about the Prince of Wales. In 1840 he was a founder of the Granger Society, whose object it was to publish previously unengraved historical portraits. After this group dissolved, Harding published fifteen portraits on his own account. In 1839 he was elected a fellow of the Society of Antiquaries. A group of his works can be found in the Print Room of the British Museum.

Miniature, etching (probably aquatint), hand-painted with opaque watercolor; 6 3/8 x 4 7/8; signed and dated at lower left, "G. P. Harding 1815." Presented by John Kearsley Mitchell in 1908. Pencilled inscription below the miniature, "Andreas Vesalius/ from an original by I. Calcar in the College of Physicians." Jan Stephan Van Calcar (1499–1546) was a pupil of Titian who is said to have illustrated Vesalius's Tabulae Anatomicae *and possibly the* Fabrica. *Harding's copy resembles a painting supposedly of Vesalius and attributed to Calcar at the Royal College of Physicians in London and another portrait with similar pose at the Académie de Médecine in Paris, attributed to Titian or Calcar. M. H. Speilmann, the author of* The Iconography of Andreas Vesalius *(London, 1925), questions the identity of both subject and artist in both paintings and suggests that the London portrait may be a copy of the Paris portrait.* *PH 261*

Vesalius is shown half-length, his body and face slightly to the right. He stands with his left arm bent slightly and his right arm akimbo. The stippled background is a medium-toned greenish-brown. The face is rectangular. The subject has brown hair, side-whiskers, moustache, and a full, round beard. His round brown eyes look out of their corners toward the left. His long thin nose is seen almost in profile. His small mouth has a full lower lip. The complexion is pink. The lips are red, and there are greenish-gray shadows and white highlights. The subject wears a fur-edged black gown over a brown doublet which has a linear black pattern. White cuffs show at the sleeve. The background, hair, fur, and doublet have the grainy quality of the aquatint print, while the face and gown show the heavy opaque watercolor. The whole portrait is rendered in a linear style with precise contours and details of all elements. The head is fairly well modeled in three dimensions, but the hand is flat and awkward. There is no suggestion of the body under the folds of the costume. Both pose and costume are those seen in conventional portrayals of aristocratic and celebrated Renaissance subjects.

John Collins Warren (1778–1856)

Born in Boston, Dr. Warren was the son of a physician. After graduating from Harvard College in 1797 as Latin valedictorian of his class, he entered his father's office as an apprentice. Then he studied with Astley Cooper in London, Dubois in Paris, and Monro *Secundus* and John and Charles Bell in Edinburgh. He received an honorary M.D. degree from St. Andrews University, Scotland, in 1802. After his return to Boston he entered partnership with his father and assisted in the anatomical dissections for his father's lectures at the Harvard Medical School. On his own initiative he gave private lectures on anatomy and physiology, organized a private medical society, and was a founder of the Anthology Club. With James Jackson he prepared a *Pharmacopoeia* for the Massachusetts Medical Society. In 1809 he was appointed adjunct professor of anatomy and surgery at Harvard Medical School, and after his father's death in 1815 he became full professor, a post he held until 1847, when he was named professor emeritus. He was dean from 1816 to 1818 and received an honorary M.D. degree in 1819. With Jackson, Warren was a prime mover in founding the *New England Journal of Medicine and Surgery* in 1812, in relocating the

Medical School from Cambridge to Boston in 1815, and in raising money for the establishment of the Massachusetts General Hospital, which opened in 1821. Warren was one of the most celebrated surgeons of his day and the first in the United States to operate for strangulated hernia. He is best remembered for his courage in allowing William Morton to perform the first public demonstration of ether anesthesia by inhalation in 1846. His most important contribution to the medical literature was *Surgical Observations on Tumours with Cases and Operations* (1837). He was a leading figure in New England civic life and was co-editor of the monthly, *Anthology*, president of the Massachusetts Temperance Society, a fund-raiser for the Bunker Hill Monument, the author of books on the virtues of physical education, president of the Boston Society of Natural History, and author of a book on the mastodon *Giganteus*. His medical specimens, left to the Harvard Medical School, formed the Warren Anatomical Museum. Late in his career he was active in establishing the American Medical Association, and he served as its president in 1850.

Artist: Robert Ball Hughes (1806–1868)

Hughes, a native of London, studied sculpture with Edward H. Baily at the Royal Academy School. There he was such an outstanding student that he won prizes at the Royal Academy exhibitions between 1822 and 1828. He was famed for his portrait busts of the Prince Regent and for his neoclassical reliefs and idealized sculptures in the round. In 1829 he arrived in New York, where he quickly established himself at a sculptor of portrait busts of prominent members of society as well as of fellow artists, including Washington Irving, Henry Inman, and John Trumbull. He showed his sculpture at the annual exhibitions of the Pennsylvania Academy of the Fine Arts, the Artists' Fund Society of Philadelphia, the American Academy of Fine Arts, and the Boston Atheneum. In 1831 he was elected an honorary member of the National Academy of Design. In addition to portrait busts, Hughes was commissioned to produce public works, including a statue of DeWitt Clinton for the Clinton Hall Association and a marble bas-relief of Bishop Hobart for Trinity Church. His marble statue of Alexander Hamilton, made for the New York Merchants' Exchange in 1834, was destroyed by fire the following year. He also made a life-size bronze statue of Nathaniel Bowditch for Mount Auburn Cemetery in Boston. He was in Philadelphia from 1838 to 1840 to prepare an entry in a competition for an equestrian statue of George Washington, sponsored by the Society of the Cincinnati. This project was doomed by the failure of the Bank of the United States. After his removal to Boston in 1840 and then to Dorchester, Massachusetts, he received fewer important commissions and was reduced to turning out minor works such as wax medallions and cameos.

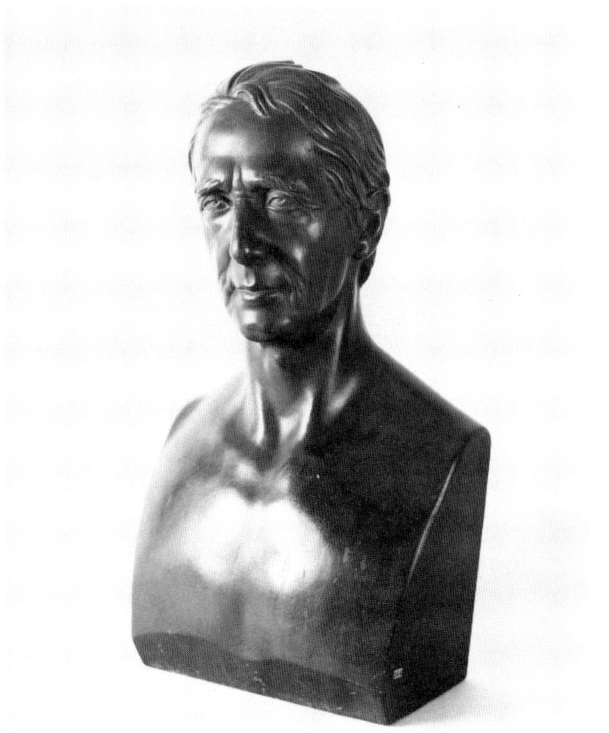

John Collins Warren *ST 544*

Plaster, painted black; 22 x 13 x 10 1/4; no base; signed and dated on the left side, "J.C. Warren, M.D./Ball Hughes/Sculp 1856." Neither the donor nor the date of the donation is on record, but the work is mentioned in the College of Physicians Inventory of 1898–1915. *ST 544*

Dr. Warren is shown bust length, with body frontal and head turned to the right and slightly down. (The head turn is not so apparent in this photographic view.) His face is thin and rectangular. He has long strands of wavy hair, a prominent eyebrow ridge, and narrow eyes with crinkles at the corners and with carved irises and pupils which look upward. The nose is prominent and aquiline. The cheeks are hollow and there are deep furrows next to the nose, mouth, and pointed chin. Below his neck, which has prominent muscles, the anatomy of the torso is only vaguely suggested. The surface of the bust has the slightly irregular texture characteristic of plaster. The head is well modeled with good understanding of anatomy. Although the form and concept of the bust originates in neoclassical idealism, the subject's features have been individualized to a great extent; they are perhaps somewhat too firm and strong for a man of 78 years. Executed in Warren's last year, it is not known whether the bust was done from life or copied from another source posthumously.

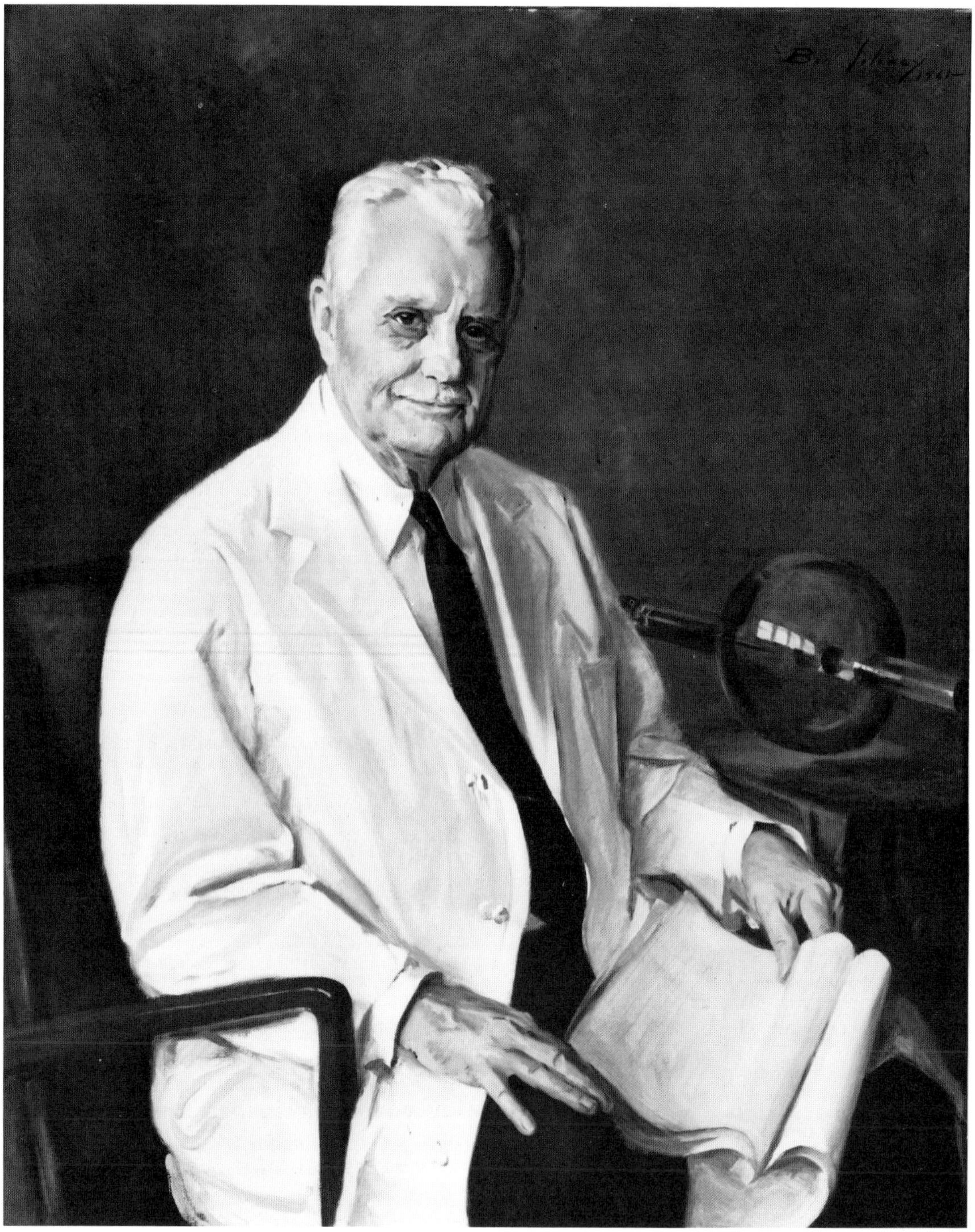

Bernard Pierre Widmann *PA 41*

Bernard Pierre Widmann (1890–1971)

Born in Johnstown, Pennsylvania, Dr. Widmann was the eighth in a Swiss-German family of thirteen children. His undergraduate degree was from St. Vincent's College in Latrobe, Pennsylvania, and his medical degree from the Medico-Chirurgical College in Philadelphia (1916). During World War I he was a first lieutenant in the United States Army Medical Corps, where he was assigned to the Army X-ray School at Camp Greenleaf. He continued his specialized interest in radiology by serving for ten years as the full-time office and hospital assistant to Dr. George E. Pfahler (q.v.), the pioneer radiologist. His academic career began at the Graduate School of Medicine of the University of Pennsylvania, where he was appointed assistant professor of radiology in 1922 and then rose to the rank of professor in 1934. He was chairman of the department from 1945 until he was named professor emeritus in 1957. He was also chief of the department of radiology at Philadelphia General Hospital from 1928 to 1960 and supervising consultant in radiology at Fitzgerald-Mercy Hospital in Darby, Pennsylvania, and at Our Lady of Lourdes Hospital in Camden, New Jersey. During World War II he was consultant in radiology at the Philadelphia Naval Hospital. He wrote more than 100 scientific articles and received world-wide renown for his work on radiation therapy in skin cancer. He was well known also for his studies of leukemia survival time and pulmonary metastases in the irradiated lung and for diagnostic gastro-intestinal X-ray examinations. He was president of the Philadelphia Roentgen Ray Society and the American Roentgen Ray Society, a trustee and chairman of the American Board of Radiology, and chairman of the residency review committee on radiology of the American Medical Association. He was a fellow of the College of Physicians. He received honorary degrees from St. Vincent's College, Hahnemann Medical College, and St. Joseph's College. He received the Schaffrey medal from St. Joseph's College, the Strittmatter award from the Philadelphia County Medical Society, and the gold medal of the American College of Radiology for "outstanding service to radiology."

Artist: Ben Solowey (1900–1978)

For biography, see page 152.

Oil on canvas; 35 1/4 x 29 1/4; signed and dated at upper right, "Ben Solowey 1961." Commissioned by the Blockley Radiological Society and presented to the radiology department of Philadelphia General Hospital. Transferred to the College of Physicians in 1977 as a permanent loan from the City of Philadelphia. *PA 41*

Dr. Widmann is shown two-thirds length. His body is turned to the right; his head is turned slightly to the right and tilted diagonally down. He is shown seated in a green upholstered armchair, with his right hand resting on his knee and his left hand holding an open hospital chart with white, yellow, blue, and pink pages. The interior setting includes a green wall which is darker on the left. At the right a table covered with orange cloth has an X-ray tube on its top. The subject's face is square. He has white hair brushed back from his forehead, blue eyes which look in the direction of the head turn toward the viewer, and a slender nose with a flat upper surface. The cheeks are full. There is a white moustache over a wide mouth, and the thin lips form a pleasant smile. The chin is square. Age is indicated by lines on the forehead, under the eyes, next to the nose, and in the folds of skin in the jowls and the neck. The subject wears a white shirt, a maroon tie with clip, a white laboratory coat, and dark gray trousers. The surface of the portrait is painted fluidly. The head and hands are well constructed in solid and three-dimensional volumes, and the ripples and folds of the costume give a sense of the underlying bodily forms. Although the glass X-ray apparatus appears to be floating, its symbolic message is unmistakable. Widmann appears as the paradigm of a dignified but kindly physician who takes a moment from reading a patient's history to glance up engagingly and encouragingly toward an unseen visitor, perhaps the patient.

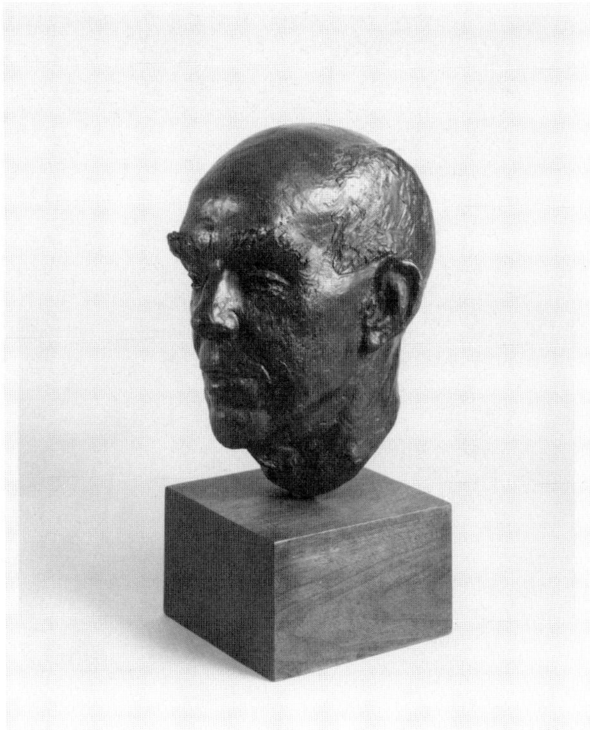

Philip Francis Williams *ST 571*

Philip Francis Williams (1884–1970)

Williams was born in Martin's Ferry, Ohio, the son and great-grandson of physicians. He was graduated from Lafayette College in 1905 and from the medical school of the University of Pennsylvania in 1909. After internship at the Philadelphia General Hospital and the Hospital for Contagious Diseases and a residency at the New York Lying-in Hospital, he established a practice in obstetrics in Philadelphia. His academic career at the University of Pennsylvania started in 1912, when he was appointed demonstrator in obstetrics in the school of medicine and an assistant in the maternity dispensary of the hospital. After a long succession of appointments, he was made professor of clinical obstetrics and gynecology at the school of medicine (1940) and emeritus professor (1952). He was also appointed clinical professor of obstetrics and gynecology at the Graduate School of Medicine in 1949 and emeritus professor in 1952. He was chief of obstetrics at Philadelphia General Hospital, Presbyterian Hospital, Abington Memorial Hospital, and the Jewish Hospital (now the Albert Einstein Medical Center–Northern Division). He was the first chairman of the maternity mortality committee of the Philadelphia County Medical Society, which made investigations into each maternal death in Philadelphia. The results were published in a bold report that made urgent recommendations for improvements in maternal care, seminars for practicing obstetricians, residencies, and regulation of their staff members by hospitals. For this work, which contributed greatly to the decline of maternal mortality, Williams received the Strittmatter award of the Philadelphia County Medical Society in 1933. He served as president of the Obstetrical Society of Philadelphia, the Federation of Obstetric and Gynecologic Societies, and the American College of Obstetrics and Gynecology, and he was the chairman of the section on obstetrics and gynecology of the American Medical Association. He was a founder of the American Board of Obstetrics and Gynecology. He was a fellow of the College of Physicians. During World War I Williams attained the rank of major and served in France with the unit of the Hospital of the University of Pennsylvania (Base Hospital No. 20) as head of the laboratory of clinical pathology. In addition to writing the chapters on nutrition and toxemia of pregnancy in seven textbooks, Williams was the unofficial book review editor of the *American Journal of Obstetrics and Gynecology*, for which he wrote 500 book reviews between 1912 and 1955.

Artist: Harry Rosin (1897–1973)

Rosin, the son of an immigrant Russian shoemaker, was born in Philadelphia. Between 1914 and 1917 he worked for Samuel Yellin, a master craftsman in wrought iron, and executed the iron gates of the Curtis Institute of Music in Philadelphia. After taking night classes at the School of Industrial Art, he taught pottery and modeling at the Trenton Art School. In search of further training, he spent the years from 1923 to 1926 studying sculpture with Charles Grafly (see Joseph Price entry) at the Pennsylvania Academy of the Fine Arts, where he won a Cresson traveling scholarship. He spent the next five years in Europe, chiefly in Paris, and then carried out a commission for a twenty-foot concrete figure of Christ for the façade of the cathedral at Guadeloupe. From 1932 to 1936 he lived in Tahiti, where he executed portrait commissions and did well-known sculptures of nude native women. Upon returning to Philadelphia he divided his time between his Bucks County studio and the Pennsylvania Academy, where he was an instructor of sculpture from 1939 to 1972. He participated in the International Sculpture Exhibition at the Philadelphia Museum of Art in 1933 and at the Chicago World's Fair in 1934. His awards include the Widener gold medal (1939) and the Fellowship prize (1941) at the Pennsylvania Academy, the Regional gold medal (1950), and a Distinguished Pennsylvania Artist Award (1964). He was made an associate of the National Academy of Design in 1970. He had one-man shows at the Gimbel Galleries in 1936, the Pennsylvania Academy in 1945, and the Peale House of the Pennsylvania Academy in 1965. In addition to his portraits and other works in private and museum collections, his work includes many public sculptures. Those in the Philadelphia area include two large limestone figures of *The Quaker* and *The Puritan* in Fairmount Park; an over-life-sized bronze figure of Connie Mack, "Mr. Baseball," at Veteran's Stadium; a bronze figure of John B. Kelly, the Olympic rowing champion, in Fairmount Park; four carved limestone panels for the façade of the West Chester County Court House; and a series of commemorative coins for the 1974 centennial of the Philadelphia Zoo.

Fiberglass; 10 3/4 x 73/4 x 91/2; no base; held by metal rod inserted in wooden pedestal, 37/8 in high; signed and dated on beveled edge on back of head, "Rosin 67." Commissioned in 1967 by the Obstetrical Society of Philadelphia and presented to the College in 1968. *ST 571*

Dr. Williams is shown head-and-neck length. The subject's face is slender. He is totally bald except for a fringe of hair at the sides. Under thick, wavy eyebrows his narrow eyes with carved pupils look straight ahead. His nose is short and thick. The lips of the small mouth are parted and the chin is narrow and pointed. The surface of this portrait bust is very irregular and has visible tool marks throughout. The planes of the face are rather shallow, emphasizing textured surface at the expense of underlying anatomical structure. Nevertheless, the likeness is naturalistic and the facial expression is somewhat pugnacious, almost ominous.

James Cornelius Wilson (1847–1934)

Dr. Wilson was born in Philadelphia, the son of a physician and the descendant of English Quakers on his father's side and of Scotch-Irish forbears on his mother's side. He received the A.B. degree in 1867 and the A.M. degree in 1870 from Princeton and the M.D. degree in 1869 from Jefferson Medical College, where he was a private pupil of W.W. Keen (q.v.). After residencies at Wills Eye and Pennsylvania Hospitals, he continued his education in Vienna and Dresden for a year and then returned to Philadelphia. He began his academic career at Jefferson Medical College, where he was named in rapid succession chief of the medical clinic, chief clinical assistant to Dr. Jacob Mendez Da Costa (q.v.), lecturer in physical diagnosis, and attending physician at Jefferson Hospital. In 1891 he succeeded Da Costa in the chair of the practice of medicine and clinical medicine, a post he held until he was made emeritus professor in 1911. He was also physician-in-chief to the German (now Lankenau) Hospital from 1897 to 1924, attending physician to Philadelphia General Hospital from 1876 to 1890, physician to the Pennsylvania Hospital, and consulting physician to the Philadelphia Lying-in Charity Hospital, the Rush Hospital for Consumptives, the Jewish Hospital (now Albert Einstein Medical Center-Northern Division), Bryn Mawr Hospital, the Amer-

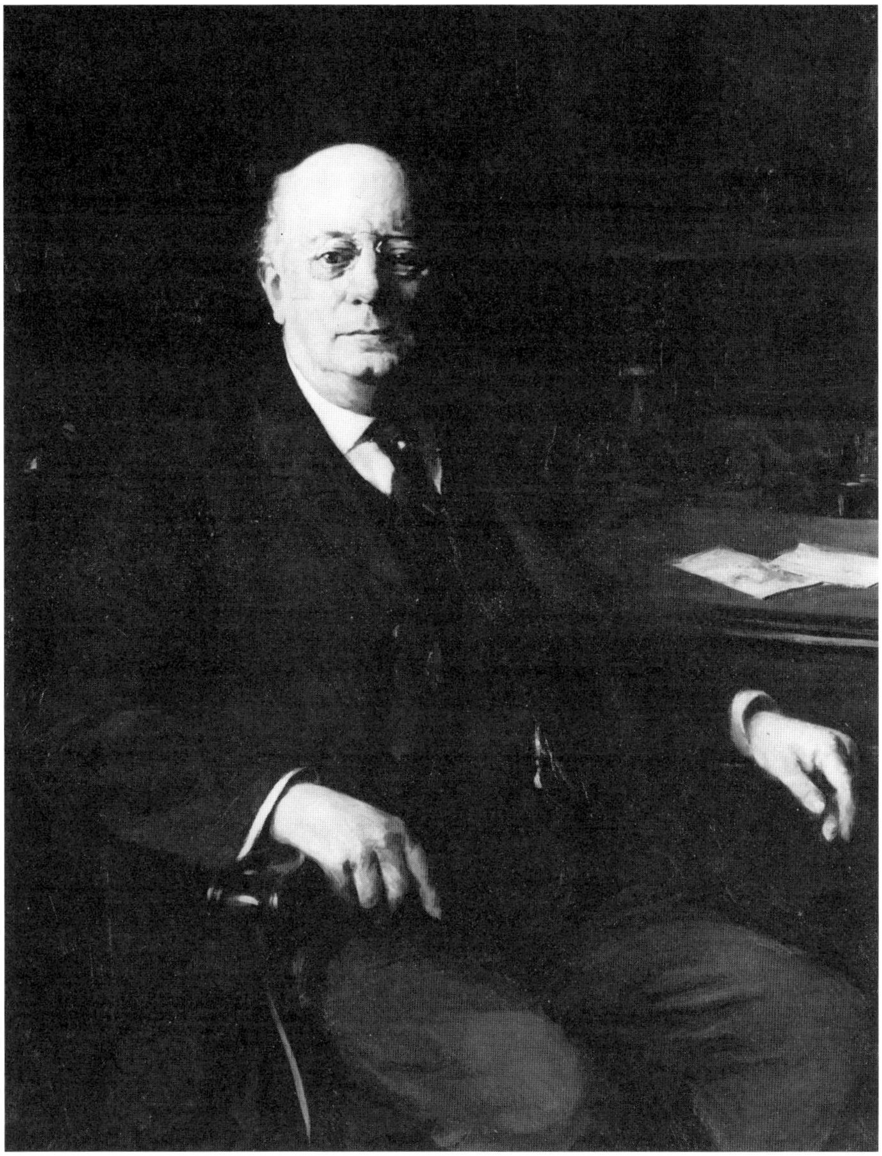

James Cornelius Wilson *PA 30*

ican Hospital for Diseases of the Stomach, and the Widener Memorial Home for Crippled Children. He was president of the College of Physicians (1913–1916), the Philadelphia Medical Club, the Philadelphia Pathological Society, the Philadelphia County Medical Society, the American Academy of Medicine, the Association of American Physicians, the American Climatological and Clinical Association, and the American Therapeutic Society, and he was vice-president of the American Pediatric Society. He wrote more than 100 articles, especially on the treatment of typhoid fever and tuberculosis. He edited *An American Text-book of Applied Therapeutics* (1896) and was author of the following books: *The Summer and Its Diseases* (1879), *A Treatise on the Continued Fevers* (1881), *A Manual of Fever Nursing* (1887), and *A Handbook of Medical Diagnosis* (1909). Through his efforts, the Sarah Magee chair of medicine was endowed at Jefferson Medical College and the Magee Memorial Hospital for Convalescents was founded.

Artist: Frank Benton Ashley Linton (1871–1943)

Born in Philadelphia, Linton studied at the Pennsylvania Academy of the Fine Arts under Thomas Eakins, who painted his pupil's portrait in 1904. He also studied in Paris at the École des Beaux Arts and the Académie Julien under Jean-Léon Gérôme, Jean Joseph Benjamin-Constant, William-Adolphe Bouguereau, Léon Bonnat, and Jean Paul Laurens. He was a well-known painter of portraits and figural scenes both in America and in Paris. He exhibited frequently at the Pennsylvania Academy annuals, the Art Club of Philadelphia (where he won an honorable mention), the Chicago Art Institute, the Society of American Artists (where he won a silver medal), and the Paris salons. He had a one-man show at the Corcoran Gallery of Art in Washington. Among the distinguished subjects of his portraits are Ruth St. Denis, Admiral Benson, and Cardinal Dougherty. In 1921 his painting of General John J. Pershing was commissioned by the Knights

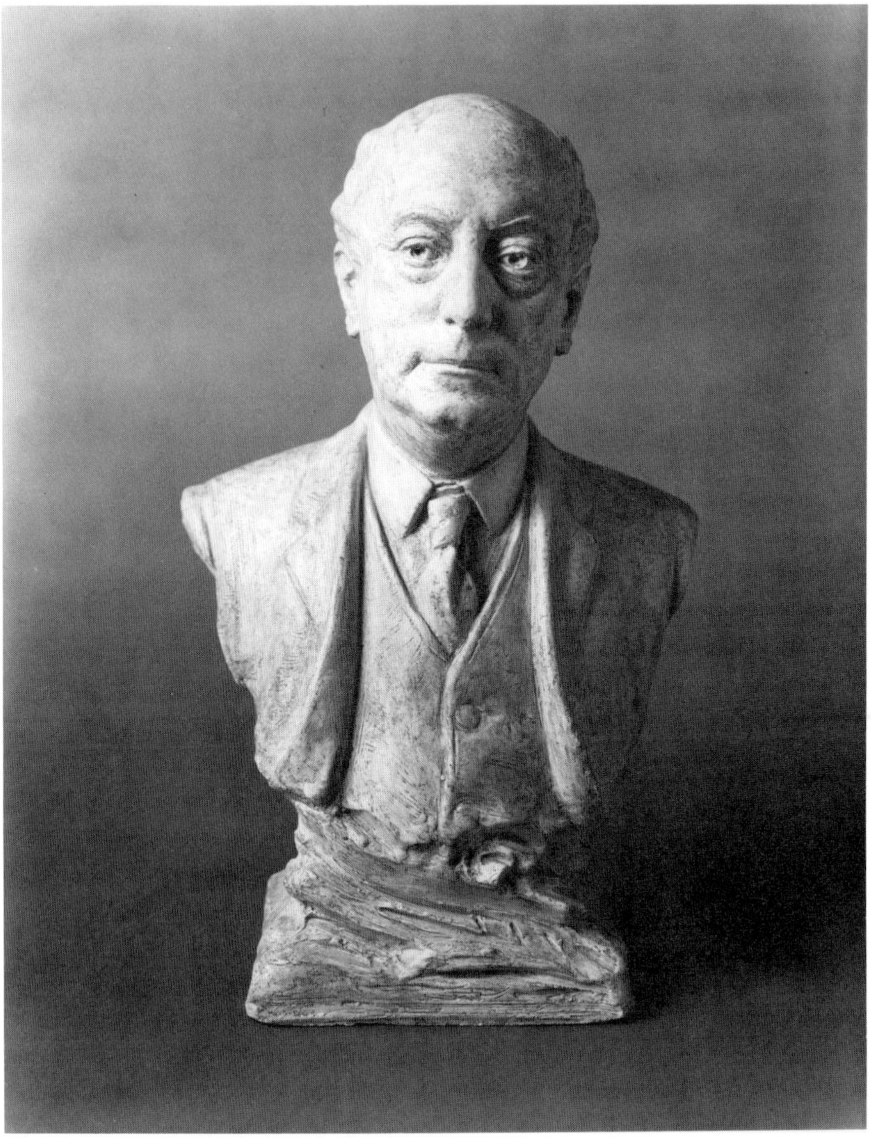

James Cornelius Wilson *ST 558*

of Columbus and presented by the U.S. War Department to the government of France; it was hung in the Palace of the Invalides. Perhaps better appreciated and recognized in Paris than in his native city, he was elected a member of the prestigious Société Internationale des Beaux Arts et des Lettres in 1914. This award, the commission of the Pershing portrait, and the ironic circumstances regarding the purchase of a painting, *The Last Touch,* were fully described in contemporary Philadelphia newspapers. The last-named painting, which shows a clown applying makeup, had been rejected by the Pennsylvania Academy jury for the exhibition of 1922. It was subsequently exhibited in galleries in Philadelphia, New York, Washington, Baltimore, and Dallas. It was sent to the Paris salon of 1927, where it won a bronze medal, was purchased by the French government, and hung at the Luxembourg Galleries and then at the Louvre. Linton died insolvent. His effects were sold at auction to pay creditors, even though at one time his portraits allegedly had sold for $5,000 to $10,000 each.

Oil on canvas; 45 1/2 x 36 1/2; signed and dated at lower left, "Frank B.A. Linton 1917." Presented by Mrs. James Cornelius Wilson in 1917. *PA 30*

Wilson is shown two-thirds length, his body turned to the right, head frontal. He is seated in a Chippendale-style armchair, with his arms resting on the chair arms and his hands pendent over the volute hand holds. The interior setting has a broadly brushed brown background at the left and center and a slant-top, Chippendale-style desk with a green writing surface on which are two stamped envelopes, a lamp, an inkwell, and a round bowl. The space is rather cramped and does not show great depth. The subject has an oval face, a dome-shaped, bald head with a fringe of white hair at the sides, blue eyes which look straight toward the spectator through a pince-nez, puffy lower lids, a full nose with a bump at the bridge, a wide mouth with thin lips, a prominent jawline, a cleft and rounded chin, and a full throat. He wears a white shirt, a black necktie with white tie-pin, a black vest, a gold watch chain, a black single-breasted cutaway coat, and black trousers. The surface of the portrait is brushed fluidly throughout. The head and hands have been modeled strongly in three-dimensional and solid volumes.

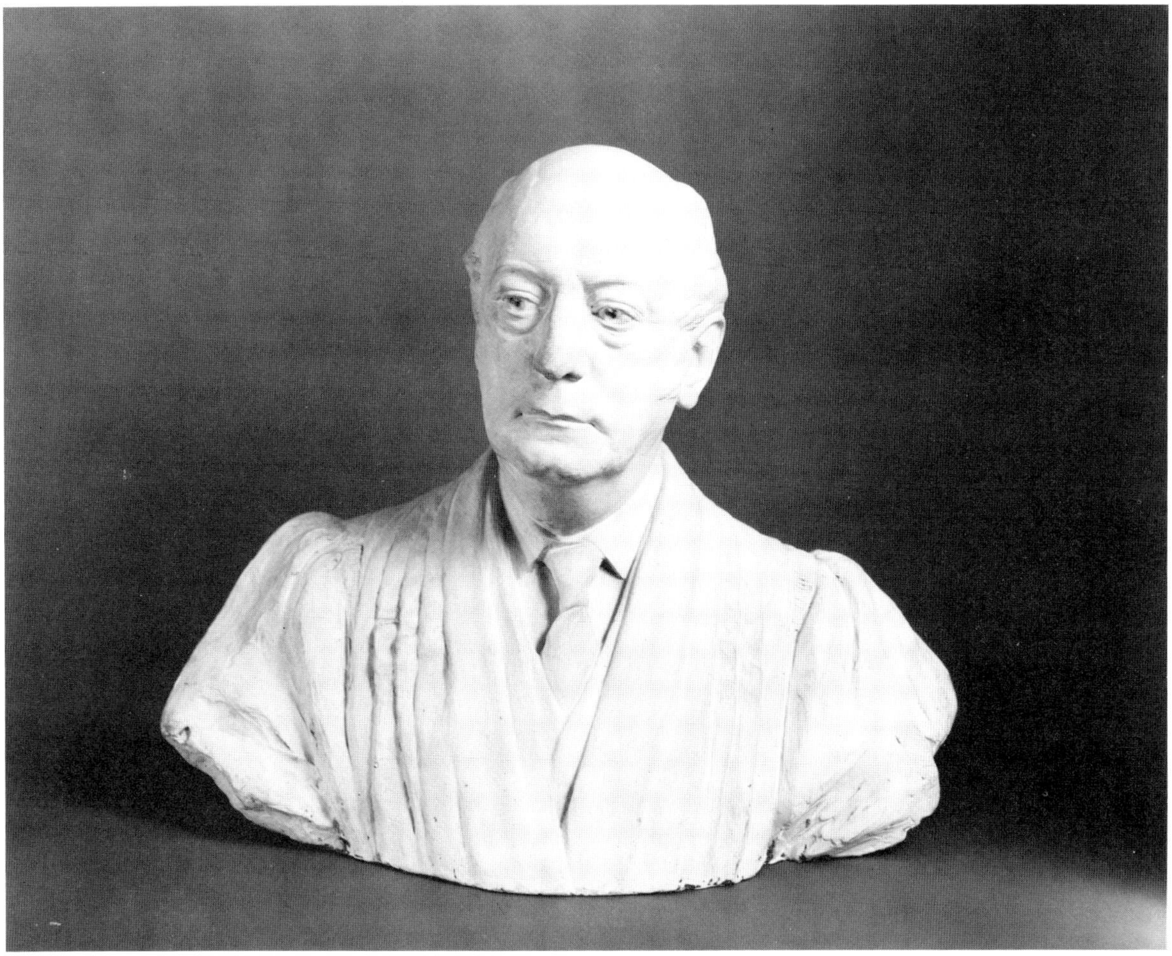

James Cornelius Wilson *ST 559*

The costume emphasizes the ample girth of the body. The portrayal is dramatic, with the spotlighted head and hands emerging from the dark background. The thighs are disproportionately short in order to show the knees and legs. The posture shows much animation, as though the subject has just moved his chair away from the desk and turned his head even further in order to face the viewer. His facial expression is serious and almost challenging.

Artist: Samuel Aloysius Murray (1870–1941)

For biography, see page 3.

Plaster, varnished; 12 x 7 5/8 x 4 7/8; base integral with sculpture, 3/4 in. high; signed and dated on rear at center of the shoulder line, "Murray, 1924." Presented by Mrs. Samuel A. Murray through Dr. William N. Bradley in 1944. *ST 558*

Dr. Wilson is shown bust length, body frontal, with head very slightly to the left and tilted diagonally to the left. His face is oval. He has a bald crown with a fringe of hair at the sides. Under arched brows his eyes have very deeply carved pupils and irises, puffy lower eyelids, and wrinkles at the corners. His cheeks are hollow, and there are age lines next to his prominent nose with its bump at the bridge and next to his wide mouth with its pursed lips. He has a prominent jawline and a square cleft chin. The subject wears a shirt, a necktie slightly askew, a vest, and a coat. The surface of the bust is rough and irregular, with visible tool marks cut into the plaster. Below the jagged bottom of the vest there is a transitional area between the costume and the base that has deeply cut, agitated, angular and curved lines, which create an expressionistic effect. This is in contrast to the calm and serious facial expression and the somewhat stiff pose. The naturalistic rendering of the head is modeled with complete mastery of the underlying anatomy. The costume does not suggest the underlying bodily forms. Compared with the painting by Linton, discussed previously, the subject's face is thinner and his body more slender.

Plaster, painted white; 19 5/8 x 22 7/8 x 11 1/8; no base; not signed or dated. Presented by Mrs. Samuel Murray through the efforts of Dr. William N. Bradley in 1944. According to Michael Panhorst (doctoral candidate in art history at the University of Delaware, authority on Murray, and author of the exhibition catalogue, Samuel Murray at the Hirshhorn Museum and Sculpture Garden, *1982), a bust of Wilson in academic robes by Murray was pictured in the* Philadelphia Public Ledger *on January 6, 1918. There is a bronze bust of Wilson by Murray at Jefferson Medical College dated 1917, but it could not be found for comparison.* *ST559*

Wilson is shown bust length, with body frontal and head turned to the left and slightly tilted. His dome-shaped head is bald except for sparse hair at the sides and low sideburns. Under arched brows, his eyes, which look in the direction of the head turn and tilt, have puffy lower lids and deep wrinkles at the outer corners. The prominent nose has a bump at its bridge. The wide mouth has thin, pursed lips. The subject has a prominent jaw line, a cleft, rounded chin, and a full neck. He wears a shirt, a necktie whose knot is offset to the right, and an academic gown with diagonal soft, rippling folds at the shoulders and tighter, flatter, vertical folds over the chest. The surface of the bust is smooth, except for the rougher, expressionistic treatment of the irregularly contoured sleeves which contrasts with the stiff sobriety of the pose and facial expression. The planes of the head have been modeled with skillful understanding of anatomy. The costume suggests the width and depth of the bodily forms underneath. The naturalistic rendering of the head bears a close resemblance to that in the small bust by Murray already mentioned, but here the face is fuller and the body is more expansive. Here the subject looks off to the side with a morose expression, so that the direct engagement between the subject and viewer seen in the other bust is lacking. However, the fullness of face and body resembles that in the painted portrait by Linton.

Caspar Wistar (1761-1818)

Dr. Wistar was born in Philadelphia. His parents were members of the Society of Friends, and he was the grandson of the founder of the first glassworks erected in this country. During the battle of Germantown he attended the wounded troops. He spent three years as a private pupil of John Redman (q.v.) and also attended the practice of John Jones (q.v.). After this, in 1782, he received the M.B. degree at the University of the State of Pennsylvania. He continued his education in London and then under William Cullen (q.v.) at the University of Edinburgh, where he received the M.D. degree in 1786. On returning to Philadelphia he established a practice in medicine and surgery with the help and patronage of John Jones. He was appointed physician to the Philadelphia Dispensary in 1787 and professor of chemistry in the College of Philadelphia in 1789. He was physician to the Pennsylvania Hospital from 1793 to 1810. He was a junior founding fellow and a censor of the College of Physicians and a founder of the Society for the Promotion of Vaccination. He was elected president of the American Philosophical Society in 1815, succeeding Thomas Jefferson. Wistar was instrumental in effecting the merger in 1791 of the medical school of the University of the State of Pennsylvania with its rival, the College of Philadelphia. In the resulting University of Pennsylvania, he was associated with William Shippen, Jr. (q.v.) as adjunct professor of anatomy, midwifery, and surgery. In 1808, after the death of Shippen, Wistar was made professor of anatomy. His most important medical writing was *A System of Anatomy for the Use of Students of Medicine* (1811-14) in two volumes, the first comprehensive treatise on the subject prepared by an American and published in this country. He is credited with the first observation and description of the posterior portion of the ethmoid bone with the triangular bones attached to it. An innovative teacher, he supervised the preparations of large-scale anatomical models carved in wood by William Rush (q.v.). He also amassed a large collection of anatomical preparations, drawings, and models, which his family presented to the University of Pennsylvania for an anatomical museum. The assemblage was enlarged by the specimens prepared by his former prosector, William E. Horner (q.v.), who became professor of anatomy in 1831. After Horner's death, it was known as the Wistar and Horner Museum until 1892, when it was endowed by a great-nephew of Wistar and became the Wistar Institute of Anatomy and Biology. Wistar was a devout Quaker and a civic-minded and charitable citizen. He succeeded Benjamin Rush (q.v.) as president of the Society for the Abolition of Slavery. He was the founder of the so-called Wistar parties, held at his home on Sunday, later Saturday, evenings for the local intelligentsia, students, members of the American Philosophical Society, and visiting scientists and foreign dignitaries. An honor was accorded him when Thomas Nuttall, a botanist friend, named a flowering vine "wistaria" after him.

Artist: William Rush (1756-1833)

For biography, see page 169.

Plaster; 20 1/4 x 17 3/8 x 12; round base integral with sculpture, 4 3/4 in. high; not signed or dated. Presented by the Wistar Institute of Anatomy in 1958. A plaster cast after the original terra-cotta of 1812-13 is located at the Pennsylvania Academy of the Fine Arts. A description of the piece-mold casting technique is given above, in the entry on Rush's bust of Philip Syng Physick. Probably the present work was made by Rush shortly after the original terra-cotta; a letter from Rush about his preparation of plaster casts of Physick, Rush, and Wistar is mentioned above, in the entry on his bust of Benjamin Rush. Other plaster replicas are to be found at the American Philosophical Society and the Pennsylvania Hospital. Virginia Norton Naudé, sculpture conservator at the Pennsylvania Academy of the Fine Arts, has observed that the bust at the College of Physicians was heavily coated with three layers of paint over a layer of varnish or shellac, with no intervening layer of gesso. When all three layers of paint were removed, it was found that the varnish had been applied after minor damages had been repaired. Hence it was surmised that the bust had left Rush's studio without this layer of varnish. An inscription, "R W," in script capital letters was found painted on the back of the base. The bust at the College of Physicians was included in the exhibit, William Rush, American Sculptor, *at the Pennsylvania Academy of the Fine Arts, 1982.* *ST 562*

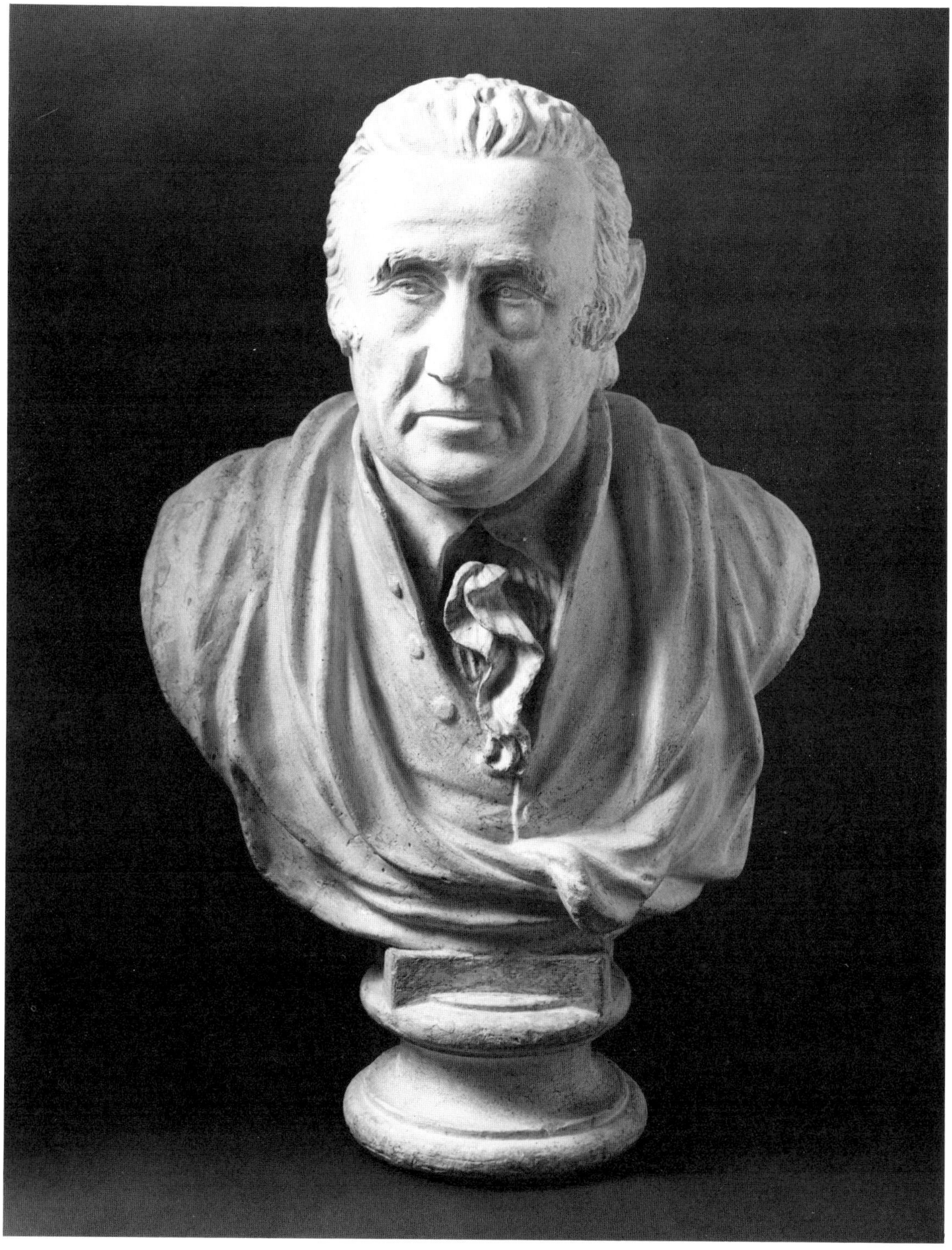

Caspar Wistar *ST 562*

Wistar is shown bust length. His body is frontal, and his head is turned slightly to the left. His face is round. His thick, wavy hair has been brushed back from his forehead. He has long, curly side-whiskers and a long queue at the back tied with a bow. Under thick, wavy eyebrows, his small, narrow-set eyes with their carved irises and pupils look upward in the direction of the head turn. There are wrinkles in the outer corners, and the lower lids are deep and puffy. The prominent nose has a bump at its bridge. The lips are thin and straight. There are deep lines next to the nose and mouth, and a deep U-shaped curve separates the round double chins. The subject's shirt has its collar pointed down, the jabot has rippling curves, and there are a waistcoat with stand-up collar and a coat with deep curving folds tied at the bottom. The surface of the bust has the irregular texture characteristic of plaster. The head is modeled in convincingly solid, anatomical planes. The costume conveys minimal suggestions of the subject's portly body. The facial expression is one of sober dignity. The animation in the portrayal comes from the contrast of light and dark on the sculpted forms and from the movement in the folds and curves of the costume and hair. Compared with the terra-cotta original, the carving is not as deep and its contours not as well defined.

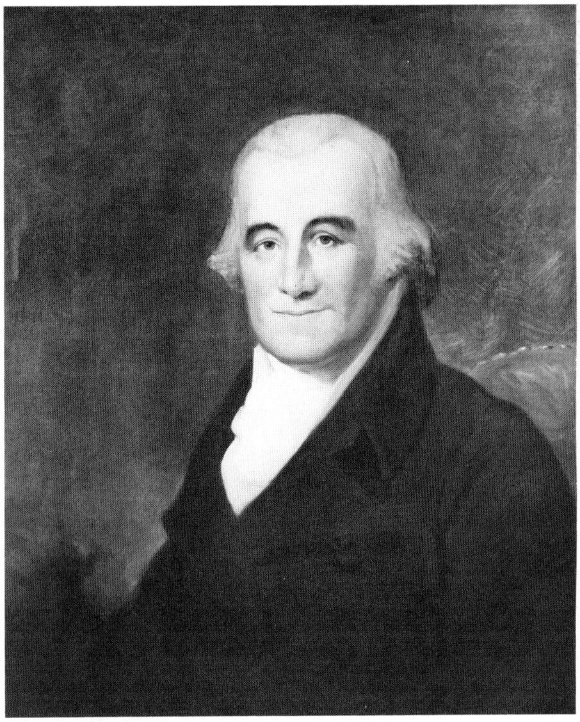

Caspar Wistar *PA 34*

Artist: Attributed to Waugh.

For biographies, see page 44.

Oil on canvas, mounted on wood; 29 1/4 x 24 1/4; not signed or dated. Presented by Mrs. Mifflin Wistar in 1874. When the portrait was included in the College of Physicians' Centennial Celebration Loan Collection of Portraits, *the artist was listed as "Waugh, after Bass Otis." Later inventories, lists, and the Bradley File attribute this portrait to "Waugh" or "Ida Waugh, after Bass Otis." There are probably at least three original portraits of Wistar by Bass Otis. One is in the possession of the Wistar family, another is at Pennsylvania Hospital, and a third was made in 1816 for Joseph Delaplaine's* Repository of the Lives and Portraits of Distinguished Americans. *In addition to the copy at the College of Physicians, there are other copies of Otis originals, including one by Thomas Sully (1830) at the American Philosophical Society, one by Samuel Bell Waugh at the Historical Society of Pennsylvania, and ones by Samuel Bell Waugh and Lucy D. Holme at the University of Pennsylvania. Another portrait of Wistar, attributed to Otis and dated ca. 1816, is located at the Green Tree Collection of the Mutual Assurance Company and shows the subject in the same pose but includes a table with books in the background. For discussions of these portraits, see catalogues of the art collections of all the above institutions, especially that by Anthony N.B. Garvan and Carol A. Wojtowicz,* Catalogue of the Green Tree Collection, *Philadelphia, 1977. See also the exhibition catalogue,* Bass Otis: Painter, Portraitist and Engraver, *Historical Society of Delaware, 1976, with essays by Gainor B. Davis and Wayne Craven, and an essay by Robert G. Stewart in the exhibition,* A Nineteenth-Century Gallery of Distinguished Americans, *National Portrait Gallery, 1969. Further research will be necessary before secure attribution of the portrait of the College of Physicians can be made.* *PA 34*

Dr. Wistar is shown bust length, body turned to the left and head slightly to the left. He is seated in a red upholstered chair. The thinly painted, mottled background is greenish-brown at the right and warm reddish-gray at the left, with a dark shadow below. The subject has an oval face. His gray hair is worn full over the ears and tied in a queue. He has thick, black, arched eyebrows, brown eyes which look out toward the viewer, a prominent nose with a bump on its flat bridge, a wide mouth with thin lips and a trace of a smile, full cheeks, and a round chin. His complexion is ruddy. The subject wears a white stock, a white jabot, a white waistcoat with stand-up collar, and a black double-breasted coat with M-notched lapels and a high collar. Except for the mottled background, the surface of the portrait is smoothly painted and the forms have soft edges. The head is rendered in solid and three-dimensional planes, while the costume is flat and does not suggest the underlying body. Although the subject regards the viewer directly and has a pleasant expression, his bearing lacks the energy and animation of a portrait painted from life.

George Bacon Wood (1797–1879)

Descended from forbears who came to America from Bristol, England, in 1682, Wood was born to a prosperous farmer in Greenwich, New Jersey. He was graduated from the University of Pennsylvania with an A.M. degree in 1815 and an M.D. degree in 1818, after having studied with Joseph Parrish (q.v.). His earliest academic appointments were at the Philadelphia College of Pharmacy, where he was professor of chemistry from 1822 until 1831 and professor of materia medica from 1831 to 1835. He was attending physician at the Pennsylvania Hospital from 1835 to 1859. At the University of Pennsylvania he was professor of materia medica from 1835 to 1850 and of the theory and practice of medicine from 1850 to 1860, when he was named professor emeritus. In 1863 he became a trustee of the University and held that position until his death. In 1865 he endowed an auxiliary faculty of medicine composed of five chairs—zoology and comparative anatomy, botany, mineralogy and geology, hygiene, and medical jurisprudence and toxicology. He bequeathed to the University Hospital funds to build the Peter Hahn ward in honor of his father-in-law. He was president of the College of Physicians from 1848 to 1879 and bequeathed to it his library and $15,000. He was president of the American Philosophical Society from 1859 to 1879 and of the American Medical Association from 1855 to 1856. His most important literary work is *The Dispensatory of the United States,* written in 1833 with Franklin Bache. He also wrote *A Treatise on the Practice of Medicine* (1847), *A Treatise on Therapeutics* (1856), and histories of the University of Pennsylvania and of Pennsylvania Hospital. He received an honorary LL.D. degree from Princeton University in 1858.

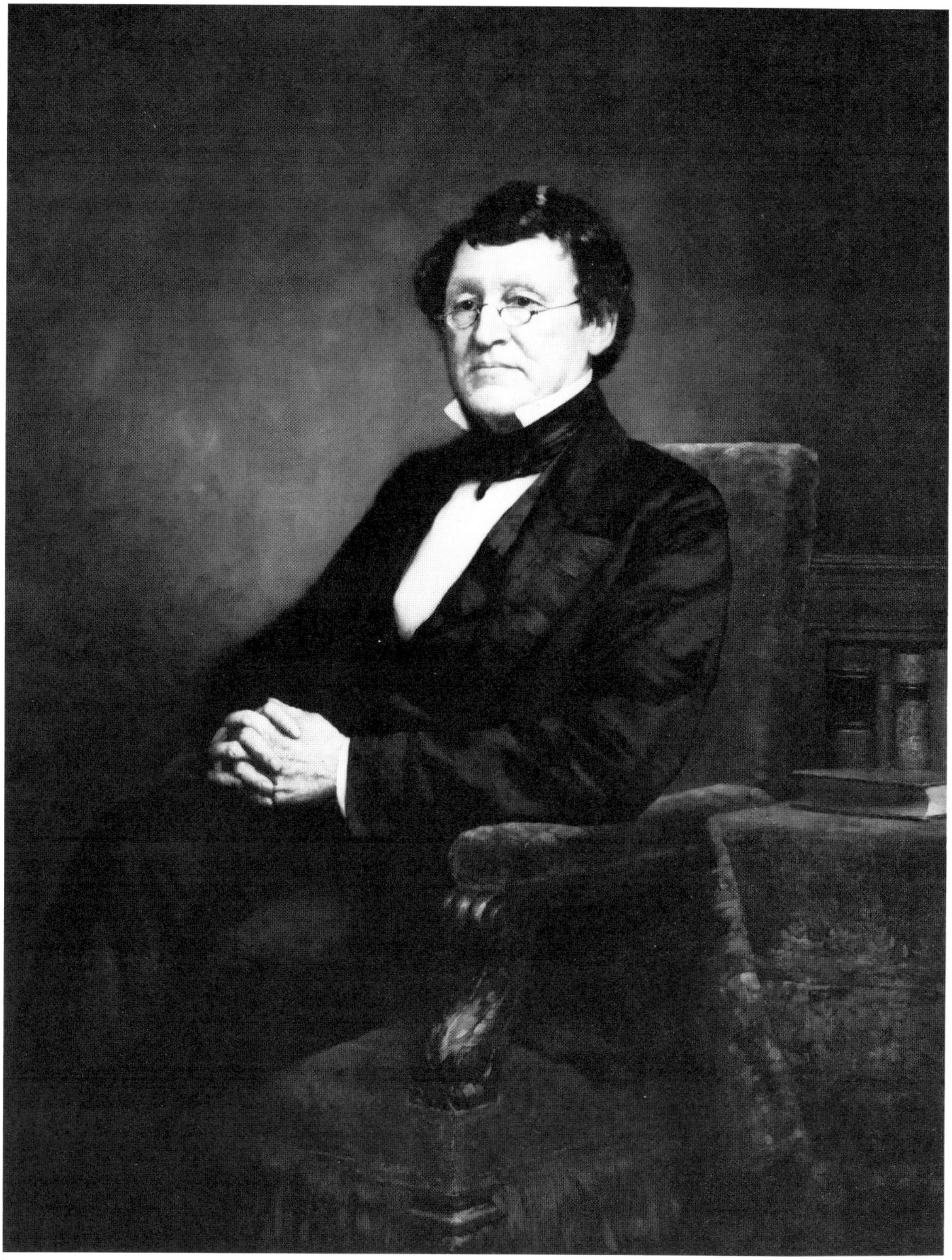

George Bacon Wood *PA 28*

Artist: Bernard Uhle (1847–1930)

For biography, see page 3.

Oil on canvas; 51 1/2 x 40 1/2; not signed or dated. Presented by Richard Wood on behalf of Mrs. George Bacon Wood in 1887. When it appeared in the College of Physicians' Centennial Celebration Loan Collection of Portraits, *the artist was listed as "B. Uhle." Because of the chronology of Uhle's career, this portrait was very probably copied from an earlier source. After his student days, Uhle is known to have been a photographer from 1867 to 1875. Although he opened a portrait studio in Philadelphia in 1877, he was abroad twice between 1875 and 1879, the year of Wood's death, and was not steadily employed in making portraits until 1880. The collection at the College contains a photograph taken by Frederick Gutekunst and dated 1870 that is almost identical to the Uhle painting in pose, position, and costume, and it is a likely source of this portrait. The painting shows evidence of having been enlarged 3 1/4 inches on all sides.* *PA 28*

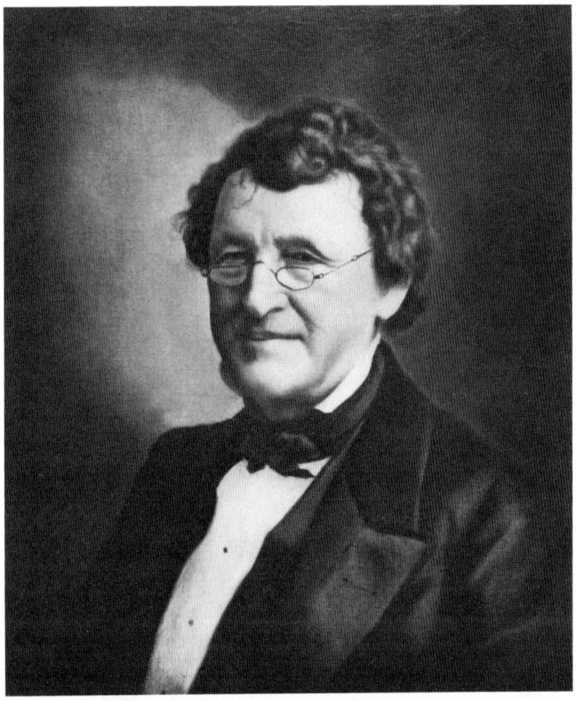

George Bacon Wood *PA 118*

Dr. Wood is shown three-quarter length, with body and head turned to the left. He is seated with forearms resting on the padded arms of a red velvet upholstered armchair that has volute-carved arm supports. His hands are clasped together and rest above his legs, which are crossed at the knees. The atmospheric background is grayish-umber, lighter in the center around the head of the figure, and darker at the upper right and lower left. Next to the chair on the right are a bookcase containing four volumes and a table covered with a "turkey" carpet in red, green, and yellow; a closed book is lying on it. The subject's face is triangular. His thick, reddish-brown hair is known to be a wig. Under almost hairless eyebrows, his heavy-lidded blue eyes look over metal-rimmed spectacles into the distance in the direction of the head turn. His nose has a bump at its bridge and a long tip that points down to a wide mouth with full red lips and a rounded, narrow chin. His face is wide across the cheeks and has age lines encircling the eyes and next to the nose and mouth. The subject wears a white shirt with stand-up collar, a black neckcloth tied into a bow, and a black vest, coat, and trousers. The surface of the portrait has been brushed meticulously with small, visible strokes. The costume, chair, and carpet show skillful depiction of their various textures. The head and hands have been extremely well modeled in convincingly solid volumes. There is a suggestion of the bodily masses under the costume. The posture of the subject is erect and formal. The expression is dignified and bland, as though the doctor were posing for a photograph. There is a disparity in focus between the contours of the near and far shoulders and arms, such as is often seen in contemporary photographs. In comparison with the photograph by Frederick Gutekunst, the portrait shows that the painter has retained the composition but has effected subtle changes by softening the angularity of the face, elongating the legs, changing the style of the chair and table, and eliminating a curtain and bellpull from the background.

Artist: Unknown

Oil on canvas; 23 1/2 x 19 1/2; not signed or dated. Presented by Dr. George B. Wood in 1948. Although it has a photographic appearance, investigation has shown that it is not a painted-over photograph, as was once suggested. In all probability it was copied after Uhle's portrait of Wood, mentioned above, or from its probable source, the Frederick Gutekunst photograph of 1870, also mentioned above.
PA 118

Dr. Wood is depicted bust length, head and body turned to the left. The atmospheric background is dark brown to dark red on the right and dark brown to yellowish-umber on the left. The face is oval. The subject is wearing a dark brown, curly wig with several loose strands on his forehead. The dark brown eyebrows—Wood was totally bald and lacked brows—have an exaggerated diagonal curve; they parallel the extremely narrow, hooded brown eyes, which gaze over metal-rimmed spectacles directly toward the viewer. The long nose has a bump at its bridge and a tip that points down to a wide mouth whose red lips form a tense smile. There are deep lines in the forehead and next to the nose and mouth. The lines of the chin and jowls are soft. The subject wears a white studded shirt with one collar tip up and one down and a dark brown tie, vest, and coat. The style of this portrait is smoother than that of Uhle described above, and shows no brush strokes. All contour lines are softer. Although well modeled, the figure is less convincingly solid than Uhle's. Here the face is longer and the expression more amiable and direct. In addition to changes in the size, colors, background, and costume, the artist has reversed the focus; here the far shoulder and arm are clearer and the near shoulder line is blurred.

Artist: Edward Stauch (b. ca. 1830)

Born in Saxe-Coburg, Germany, Stauch emigrated to the United States and was active in Philadelphia in the late 1850s and 1860s. He exhibited sculpture at the Pennsylvania Academy of the Fine Arts from 1856 to 1860, where records show that he was nominated associate in 1859 and elected prior to 1860.

Marble; 27 1/4 x 17 1/4 x 11 5/8; rectangular base integral with sculpture, 5 1/2 in. high; signed on the back below the coat collar, "E. Stauch Phila." The plaque at the College of Physicians reads, "This bust was executed by order of/J.B. Lippincott/on account of his admiration for/Doctor George B. Wood/and presented to the/College of Physicians/ by his sons/Craige, Walter and J. Bertram Lippincott." The College of Physicians Inventory of 1898–1915 confirms the donors and adds that the sculpture was presented in 1910. Although there is a marble replica at the American Philosophical Society, it was probably the present bust that was exhibited at the Pennsylvania Academy of the Fine Arts annuals in 1857 and 1858, the owner being listed as J.B. Lippincott. The work closely resembles marble busts of Dr. Wood at the University of Pennsylvania and at the American Philosophical Society. *ST 551*

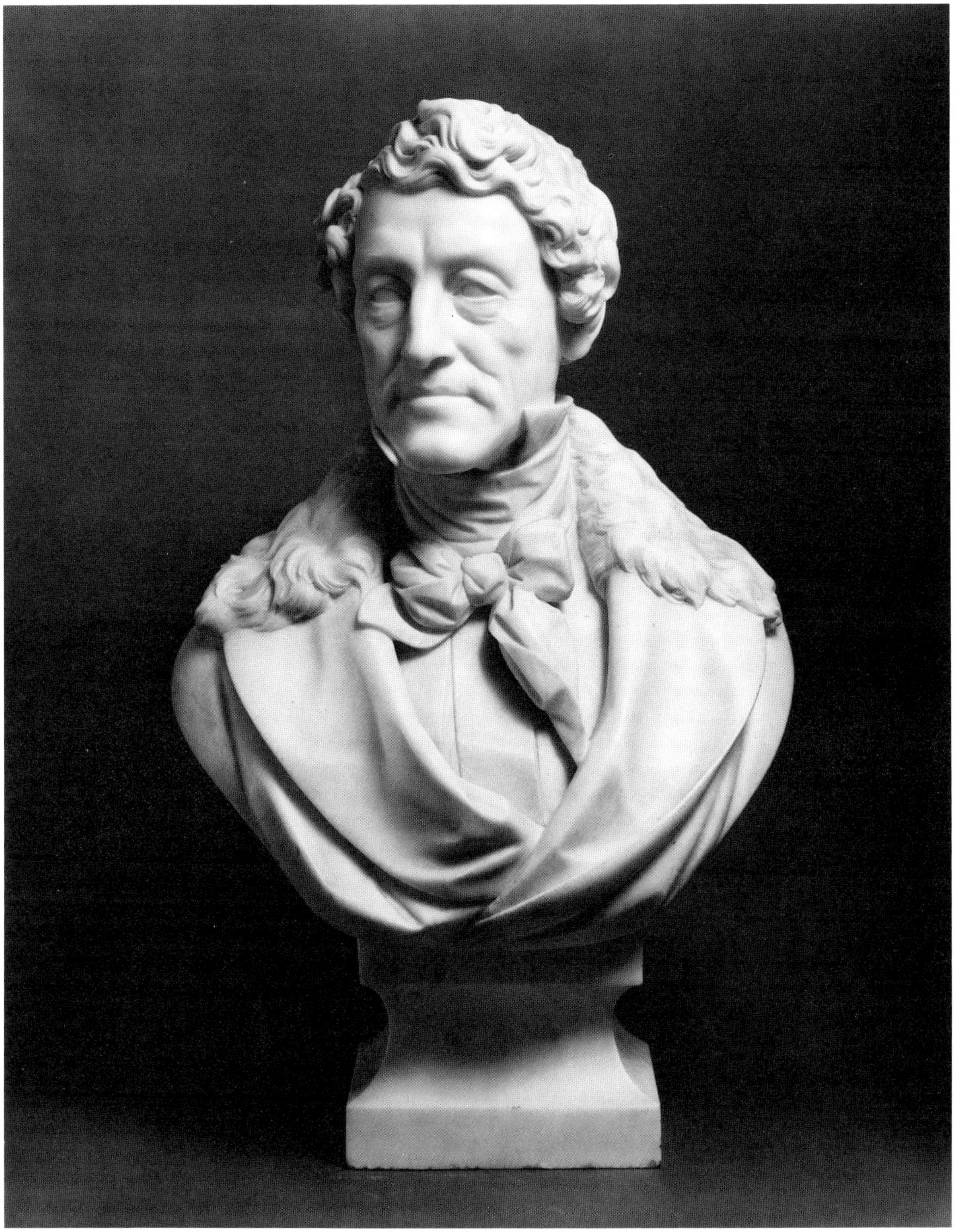

George Bacon Wood *ST 551*

Dr. Wood is shown bust length, with body frontal and head turned to the left. His face is rectangular. He has very thick, wavy hair, worn full at the top and sides. There is a vertical wrinkle between the hairless eyebrow ridge. The hooded and slanted eyes are blank; there are wrinkles at the outer corners and the lower lids are puffy. The nose, wide at the bridge, has a long tip which points down to a wide mouth with full lips and a jutting square chin. The subject has high cheekbones, hollow cheeks, and deeply incised, asymmetrical age lines next to his nose and mouth. He wears a shirt whose stand-up collar has one tip up and one down, a wide neckcloth tied in a large bow whose ends trail off in different directions, and a coat with a fur-trimmed, shawl collar and overlapping lower sections. The surface of the marble is smooth. The head is modeled convincingly with subtle depiction of anatomical planes. Even though the eyes are blank and the expression neutral in the usual neoclassical manner, the bust radiates a sense of energy and strength. There is abundant animation in the wavy hair, fur-trimmed collar, and jauntily tied bow and a contrast of light and dark which is caused by the light falling on the deeply carved forms of the head and costume. Although there is an unmistakable resemblance to the painted portraits above, the marble bust presents a somewhat more idealized face, with longer, thinner, and more angular conformation.

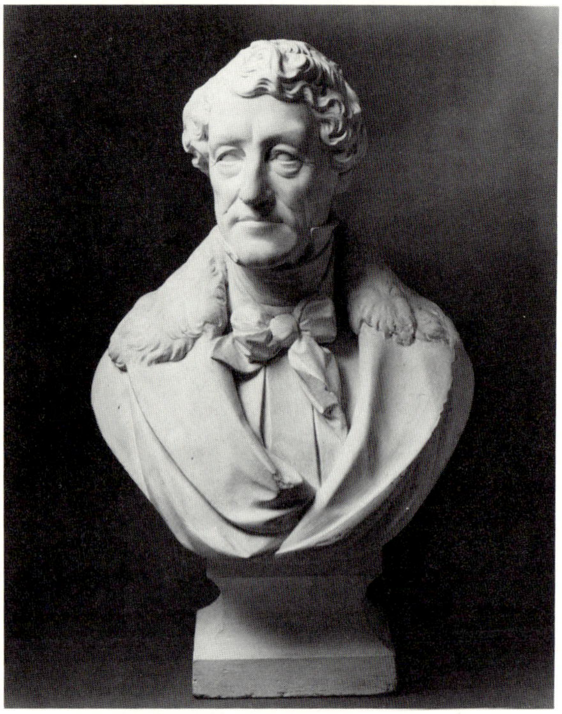

George Bacon Wood *ST 520*

Artist: Unknown

Plaster, painted white; 27 x 17 1/2 x 16/8; rectangular base, integral with sculpture, 6 in. high; not signed or dated. Neither donor nor date of donation is on record. *ST 520*

This plaster figure is obviously related to the marble bust of George Bacon Wood by Edward Stauch, described above. It has not been ascertained whether the plaster is a copy or a cast of the marble version or if it served as a source from which the marble was copied. When the two are placed side by side, one notices subtle differences in the texture and folds of the hair, fur collar, neckcloth, and face. Not all of these dissimilarities need be due to inherent qualities of the media or to the processes of casting or copying.

Artist: Edward Dufrène (b. 1836)

For biography, see page 80.

Plaster, painted white; 26 1/2 x 16 3/4 x 10; rounded base integral with sculpture, 5 in. high; signed on rear on beveled edge below collar, "Edward Dufrène Philada."; dated below signature on columnar part of base, "sculp 1851." Neither donor nor date of donation is on record. Included in the College of Physicians Inventory of 1898–1915 is mention of a plaster bust of George Bacon Wood, "bronzed." The catalogue of College Collections of 1940 contains the report of a bronze bust of George Bacon Wood by "Edoard Dufrene, 1851." In both cases, "bronze" refers to the color. It is not uncommon for plaster busts of this kind to have received multiple layers of different colors of paint, in the fashion of the day. It is improbable that the entry in the Inventory of 1898–1915 refers to plaster bust ST 520, described above. *ST 513*

Dr. Wood is shown bust length. His body is frontal, his head is turned slightly to the right. His face is triangular. He has thick strands of wavy hair, a vertical crease in his forehead, hairless eyebrow ridges, narrow and slanted, blank eyes with linear upper lids and puffy lower lids, a long aquiline nose, a wide mouth with thin upper lip and protruding lower lip, and a narrow chin which juts forward. He has hollow cheeks and high cheekbones. There are creases next to his nose. He wears a shirt with stand-up collar, a very thick neckcloth tied in a large bow, a waistcoat, and a coat with M-notched collar. The surface of the bust has the slightly irregular texture characteristic of plaster. The modeling of the planes of the head is relatively shallow and the costume does not suggest underlying bodily forms. The facial expression is austere but bland. Compared with the Stauch marble bust and the other plaster bust of Wood discussed above, this portrayal is less energetic and the costume less animated, yet the shape of the face, especially the width across the cheeks and the narrow chin, bears a closer resemblance to the two painted portraits of Wood that are discussed on previous pages.

Horatio C Wood (1841–1920)

Born in Philadelphia, Wood was a ninth generation descendant of English Quakers who arrived in America with William Penn. He was graduated from the medical school of the University of Pennsylvania in 1862. After interning at the Pennsylvania and Philadelphia General Hospitals, he enlisted in the United States Army Medical Corps and served in a front line hospital in Virginia during the Civil War. Upon his return to the University he became a quiz-master of therapeutics, the practice of medicine, and chemistry. In 1873 he became lecturer on nervous diseases and, in 1875, clinical professor of nervous diseases. The latter position he held until 1902. He was made professor of materia medica and pharmacology in 1876, professor of general therapeutics in 1877, and professor emeritus in 1907. At Philadelphia General Hospital, he served on the medical staff from 1870 to 1883 and on the neurological staff from 1883 to 1887. He was president of the Philadelphia Neurological Society (1890–1901), the Pharmacopoeial Convention of the United States (1890–1910), and the College of Physicians (1902–04). He also was a charter member of the American Physiological Society. He was not only a captivating teacher, a forceful lecturer, a skillful diagnostician, and an original investigator, but he was also the clear and fluent writer of more than 300 scientific publications. He wrote a series of papers on botany, entomology, and zoology, was an assiduous collector, made two expeditions for the Smithsonian Institution, filled the chair of botany in the auxiliary faculty of medicine at the University of Pennsylvania, and wrote treatises on natural history, such as *The Myriapoda of the United States* (1865) and *The Fresh Water Algae of North*

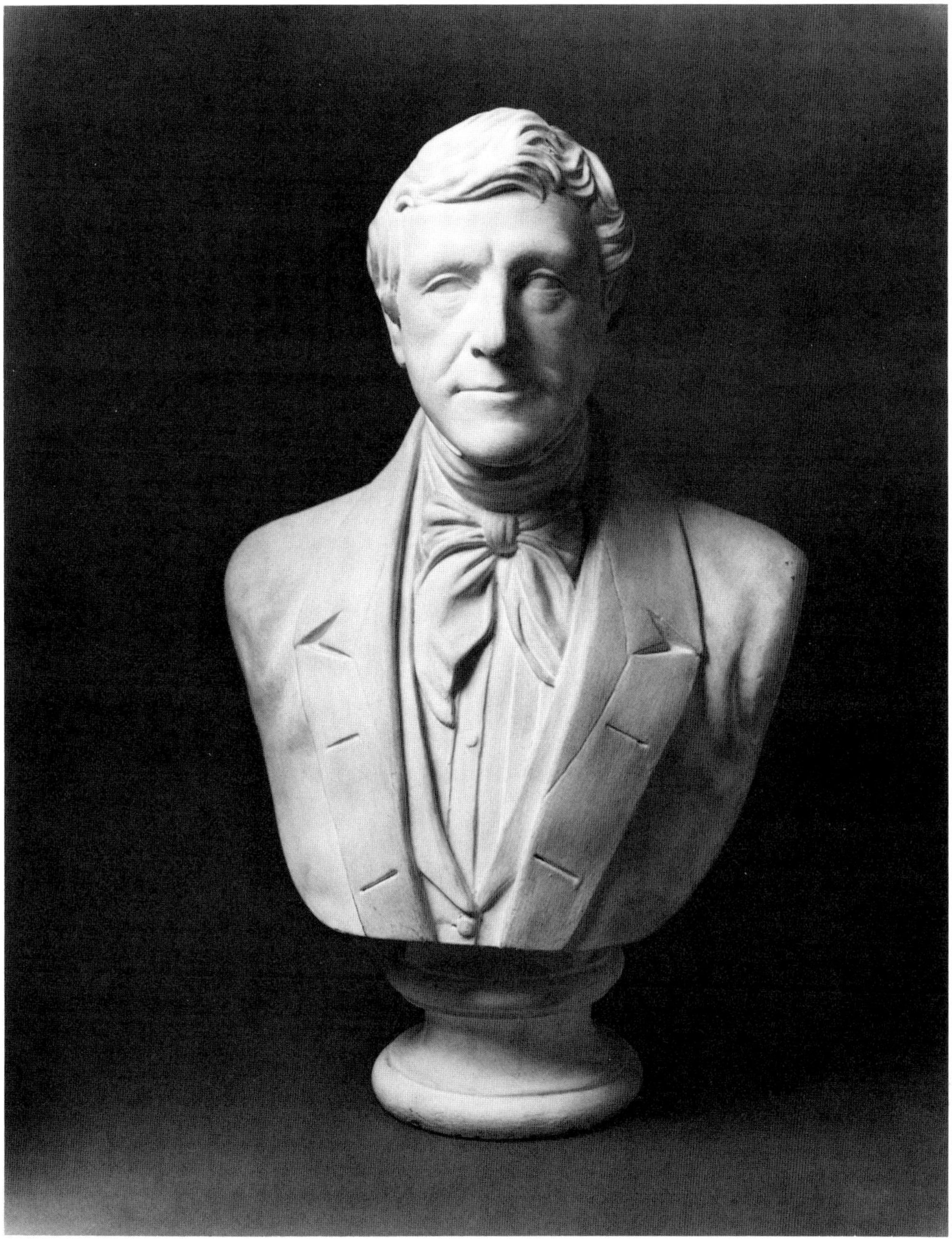

George Bacon Wood ST 513

America (1872). Among his numerous publications in neurology are *Nervous Diseases and their Diagnosis* (1887) and *Syphilis of the Nervous System* (1889). He investigated sunstroke, and his treatise, *Thermic Fever, or Sunstroke*, won the Boylston prize of Massachusetts General Hospital in 1872. With funds from a Smithsonian grant he did further research on the nature and causes of fever, which established the scientific basis of cold bath therapy and made the treatment universal. His most enduring work, *A Treatise on Therapeutics, Comprising Materia Medica and Toxicology, with Especial Reference to the Application of the Physiological Action of Drugs to Clinical Medicine* (first published in 1874; 13 editions), helped to lay the foundation for the modern practice of therapeutics based on known physiological effects rather than on empiricism or clinical experience. Other significant contributions to the medical literature are his works on medical jurisprudence and the books, *Brain-work and Overwork* (1880) and *The Practice of Medicine* (with Reginald Fitz, 1896). He was editor of *New Remedies, Philadelphia Medical Times, Therapeutic Gazette*, and the fifteenth edition of *The Dispensatory of the United States* (with Joseph P. Remington and Samuel P. Sadtler). Advocating the elevation of medical requirements and the improvement of medical instruction, he was a prime mover in the University of Pennsylvania's adoption of a three-year course in medicine and in the fund-raising and erection of the University Hospital. He was awarded honorary degrees from Yale, Lafayette, and the University of Pennsylvania.

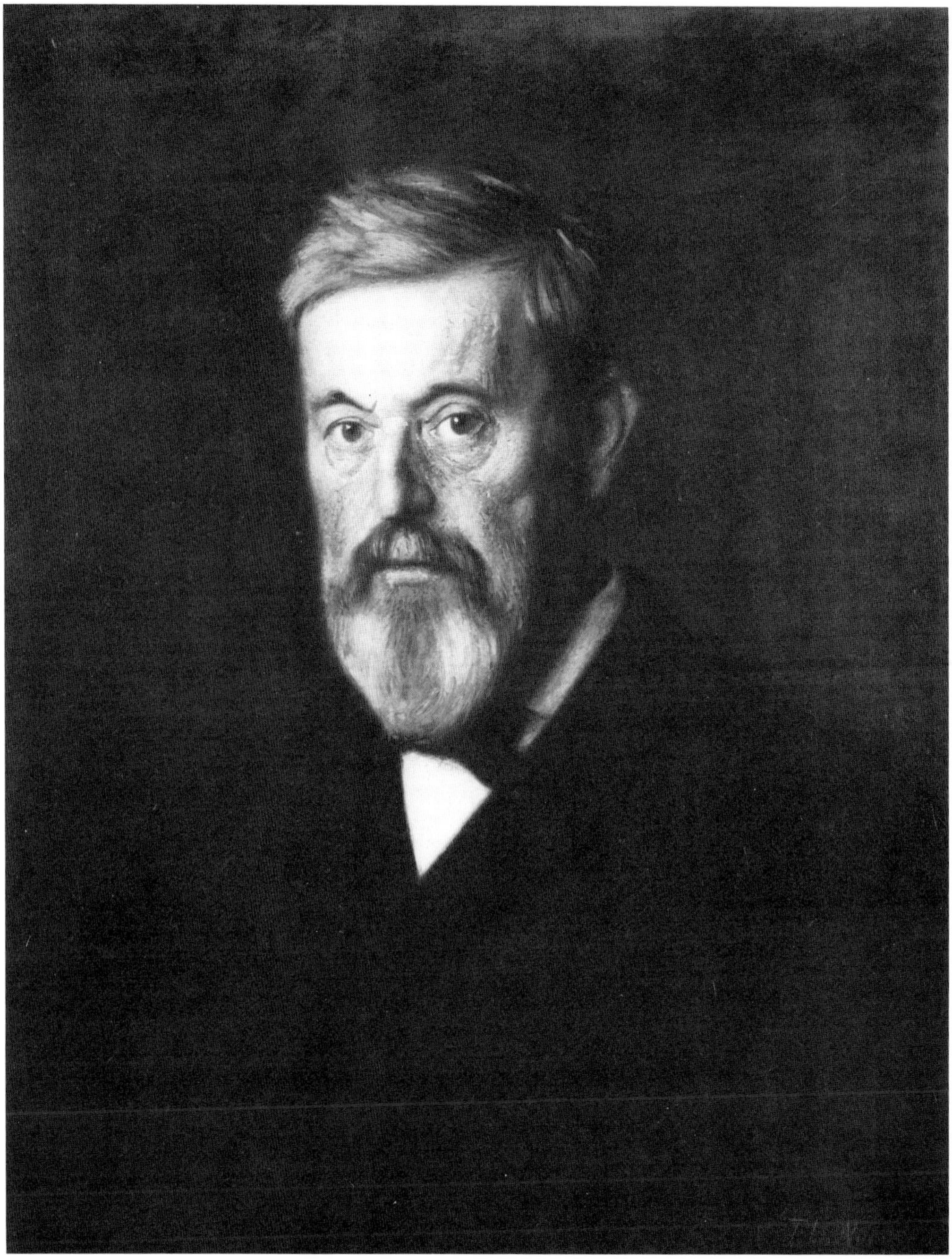

Horatio C Wood *PA 20*

Artist: James Longacre Wood (1867–1938)

For biography, see page 96.

Oil on canvas; 28 1/4 x 22 3/4; signed and dated at lower right, "James L. Wood/1905." Presented by friends and former students in 1905. *PA 20*

Dr. Wood is shown bust length, with body turned to the left and head slightly to the left and downward. The background is dark greenish-gray. The subject's face is slender. He has steel-gray short hair, black eyebrows, a dark gray moustache, and a medium-gray pointed beard. His brown eyes, which look out of their corners and upward toward the viewer, are surrounded by creases and puffy lower lids. His nose has a bump at its bridge and a sharp tip which points down to a small mouth with a full lower lip. The flat cheeks add to the elongation of the face. The subject wears a white shirt, a black bow tie, a black vest buttoned high, and a black coat. The surface of the portrait combines a painterly style in the head and a smoother style in the costume and background. The head has been modeled extremely well in convincingly solid, three-dimensional forms. The costume is so flat and dark that it almost merges into the background. This portrait is a poignant statement about a once-powerful member of the medical elite, now sick and depressed and one year away from forced retirement. It was painted by Dr. Wood's artist son, who in his father's opinion never lived up to family expectations. The haunting quality of the image is derived from the luminous eyes, the brooding facial expression, and the dramatic contrast of light and dark, so characteristic of this painter's finest work.

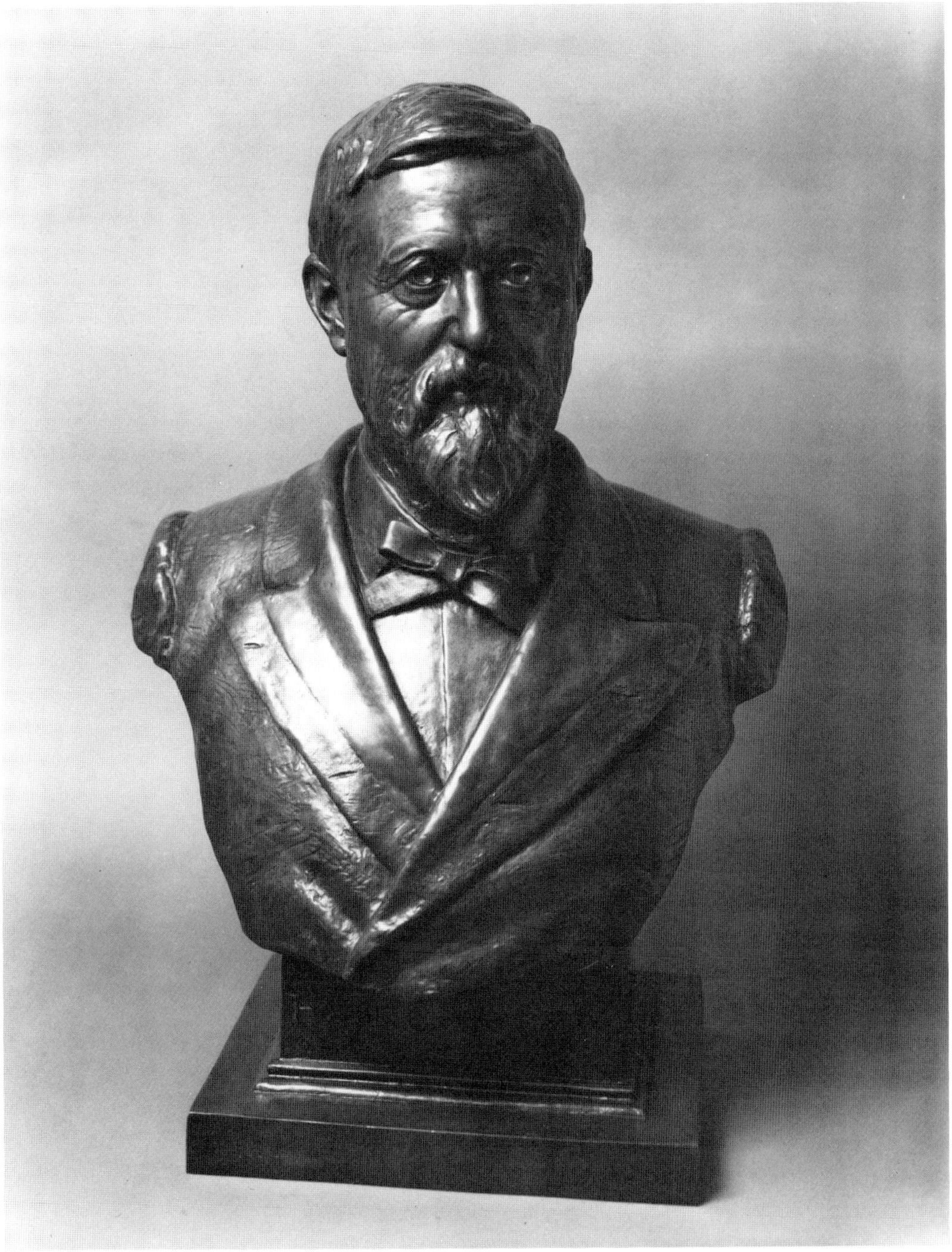

Horatio C Wood *ST 549*

Artist: Samuel Aloysius Murray (1870–1941)

For biography, see page 3.

Bronze; 26 1/4 x 18 x 11 1/2; rectangular base integral with sculpture, 4 3/4 in high; signed and dated on back, below shoulders, "S. Murray May, 1898"; inscription on front of upper tier of base, "Horatio C. Wood M D"; identity of foundry is stated in the rear, at the bottom of the base, "Roman Bronze Works N Y." Presented by George Wood and George Wood Bacon in 1910. *ST 549*

Dr. Wood is shown bust length, body frontal and head turned to the right. His face is oval. He has smooth hair and furrowed brows. His large round eyes, with irises and pupils carved, look out in the direction of the head turn. There are wrinkles at their outer corners and puffy lower lids. His nose has a bump at its bridge. The small mouth is almost hidden by the moustache, which connects side-whiskers with the Vandyke beard. The subject wears a shirt, a narrow bow tie slightly askew, and a coat with wide, notched lapels. The surface of the bronze is smooth on the face and shirt. A rougher texture is shown by incised lines on the coat. The head is skillfully modeled with convincing anatomical depiction. The costume suggests the underlying bodily forms. The subject looks energetic, confident, and strong. The sculpture was made two years before illness struck the subject, when he was still at the height of his great ability. Adding to the power of the image is the dramatic contrast of light and shadow falling on the deeply carved surfaces of the head and costume.

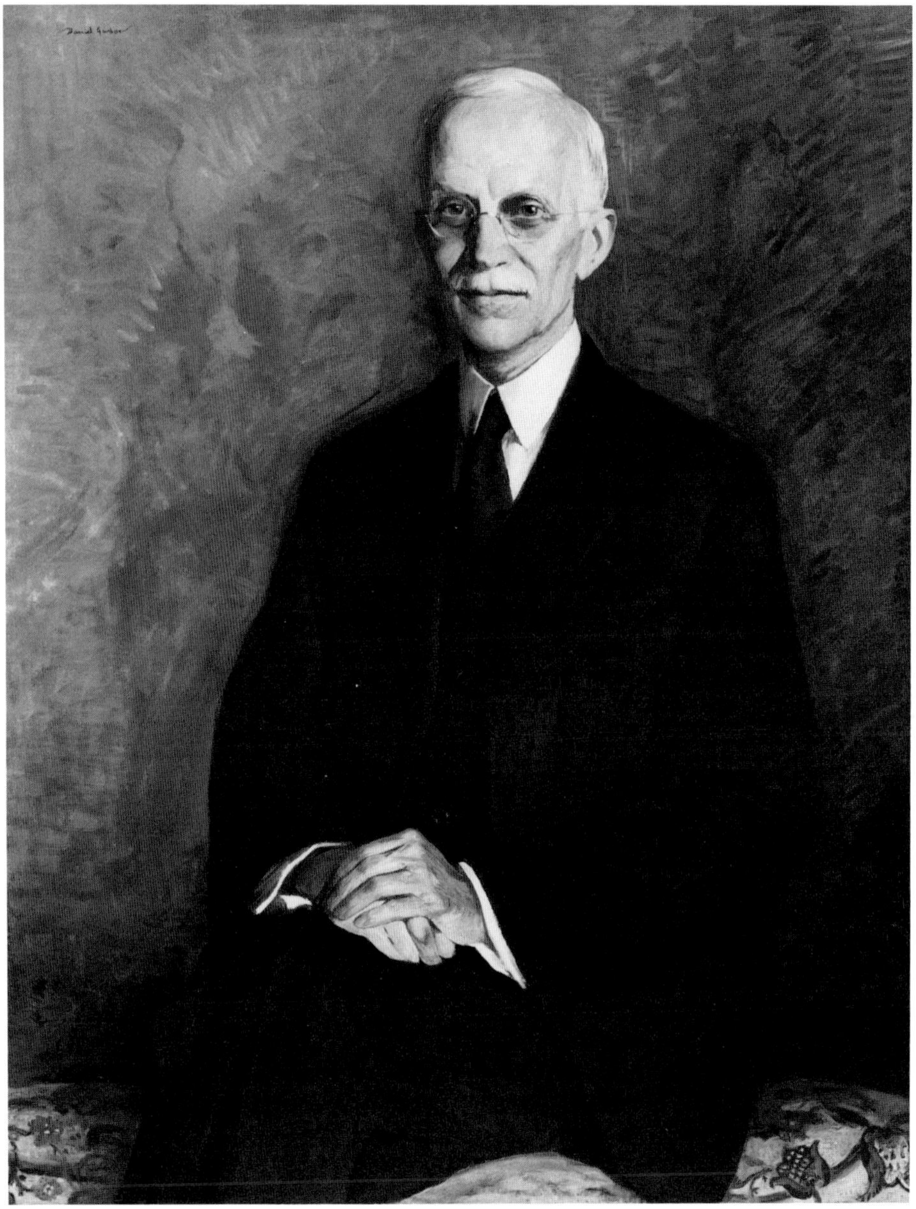

William Zentmayer *PA 106*

William Zentmayer (1864–1958)

Born in Philadelphia, William Zentmayer was the son of Joseph Zentmayer, a German-born optician and manufacturer of precision instruments who won world-wide renown for his work and inventions on microscopes. For them he won gold medals from the Franklin Institute, the Paris Exposition of 1878, and the Centennial Exposition in Philadelphia in 1876; the latter award-winning microscope is in the Mütter Museum of the College of Physicians. William Zentmayer was graduated from the medical school of the University of Pennsylvania in 1886. He began his clinical experience in the outpatient department of Children's Hospital. In 1890 he became assistant surgeon at Wills Eye Hospital, and as successor to Dr. William F. Norris (q.v.), he served as attending surgeon from 1901 until 1928, when he became consulting surgeon. He was professor of ophthalmology at the Graduate School of Medicine of the University of Pennsylvania and surgeon to St. Mary and St. Agnes Hospitals. Zentmayer was elected president of the American Ophthalmological Society in 1926, chairman of the section on ophthalmology of the American Medical Association in 1916, and chairman on the section of diseases of the eye, ear, nose, and throat of the Pennsylvania State Medical Society in 1935. He was editor of the *Archives of Ophthalmology* from 1950 to 1958 and editor of the *Transactions of the College of Physicians of Philadelphia* from 1899 to 1913. He bequeathed $15,000 to the College library for a book fund and made other bequests to the section on ophthalmology and to general College funds. Dr. Zentmayer was awarded the Leslie Dana gold medal of the St. Louis Society of the Blind in 1945 and the Lucien Howe gold medal of the American Ophthalmological Society in 1948.

Artist: Daniel Garber (1880–1958)

For biography, see page 16.

Oil on canvas; 39 1/2 x 31 1/2; signed at upper left, "Daniel Garber." Presented by the section on ophthalmology of the College of Physicians in 1940. *PA 106*

Dr. Zentmayer is shown three-quarter length, with body and head turned slightly to the left. He is seated with his left hand placed on top of the right and both hands resting on his right knee, which is crossed over the left. The background is composed of loosely brushed diagonal or horizontal strokes in lavender, blue, umber, gray, and pale green, with darker tones on the right and lighter on the left. He sits on a soft floral-patterned cushion. No explanatory details of furniture are shown. The subject's face is triangular, the forehead high. He has fine white hair, blue eyes which look straight ahead through rimless glasses, a slender nose with a bump at its bridge, a wide mouth with thin lips under a neat, white, brush moustache, hollow cheeks, a narrow jaw, and a pointed chin. The tapering face has creases in the forehead and next to the nose and mouth. The subject wears a white shirt, a dark blue-black necktie, and a dark purplish-blue three-piece suit. The surface of the portrait is painterly, with impressionistic, visible brush strokes. The head and hands are well-constructed in solid and three-dimensional forms. The costume gives a suggestion of underlying body structure. The painting is a lyrical study of cool colors—the blues, greens, and violets of the background and cushion relate to the colors of the costume and the shadows of the face and hands. Although of slender build, the doctor radiates a feeling of good health and strength as he sits erect without visible back support. His pleasant facial expression and calm demeanor communicate an open and attentive attitude toward the viewer, who responds in kind.

INDEX I
The Subjects

* * *

INDEX II
The Artists

* * *

The page number following each artist's name indicates the location of the biographical entry. Each artist's work is listed by subject, accession number, and page in the catalogue on which it appears.

The artists of the following works are unknown.

Paintings

Sculpture

Miscellaneous Works